Medical Tribune

MEDICINE
The Year in Review©

1992 Medical News and Events

1993 EDITION

A Medical Tribune · Mosby Year Book Publication

First published by Medical Tribune, Inc., 257 Park Avenue South, New York, New York 10010
Distributed by Medical Tribune, Inc.
© 1992 Medical Tribune, Inc.
A catalog record for this book is available from the U.S. Library of Congress
ISBN 0-931861-81-0
ISSN 1066-4149
Printed in the United States by Quebecor Printing Co., Semline Inc., 270 University Avenue, Westwood, Massachusetts
For inquiries about subscribing to Medical Tribune or about this publication, please contact:
Medical Tribune, Subscription Manager, 257 Park Avenue South, New York, NY 10010
Tel. (212) 674-8500 FAX (212) 529-8490

Medicine: The Year in Review

As a corporation committed to health care, Bristol-Myers Squibb is particularly proud of our role in the nation's steady progress toward improving health. We have a continuing research commitment to meet the important challenges the medical profession faces in understanding and treating cardiovascular diseases, infectious diseases, CNS disorders, AIDS and many other problematic diseases.

In this spirit, Bristol-Myers Squibb is pleased to send you *Medicine: The Year in Review.* This volume, prepared by the editors of the *Medical Tribune*, provides a concise review of scientific and clinical events in the medical field during 1992. In these pages you will learn about the progress made, as well as the new challenges we face in the years ahead.

Progress in health care is measured not only in research and development of new compounds, but also in the assurance that these therapeutic advances will be made available to all patients who need them. Toward this end, Bristol-Myers Squibb has been at the forefront of making medications available at no cost to patients who, because of their inability to pay, might otherwise go without treatment. These programs cover a wide array of therapeutic categories, including oncology, cardiovascular medicine, and AIDS.

We hope that this informative book will serve as a small reminder of our commitment to the goal of a strong partnership with the medical profession and to the needs of the patients served.

Bristol-Myers Squibb Company

Contents

6
Year's 'best' stories not
always glories

PRIMARY CARE
12
Overview:
The amazing, expanding
primary-care visit

14
Month-at-a-glance

26
Reported at the Time

39
Commentary:
Regulated into despair

PEDIATRICS
42
Overview:
Strides made in preventing and
treating genetic disorders

44
Month-at-a-glance

56
Reported at the Time

67
Commentary:
Pushing for teen immunization

CARDIOLOGY
72
Overview:
The year of the ACE
inhibitor

74
Month-at-a-glance

86
Reported at the Time

103
Commentary:
Drug trials shed light
on CHD mechanisms

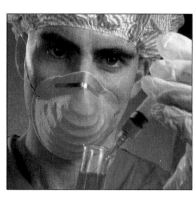

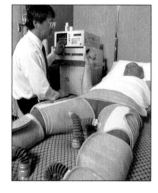

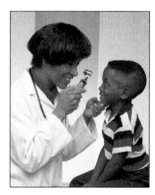

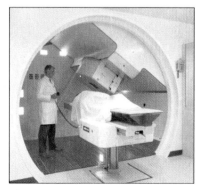

OBSTETRICS/ GYNECOLOGY
108
Overview:
Obstetric advances ranged
from preimplantation to
postmenopause

110
Month-at-a-glance

122
Reported at the Time

131
Commentary:
Treatment advancing,
diagnosing lagging

CENTRAL NERVOUS SYSTEM
135
1992 Highlights

139
Reported at the Time

NUTRITION
144
Overview:
Despite new insights on
nutrient-disease links, advice
the same: less fat,
more veggies

146
Month-at-a-glance

158
Reported at the Time

171
Commentary:
Dietary research
is bearing fruit

Contents

UROLOGY

172
1992 Highlights

175
Reported at the Time

**CLINICAL
MEDICINE**

182
Overview:
Drug resistance, some
infectious diseases on
the rise in 1992

184
Month-at-a-glance

196
Reported at the Time

211
Commentary:
Building bone with
drugs and diet

SURGERY

212
1992 Highlights

215
Reported at the Time

ONCOLOGY

222
Overview:
Despite diagnostic and preventive
strides, war on cancer
is far from won

224
Month-at-a-glance

236
Reported at the Time

247
Commentary:
Molecular biology is the
wave of future

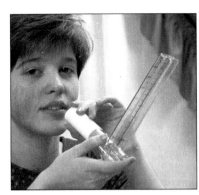

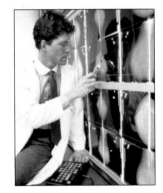

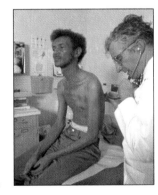

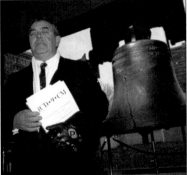

**DERMATOLOGY/ ALLERGY/
RHEUMATOLOGY**

250
Overview:
As skin-cancer, asthma rates
rise, research takes on urgency

252
Month-at-a-glance

264
Reported at the Time

271
Dermatology Commentary:
No longer just skin deep

272
Allergy Commentary:
Breathlessly awaiting new drugs

AIDS

276
Overview:
AIDS penetrates the heartland

278
Month-at-a-glance

290
Reported at the Time

303
Commentary:
AIDS-like illness remains elusive

HEALTHCARE POLICY

308
Overview:
Is reform a Gordian knot?

310
Month-at-a-glance

322
Reported at the Time

335
Commentary:
3 battles to watch in the 1990s

INDEX 336

Year's 'best' stories not always glories

BY BILL INGRAM

1992, like every year before it since Canada's Marc Lalonde launched the watershed "Operation Lifestyle" in 1978, reached a new high in health consciousness-raising and a new high in the pure volume of medical information.

How do you sift through scores of the most publishable medical chronicles in captivity, which comprise *Medicine: The Year in Review*, surmount a word-count that rivals *War and Peace* and come up with the "Stories of the Year"?

Would that it were as simple as judging tiebreaking essays in those giveaway contests of yore, based on "neatness, conciseness and originality." It isn't. It's a high-flown, hair-tearing consideration, and the staff has some bald patches to show for it.

In part, selections are based on the extent to which the premise of a "running story" demonstrably grabbed the attention of doctors and health consumers—often the "badder," the "better." Mainstream feedback and repercussions, even the Larry ("All I do is ask questions") King show, can dictate prominence. Witness the silicone breast-implant imbroglio.

Though more prosaic, the actual importance to healthcare of a new development, approach, treatment or trend perforce counts in terms of numbers of beneficiaries, years of benefit and quality of life. The unexpected has pulling power. So do the narrative and the internal dynamics.

The heart dominated research and media reports in 1992, just as it has for decades. And rightfully so. About 70 million Americans have "some form" of cardiovascular disease, and it's "the nation's number one killer" (IF you throw in stroke and hypertension).

There were the usual comforting communiques. The downtrend in heart disease deaths continued, exemplified by a 1988 rate 24% lower than in 1980. The stroke death rate has declined by more than 50% in the last 30 years. (The literature and public prints were strewn with findings on lifestyle and nutrition, putative contributors to the downtrend. But store sellouts of oat bran, broccoli and red wine were not accompanied by firm links to heart health.)

Antihypertensives, thrombolytics, anticoagulants, aspirin, angioplasty and CABG formed the broad front of treatment, as they have for some years now. But there were strong signs that ACE inhibitors, already antihypertensive standbys, were coming into their own versus heart disease.

ACE inhibitors draw the high cards (p. 99) described how captopril (Capoten, Squibb), the first and best-known of the class, brightened the picture for the "left-out bunch"—older MI victims with compromised left-ventricular function. Other studies showed that people over 75 are just as likely to benefit from thrombolytic therapy as younger people.

Marring these gains, elder bias reared its unpretty head. And of course, all year, wherever cardiovascular treatment went, gender bias seemed sure to follow.

In **Women and elderly often underrepresented in cardiac trials** (p. 100), one of the most damning investigations, out of Canada, discovered that of 2,546 CCU admittees,

8.2% of females had died by the 28th day, as compared with 4.8% of their male correlatives.

Moreover, a separate meta-analysis showed that in more than 60% of 214 studies of drug therapy for MIs that were examined, no patients over 75 had been enrolled; overall, fewer than 20% of the patients were women.

The therapeutic approaches taken in cancer, responsible for a greater toll (520,00 deaths expected in 1992) than heart disease per se (about 500,000), would appear to be innocent of bias at this point.

Not so the cancer establishment. In **Cancer 'strides' challenged as spurious** (p. 236), the American Cancer Society and the National Cancer Institute were taken to task by a group of 60 scientists for "confusing the public with repeated claims that we are winning the war against cancer [when we are not]."

The philippic was unparalleled.

With the overall cancer incidence rising relentlessly 1% a year, the cancer establishment has "repeatedly grossly exaggerated the ability to treat and cure cancer," charged an occupational and environmental medicine expert speaking for the group of 60. He noted that the low five-year survival rates for nonlocalized breast (18%) and lung cancer (13%) have persisted for decades.

"Millions have died from what should be a preventable disease," he proclaimed, while NCI skimps on initiatives.

ACS and NCI officials lashed back, asserting that a third of the NCI budget is spent on causation and prevention-related research and citing gains in the fight against colon, rectal, bladder and ovarian cancer. Officials did concede, however, that the ACS president was exaggerating when he attributed two thirds to three quarters of cancers "to external things we might modify."

With smoking and longevity at the top of the cancer-causation list, diet has been judged a clear contributor to colon and stomach cancer. The jury is still out on others.

Fat, fiber don't affect breast-cancer risk (p. 170) portrayed the fairer sex as having a longer dietetic leash than many think. At eight-year follow-up of 89,494 women, breast cancers could not be related to the fat in their diet, which ranged from 27% to 50% of total calories.

Another prevention equivocality, this one highly disputatious, was detailed in **Do tamoxifen benefits outweigh its risks?** (p. 245). The National Women's Health Network inveighed against the forthcoming five-year government-sponsored trial of tamoxifen (Nolvadex, ICI Pharma) as a threat to the health of enrollees, who are women at high risk of developing breast cancer.

Early in the year, a meta-analysis of adjuvant therapy for early breast cancer in 74,652 women found that 59% of those receiving tamoxifen were alive ten years later, compared with 53% of controls. But protesters wouldn't buy the drug's track record on survival vis-à-vis its association with an increased risk of blood clots, uterine and liver cancers and ocular toxicity.

Still another prevention modality, mammography, was shaken by news leaks to the effect that a Canadian study had found that routine mammograms before the age of 50 paradoxically increased the risk of developing breast cancer.

Mammography called neither a risk nor a help (p. 242) cleared away some of the clouds. Revised data showed the risk margin was not significantly higher in the mammography group, said the chief investigator. Nonetheless, younger women do not benefit in terms of reduced mortality, she said.

In terms of bitter polemic, none of the breast-cancer issues could equal the controversy over silicone implants.

Plastic surgeons still swear they can and do bounce the implants on the office floor and stomp on them, with the patient looking on, so confident are they of leakproofing. But largely anecdotal testimony anent dozens of cases of toxic, systemic reactions to leaking silicone, and stout defenses from makers, had the media hopping for months.

FDA places strict limits on silicone-gel implants (p. 326) had FDA Commissioner David Kessler, M.D., reaching the Solomonic decision to allow use of the implants for all women who want them for breast-cancer surgery but to sharply restrict their use in women seeking breast enlargement.

The prostate to men is what breasts are to women—the biggest "big C" threat.

When urologists announced early in the year that the prostate-specific antigen test, combined with a digital rectal exam, can detect most cases, the question became how to distinguish indolent cancers from aggressive ones.

PSA screen and ultrasound favored in prostate test (p. 239) explored a diagnostic formula that might at least help point to substantial cancers: a normal PSA in nanograms is roughly one-tenth the size of the gland in cubic centimeters. If a man's PSA is 10 ng/ml and his prostate is over 105 cc, the gland is probably normal. But if the gland is only 25 cc, he almost certainly has cancer.

On a procreative note, the ability to screen out "bad genes" reached technologic heights and descended into ethical valleys.

Cystic fibrosis identified in three-day-old embryos (p. 129) chronicled in appropriately measured cadences an Orwellian advance: the isolation of a single cell from three-day-old embryos and elaboration by polymerase chain reaction to cull out those carrying cystic fibrosis genes.

Out of the first small trial came an apparently normal baby.

The technique circumvents abortion and can be applied to hemophilia, sickle-cell disease, Tay-Sachs disease and muscular dystrophy. But the idea of couples sitting down to pick and choose from an array of embryos is a bit unsettling.

If the gene story was the most futuristic, **Peptide in albumin of cow's milk may trigger onset of diabetes in children** (p. 61) was the most surprising. A Finnish-Canadian team found that a group of 142 children with recently diagnosed Type 1 diabetes all had highly elevated serum concentrations of antibodies against bovine serum albumin. Fewer than 3% of controls had these antibodies. The implication: Take cow's milk off the table and you can prevent diabetes in genetically susceptible infants. An udderly exquisite strategy.

For the explication of a single solid advance in 1992, it would be hard to top **Enzyme eases breathing in cystic fibrosis crises** (p.199). Patients experienced a 10% to 20% improvement in forced vital capacity after a six-day regimen of aerosolized recombinant human deoxyribonuclease I, or rhDNase.

Easily the most powerful pathogenetic insight, with the most profound therapeutic implications, was set forth in **Canadian study backs corticosteroids as Rx for moderate asthma** (p. 33). Using computer simulations of the lung, a Canadian team determined that thickening of the airway wall by inflammation, dramatically reducing airflow, is the critical factor in asthmatic constriction.

The insight provided a rationale as to why the use of bronchodilators has failed to slow asthma deaths and hospitalizations, why beta-agonists may be contributing to morbidity and why corticosteroids are the therapeutic answer.

If the inflammation communication had the most answers, **Reports of AIDS-like illness baffle researchers** (p. 295) posed the most questions. Catalyzed by researchers at the 8th International Conference on AIDS in Amsterdam, it was a mystery story worthy of Berton Roueche or Hans Zinsser: 26 cases of people with AIDS symptoms and low or borderline CD4 cell counts, but negative for HIV. Many had potential AIDS risk factors .

Was this THE DAY OF THE MUTANT VIRUS?

"The cases were blown all out of proportion to the overall magnitude of the AIDS tragedy," commented David Rogers, M.D., vice chairman of the National Commission on AIDS. Let's get down to brass tacks and deliver the AIDS preventive message, he urged.

Keyhole surgery linked to deaths; aggressive marketing blamed (p. 215) had nothing overblown about it. The surgery story of 1990 became the professional misfeasance story of 1992 when the New York State Health Department documented 128 injury-causing incidents at 73 hospitals, including six deaths. Three months later, a National Institutes of Health panel recommended that training guidelines be formulated. New York State's now stipulate that doctors assist in laparoscopic cholecystectomy at least 10 times and perform the technique under supervision another 15 times before tackling it on their own.

Surgery's black eye aside, **Baboon transplant may open xenograft era** (p. 216) told how frontiers were rolled back by the grafting of a baboon liver into a 35-year-old man dying of hepatitis, presaging the day when genetically engineered pig organs may help solve the tragic shortage. Six patients a day die while awaiting a human one.

Need is what tuberculosis is all about, too. The need for patients to take their medicine.

Step-care for TB proposed (p. 200) relayed a leading pulmonologist's call for a step-by-step system to ensure compliance: friendly urging, incentive payments, mandatory observation, court-ordered treatment and hospital detention.

"Like the Framm oil-filter TV ad says, 'Catchya now...or catchya later [when the multi-drug-resistant epidemic hits],' " says the pulmonologist.

Finally, **Candidates lure MDs with different health plans** (p. 327) presented 500-word healthcare statements by President Bush and then-Governor Clinton for doctors' eyes alone, kicking off a six-month Presidential straw vote.

The straw vote drew one of the heaviest responses in this newspaper's history. Doctors chose the wrong man by a lopsided margin, 47% to 19%, but may yet make their peace with the New Covenant's managed competition.

The voice of healthcare remains loud and clear, if a little hoarse.

Notes

Notes

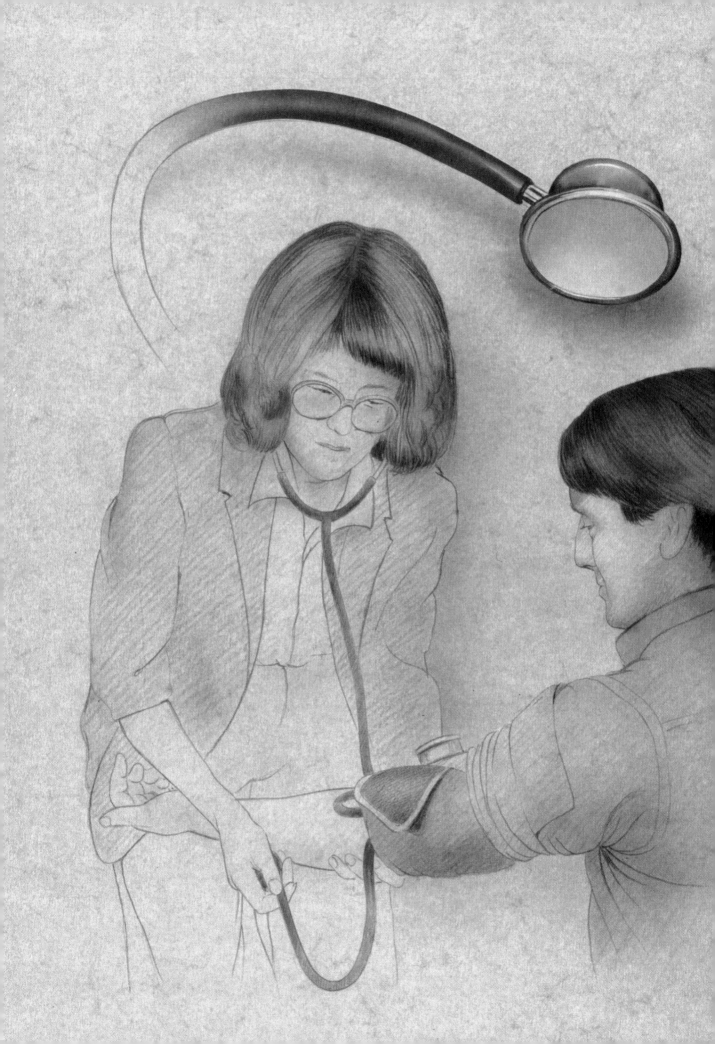

Overview 12
The amazing, expanding
primary-care visit

Month-at-a-glance 14

Reported at the Time 26
About one quarter of physicians
would choose another
profession...buspirone helps
smokers quit...CTS eased with
estrogen...preparing patients for
pregnancy...asthma news: home
checks urged, study backs
corticosteroids for moderate
disease...HSV most infectious in
first three months...more-frequent
mammograms catch cancer
early...the latest on weight
loss...Lyme disease reports: new
test detects antibody, early
antibiotics advised...physicians
cope with California earthquake,
Hurricane Andrew...cholera watch

Commentary 39
Regulated into despair
By Michael Victoroff, M.D.

The amazing, expanding primary-care visit

In 1992, researchers and government agencies added the detection of a host of medical and social ills to the agenda of the primary-care visit.

During a year when physicians were often in doubt about whether they would be reimbursed for comprehensive patient examinations, new scientific evidence showed that such primary-care evaluations can have a major impact on the incidence and outcome of leading killers, such as heart disease, cancer and stroke.

In 1992, striking benefits were revealed for a thorough physical, life-style and laboratory check on the patients least likely to receive one—healthy adults.

To aid prevention of heart attacks, a National Institutes of Health consensus panel recommended that all patients receive at least two routine HDL checks, with appropriate risk counseling for all patients in whom the ratio of total cholesterol over HDL tops 4.5.

The NIH panel stopped short of recommending triglyceride screening for everyone, but new data from Finland demonstrated the importance of lipid-lowering efforts in men with triglyceride levels over 203 mg/dl and LDL/HDL ratios greater than 5. At the start of the study these men faced almost a fourfold risk of heart attacks, but their risk was reduced 71% after treatment with gemfibrozil.

The wisdom of cajoling nonathletic patients into moderate exercise, such as gentle bicycling, gardening or golf, was confirmed in a nine-year British study of 7,735 healthy middle-aged men. Those who exercised moderately had less than half the stroke rate of their inactive counterparts. Exercise also reduced blood pressure and blood coagulability.

On this side of the Atlantic, analysis of the Physicians' Health Study showed that a weekly workout reduced the risk of

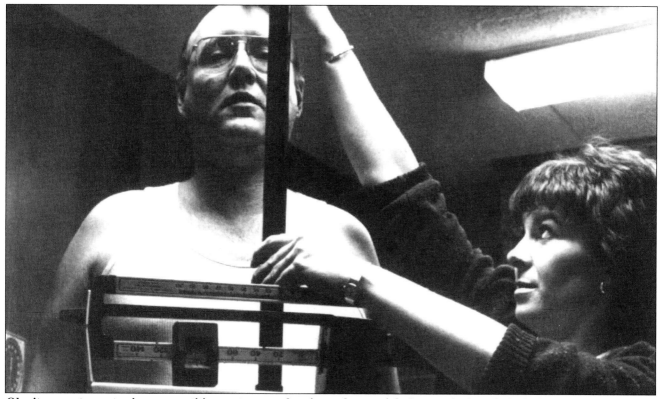

Obesity experts want primary practitioners to counsel patients about weight-loss methods and obesity's health risks.

non-insulin-dependent diabetes by 23%, with those exercising five or more times a week showing a 42% reduction.

In light of new data from Hawaii on the reduction of disease risk in patients who successfully quit smoking—quitting cuts lifetime lung cancer risk by 75% and helps prevent several other cancers—physicians were asked to become familiar with the most effective smoking-cessation programs.

This year, physicians could add pharmacologic aids to behavioral smoking-cessation strategies. Several nicotine patches were available. In a study from Creighton University in Omaha, Neb., the antianxiety agent buspirone boosted short-term quitting rates from 50% to 79% and was associated with less recidivism at one year.

Obesity experts, while recognizing individual responsibility for controlling weight, nevertheless announced that it is the duty of the primary-care physician to warn patients about the health risks of obesity. And the information must be specific, according to Theodore Van Itallie, M.D., professor emeritus at St. Luke's-Roosevelt Hospital Center in New York.

He wants physicians to heed a patient's family history (obesity-related diseases such as diabetes, gallbladder disease, hypertension, hypercholesterolemia and heart disease) as well as body shape (fat in "pot bellies" has more of an impact on lipid and insulin metabolism than fat in hefty hips and thighs). Even more: A physician must work in concert with dietitians in order to guide the patient, not just take the "easy way out" and make a referral to a commercial program.

Recognizing that primary-care doctors represent the first line of defense against illness, several agencies called on the phy-

sicians to sharpen their lookout for medical and social problems that often reach debilitating proportions before they are diagnosed. Counseling sexually active patients continued to be a high priority, and family physicians learned that it is not just naive, but statistically a poor bet, to assume that teenage patients are not sexually active.

After a study revealed that most persons with dystonia consult between four and 25 different doctors prior to diagnosis, advocacy groups asked generalists to pay more attention to signs and symptoms of movement disorders.

In early 1992, an NIH panel issued guidelines asking primary-care physicians to improve skin examinations in order to detect melanomas earlier. And monitoring for cutaneous signs of Lyme disease is not enough following a tick bite; Denver physicians suggested prophylactic antibiotics in some endemic areas.

In January, Surgeon General Antonia Novello, M.D., asked primary-care physicians to routinely check patients for signs of abuse. The American Medical Association followed up last summer with specific protocols to help doctors detect signs of abuse in children, women and the elderly. At the October meeting of the American Academy of Family Physicians, attendees were told to use medical clues—such as frequent sprains—to identify the estimated one in six patients with an alcohol or substance-abuse problem.

So 1992 was a year for primary-care physicians to be acknowledged for their special role in protecting the health of patients—even while many feared for the health of their medical practices.

JANUARY

Jan. 1
Smokers learned that their lifetime risk of getting lung cancer is 12 times that of non-smokers, and that that rate dropped to a threefold risk if they abandoned the habit. In a study of 8,006 Japanese-American men in Hawaii, smokers also faced increased risk for cancers of the bladder, esophagus, kidney, mouth and pancreas. In the American Journal of Public Health, Honolulu researchers suggested that physicians support smoking-cessation programs that enable current smokers to quit permanently within the shortest time period.

Jan. 3
Unless told differently, physicians should assume that their high-school-aged patients are sexually active, according to statistics released by the Centers for Disease Control. By 1990, being a virgin put an American high-school student in a distinct minority, according to a survey of 11,631 teens in grades nine through 12. Fifty-four percent had had sexual intercourse at least once, and more than 75% had used contraception the last time they had sex.

Jan. 4
Headache experts at London's Charing Cross Hospital reminded physicians to consider migraine when men complain of weekend headaches. Although migraines affect three times as many women as men, men are more likely to suffer weekend attacks, the team wrote in a letter to The Lancet. Friday-night drinking, stress withdrawal, reduced caffeine consumption and changes in sleep patterns have been considered as triggers for the weekend headache pattern.

Jan. 7
Physicians could bolster teenagers' use of sunscreens if they explained how sun exposure causes skin cancer and prematurely ages the skin, claimed researchers from Johns Hopkins University. Most adolescents fail to use sunscreen, even if they have a family history of skin cancer, according to a survey of 220 Virginia teens, 81% of whom spent most weekends in the sun. One third said they never used a sunscreen and 9% said they always used one, according to a report in Pediatrics. Teens were more likely to use a sunscreen if their parents had insisted on it when they were young, and also if their close friends used sunscreens.

Jan. 10
The Coalition for Consumer Health and Safety announced that while more Americans are buckling up when driving cars, they need to be reminded to observe safety warnings on leisure vehicles. In 1990, the number of injuries involving bicycles was up 11% over 1989. Accidents involving all-terrain vehicles were up 12.7%, and skateboards injured 82,248, up 25.2%, according to the alliance of medical and insurance groups. Also on the rise: injuries involving bunk beds, playground equipment, stairs, swimming pools, toys and windows.

• • •

Americans did not even come close to achieving the recommended levels of dietary fat, according to a new national report. On average, Americans obtain 36.3% of their daily calorie intake from fat, well above the FDA recommendation of no more than 30%, said the Coalition for Consumer Health and Safety. Meanwhile, other healthy life-style messages seem to be getting across, since levels of smoking and alcohol use decreased.

Jan. 11
Dizziness and tiredness were linked with low systolic blood pressure in a health analysis of 10,314 British civil servants. In the British Medical Journal, London researchers suggested that more attention be focused on the health effects of hypotension, which is usually only treated if dizziness is sufficient to cause falls.

Jan. 13
Officials at the Centers for Disease Control declared the year's flu outbreak a nationwide epidemic. The A-Beijing strain of influenza began in November, affecting children first and then spreading to the elderly, who suffered the most complications and deaths. Fourteen states reported outbreaks in more than 50% of their populations.

Jan. 16
Calling domestic violence a major public health problem, Surgeon General Antonia Novello, M.D., urged the nation's physicians to check their patients routinely for signs of domestic abuse. The medical setting may be the first and only place an abused person seeks help, she said. As many as 35% of injured women who seek care in emergency rooms have been abused, yet as few as 5% are identified as victims of family violence.

Jan. 18
British researchers cautioned that influenza vaccine should not be administered to stable asthmatic patients because it can increase bronchial reactivity and worsen symptoms. Three of their patients were hospitalized after receiving the vaccine, physicians from the Royal Infirmary in Sunderland reported in The Lancet. However, U.S. health officials advise that asthmatics on regular medication receive the vaccine because asthma flare-ups can be triggered by upper-respiratory-tract infections.

Jan. 20
Pending FDA action on Halcion (Triazolam, Upjohn), sleep specialists urged physicians to prescribe the popular benzodiazepine only to carefully selected patients, and to adhere strictly to proper dosages. Halcion should not be given to elderly people or to those prone to depression, anxiety, or alcohol or drug abuse, cautioned some sleep disorders experts. When prescribed to treat short-term insomnia, the maximum suggested starting dose should be 0.125 mg.

Jan. 23
A simple test revealed which elderly patients were likely to die or become severely disabled in the year following hospital discharge. Patients discharged with the most prescriptions and with the least ability to independently carry out the activities of daily living (bathing, toileting, dressing, continence, feeding and transfer) were most likely to die, according to a study of

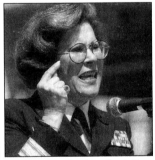

Dr. Novello: check patients for signs of domestic violence.

178 Italian patients. Disability and medication use predicted mortality as well as a diagnosis of neoplasia, the researchers report in the Journal of the American Geriatrics Society.

Jan. 30
Twenty-seven percent of primary-care doctors said they would not choose medicine as a career if they had it to do all over again. One in 10 were preparing to abandon solo practice and less than half were likely to recommend a medical career to their children, declared the 2,264 physicians (mostly FPs, GPs and internists) who responded to a national Medical Tribune survey. Biggest headaches: paperwork, government regulation and Medicare reimbursement.

FEBRUARY

Feb. 3

The antianxiety drug buspirone (Buspar, Mead Johnson) blunted nicotine withdrawal symptoms in long-term smokers trying to quit, reported researchers from Creighton University in Omaha, Neb. In a four-week study, 40 people who smoked at least a pack a day were told to continue smoking for the first three weeks. Half received buspirone three times a day, starting with the pre-quitting weeks and continuing through the quitting week; others received a placebo.

In the withdrawal week, 79% of the buspirone group completely abstained from smoking, compared with 50% of smokers given a placebo. Placebo-treated patients had significantly higher ratings for craving, anxiety, irritability, restlessness and sadness during tobacco withdrawal, according to data published in the Archives of Internal Medicine.

Feb. 6

Elderly patients with osteoporosis reduced their risk of spinal fractures by taking the hormone calcitriol, observed New Zealand researchers. In a study of 622 women who had received either calcitriol or calcium for three years, women who took calcium had three times as many new bone fractures as those who took the hormone, the investigators reported in The New England Journal of Medicine.

Feb. 8

Estrogen replacement therapy was found to decrease symptoms of many common painful disorders in menopausal women, researchers from St. Bartholomew's Hospital in London reported in the British Medical Journal. Examination of 42 menopausal women revealed that seven women had carpal tunnel syndrome and six women had fibromyalgia. Women with both conditions improved significantly after six months of hormone replacement therapy.

Feb. 12

Injuries caused by repetitive movements account for more than 50% of all occupa-

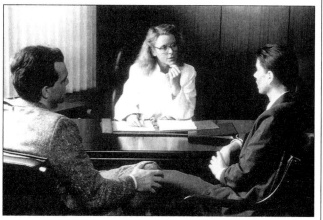

Counseling by primary-care doctors improves pregnancy outcome.

tional illnesses in the United States, claimed researchers from the University of California, San Francisco. They recommended that physicians prescribe resting the affected part of the body for at least two weeks, during which time patients should be provided with specific job adaptations. Affected joints should be immobilized, especially at night. Anti-inflammatory drugs and icing of the affected area may also be therapeutic, the team stated in The Journal of the American Medical Association.

Feb. 14

Patients suffering from specific problems due to drug addiction or grief may benefit as much from referral to short-term psychotherapy as from long-term psychological counseling, University of Pennsylvania researchers determined. They reached that conclusion after comparing findings from 12 studies that examined treatment of people suffering from depression, drug addiction, personality disorders, post-traumatic stress disorder or grief. The analysis,

in the American Journal of Psychiatry, encompassed various types of psychotherapy, such as hypnotherapy, self-help groups and cognitive or dynamic therapy.

Patients found most likely to benefit from short-term therapy: those with specific problems relating to substance abuse, rape or other physical injury, property loss or death.

Feb. 20

McGill University researchers warned that regular use of beta-agonists can lull both physicians and patients into believing that asthma is under control when it is in fact worsening and may become life-threatening. In a study of 784 people with asthma, those who used an inhaler of a beta-agonist every month faced a 2.6-times higher risk of death or of a near-fatal asthma episode than asthma patients who never used an inhaler, they reported in The New England Journal of Medicine.

A patient's increasing need for beta-agonists should be considered a sign of worsening disease and an indication for anti-inflammatory therapy, researchers concluded

Feb. 24

Sleep-disordered breathing usually does not affect day-

time functioning, concluded a study from the University of Kentucky in Lexington. The study of 92 healthy volunteers aged 50 to 80 revealed that more than 15% experienced five or more SDB events (apnea, hypopnea and oxygen desaturation) per hour of sleep. However, testing revealed their daytime functioning to be no different than that of subjects without SDB, they stated in Chest.

• • •

California researchers reported that elderly patients who complain of sleeping problems may be victims of nocturnal myoclonus. In a study of 427 elderly San Diego residents published in Sleep, 45% were found to suffer from periodic leg jerks. The problem was associated with insomnia, motor restlessness and excessive daytime sleepiness.

Feb. 27

Preconception counseling and a thorough physical examination by the primary-care physician can improve pregnancy outcomes and reduce infant-mortality rates, an obstetrician at Upstate Medical Center in Syracuse, N.Y. advised in Medical Tribune.

• • •

Oral prednisone alone was worse than ineffective in the treatment of acute optic neuritis: It also appeared to increase the risk of new attacks, concluded the National Eye Institute's Optic Neuritis Trial. In a comparison of 457 optic neuritis patients who received oral prednisone, intravenous methylprednisolone followed by oral prednisone or placebo, oral prednisone alone was found to be ineffective, and 27% of patients in that group suffered at least one recurrence during the next two years. Those on combination therapy recovered their vision slightly faster than placebo patients, but their vision six months later was only slightly better than that of the untreated patients, the researchers reported in The New England Journal of Medicine.

MARCH

March 1

The use of restraints on elderly people may cause more injuries than it prevents, warned a Yale internist after studying nursing-home residents. The researchers followed 397 nursing-home residents who had never been restrained. After one year, 31% were being strapped into chairs to prevent falling or wandering. But 17% of restrained residents sustained a

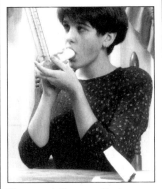

Home peak-flow monitoring urged to cut asthma deaths.

serious fall-related injury during the year, compared with 5% of unrestrained residents, according to data presented in the Annals of Internal Medicine. Instead of restraints, unsteady elderly persons may need supervision when walking, training for improved balance and examinations to detect underlying medical problems, the researchers advised.

March 5

Vaccinating the elderly against the flu protects them against potential infections and helps contain healthcare costs, the Centers for Disease Control reported. But because immunizing these patients does not always prevent infections, the CDC also recommended that some elderly be prescribed amantadine, particularly if they reside in nursing homes.

March 7

An international panel of experts advised that anti-inflammatory drugs be used as first-line therapy for the chronic care of all but mild, intermittent cases of asthma. Daily inhaled corticosteroids or cromolyn sodium (Fisons Pharmaceuticals) is needed to reduce and prevent recurrence of inflammation, the panel reported at the annual meeting of the American Academy of Allergy and Immunology in Orlando.

• • •

March 8

Physicians should recommend home peak-flow monitoring as a potentially lifesaving measure in asthmatic patients who receive daily medications, an international panel of experts at the Orlando meeting of the American Academy of Allergy and Immunology recommended. Even children as young as five years old can use a peak-flow meter adequately, according to their consensus statement.

March 9

A prominent allergist advised persons with asthma to pay attention when weather forecasters announce ozone levels. When ozone levels are high, asthmatics are more likely to have difficulty breathing and to require hospital treatment, the president of the American Academy of Allergy and Immunology told colleages at their annual meeting in Orlando. Ozone also may worsen hay fever and ragweed allergy, he said.

March 10

Yoga may help asthmatic patients to relax and control their breathing when an attack appears imminent, said researchers from the University of Colorado. A study of 17 asthmatics showed that those who were instructed in breathing exercises and meditation three times a week for 30 to 40 minutes reduced their use of beta agonists and felt less panic during attacks, they reported at the meeting of the American Academy of Allergy and Immunology.

• • •

A humidifier may help when elderly people complain of sneezing and nose irritation, suggested a Johns Hopkins allergist. Non-allergic rhinitis, which often results from aging of the nasal mucosa, is eased when patients breathe moistened air. However, patients with asthma or other allergies should seek medical advice before trying a humidifier, he told the American Academy of Allergy and Immunology.

• • •

Migraine headaches are not only treatable but are preventable in some cases, a migraine expert said at a symposium on the subject. Medications, behavioral therapy and diet changes can all offer relief, the Albert Einstein College of Medicine neurologist asserted. Among the drugs that help sufferers: beta-blockers, calcium-channel blockers and tricyclic antidepressants. Sumatriptan (Imitrex, Glaxo) has also been shown to provide relief, but is awaiting FDA approval, he noted.

March 11

The upper age limit for semen donors was lowered from 50 years to 40, the director of the American Fertility Society announced at an American Medical Association meeting. He cited evidence that the incidence of serious genetic mutations in sperm from men over 40 was four times higher than the rate among men under 35.

March 15

Infectious disease experts cautioned that persons infected with herpes simplex virus must use condoms to avoid transmission of HSV during the three months after initial lesions have healed. When University of Washington researchers followed 306 women for 63 weeks after their first episode of herpes, one in five women with type 2 HSV and one in 10 women with type 1 HSV had asymptomatic shedding of virus from the cervix or vulva. Cervical shedding of type 2 HSV was three times more likely to occur during the first three months after lesions resolved than during later months, they reported in Annals of Internal Medicine.

March 21

Athletic patients can take single doses of the antihistamines terfenadine (Seldane, Marion Merrell Dow) or diphenhydramine without fear of compromising their performance, announced a team from the Uniformed Services University of the Health Sciences in Bethesda, Md. In a randomized, double-blind study, 12 healthy active subjects were given either placebo, 50 mg diphenhydramine or 60 mg terfenadine. Maximum exercise testing produced no significant differences in oxygen consumption, carbon dioxide production, ventilation, core body temperature and plasma concentrations of lactate, they reported in Medicine and Science in Sports and Exercise.

March 27

Postmenopausal women who experience hot flashes may cut their suffering in half by practicing deep breathing exercises, a Detroit researcher told a meeting of the Society of Behavioral Medicine. This treatment can be especially helpful for those patients for whom estrogen replacement therapy is contraindicated, said the Wayne State University expert. He studied 33 postmenopausal women randomly assigned to eight-hour sessions of slow, deep abdominal breathing, muscle relaxation techniques or a placebo drug. The women who practiced deep breathing experienced 50% fewer hot flashes than any of the others, he said.

April 3

An outbreak of Legionnaires' disease in Bogalusa, Louisiana, was traced to a contaminated ultrasonic mist machine in a local grocery. Thirty-three persons were hospitalized after working or shopping in the grocery's produce department, where an infrequently cleaned mist machine was used to keep vegetables looking fresh, Centers for Disease Contol investigators stated in the Journal of Infectious Diseases.

April 6

A Canadian study concluded that asthma patients need better advice on pre-exercise medication in order to break out of a vicious circle of increasing breathlessness and exercise avoidance. A study of 27 asthma patients found that most of the subjects mistakenly thought their disease prevented them from exercising; 75% reported having suffered postexercise wheezing in the past and 80% said that their physicians had not recommended prophylactic medication. However, when premedicated, none showed symptoms during exercise testing conducted at Toronto Hospital in Ontario.

When the report appeared in the American Review of Respiratory Disease, commentators reminded asthma patients that exercise-induced breathlessness gets worse as fitness decreases and deconditioning also raises the risk for other health disorders.

April 8

Antihistamines are not only completely ineffective against colds, but the medications have potentially dangerous side effects, experts testified to Congress. A Johns Hopkins researcher said she had found no difference in symptoms among 96 children, regardless of whether they had been given no medication, a placebo or standard over-the-counter medication, including an antihistamine.

The antihistamines did, however, cause sedation and hyperactivity, and might also induce a seizure in a susceptible child, the investigator testified.

• • •

Houston researchers announced that a new drug treatment for travelers' diarrhea was found to be more effective and safer than current therapies. In a study of 191 students visiting Mexico, the antibiotic aztreonam (Azactam, Squibb), taken orally, quelled diarrhea in an average of 44 hours. Those on placebo averaged 84 hours to recover, the University of Texas team reported in The Journal of the American Medical Association. The drug should cause fewer side effects than other antibiotics because oral aztreonam kills bacteria in the intestine without being absorbed in the bloodstream, the researchers added.

April 13

An Oregon researcher suggested that obesity, not work-related strain, is the main cause of carpal tunnel syndrome. In a controversial report in the Journal of Occupational Medicine, the director of the Portland Hand Surgery and Rehabilitation Center found no consistent relationship between the disease and any work activity. However, he did find that obese workers have a four times greater risk of developing carpal tunnel syndrome than nonobese workers.

• • •

Overweight women were advised that they can reduce their risk of osteoarthritis of the knee by losing weight. Boston University researchers performed a retrospective study of 64 women who had early symptoms of knee arthritis and 728 who did not. Over an eight- to 12-year period, women who lost an average of 11 pounds cut in half their odds of developing arthritis of the knee, the team reported in the Annals of Internal Medicine.

In a related study in the same journal, a Hospital for Special Surgery team found that women who already suffer from the disorder can markedly reduce pain and increase mobility through a program of fitness and patient education. The New York team reported that 102 women with advanced knee arthritis who underwent an eight-week trial of fitness walking and education counseling had a 70-meter average increase in walking distance and averaged 27% less pain.

April 15

Physicians were reminded that diabetic patients need an eye examination every year in order to detect retinopathy

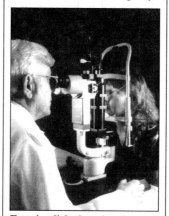

Examine diabetic patients' eyes annually for early retinopathy.

early enough to perform blindness-preventing laser surgery. Laser surgery can cut the rate of vision loss by half, claimed a Harvard physician in the Annals of Internal Medicine.

April 18

Microwaved eggs can explode and cause severe eye injuries, warned physicians from the Birmingham and Midland Eye Hospital in England. A woman entered the hospital with first-degree burns to the eyelids and epithelial loss affecting the conjunctiva and cornea in both eyes. She had followed safety instructions to crack the eggshell before microwaving; however, she had not pierced the yolk and it exploded in her face when the egg was removed from the oven. Her physicians cautioned in the British Journal of Medicine that damage can be long-lasting.

April 20

The U.S. Department of Health and Human Services announced the formation of a 23-member expert panel to determine the best way to diagnose and treat lower back pain. Government officials said they hope to reduce the $18-billion annual cost of treating back pain.

April 28

Contrary to some widely publicized clinical findings, physicians from Massachusetts General Hospital claimed that women under 50 do benefit from mammography screening. In a study of 1,039 breast-cancer patients in their 40s, the five-year survival rate stood at 94% among women whose disease had been detected with mammography, compared with 74% among those whose cancer was detected by palpation, the physicians reported at the American College of Radiology's 25th National Conference on Breast Cancer in Boston.

April 29

A newly developed plastic plate, designed at the Breast Clinic in Wichita, Kansas, improved screening for breast cancer in women with breast implants. The plate, which has a cutout area placed over the implant, relieves pressure exerted by the implant. The device has so far been used in 300 to 400 women with implants, its developer told the American College of Radiology's 25th National Conference on Breast Cancer.

May 1

Moderately obese people were reported to have lost weight and not regained it, with the help of prescription appetite-suppressing pills. In a multipronged program that also included diet, exercise, behavior modification and counseling, about 20 male and 40 female patients (average weight, 200 pounds) were given a combination of phentermine (Ionamin, Fisons Pharmaceuticals) and fenfluramine (Pondimin, A.H. Robins). The patients lost an average of 30 pounds and maintained the loss as long as they took the drugs, which for some people was as long as three and a half years, University of Rochester researchers reported in the journal Clinical Pharmacology and Therapeutics.

• • •

The best way to avoid the bite of encephalitis-infected mosquitos is by wearing protective clothing and using topical mosquito repellents, advised a physician at Thomas Jefferson University in Philadelphia. His advice followed an earlier report from the Centers for Disease Control that the Asian tiger mosquito, an aggressive mosquito that carries eastern equine encephalitis, had spread to 61 of Florida's 67 counties since 1986. While it is rare for people bitten by infected mosquitos to contract the disease, the Philadelphia physician told the Medical Tribune News Service that people living in infected areas should still take special precautions to avoid being bitten.

May 4

A relaxation technique can help eliminate bad dreams among people who have suffered from repetitive nightmares for many years, reported a group of researchers from Albuquerque. The technique—imagining the nightmare ending happily before going to sleep—helped relieve or eliminate bad dreams in 12 nightmare sufferers, the

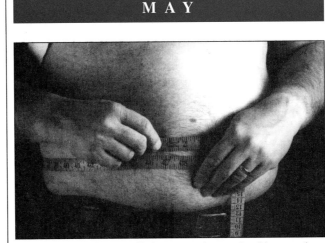

MAY

Shedding pounds is especially important for people with spare tires.

researchers wrote in the American Journal of Psychiatry. About 5% to 6% of American adults are tormented by frightening dreams that occur at least once a week for six months or more, and may continue for decades, the researchers told the Medical Tribune News Service.

May 7

Men with beer bellies are the patients who most need a physician's nudge to diet, advised a weight-control expert from the Department of Health and Human Services. People with pot bellies risk illness because abdominal fat releases fatty acids into the portal vein and, ultimately, into the liver, where it interferes with insulin metabolism, he told Medical Tribune.

May 13

Ursodiol (ursodeoxycholic acid) can prevent gallstones in obese people on rapid weight-loss programs, announced a researcher at Cedars-Sinai Medical Center in Los Angeles.

Ursodiol (Actigall, Summit Pharmaceuticals) should be given only to very obese patients who have high triglyceride levels, he reported at the Digestive Disease Week meeting in San Francisco.

About 25% of obese patients on a 520-calorie-a-day diet develop gallstones within 16 weeks, he said.

May 18

Researchers at the Gundersen Medical Foundation in La Crosse, Wisc., announced that they had developed the first definitive test for Lyme disease. The laboratory kit detects a borreliacidal antibody active in the body seven days after exposure.

• • •

An advisory committee to the Food and Drug Administration concluded that the widely used sleeping pill triazolam (Halcion, Upjohn) is safe and effective. Critics have claimed that the drug induces anxiety, depression and short-term memory loss. The committee recommended that the drug be kept on the market and called for warning labels to be strengthened and simplified. Last year, the drug was banned in the United Kingdom after a drug advisory group there concluded that adverse psychological effects were associated with its use.

May 20

Changes in stress levels and sleeping patterns may provide advance warning of depression, reported a researcher from the University of Pittsburgh School of Medicine.

Over time, repeated stress may produce changes in neurotransmitters that can lead to depression, he reported at the Decade of the Brain symposium in Washington, D.C.

May 27

The spigots of water coolers should be rinsed with bleach and flushed with water every four weeks to rid them of bacteria that could cause diarrhea and stomach distress, advised a Northeastern University researcher at the American Society for Microbiology meeting in New Orleans.

May 28

Ice skaters and their fans may be at risk for respiratory or nervous-system disorders caused by breathing toxic air trapped in enclosed ice rinks, warned the Centers for Disease Control.

At least 60 of 130 Wisconsin students who attended an ice hockey tournament re-

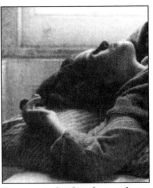

Stress may lead to depression and neurotransmitter changes.

ported headaches, nausea, dizziness, vomiting or coughing spells within a day or two of the games.

Health officials attributed the illnesses to toxic doses of nitrogen dioxide and carbon monoxide released by the Zamboni ice-cleaning machine as well as the heaters used to heat the stands.

• • •

Lifting weights may help women lose weight without losing bone density, reported a Tufts University researcher who is conducting an ongoing study of 100 postmenopausal women. He told a conference on nutrition and aging in New York City that he had previously found that frail 90-year-olds tripled muscle strength in eight weeks of weight lifting.

June 1

A skin patch may suppress some of the symptoms that accompany menopause by combining estrogen and progesterone, researchers told the Medical Tribune News Service. The patch, called Estracombi (Ciba-Geigy), went on the market in Britain and is designed to improve compliance by countering the side effects many women experience on progesterone.

• • •

A sleep disorder consultant claimed that patients who take one lesson in a technique called imagery rehearsal can get rid of their nightmares.

When patients have a bad dream, have them write it down and then change it or imagine it has a different ending, he told the American Sleep Disorders Association meeting in Phoenix. The University of New Mexico researcher presented the results of a study showing that four of ten people who reported nightmares had complete relief after a single session of imagery rehearsal. The average number of nightmares per month dropped from seven to two for the other patients.

• • •

Older people who exercise regularly will sleep better and perform better during the day, Duke University researchers told the American Sleep Disorders Association meeting in Phoenix. They found that 12 healthy men over 60 who exercised regularly fell asleep in half the time, woke up less during the night and had longer periods of slow-wave sleep than 12 sedentary counterparts.

June 2

Physicians were told that a new, more convenient form of light therapy may be as effective in the treatment of seasonal affective disorder as conventional light treatment. The new treatment is a low-intensity light that simulates the dawn by gradually increasing in intensity while the person is asleep, a University of Washington psychiatrist reported at the Association of Professional Sleep Societies meeting.

In a preliminary study, 13 SAD patients who received two hours of the gradual light treatment between 4 a.m. amd 6 a.m. showed a significant improvement in their symptoms.

June 5

Abbott Laboratories recalled the antibiotic temafloxacin (Omniflox) after the drug was linked to three deaths and 47 cases of severe adverse reactions, including hypoglycemia, liver and kid-

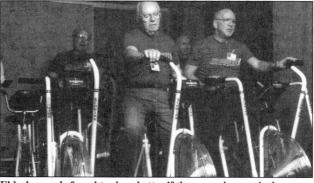

Elderly people found to sleep better if they exercise regularly.

ney dysfunction and hemolytic anemia and other blood-cell abnormalities. The drug was approved in January by the Food and Drug Administration, and, like other fluoroquinolones, was used for infections of the lower respiratory tract, urinary tract, bone, skin and prostate. The FDA halted further distribution of the drug, and advised patients to return any unused portion of the medication to the pharmacy. About 300,000 prescriptions had been written for Omniflox since it was approved, the FDA said.

June 10

A Canadian study strengthened the Federal recommendation advising physicians to treat moderate asthma with such anti-inflammatory drugs as inhaled corticosteroids.

Using computer simulations of the lung, researchers at the University of British Columbia showed that airway constriction alone had little effect on airflow, unless the airways were inflamed. Once the airways were thickened by inflammation, even minor muscle constrictions produced dramatic reductions in airflow, they reported in the American Review of Respiratory Disease.

June 15

Maintaining a close physician-patient relationship is an important part of helping patients live comfortably with irritable bowel syndrome, reported University of North Carolina researchers. Mild disease can usually be controlled by increasing fiber in the diet and avoiding fatty foods, caffeine and alcohol; moderate disease may necessitate behavior therapy, hypnosis or education about possible triggers, the researchers declared in the Annals of Internal Medicine. More severe cases with coexistent symptoms of depression or impaired daily functioning may require antidepressant medication, they said.

June 17

Physicians were urged to be alert to the possibility of domestic violence in female patients being treated for injuries. Although at least one in five women seen in the emergency room may have symptoms of abuse, a survey in The Journal of the American Medical Association reported that most physicans were too busy or too afraid of offending patients, or felt inadequately trained to deal with the problem. Routine screening for emotional and physical signs of battering, careful record-keeping and referrals to persons trained in handling domestic violence were recommended.

June 20

A diagnosis of osteoporosis evoked both negative and positive behavioral changes in female patients, said California researchers who surveyed 261 women. Those with subnormal bone density measurements on spine densitometry were significantly more likely to initiate estrogen replacement therapy, to start or increase intake of calcium and vitamin D, to start or increase exercise and to quit smoking, according to investigators from the University of California at San Francisco. However, these women were also more likely to become overly fearful of falling and to curtail their activities to such an extent—avoiding unnecessary activities outside the home and increasing use of a cane or handrails, for example—that bone loss might be accelerated, the team reported in the Annals of Internal Medicine.

June 24

Physicians often fail to diagnose migraine headaches and thus their patients do not benefit from the latest treatments, suggested New York and Baltimore researchers. Their survey of 20,468 people aged 12 to 80 found that migraines were only diagnosed in 41% of female and 29% of male sufferers. Older, high-income migraine patients are more likely to be diagnosed and treated than younger, poorer ones, the researchers stated in the Archives of Internal Medicine.

Primary Care

July 1

Physicians were advised to include an assessment of their patients' exercise habits in their medical histories. A Philadelphia cardiologist who believes that exercise habits are as important as cholesterol levels, family medical history and smoking habits made the recommendation at a press conference sponsored by the American Heart Association. It followed the release of a new AHA position paper stating that in addition to smoking, hypertension and hyperlipidemia, physical inactivity is a major risk factor for heart disease. A weekly exercise total of 90 minutes to four hours was

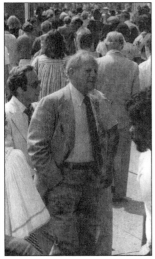

Swedish data suggest that city life breeds schizophrenia.

recommended, and exercise testing was advised for sedentary patients, those over the age of 40 and those with significant coronary risk factors or a history of heart problems.

• • •

University of Virginia researchers reported that a nonsteroidal anti-inflammatory may reduce cold symptoms by almost a third. The Charlottesville researchers exposed 79 healthy, college-age people to a rhinovirus; half the cohort were given a loading dose of 400 mg of naproxen (Naprosyn, Syntex) followed by 200 mg three times a day for five days. The other half of the cohort received a placebo.

Those taking the drug experienced a 29% reduction in cold symptoms, particularly headache and cough, compared with those in the placebo group, with no apparent difference in sneezing, the researchers reported in the Annals of Internal Medicine.

July 4

Hypnosis was effective in easing the symptoms of 18 patients suffering from irritable bowel syndrome, researchers from Manchester, England, reported in The Lancet. Using solid-state rectal catheters to measure bowel activity during the hypnotic state, the researchers found that pleasant thoughts during hypnosis produced an improvement of symptoms, while hypnosis-induced anger aggravated the bowels.

July 14

The Alzheimer's Association released the first guidelines for the nursing home care of Alzheimer's patients. The guidelines, issued at the annual meeting of the Alzheimer's Disease and Related Disorders Association in Chicago, called for ongoing training of staff; preadmission examination to assess care requirements; and reevaluation of care as the disease progresses.

July 18

People who grew up in an urban environment were found to have a greater incidence of schizophrenia than their country counterparts. Researchers from London's Institute of Psychiatry studied 49,191 Swedish men and found that schizophrenia was 1.65 times more likely to occur among those who were born and raised in an inner city than among those reared in the country. The study,

reported in The Lancet, identified 268 schizophrenics among the participants.

July 25

Maryland researchers warned that assembly-line welders who fail to wear protective goggles may be at risk of developing red-green color blindness. Exposure to the intense light created

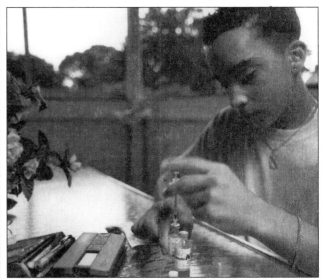

Latest trial: Tight diabetic control shows no benefit.

during arc welding or when electricity arcs between two circuits was found to affect the eye's ability to distinguish between red and green, researchers from the Braddock Medical Group, in Cumberland, reported in The Lancet. The color blindness appeared to be permanent in the workers exposed to the welding light.

• • •

A team of international researchers revealed that exposure to solvents used in the dry-cleaning industry may produce kidney damage and eventual renal failure. Researchers at the University of Parma, Italy, studied 50 employees who worked an average of 10 years in the dry-cleaning business and 50 healthy volunteers. Abnormal proteins and cell fragments were found in the employees'

urine and blood samples, indicating structural and functional damage at the glomerular and tubular proximal and distal levels of the kidney, the team reported in The Lancet. The abnormalities were associated with perchloroethylene, the most commonly used dry-cleaning solvent.

July 26

Tight control of insulin-dependent diabetes mellitus poses significant hazards to diabetics, with no conclusively proven benefits as yet, the physician leading the largest U.S. study ever on the topic reported at the annual meeting of the Endocrine Society in San Antonio.

Until such time as there's a proven benefit, physicians should be cautious in urging patients to seek excessively tight control, warned the head of the Diabetes Control and Complications Trial. Risks include dangerously low blood glucose levels and excessive weight gain, he said.

But physicians from the Joslin Diabetes Center in Boston and the University of California at San Francisco maintained a seemingly unshakable faith in the benefits of tight control, even while acknowledging the difficulties the treatment poses to patients and physicians alike.

AUGUST

Aug. 1

British physicians advised that abuse of the designer drug "ecstasy" can be the cause of chest pain or hepatitis in some patients. As reported in the British Medical Journal, a Manchester doctor reported three cases of chest pain in teenagers who admitted themselves to an emergency room. All three had taken ecstasy and drunk alcohol at all-night parties. The chest pains subsided after several hours.

In other case reports appearing in the same issue, a 27-year-old housewife developed non-A non-B hepatitis after taking ecstasy every weekend for about three months.

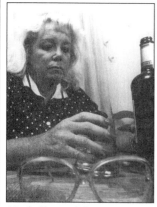

Alcoholics took longer to heal after surgery than teetotalers.

The National Institute on Drug Abuse said the amphetamine-derived drug is available in at least 21 states and is popular with college students and young professionals.

Aug. 6

In the wake of the June 28 earthquake in California, physicians in the area of Big Bear Lake, Landers and Joshua Tree told Medical Tribune that they were seeing a steady stream of patients unnerved by the massive trembler. One family practitioner said he had been seeing three to five patients a day who came seeking tranquilizers, a shoulder to cry on or just someone to tell their fears to.

As continuing aftershocks kept people awake at night, physicians said fatigue became a major problem. A group-counseling session and special courses on dealing with postearthquake stress were held.

Aug. 8

Patients who habitually consume large amounts of alcohol should be warned that they face higher rates of complications and longer recovery periods after major surgery than teetotalers, suggested a study from the University of Copenhagen.

The postoperative progress of 15 patients who had consumed four or more drinks daily for an average of 27 years was compared with that of 15 nondrinkers. Nondrinkers averaged about half as much time in the hospital after surgery as the alcoholics and had lower blood pressure and higher lymphocyte counts 24 hours after surgery, it was reported in The Lancet. Although neither group had a previous history of heart disturbances, 50% of the alcoholics developed arrhythmias immediately after surgery, compared with 10% of the nondrinkers.

• • •

Smokers may have an easier time quitting if they use an experimental nasal nicotine spray combined with group therapy, suggested London researchers. The spray, which had not been approved by the U.S. Food and Drug Administration, appeared to be particularly effective in helping the heaviest smokers quit, investigators from the Institute of Psychiatry reported in The Lancet. In a study of about 200 smokers, half used the spray up to 80 times a day, which would deliver the amount of nicotine in 40 cigarettes, and half used a placebo nasal spray. About 25% of the nicotine-spray users refrained from smoking for one year, compared with one tenth of the smokers using the placebo spray.

Aug. 20

Physicians who practice in areas where Lyme disease is endemic should, under certain circumstances, begin patients on antibiotic therapy soon after they are bitten by a deer tick rather than waiting for the characteristic "bull's-eye" rash to appear, advised a Colorado physician in The New England Journal of Medicine. The Denver General Hospital physician and colleagues based their advice on a calculation of the health outcomes and costs of a

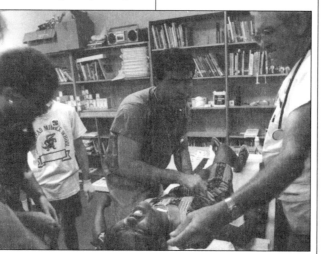

Physicians scrambled for supplies after Hurricane Andrew struck.

hypothetical cohort of 100,000 patients bitten by ticks. They concluded that early, empirical treatment is the least expensive strategy, and results in the fewest cases of Lyme disease—but only if the probability of infection after a bite is 3.6% or higher. Physicians were advised to contact their local health department to find out tick infection rates in their area.

Aug. 24

About 200 physicians in southern Florida had their practices totally destroyed by Hurricane Andrew, Medical Tribune reported. One primary-care physician who lost two offices in the hurricane treated his patients at the office of Miami colleagues who offered temporary accommodations.

In the days following the storm, about 100 physicians volunteered to help out in the migrant camps and tent cities erected by the military, but conditions were rocky. Medical equipment was destroyed by the high winds and rain, and physicians were left to scramble for EKG machines, crash carts and intravenous medications.

Aug. 26

Smoking cigarettes increases the risk of cataracts, two separate studies in The Journal of the American Medical Association revealed. Researchers from Harvard Medical School found that men who smoked more than 20 cigarettes a day were twice as likely as nonsmokers to develop cataracts. The results were derived from the Physicians' Health Study of 22,000 American doctors. The second study found that women who smoked at least 35 cigarettes a day were at a 63% increased risk of developing a cataract compared with nonsmokers. The results were derived from the Nurses' Health Study, an ongoing Boston study of 122,000 female registered nurses.

Sept. 1

Early oral acyclovir (Zovirax, Burroughs Wellcome) therapy was found to decrease cutaneous healing time of adult varicella, shorten the duration of fever and ease symptoms, reported investigators from the U.S. Naval Hospital in San Diego. Starting therapy after the first day of illness was of no value for 36 uncomplicated cases of adult varicella, however. In the study, published in the Annals of Internal Medicine, 148 sailors and marines were given 800 mg of acyclovir, five times daily for seven days, or a placebo. For 38 uncomplicated cases treated with acyclovir within 24 hours of rash onset, time to 100% crusting was reduced by nearly two days, and the maximum number of lesions was cut in half. Length of fever was reduced by a half-day.

Sept. 5

Danish researchers announced that nasally delivered calcitonin derived from salmon can reduce the rate of bone fractures in women with osteoporosis. They studied 164 women, aged 68 to 72, with moderate osteoporosis and found that those who used the spray and took calcium supplements had two-thirds fewer bone fractures than women who took calcium alone. The spray, which despite its source does not smell fishy, also increased spinal bone density by 3%, they reported in the British Medical Journal.

Sept. 11

The Centers for Disease Control advised doctors to tell patients planning to travel to countries where cholera is endemic to take some simple steps to lessen the chance they will contract the disease. In the Morbidity and Mortality Weekly Report, the CDC noted that approximately one new case of cholera is reported in the United States each week, and most of the cases have been acquired during travel to Latin American countries. Cholera prevention should include avoiding unboiled or untreated water, ice made from untreated water, food and beverages from street vendors, uncooked vegetables and raw or partially cooked fish and shellfish.

Sept. 15

Physicians at the Palo Alto Veterans Affairs Hospital warned that treating elderly depressed people with fluoxetine (Prozac, Dista) can result in significant weight loss, nausea and anorexia. Seven of 15 patients who were over 75 years old lost more than 5% of their body weight during four months of fluoxetine therapy,

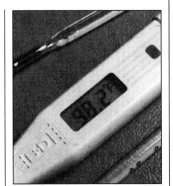

Normal body temperature may be lower than 98.6 F.

the team revealed in the Journal of the American Geriatrics Society. In contrast, only two of 20 fluoxetine-treated patients between the ages of 60 and 71 lost more than 5% of their body weight. Twenty patients over 75 years of age achieved an average weight gain of half a pound during treatment with tricyclics.

Sept. 18

Primary-care physicians were advised to keep their eyes open for back injuries from windsurfing. Researchers at the Australian Sports Medicine Clinic in Brisbane studied five men and two women aged 20 to 40 who windsurfed competitively. All were healthy, but reported lower back pain while windsurfing. Further investigation showed that prolonged surfing in light wind conditions was most taxing on the back, the Australian team reported in Medicine and Science in Sports and Exercise. They found that the best way to avoid the discomfort was to use a seat harness that attaches to the boom on either side of the sail and supports the surfer's rear end.

Sept. 23

A Veterans Affairs Medical Center research team found that normal body temperature may be slightly lower than 98.6 degrees Fahrenheit. A total of 700 oral temperature readings taken on 148 healthy men and women averaged 98.2 and ranged between 96.0 and 100.8 degrees, the Baltimore investigators reported in The Journal of the American Medical Association. Temperatures dropped in the early morning and peaked in the afternoon during the three-day study. Overall, women had a slightly higher average temperature.

Sept. 24

Patients with chlamydia, the most common sexually transmitted disease in the United States, can be successfully treated with a single oral dose of azithromycin (Zithromax, Pfizer), investigators from Louisiana State University reported. They studied 141 patients given azithromycin (1 g once orally) and 125 given doxycycline (100 mg orally twice daily for seven days) for treatment of urethral or endocervical chlamydial infection. Of the patients evaluated 21 to 35 days posttreatment, none of 112 repeat bacterial cultures were positive in the azithromycin group, compared with one of 102 in the doxycycline group, the New Orleans team reported in The New England Journal of Medicine.

Sept. 25

The National Institute for Occupational Safety and Health suggested that workers in a variety of occupations request blood-lead tests from their physicians. People who work with lead paint, who are involved in demolition of lead materials (particularly torching or sandblasting structural steel coated with lead paint), who recycle batteries for the lead or who repair radiators were said to be at high risk in an announcement in the Centers for Disease Control's Morbidity and Mortality Weekly Report.

According to NIOSH, 95% of elevated blood-lead levels in adults result from workplace exposure, but only 5% of employers who use lead materials monitor their workers' blood-lead levels.

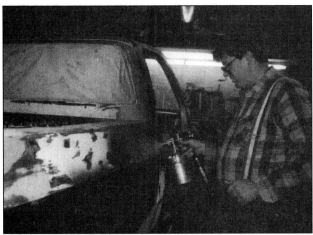

Workers who torch or sandblast steel coated with lead paint should be screened periodically for lead levels, suggested NIOSH.

OCTOBER

Oct. 2

The Centers for Disease Control warned that patients traveling to tropical areas face a small risk of contracting dengue fever. Physicians should suspect dengue in all patients who have recently returned from tropical areas and present with classic dengue symptoms: fever, rash, headache and myalgia, a CDC epidemiologist advised. In its Morbidity and Mortality Weekly Report, the CDC reported 25 confirmed cases of dengue fever in 1991, acquired by Americans traveling in tropical areas. The disease is spread by mosquitoes.

Oct. 8

A Chicago neurologist cautioned that exposure to trichloroethylene, a chemical solvent used in a variety of industries and found in numerous water supplies, may be a cause of severe, chronic headaches. He told the American Academy of Pain Management convention in Albuquerque that of 106 Illinois residents whose wells were polluted with TCE, 62% had severe or frequent headaches. After excluding migraines, the Rush-Presbyterian-St. Luke's Hospital researcher attributed the 57 unexplained headaches to TCE pollution.

Oct. 15

The U.S. Public Health Service advised physicians that the best time to administer flu shots to high-risk patients had arrived and would continue through Nov. 15. An article in American Lung Association Influenza News '92 suggested that both influenza A and influenza B could circulate during what is predicted to be a mild to moderate 1992-1993 flu season. The influenza strains expected to dominate this season are A/Texas (H1N1), B/Panama and B/Qingdao. About 10% to 20% of Americans get the flu each year, according to the CDC.

Oct. 17

Physicians were told that elderly patients who have trouble sleeping may benefit from light therapy to help regulate their circadian cycle. Boston researchers made the suggestion after finding that age-related changes in circadian rhythm and adjustments in mean body temperature may be the reason that elderly people wake often in the night and feel the need to get up early. The Brigham and Women's Hospital team reported in The Lancet that people over age 65 experienced a drop in body temperature an average of one hour and fifty-two minutes earlier than people in their 20s. This difference correlated with the sleeping patterns of both groups.

• • •

Primary-care physicians who have patients with lower-back pain can treat it with a few relatively simple procedures, doctors were told at a seminar at the 44th annual scientific assembly of the American Academy of Family Physicians in San Diego. These patients often can avoid the need for surgery or referral to a specialist, said a family physician in Lewiston, N.Y. Doctors can use manipulation, caudal epidural injections or a technique called prolotherapy to successfully treat patients with herniated discs or other lumbar disorders, he said.

Oct. 18

Family physicians were told that they should learn to recognize the symptoms of alcoholic or drug-addicted patients, and be willing to offer them treatment, in hopes of deterring the addiction before it consumes the patient. One in six patients that a primary-care physician will see has an addiction problem, and doctors should use clues, such as patients who are noncompliant, have foggy memories or who have frequent bruises or sprains, to spot alcoholics or addicts, a treatment expert advised during the American Academy of Family Physicians annual scientific assembly. Doctors can consult Alcoholics Anonymous for advice on supporting addicted patients through their recovery, he added. He advised against prescribing antidepressants or other drugs to help the patient recover.

Oct. 22

A new interactive computer software package that teaches patients the risks and benefits of various medical procedures may also protect against malpractice lawsuits, the maker of the package told Medical Tribune. The program, made by Medi-Disc Inc., of Carrollton, Texas, requires patients to answer questions about what they have read on the screen, and records any questions they missed so a doctor can later review that material with the patient. This helps establish informed consent, and thus may protect the doctor from being sued in the future, a company official said.

• • •

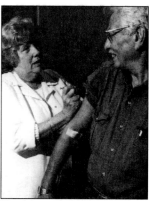

Physicians advised to start influenza shots in October.

The American Academy of Orthopaedic Surgeons introduced a program designed to reduce the estimated 280,000 hip fractures in elderly people each year in the United States. The program, called "Live It Safe," provides information to older patients and their doctors on how to make homes more fractureproof, such as using slip-resistant rugs and installing grab bars in bathtubs. The program also suggests including considerable calcium in the diet and weight-bearing exercises to keep bones strong.

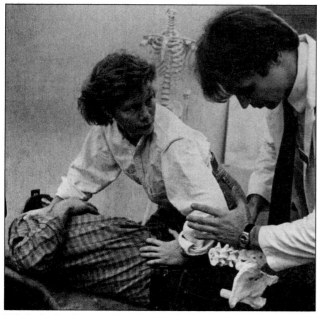

Relatively simple procedures can ease back pain, said N.Y. physician.

NOVEMBER

Nov. 2

Physicians were told that frightening a person works as well as any other treatment for garden-variety hiccups. A specialist in head and neck surgery said that he could not provide a scientific explanation for why the fright technique works. However, when hiccups occur because there has been a release of the central nervous system's normal inhibitory tone on the hiccups reflex arc, any change in CNS stimulation could allow restoration of normal inhibition, stated the physician from the Manhattan Eye, Ear and Throat Hospital in New York.

Other hiccup cures include swallowing granulated sugar, breathing into a bag, gargling with ice water, smelling or tasting something noxious, pressing against the eyes, holding one's breath, concentrating on something other than the hiccups or drinking from the opposite side of a glass, the investigator stated in the Archives of Otolaryngology-Head and Neck Surgery.

Nov. 4

Physicians who prescribe methylene-blue-containing medications to patients who may be subject to random urine drug testing were told to advise their patients to alert collection-site personnel that their urine will be discolored.

To discourage workers from substituting or diluting their urine specimens with toilet water during drug testing, drug-testing programs sanctioned by the U.S. Department of Transportation are required to have any water at the testing site colored blue.

Certain medications prescribed to relieve temporary urinary discomfort (such as Urised, Webcon Pharmaceuticals, or Prosed and Urolene Blue, Star Pharmaceuticals) contain methylene blue, which can turn urine blue within an hour after being taken and for at least 24 hours afterward, two physicians from the Veterans Affairs Medical Center in

San Francisco wrote in The Journal of the American Medical Association.

Nov. 7

Headaches during intercourse were found to be a temporary problem in half of the people who experience them, reported Danish researchers. They surveyed 26 people between six months and 14 years after they had first complained of headaches during intercourse. All the patients had suffered intense headaches that lasted from five to 15 minutes. Thirteen patients experienced only one headache or one cluster of coital headaches. In the other 13 patients, the coital headache pattern reappeared after a headache-free period of up to 10 years.

People with no history of regular headaches and only one sex-related headache can be reassured that they are not at risk of continued episodes, the researchers wrote in the British Medical Journal. But patients who also suffer from migraines or tension headaches and experience benign coital headaches are at great risk of recurrent attacks, said the team from University Hospital of Arhus.

If the headaches become chronic, beta-blockers may be indicated, according to one researcher.

Nov. 16

Massachusetts physicians warned that hay fever sufferers who stay indoors in autumn to avoid ragweed pollen may actually aggravate other allergies. The allergy specialists, from the Lahey Clinic in Burlington, found that the number of house dust mites greatly increases in the early fall, coinciding with the peak ragweed season in the Northeast and elsewhere. Ragweed sufferers who are also allergic to dust mites may thus be unwittingly surrounding themselves with allergens by staying inside,

the doctors told the 50th Anniversary Meeting of the American College of Allergy and Immunology in Chicago. Patients who report seasonal allergic symptoms in August and September may be misdiagnosed as allergic to ragweed, when in fact dust mites may be the symptom trigger, the researchers suggested.

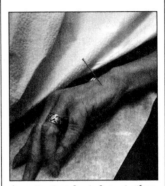

Acupuncture bested most other methods for quitting smoking.

Nov. 18

Primary-care doctors were told that they can easily measure strength and endurance in their elderly patients by having them carry successively heavy bags up and down stairs, Philadelphia researchers told a session at the annual meeting of the Gerontological Society of America. Patients who can carry 40 pounds can perform household duties requiring strength and endurance, they said. Ten of 34 women over the age of 68, and all of the young women in the study, were able to carry the maximum weight of 40 pounds up and down four steps.

Nov. 19

University of Maryland researchers warned that elderly patients may poison themselves with benzodiazepines, either accidentally or intentionally. According to data from the American Association of Poison Control Centers, 69% of benzodiazepine poisoning victims were

women, 92% of the exposures occurred in the home and 65% of the calls to poison hotlines were intentional poisonings. Since people 65 years of age and over account for a third of chronic benzodiazepine use, steps need to be taken to reduce the consequences of benzodiazepine misuse in the elderly, the researchers reported at the annual meeting of the Gerontological Society of America.

Nov. 20

Almost a third of the elderly people in a German study were found to be at serious risk of drug side effects and dangerous drug interactions. A team of researchers at the Academy of Sciences and Technology in Berlin found possible drug interactions in 60% of all multiple drug regimens reported by the elderly people; 23% of the people took more than four drugs daily. The investigators told the annual meeting of the Gerontological Society of America that clear indications were apparent in only 52% of the prescriptions; 33% were of questionable necessity.

Nov. 30

A meta-analysis of 633 studies revealed that acupuncture and hypnosis worked better than most other methods studied in helping patients quit smoking. The analysis of 23 different smoking-cessation methods, presented by University of Iowa researchers in the Journal of Applied Psychology, found that 36% of smokers who underwent hypnosis quit for at least three months, as did 30% of those smokers who underwent treatment with acupuncture needles.

By contrast, 16% of smokers who tried chewing nicotine gum were still smoke-free three months later. And just 7% of those who were simply advised by their doctors to quit, without any extra help, did so. The analysis reviewed no studies involving the nicotine patch.

DECEMBER

Dec. 6

A reference committee told the American Medical Association's House of Delegates meeting in Nashville that walkers for babies pose an unreasonable risk of injury and death and should be banned. The committee members advocated that the AMA strengthen its policy on the ambulation contrivances by urging the Consumer Product Safety Commission to ban them as a mechanical hazard. Previously, the AMA had adopted a policy acknowledging that parents should be counseled on the risk of injuries and informed that the support mechanisms do not promote ambulation.

Baby walkers resulted in at least six deaths between 1989 and mid-1991, and caused 28,913 injuries in 1991, according to the delegates.

Dec. 7

When physicians lament excessive jury awards in malpractice cases, they may be blasting the wrong target, a Chicago attorney told the American Academy of Dermatology meeting in San Francisco. In a recent study, doctors were found to win 71% of malpractice cases heard by a jury, but only 50% of the cases in which judges made the decisions, the lawyer reported.

Further, highly publicized million-dollar judgments are rare: The majority of medical malpractice cases generate little or no money for the plaintiff, stated the malpractice attorney.

Dec. 8

A New York researcher told the American Academy of Dermatology meeting that the chief risk factor for varicose veins is a positive family history. When 500 women with telangiectatic and varicose veins of the lower extremities were compared with a control group of 500 female dermatologic patients, 84% of varicose vein patients and 52% of controls reported having at least one family member with the condition. Women with varicose veins were also significantly more likely to have a vocation that involved standing more than six hours a day (18% of varicose vein patients vs. 7% of controls) and to be more than 20% over their ideal weight (15% vs. 3%).

Other proposed etiological

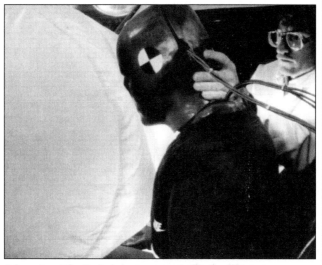

Advocates claim that air bags are cost-effective lifesavers.

factors were not supported by the study, according to the dermatologist from Cornell University Medical College. Varicose vein patients were no more likely than controls to have used oral contraceptives, been exposed to X-rays, suffered lower extremity infections or anoxia, or to have a history of thrombophlebitis.

Dec. 9

Delegates to the American Medical Association's interim meeting debated whether to recommend speeding up nationwide plans to require air bags in automobiles. Advocates of the stance told the Nashville, Tennessee, gathering that the emerging evidence is overwhelming that air bags are capable of preventing injuries as well as reducing mortality, making them a cost-effective addition to American automobiles.

Citing instances when air bags have caused injuries or failed to protect vehicle occupants, opponents of the resolution argued that the AMA should first encourage the U.S. Department of Transportation to collect and evaluate injury data related to air bag use and efficacy.

• • •

Canadian physicians reported that women who receive cosmetic breast implants are not at increased risk of breast cancer. The doctors, from the Alberta Cancer Board in Edmonton and Foothills Hospital in Calgary, looked at a population-based cohort of 11,991 women who had had cosmetic breast implantation during 1973-1986, and linked them with the population-based Alberta Cancer Registry.

The observed number of breast-cancer cases among women with bilateral implants was 41 after a mean follow-up of 10 years, the investigators told the 15th Annual San Antonio Breast Cancer Symposium. The expected number of cases was 86.2, leading the researchers to conclude that breast implants do not constitute a risk factor for breast cancer. Women with implants who developed breast cancer had five- and 10-year survival rates similar to breast-cancer patients without implants.

Dec. 18

Spanish researchers warned that people with asthma may unknowingly worsen their condition by using mint-flavored toothpaste. In a case report appearing in the Journal of Clinical Allergy and Immunology, the investigators concluded that the mint flavoring was the cause of a significant immediate bronchial response following brushing in a 21-year-old woman with a history of asthma. The woman was instructed to brush her teeth with water alone and avoid peppermint, spearmint and menthol. After four months she had not had any asthma attacks and had added 20 mg of cromolyn sodium (Fisons Pharmaceuticals) four times a day to her asthma therapy.

The report noted that since the patient was already receiving high doses of inhaled corticoids, it was unlikely that the cromolyn was responsible for her improvement. This is only the second known case in the literature of a mint- or menthol-induced asthma attack, according to the team from Hospital Universitario San Carlos in Madrid.

Dec. 30

A philosophy of medicine expert said that medical education does little to prepare health professionals to deal effectively with dying patients. Writing in the publication of the National Council for the Right to Die, he said that reading books, taking classes and discussing abstract ideas are not enough; physicians need workshops or other structured opportunities to examine their own feelings about death and dying, declared the University of Houston Health Law and Policy Institute professor.

Citing paperwork, regulations and job stress, 27% of MDs would choose another profession

JAN. 30—About a third of physicians would choose another profession, nearly 10% plan to stop practicing as solo practitioners and about half would not recommend that their children go into medicine, according to a wide-ranging survey conducted by Medical Tribune.

Physicians responded to an assortment of questions, from what are the greatest problems facing their practice to how they use computers.

Thirty-nine percent of the physician respondents seek to improve their cash flow, while 35% said they would improve their record keeping and 29% would change their staff management.

The responses reveal that 54% of our readers are still in solo practice.

Of those in groups, 24% are in practices with under 10 physicians, while 5% are in a group practice of 20 or more. Only 4% report being on staff at a health maintenance organization.

The gradual movement of physicians away from solo practice to group practice was reflected in the 44% of physicians who said they would be working in solo practice in five years.

This is 10% fewer than the number who claimed they were practicing solo.

The physicians who are planning to practice in a group of under 10 physicians totaled 29%—an increase of 5%.

Surprising, nearly a third of physicians (27%) affirmed that they would opt for another profession if they could make the choice again. Only a modest 63% of physicians said they would choose a medical career again if they were given the opportunity.

Nearly half of physicians who responded wouldn't recommend that their children or relatives pursue the medical profession as a career.

Physicians also divulged the greatest problems facing their practices. (Choices of responses were not limited.) Sixty-two percent indicated too much paperwork. Fifty-six percent cited government regulation and 49% believed Medicare reimbursement was the greatest nuisance.

Others chose job-related stress, keeping up with medical advances, malpractice premiums and the bureaucracy of managed care.

Nearly seven out of every 10 physicians use a computer in their practice, according to the Medical Tribune survey. A little over half do their billing on line, while about a third take advantage of word processing options.

The 2,264 respondents were from across the country. Forty-four percent are FPs, 29% are internists, 18% are GPs and 5% are cardiologists. Four percent are gastroenterologists and osteopaths.

Our respondents' ages are more proportional. While only 2.5% of the physicians are under the age of 30, those age 30 to 39 comprise 24% and those age 40 to 49 comprise 25%.

Almost 32% of the respondents are 50 to 64, and 17% are 65 or over. Twenty-eight percent of the readers have been practicing medicine for less than 10 years, 26% have practiced 11 to 20 years, and 18% have worked for 21 to 30 years.

Antianxiety drug helps smokers kick; alleviates cravings

Medical Tribune News Service Report

FEB. 3—An antianxiety agent may also help people quit smoking by lessening nicotine withdrawal.

In a study of 40 people, 79% of those who had smoked at least a pack of cigarettes a day for three years were able to kick the habit with the help of the drug, compared with 50% of those who took a placebo.

The drug, buspirone (Buspar, Mead Johnson Pharmaceuticals), can help smokers quit by blunting withdrawal symptoms, Daniel E. Hilleman, Pharm.D., of the Creighton University Cardiac Center in Omaha, Neb., and colleagues reported in the Archives of Internal Medicine.

In addition to craving cigarettes, people experiencing withdrawal may feel anxious, irritable, restless, hungry, sad, drowsy and unable to concentrate.

Buspirone is given to alleviate nervousness, worry, fatigue and other symptoms associated with anxiety disorders.

"The drug is not a cure," Dr. Hilleman said. "It is meant to be a boost for people who are highly addicted to nicotine. It helps you get around those symptoms so you can concentrate on quitting."

All subjects were told to continue to smoke during the first three weeks of the study, and they took either buspirone or a placebo three times a day. At the start of the fourth week, they were told to stop smoking completely while continuing to take the drug or the placebo for one more week.

Fifteen of 19 people given buspirone stopped smoking

during the fourth week, compared with nine of 18 people given placebo.

People who could not stop completely even though they were taking buspirone nevertheless were able to cut their total cigarette use by an average of 70%, compared with a drop of 39% among people who were taking the placebo.

One year after the study was completed, Dr. Hilleman said that eight of the 15 people in the study who had stopped with the help of the drug have stayed off cigarettes. Two of the nine people who quit while on the placebo have remained nonsmokers, he added.

Three people, two of whom were in the placebo group, were removed from the study because they refused to stop smoking at the start of the third week.

Dr. Hilleman said that people who quit smoking experience withdrawal within the first 12 hours and are in the most discomfort 72 hours after the last cigarette. Without intervention, the symptoms subside in about two weeks, he said.

The Creighton University researchers said that the mechanism by which buspirone reduces the severity of smoking cessation is unknown, but it may be related to its antiserotonin anxiolytic effect.

Carpal tunnel syndrome eased with estrogen

FEB. 8—Estrogen replacement therapy may lessen symptoms of carpal tunnel syndrome and fibromyalgia in menopausal women.

Of 42 menopausal women in a study, seven had CTS and six had fibromyalgia, Gerard Hall, M.D., of St. Bartholomew's Hospital in London, reported in the British Medical Journal.

Women with both conditions improved significantly with six months of estrogen replacement therapy, according to Dr. Hall.

Low estrogen levels were found in fibromyalgia patients with persistent symptoms. Estrogen withdrawal lessens rapid eye movements during sleep and heightens depression, both of which are associated with fibromyalgia, he said. Thus estrogen replacement therapy "seems a logical option."

Changes in forearm fat content that occur at menopause may be the cause of carpal tunnel syndrome in menopausal women, Dr. Hall said.

Linda Morse, M.D., chief of occupational medicine at Santa Clara Valley Medical Center, in Santa Clara, Calif., said fluid retention may be involved.

Seven times as many women as men have the syndrome, which can be triggered by pregnancy, use of oral contraceptives and gynecological surgery, Dr. Morse said.

Advice for preparing patients for pregnancy

New York Times/Medical Tribune News Syndicate

FEB. 27—Preconception counseling by the primary-care physician can help prepare patients for pregnancy, identify risk factors for a poor outcome and uncover any existing medical conditions that should be controlled prior to conception, according to obstetricians and maternal-nutrition specialists.

Such counseling, which should be accompanied by a blood workup, a thorough physical exam and a careful history, can reduce infant-mortality rates, improve pregnancy outcomes and keep perinatal healthcare costs to a minimum, the experts said.

"We can spend a lot of money on high-risk care during pregnancy that won't do a lot of good, or we can spend more time with the patient prepregnancy," said Richard Aubry, M.D., obstetrics director at Upstate Medical Center in Syracuse, N.Y.

"I believe that the latter would be more effective, in terms of preventing problems."

One of the first and most important components of preconception counseling is to educate a woman about precautions that she needs to take while she is pregnant, said Terry German, M.D., an ob/gyn and associate medical director of the Pennsylvania-based health maintenance organization U.S. Healthcare.

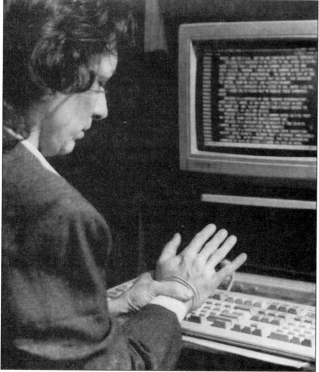

Carpal tunnel syndrome and fibromyalgia yielded to hormone.

"When a woman is trying to conceive, especially in the second half of every menstrual cycle, she should use the same precautions that she would take if she were already pregnant," he said. "Likewise, a woman needs to understand that she should stop drinking and smoking while trying to conceive."

Physicians should also discuss proper nutrition with prospective mothers, according to Judith E. Brown, Ph.D., a professor of nutrition at the University of Minnesota in Minneapolis.

Aside from stressing the importance of a balanced diet, Dr. Brown said that primary-care physicians should also advise patients to maintain a high iron status, achieve their ideal body weight (since overweight and underweight women tend to have poorer pregnancy outcomes) and reduce alcohol and caffeine intake—alcohol to no more than one drink a day; caffeine to under four cups.

Diabetic patients should be assisted in achieving glucose control prior to conception, in order to reduce the risk of birth defects and other problems, she said.

Patients with phenylketonuria should be advised to maintain a strict PKU diet for several months prior to conception and throughout pregnancy, Dr. Brown added.

Lastly, women who are trying to achieve pregnancy should never take more than the recommended daily allowance of any vitamin or mineral, according to Dr. Brown. Vitamin A in high amounts can be particularly toxic to a developing fetus, and more than 15 mg of beta-carotene per day may impair fertility, she said.

After taking a history, physicians should advise women about any special risks they may have for a poor pregnancy outcome, Dr. Aubry said. Among these may be age over 35 or under 18; a family history of illness, such as Tay-Sachs or sickle-cell anemia; hemophilia; hypertension; diabetes; or previous poor outcomes. If genetic risks exist, refer the patient to a genetic counselor, he said.

Patients who have had children with neural-tube defects should take folic acid supplements during pregnancy, Dr. Aubry said. "The bulk of evidence shows that it does help."

Contrary to earlier practice, a woman need not wait three cycles before trying to conceive after ceasing to take oral contraceptives, according to Dr. German.

Women ought to look carefully at any risks posed by their occupations, he said, including exposure to chemicals, lead or X-ray radiation. They should also avoid exercise more strenuous than what they are accustomed to, he added.

Drs. Aubry and German suggested certain tests that should be taken prior to conception.

Home asthma checks urged by expert panel

By L.A. McKeown

MARCH 8—In light of the rising number of asthma deaths, an international panel of experts has encouraged physicians to use home peak-flow monitoring as a potentially lifesaving measure in patients who receive daily medications.

According to a consensus statement released at the American Academy of Allergy and Immunology meeting in Orlando, Fla., even children as young as five years old can use a peak-flow meter adequately.

"Traditionally, we have relied on patients telling the physician how they feel and the physician listening to the patient's wheezing," said Jean Bousquet, M.D., professor of pulmonary diseases at the University of Montpellier in France. "However, these are often unreliable indicators of how much airway obstruction there is."

According to the guidelines, the physician should educate the patient and family on how and when to use the peak-flow meter, how to record peak expiratory flow (PEF) measurements, how to interpret the measurements, how to

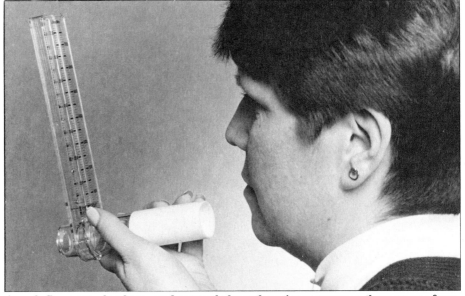

A peak-flow meter has been used correctly by asthmatics as young as three years of age.

respond to changes and what information to relay to the physician.

The resulting information may help identify patients who would benefit from anti-inflammatory medications, particularly those who use bronchodilators regularly and believe their asthma is under control while in fact they are developing potentially lethal progressive airway narrowing, according to A. Sonia Buist, M.D., head of pulmonary and critical care at the Oregon Health Sciences University in Portland.

Peak-flow measurements should be taken twice a day, immediately after rising and 10 to 12 hours later, and compared with the patient's personal best values, according to the panel's guidelines.

If the highest value is less than 80% of the personal best, more aggressive therapy and daily monitoring are indicated, according to the panel's report.

In such cases, patients may need more bronchodilators, but if they use a beta-agonist daily, they should receive anti-in-flammatory therapy—either cromolyn sodium (Fisons Pharmaceuticals) or inhaled corticosteroids, according to the panel's chairman, Albert Sheffer, M.D., of Harvard Medical School in Boston.

Australian researchers at the Orlando meeting presented data showing that peak-flow meters are invaluable because even severe asthmatics can have a "silent chest" upon examination with a stethoscope.

Another paper, from researchers at Guy's Hospital in London, showed that children as young as three years old were able to use low-range peak-flow meters.

HSV found most infectious in first three months

MARCH 15—Herpes simplex virus may be most infectious during the three months after resolution of primary disease, even if patients are asymptomatic, a study has found.

Researchers from the University of Washington in Seattle suggest that patients who have just recovered from a first outbreak of herpes sores should be counseled on the importance of condom use during that three-month period.

For 63 weeks, they followed 306 women who had recently contracted HSV primary type 1, primary type 2 or non-primary type 2 for the first time. The women were seen every other day during the initial outbreak.

After the lesions had healed, patients were tested by means of physical examination and viral culture every four to six weeks.

At three months, women with primary type 2 HSV had a rate of asymptomatic viral shedding from the cervix that was three times higher than for women with primary type 1 disease. At three months, women with primary type 2 disease were also found to have a higher rate of asymptomatic vulvar shedding than women with either primary type 1 or non-primary type 2.

Cervical shedding of type 2 HSV was three times more likely to occur during the first three months after lesions had resolved than during later months.

According to David Koelle, M.D., shedding rates did not differ between women who received acyclovir (Zovirax, Burroughs Wellcome) during their first episodes and those who did not.

Up to 23% of women in the study had no symptoms during the three-month period when they were most contagious, said Dr. Koelle and colleagues, who reported their findings in the Annals of Internal Medicine.

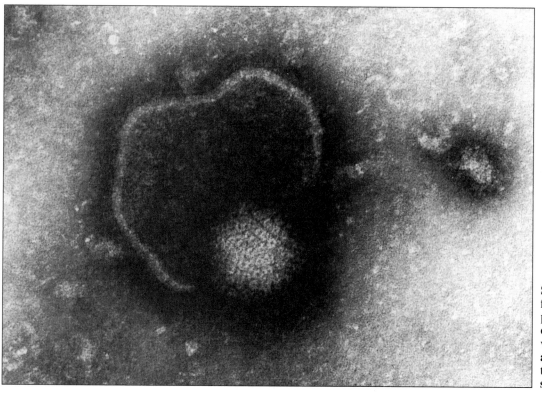

Shedding rates found to depend on precisely which type of Herpes simplex virus a patient has, as well as how much time has passed since lesions healed.

"Our data provide a rationale for recommending the routine use of condoms to prevent transmission of disease during this high-risk period," according to Dr. Koelle.

In another study, which also appeared in the Annals of Internal Medicine, New Mexico researchers found that of 14 people who acquired HSV, 70% had infected partners who were asymptomatic at the time.

Gregory Mertz, M.D., of the University of New Mexico School of Medicine in Albuquerque, said that many doctors still believe that the virus can only be transmitted when lesions are present.

He added that the use of condoms is necessary in between recurrences since there is no sure way of predicting when an asymptomatic person is shedding virus. Patients should also be educated to recognize lesions when they are symptomatic.

Approximately 30 million Americans have herpes, according to the American Social Health Association in Research Triangle Park, N.C.

ACR report: More frequent mammograms may catch cancer early, save younger women's lives

New York Times/Medical Tribune News Syndicate

APRIL 28—Although even some medical groups remain unconvinced, screening women under age 50 for breast cancer saves lives, reported researchers at the American College of Radiology's 25th National Conference on Breast Cancer in Boston.

The findings suggest that American Cancer Society guidelines, which call for screening women aged 40 to 49 every one to two years, may not be adequate, according to Daniel Kopans, M.D., director of the Breast Imaging Division at the Massachusetts General Hospital in Boston.

At least 300 45-year-old women could be saved this year, for example, if their cancer were detected early enough, according to another expert.

But women who do go for mammography often ignore their radiologist's recommendation to see a breast surgeon, reported a third group of researchers.

While physicians are united in their support of yearly mammograms for women over age 50, some medical groups do not support the screening in younger women, according to Dr. Kopans.

His study of 1,039 breast-cancer patients in their 40s found that mammograms significantly improved the chances of surviving the cancer. After five years, 94% of cancer patients who got mammograms were alive compared with 74% of women whose cancer was detected by palpation, according to Dr. Kopans.

"Mammograms are so important in the 40 to 49 age group

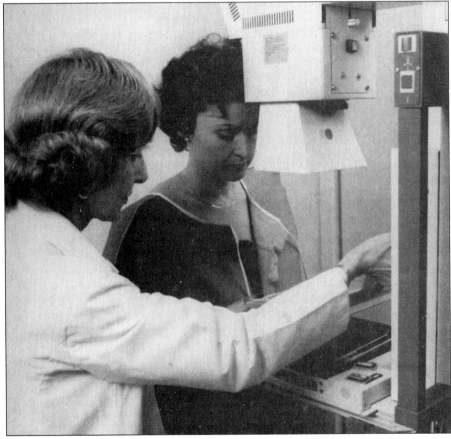

Early checkups can give doctors a lead time of one and a half years over tumor.

because cancers in younger women probably grow faster," he said. "Also, our ability to find the tumors is reduced because younger women have denser breasts."

Doctors gain a lead time of about one to one and a half years over the tumor with mammograms, Dr. Kopans said. "That's why I feel screening every two years is likely to have very little impact. Women between 40 and 49 should be screened every year."

The biggest obstacle to women getting regular mammograms may be their physicians, according to Dr. Kopans.

"When physicians recommmend them, the women go," he said. "When the doctors don't, the women don't go."

Even when women do go for a mammogram, they often ignore the radiologist's recommendation to consult with a breast surgeon, said Carole Chrvala, M.D., of the Colorado State Health Department.

In other instances, the referring physician does not refer the woman to a breast surgeon, she added.

Proper breast screening, which includes good-quality mammograms and good interpretation, could save the lives of 300 women out of a population of one million 45-year-old women, according to Stephen Feig, M.D., of the Thomas Jefferson University Hospital in Philadelphia. "We're talking about a 40% mortality reduction."

About 1,500 women out of every million develop cancer, and without screening, about 750 will die, Dr. Feig said.

Prescription diet pills help patients shed pounds

Medical Tribune News Service Report

MAY 1—Prescription diet pills can help moderately obese people lose weight, without regaining it, according to a new four-year study.

But the pills must be taken for years to maintain the weight loss, raising questions about their long-term safety, an obesity expert warns.

The new study, by Michael Weintraub, M.D., of the University of Rochester School of Medicine in Rochester, N.Y., found that a combination of two appetite-suppressing drugs helped patients lose an average of more than 30 pounds.

The study was performed using 121 patients whose weight averaged 200 pounds.They followed a program of diet, exercise, behavior modification and counseling, after which they began to lose the weight.

Six weeks later, half the patients started taking a combination of phentermine (Ionamin, Fisons Pharmaceuticals) and fenfluramine (Pondimin, A.H. Robins), and in 80%, their weight dropped even further. They maintained the loss as long as they took the drugs and followed an exercise or behavior modification routine—in some, up to three-and-a-half years.

The rest of the patients took placebo pills. They lost only a few pounds, and soon gained them back.

Many study participants who were on diet pills suffered side effects such as dry mouth, diarrhea and nervousness, according to the study, which appears in Clinical Pharmacology and Therapeutics.

"The study is long overdue," said W.L. Asher, M.D., a Denver physician and director of professional affairs for the American Society of Bariatric Physicians.

Although the diet drugs in Dr. Weintraub's study are approved only for short-term use, they aren't effective if used only for short periods, Dr. Asher said. "That's like treating hypertension in the short-term."

Dr. Asher said he has used phentermine with success, although some patients tend to build up a tolerance to it. "The drugs are a crutch, but with a crutch these people can walk," he added.

The American Society of Bariatric Physicians recommends that doctors only prescribe appetite-suppressing drugs as long as the patient responds significantly to the treatment. Doctors should carefully monitor patients who take the drugs for more than 12 weeks, according to its guidelines.

Although Dr. Weintraub's study found that the side effects from the drugs were restricted to dry mouth, diarrhea and nervousness, little data on longer-term side effects are available.

"We don't quite know what will happen to people after four, five, six years on these drugs," said Xavier Pi-Sunyer, M.D., director of the Obesity Research Center at St. Luke's-Roosevelt Hospital Center in New York City.

"Drug therapy is expensive, and it has side effects," he added. "There are some patients for whom drugs are contraindicated: those with depression, a history of GI dysfunction in the past or sleeping problems," Dr. Pi-Sunyer said in an interview.

"This is a landmark kind of study. There always has been a certain amount of room for using the drugs," Dr. Pi-Sunyer said. But the drugs should be a small component of a larger program of diet, exercise and counseling, he said.

Experts recommend weight loss for health

By Mara Bovsun

MAY 7—After losing and regaining tons of fat, overweight Americans and their doctors are still battling obesity, which affects roughly 25% of the U.S. population.

While some weary dieters are abandoning their calorie counting and scales, medical experts caution that some patients need weight-loss regimens to remain healthy.

Groups like the 3,500-member National Association to Advance Fat Acceptance of Sacramento, Calif., worry Theodore Van Itallie, M.D., professor emeritus at St. Luke's-Roosevelt Hospital Center in New York City. Its members, who range from 170 to 500 pounds, have been dieting unsuccessfully for decades and have "stopped putting their lives on hold," said Sally Smith, the group's executive director.

"People who say that they should eat what they want to eat are ignoring the fact that it puts their health at risk," said Dr. Van Itallie.

But physicians must learn to assess whether a patient needs

to lose weight for health reasons. "The questions to ask are: Does the patient have medical problems for which weight loss is indicated, is the fat in the abdomen or on the hips and thighs, and is the patient's weight acceptable for his or her height and age?" said C. Wayne Callaway, M.D., of Washington, D.C., and a member of the Dietary Guidelines Advisory Committee of the U.S. Department of Agriculture and the U.S. Department of Health and Human Services.

Physicians should look for a family history of obesity-related diseases—diabetes, gallbladder disease, hypertension, hypercholesterolemia and heart disease, he added.

People with pot bellies face a greater risk of illness than do people with fat on their hips and thighs because abdominal fat releases fatty acids into the portal vein and, ultimately, into the liver, where it interferes with insulin metabolism, according to Dr. Callaway.

To assess whether a patient is carrying too much abdominal fat, physicians can estimate the waist-to-hip ratio (WHR) by dividing the circumference of the waist (defined as a point midway between the lower rib margin and the iliac crest) by the circumference of the hip (the widest point over the buttocks). The WHR should be less than .95 for men and .80 for women.

Ironically, "men with beer bellies" have the highest WHR ratios but go on diets less frequently than pear-shaped women, who face fewer health risks, said Dr. Callaway.

The greatest predictors of successful weight loss are the patient's willingness to keep records and a commitment to exercise, according to Dr. Callaway. A patient's determination to change his or her life-style, and not just drop a few pounds, is another good way to predict diet outcome, said Dr. Van Itallie, who has been treating obese patients since 1952.

"The physician has to assess whether the patient has an understanding of the problem and the intellectual ability to change life-style and manner of eating," he said. A number of previous weight-loss attempts is a strong indicator that a new diet will fail. Another important consideration is the stress level of the patient's job.

Physicians should suggest, not coordinate, weight-loss programs for their patients, according to the Washington, D.C., physician.

There is no substitute for a registered dietitian and a professional knowledgeable in behavioral modification, said Dr. Callaway.

"The doctor should not get involved in dietetics," he said. "All people in private practice should have one or two or more dietitians with whom they can work."

Responsible and ultimately successful weight loss involves long-term changes in eating habits, according to Dr. Callaway.

"The program must be tailored to the individual," he said. "The patient's irregular eating habits and any psychiatric disorders must be taken into consideration. All patients should not be given the same 1,200-calorie diet," he added.

Referring a patient to a commercial program is "the easy way out," according to Dr. Callaway. "Physicians working at

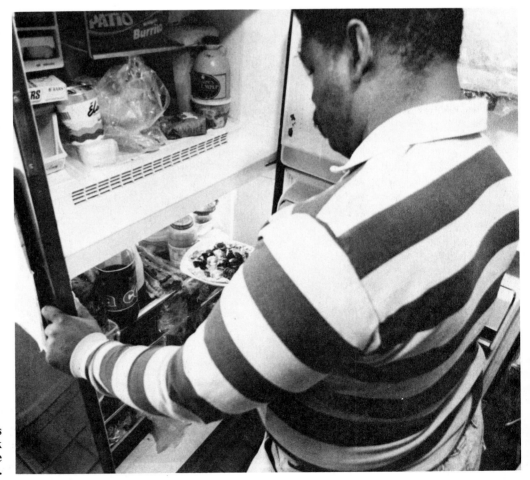

**People with pot bellies
face greater risk
of illness than do people
with fat hips and thighs.**

medical-center-based weight-loss programs are not trained in the field," he said.

It is estimated that most people who lose weight gain back those pounds and more.

Nevertheless, 48 million Americans were on a diet in 1991, and 101 million were "eating light," using fat-free foods and sugar-free sodas, according to the Calorie Control Council, a low-calorie-foods trade association in Atlanta, Ga.

Adherence to an exercise program is crucial to the success of a weight loss program.

The minimum exercise regimen for maintaining fitness—20 minutes of aerobic activity three times a week—is not enough to help people lose weight, according to Dr. Van Itallie.

He recommends that patients walk more, for as much as two hours a day.

"Walking for an hour burns 240 calories," he said. "Do that two times a day."

Alvin J. Ciccone, M.D., a family physician in Norfolk, Va., just tells his patients to get moving, and estimates that "a mile of anything burns about 100 calories."

New test detects antibody, certifies Lyme disease

By Neil Rosenberg

LaCrosse, Wis., May 18—Researchers at the Gundersen Medical Foundation here report they have developed the first definitive test for Lyme disease.

Called the Gundersen Lyme Test, it detects a bacteria-killing antibody found in the blood of people with the disease.

"Since this antibody develops only in persons with Lyme disease and kills only the Lyme organism, its detection with our test likely indicates the presence of Lyme disease," said Steven M. Callister, Ph.D., a microbiologist at the Gundersen research center who discovered the bactericidal antibody.

"When the test is positive, that physician is dealing with Lyme disease. Period. Because this antibody is very, very specific," Dr. Callister said.

Since the Lyme-killing, or borreliacidal, antibody is active in the body as early as seven days after exposure to Lyme disease, the Gundersen test also may be effective in detecting the disease much earlier than current tests, Dr. Callister added.

It also may be used to gauge whether treatment is effective, because the borreliacidal antibody disappears when treatment is successful, he said. In a preliminary study published last year, Dr. Callister and two colleagues used the test on 20 serum samples from patients diagnosed with Lyme disease, and 10 samples from healthy people.

After the test was performed, the average number of live bacteria in the healthy-patient samples was triple the average number of live bacteria in the Lyme-disease samples, a sign that the Lyme antibody was present in the diseased samples and was killing the bacteria.

When the Gundersen test is negative, it could mean the person does not have Lyme disease, or that Lyme disease is present but at too early a stage to detect it, he said.

The Gundersen test does not react to other diseases, such as Rocky Mountain spotted fever or syphilis, to create a false-positive diagnosis of Lyme disease—a decided advantage over the ELISA test currently used to detect the disease, Dr. Callister explained.

The ELISA test can result in a 25% false-positive rate at some labs, Dr. Callister said. "It picks up a lot of antibodies, maybe from past exposure [to Lyme disease] or to other, related illnesses," he said.

A lack of standardization among laboratories also can lead to false-positive results, he said.

A recent study of 70 children diagnosed with Lyme disease found that 33 of the diagnoses were incorrect, either because of faulty lab tests or of physician misdiagnosis.

The Centers for Disease Control is withholding comment on the test until it receives results from samples sent to Dr. Callister for testing.

The Gundersen clinic will perform the new test for physicians in Wisconsin, Minnesota, Iowa, Illinois and Michigan. MarDx Diagnostics of Carlsbad, Calif., will perform the Gundersen test for the rest of the United States. For information about ordering the test, call the lab at 1-800-331-2291.

The test costs about $70, about the same as many of the ELISA kits on the market, and takes three to four days to run, Dr. Callister said. Because the test depends on live Lyme disease bacteria, no kits can be developed for use in physicians' offices or clinics, he said.

Canadian study backs corticosteroids as Rx for moderate asthma

June 10—A new Canadian study has strengthened the federal recommendation advising physicians to treat moderate asthma with such anti-inflammatory drugs as inhaled corticosteroids.

Using computer simulations of the lung, researchers at the University of British Columbia showed that airway constriction alone had relatively little effect on airflow, unless inflammation was present.

Once the walls of the airways were thickened by inflammation, even minor muscle constrictions produced dramatic reductions in airflow, reported Barry Wiggs, a graduate academic assistant, in the American Review of Respiratory Disease, the official journal of the American Thoracic Society.

"No one imagined a little thickening of the airway wall would make much of a difference," said Jeffrey Drazen, M.D., of Harvard Medical School, in an accompanying editorial. "It's only in recent years that we've grasped the importance of inflammation.

"This study offers a plausible explanation of why inflammation plays so central a role," he added.

The Vancouver researchers point out that the use of bronchodilators has not slowed the recent increase in asthma deaths and hospitalizations, and some fear that beta-agonists may even be contributing to morbidity.

While European and Canadian doctors are using corticosteroids to treat moderate asthma, American physicians have been slower to switch therapies.

American physicians are naturally cautious, and the idea that asthma is an inflammatory disease is taking a long time to catch on, according to Sonia Buist, M.D., a former president of the American Thoracic Society.

Last year, the National Heart, Lung and Blood Institute issued new guidelines calling for doctors to treat moderate chronic asthma with regular, inhaled corticosteroids or other anti-inflammatory medications.

People taking inhaled steroids are less likely to react to asthma triggers, like cat dander or other allergens, according to Dr. Drazen.

The drugs can mean the difference between periodic bad attacks and a normal life, the Harvard researcher noted. As physicians see that the new guidelines work, more will institute the recommendations into their practice, he said.

About 42% of physicians are using inhaled corticosteroids for moderate asthma, according to the Asthma Report conducted by Allen & Hanburys, a division of Glaxo Inc. Roughly half of physicians are reportedly still using bronchodilators routinely.

A study published earlier this year in The New England Journal of Medicine concluded that regular use of beta-agonists may mislead both patients and their physicians into thinking that the disease is under control, when in fact it is not.

McGill University researchers in Montreal said beta-agonists should not be discontinued, but should be used cautiously.

The lung association said that beta-agonists are still recommended for asthma symptoms and for regular use in people with more severe asthma.

No 'magic pill' for irritable bowel syndrome, but partnership can boost success rates

Medical World News Report

JUNE 15—The physician-patient relationship is an important part of helping patients live comfortably with irritable bowel syndrome, according to two new reports.

An estimated 15% to 20% of the population suffer from the condition, but few seek help from a doctor, choosing instead to live with the symptoms or treat themselves, Douglas A. Drossman, M.D., of the University of North Carolina in Chapel Hill, wrote in the Annals of Internal Medicine.

Many people with IBS become frustrated because they are searching for a "magic pill" that they think will cure them, Dr. Drossman said. But the reality of IBS is that there is no proven treatment that benefits everyone.

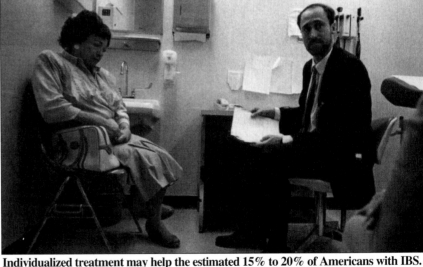

Individualized treatment may help the estimated 15% to 20% of Americans with IBS.

"The treatment can and should be individualized," Dr. Drossman said in an interview. "The vast majority of people have symptoms that are easy to manage."

He said that most cases of IBS are mild or moderate. Mild disease usually is treated by increasing the fiber content of the diet, and avoiding fatty foods, caffeine and alcohol if they trigger symptoms.

People who are suffering from moderate disease may be helped by behavior therapy, hypnosis or education to get them to avoid triggers. "It frees the physician from a sense of burden and also empowers the patient," Dr. Drossman said.

More severe cases may require antidepressants such as amitriptyline (Elavil, Stuart Pharmaceuticals) for pain when behavioral intervention fails and chronic pain persists, he explained.

The author of the second paper, Michael Camilleri, M.D.,

of the Mayo Clinic in Rochester, Minn., focuses more on relieving IBS symptoms than on the biopsychosocial approach of Dr. Drossman.

Dr. Camilleri said the diarrhea or constipation should be treated with loperamide HCI (Imodium, Janssen) or increased fiber intake, respectively, while antispasmodics should be prescribed for gas and bloating.

He reserves antidepressants for patients in whom there is a component of depression.

Patients with chronic symptoms often are the ones most likely to become depressed or anxious, Dr. Camilleri said.

In an accompanying editorial, Thomas Almy, M.D., of Dartmouth Medical School in Hanover, N.H., said that a strong doctor-patient relationship can prevent needless tests, which are uncomfortable and costly.

He added that physicians should discourage unrealistic expectations of a cure and focus instead on maintenance and supportive care.

NSAID found to ease some symptoms of colds

Axel Springer News Service

JULY 1—A nonsteroidal anti-inflammatory, typically used to treat arthritis and mild to moderate pain, may reduce cold symptoms by almost one third, according to a University of Virginia researcher.

In the study, which was published in the Annals of Internal Medicine, researchers studied the effect of naproxen (Naprosyn, Syntex) on 79 healthy college-age people exposed to a rhinovirus.

Six hours after spraying a dose of rhinovirus into the participants' noses, the researchers gave half of the cohort a loading dose of 400 mg of naproxen, followed by 200 mg three times a day for five days. The other half of the cohort received placebo.

Jack M. Gwaltney, Jr., M.D., of the University of Virginia Health Sciences Center in Charlottesville, reported that those taking the drug experienced a 29% reduction in cold symptoms, compared with those in the placebo group.

The symptoms that were most likely to be alleviated were headache and cough, while minimal differences were seen for nasal symptoms and sore throat.

No apparent difference was noted between the groups in terms of sneezing or nasal obstruction.

According to Dr. Gwaltney, naproxen may be effective for the inflammation that accompanies rhinovirus infection because it inhibits prostaglandin synthesis.

Although the effect of naproxen is considered modest on its own, Dr. Gwaltney said that in combination with two other drugs, it may eliminate the majority of cold symptoms.

Dr. Gwaltney said that naproxen, given in combination with interferon and ipratropium (Atrovent, Boehringer

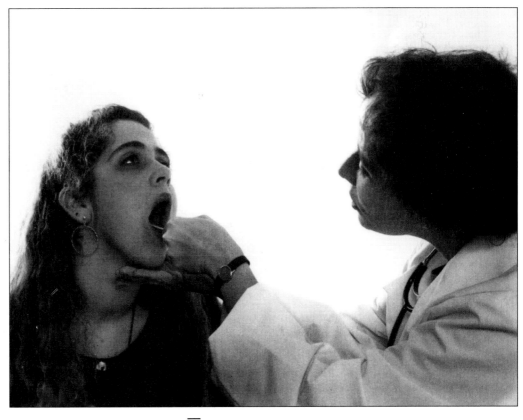

Naproxen alleviated headaches and cough, but did little for nasal symptoms and sore throats.

Ingelheim), may prove useful as a multi-ingredient cold medicine to reduce inflammation and kill the rhinovirus.

The combined three-way medication has a patent pending for development by the Center for Innovative Technology, and could be available in five to 10 years, Dr. Gwaltney said.

Another cold expert, David Proud, Ph.D., of Johns Hopkins University in Baltimore, said a potential drawback of the combined therapy is interferon's high price.

Results of a study involving the combination treatment will be published later this year, according to Dr. Gwaltney. "We've seen very beneficial effects for the combined treatment," Dr. Gwaltney said. "It's the best I've ever seen."

Physicians cope with aftershocks of earthquake

By Laura Buterbaugh

AUG. 6—Three to five times a day, W.W. Leiske, M.D., listens to reports of the fear and the suffering caused by the latest California earthquake.

The Big Bear Lake, Calif., family practitioner's patients arrive in a steady stream, seeking medication to sleep or to steady their nerves, and in some cases just looking for a sympathetic ear.

"People are just done for. They're crying. They're sobbing. They're scared," Dr. Leiske said. "In 20 years, I've never seen anything like it."

The June 28 earthquake, one of the largest in California history, shook the mountainous desert area around Big Bear Lake, Landers and Joshua Tree, leaving hundreds homeless and many more with damaged homes, offices and belongings. Aftershocks continue to rock the region.

The temblor also left a legacy of dire predictions by earthquake experts that an even larger, more devastating quake may not be far away.

"Every day there's an article that this fault is getting bigger. That kind of keeps people whipped up," Dr. Leiske said.

He and other area physicians have been busy prescribing tranquilizers to patients, to calm their fears and help them relax enough to be able to sleep.

"The fatigue is the worst problem," Dr. Leiske said. "The ground just shakes all night."

The June 28 quake and another the same day—7.4 and 6.5, respectively, on the Richter scale—increased the chance of a bigger quake happening along the San Andreas fault within 30 years, experts say. Some have predicted that a more destructive earthquake could occur in as few as two years.

Sidney Hayes, M.D., a general practioner in Joshua Tree, said some distraught patients not only come to his office, but approach him on the street for help.

"They ask me what to do," Dr. Hayes said. "What can you tell a person who's that way when you have the same thing yourself?"

Some of Dr. Hayes' office equipment was damaged, and he lost $4,000 worth of antiques in his home. He said he understands the sense of loss his patients feel, and the stress from the ongoing aftershocks.

"People want Valium. They want nerve medicine. They want Tylenol No. 3. Up at the hospital, they've had an overflow," Dr. Hayes said. "I try to give them what they ask for."

Recently, a group of psychiatrists who counseled San Francisco residents during the earthquake there came to Big Bear Lake's performing arts center, where they held a mass therapy session to help people cope.

The counseling center at Bear Valley Community Hospital in Big Bear Lake also offers special courses on dealing with postearthquake anxiety, said hospital CEO Jon Smiley.

"Some of our staff are dealing with the same anxieties as the people they're treating," Smiley said. "Even I'm on medication. I'm not from earthquake country," he said.

The earthquake has aggravated the state's existing troubles, including a high unemployment rate and state budget problems.

"The area was already economically depressed. Now it's worse," said Theresa Graham, spokesperson for Hi-Desert Medical Center in Joshua Tree. "A lot of people worked at K-Mart or Builders Emporium, and they've closed down. So now these people are out of jobs."

The state government has been issuing IOUs to all agencies that provide state services, until it resolves an $11-billion deficit and passes a new budget. Smiley said banks in his area have been accepting the IOUs the hospital deposits. "We'd be in big trouble if they didn't," he said.

Early Lyme therapy with antibiotics advised

By Saralie Faivelson

AUG. 20—Physicians who practice in areas where many deer ticks are infected with Borrelia burgdorferi should institute antibiotic therapy soon after patients are bitten, rather than waiting for a "bull's-eye" rash to appear, according to a study by a Denver physician.

But while some experts agreed with the findings of The New England Journal of Medicine study, others say it may be misinterpreted and lead to early treatment when it is not indicated.

In the Colorado study, David Magid, M.D., of the Denver General Hospital, and colleagues calculated the health outcomes and costs for a hypothetical cohort of 100,000 patients bitten by ticks.

Three treatment strategies were used: giving all patients with a tick bite two weeks of oral antibiotics; treating only those who developed the rash; and treating only those patients who have a rash or a positive serologic test one month after exposure.

Dr. Magid concluded that early, empirical treatment is the least expensive strategy, results in the fewest cases of Lyme disease and causes the fewest complications—but only if the probability of B. burgdorferi infection after a tick bite is 3.6% or higher. Empirical therapy is not warranted, he said, when the probability of infection is below 1%.

When the probability of infection is between the two percentages, the pros and cons of treatment should be discussed with the patient, he said.

To calculate the chances of a patient's developing Lyme disease, doctors must first determine tick infection rates in their area. In parts of California and Oregon, for example, the likelihood of the tick being infected with B. burgdorferi is less than 5%, according to Dr. Magid.

"Since the probability of disease transmission from any infected tick is less than 10%, this makes the probability of a person's developing Lyme disease in these areas less than 1%, so we don't recommend treatment for these patients," he said.

However, in areas of New England and the mid-Atlantic states, where infection rates among ticks may reach 50%, "we do recommend treatment."

Infection rates among ticks vary from county to county; doctors can find out the rates by calling their local health departments, Dr. Magid said.

Dr. Magid's study "puts some order into the chaos" and should be a helpful guide to physicians, according to Henry Feder, Jr., M.D., of the University of Connecticut Health Center in Farmington. "The good news is that people who get bites are not getting infected, and that if you treat at the time of rash, you're still okay," he said.

But David Volkman, M.D., of the State University of New York, Stony Brook, is concerned that doctors will miss what he considers one of the main points of the NEJM study, that empirical treatment is not warranted in areas where the prevalence of infected ticks is less than 10%.

"The right kind of tick must be infected itself, then bite you, and stay on you for two or more days," he added.

"And if it's not a deer tick, this model doesn't apply at all."

In most areas, doctors can safely wait until the characteristic rash appears before starting treatment, according to Dr. Volkman. "The really serious complications appear long after that."

In some cases, however, early therapy is warranted, Jerome Kassirer, M.D., editor-in-chief of NEJM, asserted in an accompanying editorial. "If the patient's anxiety about getting Lyme disease is great, or if the physician thinks that the patient might fail to return for a follow-up visit, prophylactic treatment is probably justified," Dr. Kassirer wrote.

Once a decision to treat has been made, physicians may want to consider cefuroxime axetil (Ceftin, Allen & Hanburys), New York researchers reported in a separate study. The antibiotic "appears to be equally as effective as doxycycline" in eliminating erythema migrans and other symptoms of Lyme disease, but causes less photosensitivity reactions, Robert B. Nadelman, M.D., of the Westchester County Medical Center in Valhalla, N.Y., reported in the Annals of Internal Medicine.

Of the evaluable patients, 51 of 55 (93%) on cefuroxime and 45 of 51 (88%) on doxycycline had resolution of erythema migrans within one to five days of beginning treatment. Satisfactory clinical responses were maintained at one year posttreatment in 90% of 48 evaluable patients treated with cefuroxime and in 92% of 38 treated with doxycycline.

Photosensitivity reactions occurred in 15% of doxycycline patients, but were not seen in any of the cefuroxime-treated patients. Diarrhea was more common, however, in the cefuroxime group (21%) than in the doxycycline group (7%), Dr. Nadelman reported.

Ousted by Andrew, doctors all pitch in

Medical Tribune Special Report

AUG. 24—When Hurricane Andrew howled its way ashore last month, it blew out the side doors of a concrete building that housed the southern Dade County practice of Wentworth Jarrett, M.D., flooding his office. The storm also wrecked the family practitioner's second office in Homestead.

Dr. Jarrett is one of about 200 physicians who have suffered the total loss of their practice, including building, equipment and patient records, according to Gerry Soud, communications director of the Florida Medical Association in Jacksonville.

Patients, overwhelmed by the loss of their homes and without telephones, transportation, power, food and clean water, have no way of reaching the physicians.

So some of the doctors are reaching out to the patients, treating them in makeshift medical facilities set amid the devastation of the hurricane.

Many of the physicians are also caring for hundreds of other patients in migrant camps and housing projects who cannot otherwise get to a doctor or a hospital.

"We are going from door to door, seeing if these people need medical care," said Cary Shames, D.O., president of the Broward County Osteopathic Medical Association. "Migrant workers distrust the military and police officers. Many of them are illegal aliens and are afraid of being taken away, so they are afraid to seek medical care."

During the first few days after Hurricane Andrew struck, there were no physicians in the migrant camps, according to Dr. Shames. Working with the Florida Osteopathic Medical Association and his Broward County group, Dr. Shames has organized a rotating group of volunteer physicians who are helicoptered daily to various areas, including Homestead, Florida City and Leisure City.

"We are working with about 100 M.D.s and D.O.s," he said. "We have between 10 and 12 in the field every day. We have doctors manning field hospitals in Homestead and working with the MASH unit of the 156th Medical Company of the National Guard."

The first few days were rocky, with a lack of equipment

hampering the delivery of care, Dr. Shames said. "We needed everything, EKG machines, crash carts, IV medications. The pictures on TV don't tell the story. There is utter devastation. Nothing was left standing."

The volunteer doctors have treated cardiac arrests, congestive heart failure, major and minor trauma and dysentery. "On Saturday we were knocking on doors in the Florida City projects when we came across a one-year-old boy covered with lacerations and infections. He was comatose,'' Dr. Shames said. The child was helicoptered to Homestead Hospital and survived.

Dozens of medical students and staff from the University of Miami School of Medicine have fanned out to four clinics in southern Dade County to help hurricane victims, according to Pedro Jose Greer, Jr., M.D., medical director of Camillus Health Concern, a medical service for the homeless. Diarrhea, heat problems, diabetes complications and minor trauma are some of the most common problems they see. "We've treated between 800 and 1,200 patients so far," he said.

Dr. Jarrett is treating his patients—but in the office of Fleur Sack, M.D., a family practitioner in Miami. Scanning the lists tacked up at Baptist Hospital of doctors whose offices had been destroyed, Dr. Sack spied Dr. Jarrett's name. She had known him as a resident, and invited him to share her office. She also has taken in a psychiatrist who lost his office to the hurricane.

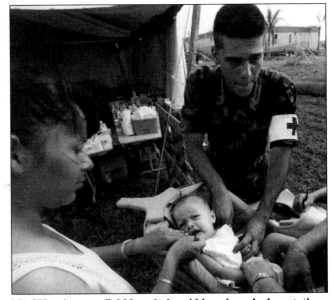

MASH unit mans field hospital amid hurricane's devastation.

"It's certainly different practicing medicine this way, but life is different in Dade County since the hurricane," she said. "I just couldn't see a doctor not have space to work out of. Everyone in Dade County is helping out."

More cholera cases brought to U.S. on the wing

New York Times/Medical Tribune News Syndicate

SEPT. 11—Approximately one new case of cholera is being reported in the United States each week, according to federal health officials, who say that most of the cases are being acquired during travel to Latin American countries.

Generalists with patients who are planning to travel to countries where cholera is endemic can advise them to take some simple steps to lessen the chance that they will contract the infection.

Most of those stricken by the potentially fatal bacterial infection were foreign-born U.S. residents traveling back to their homeland, not sightseeing tourists, said Jessica Tuttle, M.D., an epidemiologist at the Centers for Disease Control in Atlanta.

"The foreign-born may be less aware of the risks, possibly because of language barriers, and may also be less likely to seek pretravel medical advice," she said.

According to the CDC report, 96 cholera cases have been reported in the United States since Jan. 1, 1992, more than in any other year since the government began cholera surveillance in 1961.

In 1991, the first year of the current cholera epidemic in Latin America, the CDC reported 17 cases of the illness in the United States that were linked to Latin American travel, according to David Swerdlow, M.D., of the CDC.

This year, 89 of the 96 cases reported so far have been linked to exposure to food or water contamination during travel between the United States and Latin America. Seventy-five were associated with an outbreak on board an Aerolineas Argentinas flight between Argentina and Los Angeles.

Of the seven cases not associated with Latin American travel, six have been linked to travel between the United States and Asia.

The source of one patient's infection remains unknown, according to health officials.

According to the World Health Organization, 500,000 cases of cholera were reported in 1991, with 16,700 deaths from the disease.

The largest number of cases this year have occurred in Peru, followed by Ecuador, Bolivia, Brazil and Guatemala.

Physicians should advise their patients to avoid unboiled or untreated water and ice made from untreated water; food and beverages from street vendors; raw or partially cooked fish and shellfish, including ceviche; and uncooked vegetables, advised the CDC.

In addition, travelers should be advised to eat only foods that are cooked and hot or fruits they peel themselves, stated the report.

Carbonated bottled water and carbonated soft drinks usually are safe if no ice is added.

People planning to travel to Latin America or other cholera-infected areas can call the CDC's cholera hotline at (404) 332-4559 for information in English and (404) 332-3132 for information in Spanish.

COMMENTARY

Regulated into despair

By Michael Victoroff, M.D.

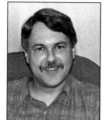

I WILL REMEMBER 1992 AS the year they took our microscopes away.

Since I first went into family practice, I have used a microscope in the office to examine vaginal wet mounts, skin scrapings and prostatic wet mounts, and to check for the presence of semen after vasectomy.

Now I can't, unless I obtain a Clinical Laboratory Improvement Act certificate, pay a few hundred dollars for someone to come and certify that I am qualified to look through a microscope, pass tests to prove that I can do what I've been doing since medical school and, perhaps, submit to random unannounced inspections. I'm not against regulation per se, and these measures would be very reasonable if I were running a blood bank or performing exacting and complicated lab work such as measuring serum lithium levels. But for the primary-care physician who wants to look through a microscope at epithelial cells, the regulations are completely insane.

As an example of how the rules will affect patients, what happens to the woman with vaginitis? I should be able to diagnose a majority of cases of vaginitis by examining a smear, but now I can't. The sample must now be examined at a specialty laboratory, and, because the smear must be viewed within minutes of obtaining it, the patient must be examined where the smear will be read. The cost of diagnosing vaginitis has just escalated from a brief office-visit charge to hundreds of dollars. And, of course, even if it takes hours of telephone calls, I must ensure that the lab I send her to is one that is acceptable to her insurance provider (and the status of various labs is likely to change in every "January shuffle" as insurers negotiate cheaper provider contracts). If I make a mistake in selecting the lab, she is subjected to belligerent denials of payment and other punitive action.

Already, half of the staff in my group practice is devoted to managing billing and the Health Care Financing Administration coding and insurance information demanded by external agencies. In some countries, where doctors and patients have to deal with a smaller number of payers and regulators, more time can be spent healing the sick.

How I wish all our computer and management knowledge could be put to use in managing the information that really matters—

clinical knowledge and specifics about our patients. Primary care sits at the crossroads between data and knowledge, where the specific patient meets the general rules of medicine. It frustrates and demoralizes me that we are asked to perform at that crossroads with pitifully inadequate informational tools and all kinds of regulatory distractions that make clear thinking extremely difficult.

The information-coordinating task of primary care is the largest of any specialty, and yet, as a nation, we've decided that primary-care physicians will be the last people to automate medical-care delivery. How many of us have even a dictated, typed medical progress note, let alone a computer-stored note that could be searched or sorted later for relevant clinical information? How many physicians routinely notify patients when follow-up examinations or procedures are due? Or can promptly identify all patients on a particular medication when an adverse drug interaction or an improved therapy becomes known? Not many. Instead, we rely on the pitifully overloaded frontal lobes of doctors to sort and recall that information at the proper time and place.

Twenty years ago, the developer of the problem-oriented medical diagnosis and records system, Larry Weed, pointed out that this type of recall is completely unreasonable to expect. And every year the task becomes more difficult. Just to see page after page of the kind of crucial tidbits that are compiled in this chapter—news items from a single year that could be translated into day-to-day practice—makes me simultaneously excited about advances in medicine and despairing of the practical obstacles we face.

So, 1992 is the year when I would have liked to expand my primary-care tools with enhanced computer capability. Instead, I watched my paperwork increase while the microscopes were taken away. Although I try not to be pessimistic, I fear that otoscopes and stethoscopes will soon follow.

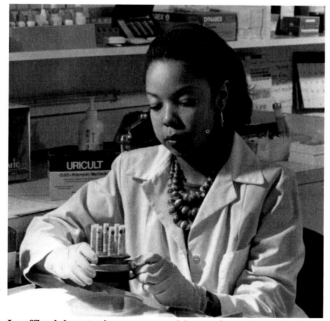

In-office laboratories are now subject to fees, "insane" CLIA regulations and, perhaps, random unannounced inspections.

Dr. Victoroff chairs the department of family practice at Aurora Presbyterian Hospital in Denver. He served on the American Academy of Family Physicians committee that issued ethical guidelines for both physicians and patients.

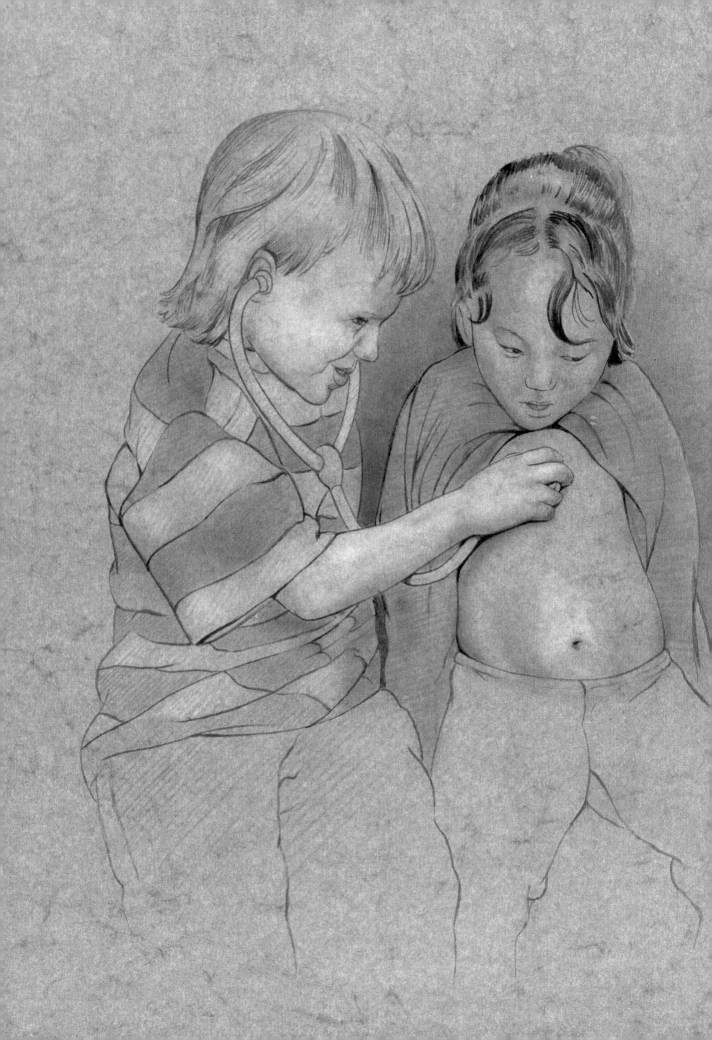

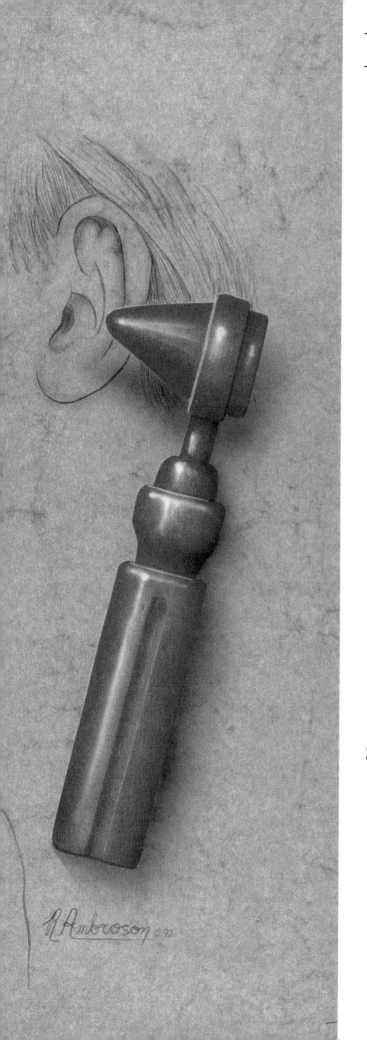

Pediatrics

Overview 42
Strides made in preventing and treating genetic disorders, vaccinating children

Month-at-a-glance 44

Reported at the Time 56
Cold virus may deliver cystic fibrosis cure...botulinum toxin for cerebral palsy...resurgent TB reaching children...immunization news: AAP, CDC, AAFP all advocate universal infant hep B shots, new easier-access vaccine rules set, one-dose vaccine for hep A...youngsters' moods and learning skills not altered by theophylline...cow's-milk peptide triggers diabetes...one in six kids has high blood lead levels...Dr. Spock and others take jabs at cow's milk...AAP faulted on SIDS warning

Commentary 67
Pushing for teen immunization
By Susan Baker, M.D.

Strides made in preventing and treating genetic disorders, vaccinating children

A host of pediatric preventive-medicine studies scrutinized the impact of early care—not only the way infants are fed, but how they are put to bed and what immunizations they receive.

In 1992, pediatricians saw great strides made toward the prevention and treatment of some of the most common genetic disorders in children.

In January, government researchers reported that a genetically engineered cold virus may hold the key to a therapy for cystic fibrosis, and said they expected to start clinical trials as early as 1993. As that advance was still being applauded, an Irish study was published that reported that botulinum toxin injections helped to relax the muscles of children with cerebral palsy. And physicians seeking to wipe out spina bifida had reason for optimism as well. Government scientists said that better nutrition—particularly increased intake of folic acid on the part of expectant mothers—may have contributed to the unparalleled drop in cases. Between 1984 and 1990, the latest year for which figures are available, the rate of spina bifida fell by half, from 59 per 100,000 births to 32 per 100,000 births.

A new strategy to prevent insulin-dependent diabetes mellitus in children may grow out of a Finnish-Canadian study that bolstered the long-held suspicion that a protein in cow's milk—bovine serum albumin—triggers the onset of the disease in genetically susceptible infants.

Based on the diabetes study and other data linking cow's milk to childhood allergies, a group of physicians—including the venerable Dr. Spock—took a highly publicized poke at cow's milk, urging moms to breast-feed or to use nondairy infant formulas instead.

A host of other pediatric preventive-medicine studies scrutinized the impact of early care—not only the way infants are fed, but how they are put to sleep and what immunizations they receive at well-baby visits.

Pediatrics

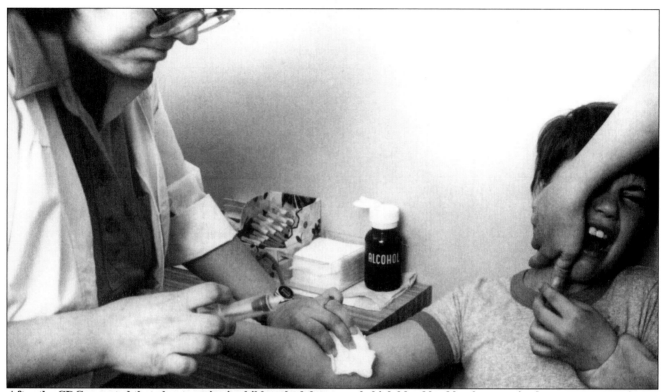

After the CDC reported that about one in six children had dangerously high blood lead levels, screening became more routine.

According to a British study, breast-feeding mothers can take steps to prevent allergy development in their children. Those moms who adhere to a strict diet devoid of known food allergens may prevent an otherwise high-risk child from developing future allergies, asthma and eczema, the research showed. A Finnish study indicated that supplementary inositol, a B-complex vitamin abundant in breast milk, may improve survival and reduce complications in premature infants with respiratory distress syndrome. Another study showed that breast-fed preemies score over 8 points higher on IQ tests at age 7 than those fed formula.

Infant formula may also indirectly lead to IQ declines when it is mixed with lead-heavy water. According to Harvard researchers, one quarter of 41 cases of lead poisoning in infants could be attributed to mixing powdered formula with contaminated water.

Lead poisoning in children was an issue that grabbed headlines all year. New research showed that lead levels as low as 10 mcg/dl will cause IQ deficiencies, growth retardation and other mental and physical problems. Using that as the danger level, the Centers for Disease Control and Prevention reported that about one in six children—as many as 17 million—potentially have threatening levels of lead in their blood.

After pondering the healthiest way to feed their infants, parents were forced to re-evaluate the sleeping position in the crib. In April, the American Academy of Pediatrics warned parents not to put babies to bed on their tummies because it increases the risk of sudden infant death syndrome. Half a year later, at the academy's annual meeting, critics charged that the warning was premature and had caused needless anxiety for all parents and unnecessary anguish for parents whose babies had died of SIDS. The AAP decided to study the issue for another year. Meanwhile, the CDC announced a 19% drop in SIDS rates among African-American babies, and a 3.5% decrease among white infants.

On the vaccination front, the AAFP and the AAP followed the lead of the CDC and recommended that all infants be vaccinated against hepatitis B—not just those at high risk for the disease (see commentary, p. 67).

In August, a study of more than 1,000 children found that a single dose of a formalin-inactivated hepatitis A vaccine is well tolerated and highly protective against the disease.

Despite advances in immunizations, a panel of experts criticized the United States for failing to deliver basic vaccines to a large portion of the country's vulnerable preschool children. The National Vaccine Advisory Council told the CDC that fewer than 60% of children, especially those in inner cities, are up to date for the recommended primary immunization series, including DTP, polio, MMR, Hib and hepatitis B.

Finally, and unfortunately, an old infectious disease is back and striking more and more children—tuberculosis. Nearly 950 children under age five had active TB in 1990, an increase of 39% from 1987. Many more are thought to be infected.

If parents felt bewildered by the bombardment of infant-care advice coming from this year's research, their confusion only mirrored that of pediatricians. Ten years after the AAP found that its members felt deficient in their knowledge of adolescent care, learning disabilities, attention-deficit disorders and psychosocial and behavior problems, a new survey revealed that they continue to feel inadequately trained in the same areas.

Jan. 3

One third of Connecticut infants failed to receive their first DTP vaccination by three months of age, according to a survey released by the Centers for Disease Control. By the time the children were a year old, 93% had received at least one dose of DTP vaccine.

Jan. 7

The Children's Defense Fund claimed that 40% of American children already lack private insurance coverage and another 10% will lose coverage by the year 2000 if healthcare reforms are not enacted. The advocacy group recommended that Congress enact a $10-billion national plan to cover healthcare for children and pregnant women.

Jan. 9

French and American researchers announced a major step toward gene therapy for cystic fibrosis. Using a genetically modified cold virus as a

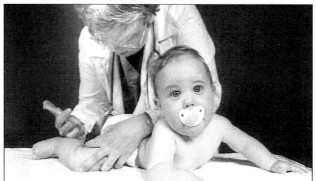

Many infants don't receive first DTP by three months: CDC survey.

vector, a normal copy of the human CF gene was introduced into the lungs of rats, researchers from the National Heart, Lung and Blood Institute reported in the journal Cell. As the adenovirus infected the lungs, the cells successfully produced the protein missing in CF for six weeks.

Jan. 13

Lederle Laboratories began shipping 10-dose vials of acellular pertussis vaccine (Acel-Imune) for use as part

of children's fourth and fifth DTP booster shots. Approved by the Food and Drug Administration last month, the vaccine, consisting of cell-free filtrates of B. pertussis, has a much lower incidence of side effects than the whole-cell vaccine. Pending the results of ongoing research, the first three immunizations will continue to employ whole-cell vaccine.

Jan. 15

Cancer specialists at New York Medical College demonstrated that parents can be taught to administer chemotherapy to children at home. A home program designed by the specialists cut time and money spent on hospital care and improved the youngsters' quality of life, they reported in Cancer. Two years of experience with the Home Intravenous Chemotherapy by Parents program revealed that the best candidates for home care are children who need consecutive doses of the same medication at frequent intervals, but who are deemed at low risk for suffering side effects or allergic reactions.

Jan. 16

Yale researchers alerted pediatricians that there may be no biological validity and no predictive value to current criteria used to diagnose dyslexia. In a follow-up analysis of 414 children presented in The New England Journal of

Medicine, they found that fewer than 50% of the children diagnosed as dyslexic in grade three were similarly diagnosed in grade five. When parents seek advice after a dyslexia diagnosis, they should be told

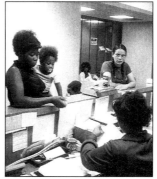

CDF claims almost half of children lack private insurance.

that dyslexia is not a permanent, all-or-none phenomenon, and that some children may simply be at the lower end of a normal curve for reading ability.

Jan. 20

Raising the legal drinking age to 21 has reduced the number of violent deaths suffered by teens and young adults. After reviewing fatal injuries in persons aged 15 to 24 between 1979 and 1984, researchers at Hunter College in New York found that young adults and teens legally entitled to drink had a 3.9% higher death rate, including a 9.7% higher rate of suicide. A higher drinking age can reduce suicides and homicides, as well as prevent deaths among motor vehicle drivers and pedestrians, they wrote in the American Journal of Public Health.

Jan. 22

North Carolina researchers cautioned that candy and gum packaged to resemble cigarettes may promote smoking among children. A study of 195 seventh-graders found that those who very fre-

quently bought candy cigarettes were three and a half times more likely to smoke than children who did not buy the candies; those who frequently bought the candies were about one and a half times more likely to smoke. About 3,000 young people become smokers every day, a University of North Carolina at Chapel Hill team wrote in Pediatrics.

Jan. 24

A Canadian study demonstrated the value of nebulized albuterol in the treatment of acute asthma in children younger than two. When treated in the emergency room with two inhaled doses of 0.15 mg/kg albuterol one hour apart, the 13 children who received the beta-agonist showed greater improvement in respiratory rate, wheezing score, accessory muscle score and oxygen saturation than the 15 children who received nebulized normal saline. The researchers, from the Hospital for Sick Children in Toronto, concluded in Pediatrics that a trial of nebulized albuterol is warranted in the treatment of acute asthma in infants and young children.

Although nebulized beta-agonists are not yet FDA-approved for use in children younger than 12, an expert panel convened by the National Heart, Lung, and Blood Institute recommended that they be used in children of all ages, including infants.

Jan. 30

An Eskimo father successfully used urine to treat frostbite. His five-year-old son licked a hand-rail in 35-degree-below-zero weather and was instantly frozen to the railing by his tongue and upper lip. With no warm water handy, the father relied on the most immediate antidote and urinated on the boy's tongue, the emergency room physician explained in The New England Journal of Medicine.

Pediatrics

Feb. 1

Mothers received news of another good reason to breast-feed: At age 7, breast-fed premature infants are smarter, scoring more than 10 points higher on IQ tests than formula-fed babies. In a British follow-up study of 300 preemies, those who received breast milk via nasogastric tube were compared with those tube-fed infant formula, so the act of breast-feeding itself was not deemed to be a factor in the IQ difference. After correcting for parental education and social class, there was still an 8.3-point difference in IQ, according to results presented in The Lancet.

• • •

An analysis of 107 measles deaths in Senegal showed that the infection is more deadly when contracted from a sibling of the opposite sex. Children in families with a boy and a girl had almost twice the mortality of children in families with two boys or two girls, a team from the Statens Seruminstitut in Copenhagen reported in the British Medical Journal.

• • •

Parents were warned that they increase the risk of sudden infant death syndrome when they put babies to sleep on their stomachs or dressed in too many layers of clothes. Every excess layer of clothing worn while asleep raises the risk of SIDS 26%, according to an analysis of 41 deaths by the University of Tasmania in Australia. Infants who died were also more likely to have been found in the prone position, researchers revealed in the British Medical Journal.

Feb. 7

Two pediatricians joined two family physicians and five orthopedic surgeons as team physicians of the U.S. Olympic team in Albertville, France. With six years of tryouts and training prior to their Olympic designation, the doctors gave up approxi-

mately 23 weeks of their private medical practices for the privilege of treating young skiers, skaters and other winter athletes.

Feb. 8

A Chinese herbal medicine proved its value in treating children with severe malaria, reported tropical medicine experts from Thailand, England and The

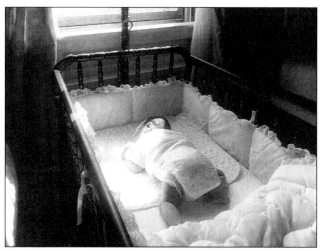

Parents are warned that sleeping position affects SIDS risk.

Gambia. Artemether, an extract of the sweet wormwood plant, cleared malaria parasites from children's bodies in 37 hours, on average, compared with 48 hours among children who received conventional chloroquine treatment, according to a report in The Lancet. The 30 Gambian children were striken by moderately severe malaria caused by the most dangerous species of the parasite, Plasmodium falciparum.

The researchers concluded that the herbal treatment would prove valuable in areas with chloroquine-resistant P. falciparum.

• • •

Carelessly discarded glass was blamed for 587 of more than 24,000 emergency room visits to a British children's hospital in 1990. Injuries

were twice as common in boys than girls, and 170 occurred in children under the age of five, according to the report in the British Medical Journal.

Feb. 12

Measles outbreaks in urban communities may be controlled by immunization coverage of 50% to 80%, the Milwaukee Health Depart-

ment reported in The Journal of the American Medical Association. Measles struck 1.2% of young children in areas where only 50% of children were immunized, compared with 0.5% in areas where 60% were immunized and no children where 81% were immunized.

Feb. 18

Pediatricians were warned that obese children are more likely than thinner children to have a family history of deaths from cardiovascular disease. Sixty percent of the deceased relatives of heavy children died from heart disease, compared with 48% of deceased relatives of lean children and 43% of relatives of a randomly selected group of children, according to a report in Pediatrics.

Obese children with elevated systolic blood pressure

had the strongest family histories, with 76% of their deceased relatives succumbing to cardiovascular disease, according to biostatisticians from the University of Iowa.

Feb. 20

Botulinum toxin injections helped relax the spastic muscles of children with cerebral palsy, Irish researchers reported at the meeting of the American Academy of Orthopedic Surgeons in Washington, D.C. All but two of 33 children who were administered toxin injections into the spastic hamstring and calf muscles showed improvement in muscle tone, and many were able to straighten their legs, said the team from Royal Belfast Hospital for Sick Children.

Feb. 24

Between 30% and 40% of fatal gun wounds, car accidents and other traumatic injuries—the leading causes of death among children—are preventable, said a child health expert at Johns Hopkins University in Baltimore. The use of child seats, seat belts and bicycle helmets, as well as such measures as locking up guns and properly fencing off swimming pools, can reduce the rate of fatal injuries, he told the National Conference on Cardiopulmonary Resuscitation and Emergency Cardiac Care.

Feb. 27

Boys who reach puberty relatively late may be at increased risk of developing osteoporosis in adulthood, suggested research from Massachusetts General Hospital in Boston. A study of 44 men aged 19 to 30 showed that those who reached puberty after age 15 had lower radial and spinal bone density than those who started puberty before age 14. Peak bone mineral density during young adulthood is a major determinant of bone density in later life, the Boston team explained in The New England Journal of Medicine.

MARCH

March 1

When adolescent girls require cancer treatment, they face an increased risk of undergoing menopause while in their twenties, a National Cancer Institute study revealed. In a 2,500-woman study detailed in the American Journal of Obstetrics and Gynecology, chemotherapy boosted the risk of premature menopause ninefold, radiation quadrupled the risk and radiation below the diaphragm combined with chemotherapy increased the risk 29 times.

Surgery was not associated with increased risk.

March 3

A survey of more than 4,000 adults and children found that children are more aware of the negative effects of their parents' smoking than are the parents themselves. Nearly 75% of children of smoking parents worried about their parents' smoking harming their own or a family member's health, compared with 64% of adults who worried about so-called second-hand smoke, according to the Louis Harris poll. And 92% of children believed that inhaling smoke in the air around them was unhealthy, compared with 87% of adults. More than 85% of the children feared that a parent would die from smoking.

March 5

Babies born to mothers infected with cytomegalovirus may be spared from debilitating effects of the infection if the mother became infected before conceiving and had the chance to mount an immune response, said University of Alabama pediatricians. They followed 125 infants born to mothers infected during pregnancy and 64 babies born to mothers infected before conception. Only infants in the former group (18%) had symptomatic CMV infection at birth, the team reported in The New England Journal of Medicine. After about five years, 13% of infants whose mothers had been infected during pregnancy

had mental impairment, compared with none of those born to mothers infected before pregnancy. Sensorineural hearing loss was found in 15% of the former group, compared with only 5% of the latter.

March 6

Voluntary daycare center guidelines that cover topics from nutritious meals to sanitary nose-blowing were released by the American Academy of Pediatrics and the American Public Health Association. Among the recommendations, which are not enforceable by law: all staff providing care to children should be certified in pediatric first aid; diapers used in daycare facilities should have an absorbent inner lining and an outer waterproof covering; and unruly children should not be hit or subjected to other forms of corporal punishment. The guidelines also gave specific nutritional recommendations for meals served at the centers, based on the children's ages.

March 13

Nearly 950 children under age 5 had active tuberculosis in 1990, an increase of 39% from 1987, according to figures released by the Centers for Disease Control. In children under age 15, the rate jumped 36%, to 1,596 cases in 1990. In addition, an increasing number of youngsters are thought to be infected, although they have not yet developed the disease. While most of the cases have been reported in poor, inner-city children, tuberculosis is also striking many youngsters who live with adults who do not belong to any of the high-risk groups, a New York pediatrician told Medical Tribune.

March 21

Children who have undergone myringotomies can swim without increasing their risk of ear infections, said French ear, nose and throat surgeons. A

study of 210 children who had ear tubes in place for an average of six months revealed that the incidence of infection was not significantly different between those who had not swum compared with those who had swum one to five

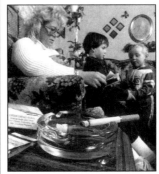

Kids know more than parents about second-hand smoke risk.

times. Children with ear tubes who swam six or more times had fewer incidences of ear discharge and infection than those who did not swim, the researchers reported in the British Medical Journal.

• • •

Canadian researchers found that children with cystic fibrosis can exercise in the heat, but must drink extra fluids to avoid dehydration and further thickening of respiratory secretions. During exercise at 78-91 degrees F in 43% to 47% humidity, eight children with cystic fibrosis were typically half as thirsty as eight healthy controls despite losing twice as much fluid in sweat, it was reported in The Lancet.

The researchers postulated that the high salt content of cystic fibrosis patients' sweat and the consequent absence of hyperosmolality during sweating deprive them of a thirst stimulus.

March 24

Pediatric researchers from Boston University reported that women with type-A personalities may pass along aspects of their intense, compulsive and impatient behavior to their babies. They studied

72 first-time mothers who were classified as type A or type B on the Job Involvement scale of the Jenkins Activity survey. Type-A moms had infants who cried more during their first week of life, and were rated as more intense and less predictable at three months than those born to type-B moms, the investigators reported in Pediatrics. The study head attributed the infants' behavior to both genetics and their mothers' childrearing techniques.

March 25

A University of Minnesota survey showed that American-Indian and Alaska-Native teenagers have a relatively high rate of suicide attempts, histories of physical and/or sexual abuse and sex without contraception. The survey of 13,454 American-Indian and Alaska-Native teens revealed that 17% had attempted suicide; 10% reported physical abuse; and about 60% had had sex by the 12th grade—with about one fourth of the boys and one third of the girls never using contraception. The survey, which was published in The Journal of the American Medical Association, also found that fewer American-Indian teens than rural white youths had visited a doctor for preventive healthcare within the previous two years, although it is provided to them on their reservations. Intervention must be grounded in the cultural traditions that promote health, commented the Minneapolis team.

March 26

A House subcommittee was told that the United States is losing the war on infant mortality, ranking 22nd among countries in the number of babies who die within a year of birth. In 1989, there were 9.8 infant deaths for every live birth in the United States, said the National Commission to Prevent Infant Mortality. The rate is highest for African-American babies, who die at twice the rate of white babies.

Pediatrics

April 8

The Centers for Disease Control announced that outbreaks of measles in the 1980s occurred most frequently in the nation's crowded inner cities, especially those with large Hispanic populations. During the decade, 56,775 cases were reported to the CDC, with many cases confined to densely populated urban areas, the CDC researchers wrote in The Journal of the American Medical Association. The researchers attributed the outbreaks to lower levels of immunization among Hispanics, particularly preschoolers. The highest number of cases were reported in Cook County, Ill., Los Angeles County, Calif., Harris County, Texas; Kings County, N.Y. and San Diego County, Calif.

April 11

British research confirmed that the best way to take an infant's temperature is rectally. Citing a new 937-infant study in which underarm temperature measurements failed to diagnose fever in 75% of cases, an Oxfordshire physician called on parents to switch to the rectal route. Writing in the British Medical Journal, he reminded parents that it is less disturbing to an infant to have a rectal thermometer inserted for two minutes than to have an arm immobilized for the nine minutes it takes to get an axillary reading.

April 13

A leading pediatrician told colleagues at the American Academy of Pediatrics that all infants and young children should be vaccinated against hepatitis B, not just those thought to be at special risk of developing the disease. The New York University pediatrician estimated that if all children received the vaccine, the number of hepatitis B cases nationwide would be reduced by at least 90% by the year 2015. The

academy and the CDC recently changed their recommendations to include all babies, not just those born to mothers who are infected with the virus.

April 15

Centers for Disease Control officials announced that they are sticking by their recently lowered estimates of safe blood lead levels for children, despite charges of scientific misconduct in one of the initial studies that documented a drop in children's IQ from exposure to small amounts of lead. Reanalysis of research data essentially confirmed the findings of the pioneering 1979 University of Pittsburgh study, and the lead risk has been well documented in subsequent studies, stated the head of the CDC's lead poisoning prevention branch. Last October, the CDC lowered its maximum safe level of lead in children's blood from 25 to 10 mcg/dl.

• • •

The American Academy of Pediatrics recommended that acellular pertussis vaccine be used for the fourth and fifth doses of childhood immunization. The acellular vaccine has proved successful in Swedish and Japanese trials, causing less redness, swelling, tenderness, fever and drowsiness than whole-cell vaccine. Until more data are available, the academy recommended that infants continue to be immunized with the whole-cell vaccine for the initial three pertussis shots.

April 16

Current methods to monitor blood oxygen levels in newborns are not sufficient to prevent the development of retinopathy of prematurity (formerly called retrolental fibroplasia), warned ophthalmologists and neonatologists from

the University of Miami. A new study of 101 premature infants requiring supplemental oxygen documented the fine line between providing sufficient oxygen to prevent brain damage and delivering so much that the eyes are damaged. In The New England Journal of Medicine, the specialists called for the creation of improved equipment to

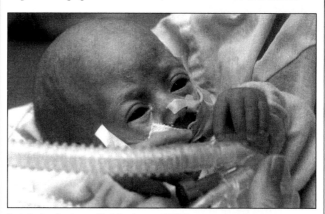

Ophthalmologists called for better NICU oxygen monitoring.

prevent fluctuations in arterial oxygen tension.

• • •

The largest study to date on congenital heart defects determined that risk factors can be identified in more than 40% of the cases, not 10% as previously thought. One third of 4,390 infants with heart defects came from families with a history of birth defects or genetic disorders, and 11% of the cases followed pregnancies complicated by diabetes, viral infection or exposure to medications or environmental toxins, a University of Maryland researcher told the American College of Cardiology meeting in Dallas.

April 22

Harvard researchers asked pediatricians to refer low-birthweight babies to early intervention programs for speech and physical therapy. A study of 1,868 children aged 8 to 10 revealed that in-

fants who weighed less than 2½ pounds at birth were more likely to have asthma, cerebral palsy, learning disabilities or multiple medical problems in the elementary school years than children born weighing more than 4½ pounds. Prompt intervention could ameliorate some of these dysfunctions, they stressed.

April 24

The Centers for Disease Control warned that babies left unattended in infant carriers can get tangled in the seats' straps or overturn, possibly causing strangulation. Infant carriers used improperly as car safety seats may not restrain babies well enough to ensure survival after a car crash, the CDC statement concluded in the Morbidity and Mortality Weekly Report. Between January 1986 and October 1991, the U.S. Consumer Product Safety Commission received reports of 26 deaths from infant carriers, most caused by strangulation and most of which involved children under one year of age, the CDC reported.

April 25

Vaccination against mumps, measles and rubella was linked to episodes of joint and limb pain in children aged five and younger, University of Manchester researchers reported in the British Medical Journal.

MAY

May 1
A California Department of Health Services statewide survey found that a significant percentage of children had blood-lead levels that exceeded government guidelines. In Oakland, 67% of children had more than 10 mcg of lead per deciliter of blood. Levels that exceed 10 mcg/dl are considered unsafe by the government. Five percent of Oakland children, 4% of Wilmington/ Compton children and 1% of Sacramento children had blood lead levels that were at least double the level considered safe, the Centers for Disease Control reported in Morbidity and Mortality Weekly Report.

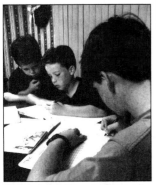

Link between theophylline and learning disabilities rebutted.

May 4
A defect of the thyroid gland was proposed as a cause of attention-deficit disorder in children. A government study found that 70% of 104 adults and children with ADD had resistance to thyroid hormone, compared with 20% of those without the disorder. A researcher from the National Institute for Diabetes and Digestive and Kidney Diseases told a meeting of the American Society for Clinical Investigation in Bethesda that some of these patients may have thyroid abnormalities that could be treated with replacement hormone.

May 5
Exposure to passive smoke was implicated by Dutch researchers as a key factor in cases of sudden infant death syndrome. Physicians attending the annual combined meeting of the American Pediatric Society, the Society for Pediatric Research and the Ambulatory Pediatric Association in Baltimore were told that infants exposed to smoke as fetuses and after birth have a SIDS rate of 219 per 100,000, compared with a rate of 140 per 100,000 for infants exposed to smoke only after birth and 63 per 100,000 for infants never exposed to smoke.

May 6
A pediatric researcher from Johns Hopkins University said a nose-drop flu vaccine can protect two- to five-month-old infants against influenza A viruses. Almost 90% of 15 infants who received a high-dose vaccine developed antibodies against the influenza strain, according to the report given in Baltimore at the combined pediatric meeting. The vaccine could be on the market in two years.

May 7
Herpes can be transmitted to a child from an infected mother with lip sores who uses her teeth, rather than scissors, to trim the child's toenails, reported two physicians from Connecticut. The unusual mode of transmission was detected in a three-year-old girl who was referred to the University of Connecticut Health Center with a toe infection days after her toenails were teeth-trimmed by her mother. The infection later spread up to her mid-foot and ankle, the physicians wrote in The New England Journal of Medicine. Many parents bite their babies' nails to avoid hurting a small finger or toe with scissors, they pointed out.

May 8
A British Institute of Child Health study of 676 children at two Bristol hospitals found that those who received vitamin K injections as newborns were two and a half times more likely to develop leukemia by age 10 than children who had received the vitamin orally or not at all. The American Academy of Pediatrics recommends that all newborns get an injection of the vitamin within the first hour after birth to prevent potentially lethal bleeding that can occur because of a lack of the vitamin. Although the study suggests that vitamin K injections may increase the risk of cancer, they are lifesaving in infancy, British researchers told Medical Tribune.

May 11
Two studies revealed that physicians who have advised parents to avoid giving aspirin to children because of concerns about Reye's syndrome now have an equally effective option besides acetaminophen: ibuprofen. In an Ohio State University study, 61 children were given multiple doses of either liquid ibuprofen or acetaminophen; there was no significant difference in the drugs' ability to reduce fever. In the second study, also published in the American Journal of Diseases of Children, doctors from Children's Hospital in Detroit reported that ibuprofen lowered temperature further and for a longer period than acetaminophen when given in a single dose to 37 children.

May 15
The Centers for Disease Control reported that children under the age of five and young adults between the ages of 15 and 24 are most at risk of drowning, the third most common cause of death from unintentional injury in the United States. Overall, the U.S. drowning rate is four times greater for males than for females, the CDC said.

• • •

Algae-laden ponds can be unhealthy to swim in, warned the CDC in a separate report on the dangers of swimming. The center reported an outbreak of pharyngoconjunctival fever, which causes sore throat and cough, fever, headaches and muscle aches, among children and counselors at a North Carolina summer camp who swam in an algae-thick pond and shared wet towels.

May 20
A University of Colorado study failed to confirm parents' accounts of learning difficulties and behavior problems in their asthmatic children following theophylline therapy. Parents could not tell whether their children took the drug or placebo in a randomized, double-blind crossover study, according to a report in The Journal of the American Medical Association.

May 21
An artificial liver device developed at Baylor College of Medicine in Houston was successfully tested on a 12-year-old girl, marking the first clinical test of such a device in a child. Physicians told Medical Tribune that the girl was placed on the device for 58 hours after she rapidly deteriorated from multiple attacks of pneumonitis and myositis into a stage 4 coma with an overwhelming liver deficit. The assist device consists of a cartridge containing hollow fibers seeded with cultured human liver cells. The patient's blood is pumped into the cartridge and through the fibers, then back into the body.

May 29
Athletes as young as 12 need to do certain strengthening and flexibility exercises to avoid future injuries, Kentucky researchers told the American College of Sports Medicine annual meeting in Dallas.

Researchers at the Lexington Clinic Sports Medicine Center studied 2,000 athletes and found that players developed an inflexibility in muscle groups adjoining those used most often in each sport. The inflexibility, they said, can put them at higher risk for injuries.

JUNE

June 1

One in three children aged 15 or younger who play ice hockey is injured during a season, warned Minneapolis Health Department epidemiologists after studying 150 boys. During the 1990-1991 season, 6% were injured to the extent that they had to cease physical activities for eight to 25 days or longer, they reported in the American Journal of Diseases of Children. Up to 15% of the injuries are intentionally inflicted by other players, the investigators noted.

They recommended that young hockey players be grouped by size and weight rather than by age, and that violent play and body checking be reduced among hockey players younger than age 16. In Canada, checking is prohibited for children under age 13, as it is in the United States for children under age 11.

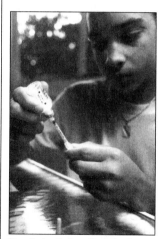

Prophylactic insulin injections may delay onset of Type I diabetes in high-risk children.

June 3

The mortality rate of Detroit children increased 50% from 1980 through 1988, while the rate remained stable in Detroit suburbs, announced researchers at Henry Ford Hospital there. Firearm homicides accounted for most of the increase in Detroit, the researchers disclosed in The Journal of the American Medical Association.

June 10

The birth rate in Russia has sharply declined due to political turmoil and the worsening economic conditions that accompanied the collapse of communism, Russian doctors told Medical Tribune. The number of births decreased about 30% from 1987, the year before Mikhail Gorbachev's policy of perestroika went into full gear, to 1991, according to the Russian Ministry of Health. In contrast, the birth rate increased by 8% between 1980 and 1987.

June 11

A panel of experts warned that current U.S. healthcare practices fail to deliver vaccines to a large portion of the country's vulnerable preschool children. Less than 60% of children, especially those in the inner cities, are up to date for the recommended primary immunization series, the National Vaccine Advisory Council told the Centers for Disease Control.

New NVAC rules include prohibition of appointment-only systems; free immunizations in the public sector; simultaneous administration of all vaccines for which a child is eligible at time of visit and institution of a tracking system to identify children at high risk of failing to complete the immunization series.

June 13

When DTP shots were bunched together earlier in infancy, compliance increased and parents reported fewer side effects, British researchers announced. When infants received DTP on a new, accelerated schedule—at two, three and four months — there were fewer fevers and less redness and swelling at the injection site, researchers from the Public Health Laboratory in London reported in the British Medi-

cal Journal. Before the new schedule was adopted in 1990, infants received DTP at three months, 4½ to 5 months, and 8½ to 11 months of age.

Compliance rose from 80% to 85% on the old schedule to over 90% with the earlier monthly shots, the investigators said.

In the United States, DTP shots are scheduled at two months, four months, six months, 15 to18 months, and four to six years.

June 18

As many as two thirds of young female athletes may suffer from eating disorders, reported researchers from San Diego State University. At particular risk are women who engage in "body-conscious" sports such as gymnastics and diving, they said. These women are also at high risk of rapid, irreversible bone loss and menstrual abnormalities, researchers told an American College of Sports Medicine conference in Washington, D.C. Amenorrhea was seen in two thirds of the women athletes who participated in one study; its prevalence among women in the general population is from 2% to 5%.

June 20

Thumb-sucking in infants may be a mechanism that compensates for respiratory insufficiency, rather than just a comforting habit, revealed researchers from Japan's Mukai Clinic and Research Institute of Biology.

They studied 40 babies with ankyloglossia, the "tongue-tied" syndrome marked by apnea and decreased arterial oxygenation during both wakefulness and sleep. When the babies sucked their thumbs, apnea disappeared and they showed normal arterial oxygenation, the investigators reported in The Lancet. Both conditions returned when the babies' thumbs were taken out of their mouths.

June 22

Harvard researchers reported that prophylactic insulin injections can delay the onset of Type I diabetes in high-risk children. Daily low-dose insulin injections (0.21 U/kg/day) plus five-day courses of additional insulin (0.52 U/kg/day) every nine months delayed diabetes for two and a half years in four of five siblings or children of Type I diabetics, according to the investigators. A control group of seven high-risk children not given insulin contracted the disease during that time, the endocrinologists told the American Diabetes Association meeting in San Antonio.

June 23

Obese teenagers have thicker, less flexible blood vessels in their forearms that are associated with increased insulin resistance, reported researchers at the University of Minnesota Medical School in Minneapolis. In a study of 135 teens, the 95 who were obese had significantly decreased forearm blood flow and increased vascular resistance; there was a significant relationship between minimum vascular resistance and fasting insulin, they found.

Both insulin resistance and vessel changes began to reverse after the obese teens entered a 20-week weight-loss program, it was reported in Hypertension.

June 30

Nearly one third of child poisoning deaths occur when young children ingest large amounts of iron supplements, announced researchers from poison control centers in Washington, D.C., and San Diego.

Antidepressants caused 19% of children's poisoning deaths in the last decade, while heart medications caused 13%, the researchers revealed in Pediatrics. Children also have died from artificial-nail remover and mouthwash containing ethanol.

Pediatrics

July 1

A Florida researcher announced that she had identified genetic mutations apparently responsible for some cases of unexplained death in newborns. The mutations result in glutaric acidemia, an inherited metabolic disorder that can lead to premature birth and low blood sugar. Affected infants often die within a day or two after birth, the University of Miami researcher told Medical Tribune. She predicted that her research could lead to the first test to determine whether a fetus has the disorder.

July 2

A University of Arizona survey of 384 pediatricians and family physicians found that doctors tend to ignore the recently revised American Academy of Pediatrics guidelines for treating infants with diarrhea. Contrary to AAP guidelines advising rehydration for four to six hours, 62% of doctors surveyed said they extend the rehydration period for 12 to 24 hours. Fewer than half said they would start babies on solid foods within 24 hours, as is currently recommended by the AAP.

For older children, the current AAP guidelines call for a normal diet after rehydration, instead of the traditional BRAT (bananas, rice, apple, toast or tea) diet. Twenty-eight percent of the doctors surveyed would still use a BRAT diet immediately after rehydration, according to the survey in Pediatrics.

July 3

Oral iron supplements may boost the mental and emotional status of teenage girls, reported researchers from the E. Wolfson Hospital in Tel Aviv, Israel.

Each day for two months, 29 girls aged 16 to 17 were given a 105-mg oral iron supplement; 30 were given placebo. All had complained of mood swings, inability to concentrate and lassitude.

Only the treatment group reported statistically significant improvements in all three parameters, according to the report in the American Journal of Diseases of Children.

July 7

Children and young adults with phenylketonuria can apparently ingest small amounts of aspartame without any ill effects, said researchers from Pennsylvania State University's Milton S. Hershey Medical Center. Five PKU patients and six normal volunteers aged 11 to 23 were given a 12-ounce can of regular cola, then a diet cola containing aspartame. The report, which appeared in Clinical Pediatrics, observed that changes in serum phenylalanine among the PKU patients were insignificant. These patients have typically been advised to avoid aspartame because it contains phenylalanine, which cannot be metabolized by people with the disorder.

July 9

A three-year study of 45 pairs of identical twins suggested that young children who consume more than the recommended dietary allowance of calcium may be protected from bone fractures later in life. The Indiana University researchers studied identical twins aged 6 to 14. All children followed a normal diet that supplied about 900 mg of calcium daily, and one twin of each pair received about 700 mg daily of additional calcium supplementation, the team reported in The New England Journal of Medicine. The children who received calcium supplementation were found to have 3% greater bone density in the spine and forearm, compared with their brothers or sisters who took placebo pills.

July 12

Michigan researchers reported that chest guards and softer-core baseballs do not sufficiently protect children from serious injuries when they are hit in the chest with a ball. The scientists fired eight types of baseballs at crash dummies and sedated swine and measured the impact with and without chest protectors. In the tests, three types of chest protectors actually increased the force of the impact, the researchers stated in the Clinical Journal of Sports Medicine. In the last 10 years, at least 25 American children have died from traumatic injuries and heart failure after they were hit in the chest by a ball, noted the team from the Institute for Preventative Sports Medicine in Ann Arbor.

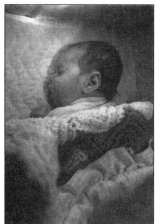

Inherited metabolic block can lead to premature birth.

July 14

A Memphis, Tenn., researcher who claims to have developed the first effective treatment for Duchenne muscular dystrophy received a U.S. patent for his technique, while the Food and Drug Administration began an investigation into whether he is following proper medical standards in his research. The investigator, who is chairman of the Cell Therapy Research Foundation, used myoblast transfer techniques to inject healthy immature muscle cells into children whose own muscle cells are wasting because they lack the gene for dystrophin. Since the injected cells contain the gene, they enable treated children to begin producing dystrophin and regain their strength, he claimed.

July 16

The Centers for Disease Control reported that the incidence of sudden infant death syndrome is declining in the United States, particularly among African-American babies. Between 1980 and 1988, SIDS rates dropped by about 19% among African-American infants and by 3.5% among white babies. The CDC researchers said that they did not know the reason for the decline.

July 20

Canadian researchers warned that exposure to adenovirus during childhood may increase the risk of developing lung disease from smoking. Polymerase chain reaction testing of lung-tissue samples from 40 smokers showed that nearly all the subjects had been exposed to the virus, which commonly affects people in childhood, according to the study in the American Review of Respiratory Disease. Smokers with chronic bronchitis had three times the amount of an adenoviral gene known as E1A. This gene renders cells less able to withstand the chemical assault accompanying inflammation, leading to scarring and thickening of the airways, said the University of British Columbia, Vancouver, researcher who led the study.

July 29

A Finnish-Canadian study provided evidence supporting the long-held suspicion that a protein in cow's milk may trigger the onset of insulin-dependent diabetes mellitus in genetically susceptible individuals. Of 142 children with recently diagnosed IDDM, all had highly elevated serum concentrations of antibodies against bovine serum albumin, the collaborators reported in The New England Journal of Medicine. Small amounts of the antibodies were found in only 3% of controls.

Pediatrics

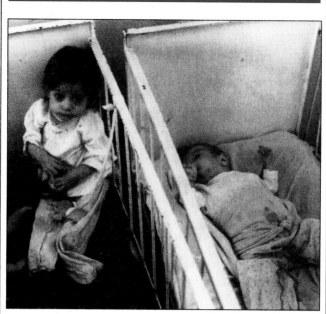

Adopted Romanian children show high rate of undetected hepatitis B.

Aug. 1

Infants less than a year old who sleep in adult beds or in unsafe baby cribs are at risk of accidental death, revealed a study in the American Journal of Diseases of Children. Small changes in a baby's sleeping environment could prevent these deaths, advised the researcher from the Kentucky Medical Examiner's Program in Louisville. She examined the records of 36 accidental infant deaths from 1979 to 1989; eight were caused by unsafe sleeping conditions. Mattresses too small for the cribs led to three deaths when infants became wedged between the crib rails and the mattress.

Aug. 5

University of Michigan pediatricians cautioned that more adopted children from Romania may be infected with hepatitis B than is indicated on their medical records. Children from Southeast Asia and parts of Africa also have a high rate of undetected hepatitis B infection. The doctors advised in The Journal of the American Medical Association that all internationally

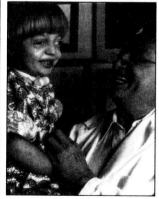

Craniofacial surgery recommended soon after birth.

adopted children be carefully screened for infectious diseases.

Aug. 10

Physicians and parents can use a few simple rules to judge whether a child's fears are normal, participants in a meeting of the National Mental Health Association in Charleston, S.C., learned.

Normal phobias, such as the fear of strangers or fear on the first day of school, will fade away after a few days or more, said a University of California child psychiatrist. But true anxiety disorders actually prevent the child from functioning and do not subside with time, he said. About 70% of four-year-olds have simple phobias that they will outgrow, he added.

Aug. 13

A team of researchers from upstate New York reported that a single dose of a formalin-inactivated hepatitis A vaccine (Vaqta, Merck Sharp & Dohme) is well tolerated and highly protective against the disease.

Investigators from the Kiryas Joel Institute of Medicine studied 1,037 uninfected children aged 2 to 16 in a Hasidic community that had had recurrent outbreaks of the disease. From the seventh week after the injection until the trial ended about four and a half months later, 25 cases of hepatitis A occurred in the placebo group and none in the vaccine group.

The early protection afforded by the vaccine, which is not yet approved by the Food and Drug Administration, should benefit people at high risk, the researchers pointed out in The New England Journal of Medicine.

An accompanying editorial recommended that all children be given the vaccine.

Aug. 14

The American Academy of Family Physicians followed the lead of the Centers for Disease Control and the American Academy of Pediatrics in recommending that infants and toddlers routinely receive immunization against hepatitis B. The recommendation is not based on any known risk of widespread hepatitis among children, but is simply a way to ensure that more people will be protected as adults.

Aug. 20

A Tampa surgeon recommended operating on children with facial deformities as soon as possible after birth. Adding computer software to sonographic equipment allows facial defects to be detected in utero, so the family and surgical team can be prepared almost immediately after birth, the director of the Tampa Bay Craniofacial Center told Medical Tribune. Three-dimensional CT-scan technology can be used to create a detailed topographic map to plan and monitor corrections while in the operating room, he said. While other surgeons see no advantage to newborn surgery over surgery at four to six months, the Florida physician believes there is far less scarring and children confront fewer psychological problems with early correction.

Aug. 21

The government announced plans to tighten the reins on vaccine injury awards and to revise the table of illnesses thought to be linked to vaccines. The announcement came in the wake of a report by an Institute of Medicine committee that looked at 17 possible health problems suspected of stemming from the DTP vaccine. The committee concluded that only anaphylaxis is linked to DTP. Since 1986, 490 awards, totaling $250 million, have been made under the Vaccine Injury Compensation Program.

Aug. 26

Negative press reports about the stimulant methylphenidate (Ritalin, Ciba-Geigy) contributed to a nearly 40% drop in its use since the late 1980s in the Baltimore area, revealed a report in The Journal of the American Medical Association. The study, based on a survey of Baltimore County schoolchildren, attributed the decline to concerns about side effects among parents, nurses and physicians. The decline in methylphenidate use may be depriving many hyperactive children of an effective treatment, said one of the report's authors from the Johns Hopkins School of Medicine in Baltimore.

Pediatrics

Sept. 1

Israeli researchers reported that children conceived through in-vitro fertilization who are healthy at birth are as likely to develop normally as naturally conceived children. The Haifa team matched 66 naturally conceived singleton births with 66 IVF singletons; 19 naturally conceived pairs of twins with 19 IVF twin pairs; and four naturally conceived sets of triplets with four IVF triplet sets. About two years after birth, the children's size, weight, physical dexterity and mental development were similar, the team reported in Pediatrics.

Sept. 4

Pediatricians from the University of Rochester, N.Y., suggested that children's behavior problems should be added to the growing list of adverse health effects linked to maternal smoking. They performed a retrospective study of 2,256 children aged 4 to 11, and found that the more a mother smoked, either during or after pregnancy, the greater the chance that her children would develop behavior problems. Some children of women who smoked showed antisocial behavior, anxiety, depression, hyperactivity, social withdrawal and immaturity, the researchers reported in Pediatrics.

Sept. 8

Philadelphia pediatricians warned that home fitness devotees need to protect curious children against injury from stationary exercise bicycles. In the American Journal of Diseases of Children, 41 injuries were analyzed; 75% involved the amputation of fingers as unsupervised youngsters played with bicycle spokes or chains, the Thomas Jefferson University team found.

Many stationary-bike manufacturers are changing to spokeless wheels and covered chains and sprockets, and installing pedal and wheel locks to engage when the bicycles are not in use. However, a recent Consumer Reports survey found that 16 of 20 popular models had holes around the wheel in which children could stick their fingers.

Sept. 10

Tests indicated that a New York elementary school did not have harmful lead levels, as had been widely publicized, but lead-poisoning experts told Medical Tribune that dangerous levels in many locales still call for constant vigilance. The chairman of the American Academy of Pediatrics Committee on Environmental Health said that all children who live in older neighborhoods or attend schools painted with lead-based paint should be screened. Parents should also check to be sure that the water supply at their child's school has been tested for lead, as required by the Environmental Protection Agency, he said.

Sept. 14

The Department of Health in the United Kingdom withdrew from the market two of three brands of measles, mumps and rubella vaccine used in that country. The abrupt withdrawal followed reports of mild, transient meningitis caused by the Urabe strain of virus contained in the two affected brands of mumps vaccine. The vaccine that remains on the market—Merck Sharp & Dohme's MMR II—is the only vaccine approved in the United States. Incidence of meningitis from the Urabe strain was as high as one in 6,000 inoculations, but still much lower than what would be expected without vaccination, said the Department of Health.

Sept. 16

Dutch researchers found that children with asthma may breathe easier if they receive anti-inflammatory medications in addition to standard asthma therapy. As described in the American Review of Respiratory Disease, 116 children with asthma were given an inhaled beta-agonist (salbutamol 0.2 mg) plus either an inhaled cortico-

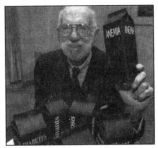

Dr. Spock advocates breast milk during the first year of life.

steroid (budesonide 0.2 mg) or placebo three times a day. Forced expiratory volume increased by 7% after two months of beta-agonist/steroid therapy, compared with a decrease of 4% after beta-agonist therapy—an 11% difference that was maintained throughout the 22 months of follow-up, reported the investigators from the Sophia Children's Hospital in Rotterdam. The study was halted after 22 months so that all the children could be given anti-inflammatory therapy.

Sept. 19

The Health Care Financing Administration instructed states to screen all children age six months to six years who are covered by Medicaid for lead levels.

Sept. 24

University of Iowa researchers found that asthmatic children given theophylline do not have more learning problems in school, on average, than their siblings without asthma. They studied 255 children with asthma who had taken standardized achievement tests. The Iowa children with asthma scored an average of 57 points, compared with a national average of 50 points, the researchers wrote in a recent issue of The New England Journal of Medicine. Of 72 asthmatic children receiving daily theophylline, the average test score was 58.5, compared with 58.4 for their siblings.

The Iowa team hypothesized that previous studies linking theophylline to poor academic performance did not adequately control for such variables as family background, intelligence and socioeconomic status.

Sept. 26

Australian researchers announced that steroid therapy reduces both the duration of intubation and the need for reintubation in children hospitalized with the croup. In a study of 70 children (six months to eight years of age) at the Royal Children's Hospital in Melbourne, children receiving prednisolone by nasogastric tube every 12 hours could be extubated 40 hours earlier than the children on placebo, the team reported in The Lancet. Only 5% of the children on steroids required reintubation after accidental or elective extubation, while 34% of the placebo-treated children were reintubated.

Sept. 29

"We need to leave cow's milk where it belongs—in cows." So advised the president of the Physicians Committee for Responsible Medicine during a recent press conference in Boston at which parents were urged to give their youngsters calcium-rich foods such as broccoli and tofu instead. One pediatrician noted that researchers are finding that infants and children who are not exposed to dairy products are less likely to contract ear infections, asthma and allergies. And Benjamin Spock, M.D., who once encouraged all parents to give their children cow's milk, urged mothers instead to breast-feed, or use nondairy infant formulas, evaporated milk or heat-treated milk, which contain modified cow proteins, during the first year of life.

Pediatrics

Oct. 1

Chronic fatigue syndrome can be difficult to diagnose in children, a pediatrician at Cambridge Hospital in Boston reported at an international meeting on CFS. Young children may not be able to describe their level of fatigue well, but parents may notice a lack of stamina, said the specialist. In some cases, CFS may even be confused with learning disabilities, he said at the Albany, N.Y., meeting. Young children tend to develop symptoms gradually, while children age 10 and older and adults often develop CFS quickly and severely, with flulike symptoms, he added.

Oct. 3

British researchers reported that a chemical compound that failed as an herbicide is being tested as a treatment for tyrosinemia, a hereditary liver illness in children. The chemical, called NTBC, could prevent the buildup of toxic compounds found in the livers of children suffering from tyrosinemia, the specialists at Imperial Chemical Industries wrote in The Lancet. The finding may enable children suffering from the disease to avoid a liver transplant, the only currently available treatment, company scientists said.

Oct. 5

Two pediatricians from the Medical College of Georgia advised that adolescents be screened periodically for iron deficiency and anemia. The major cause of anemia in adolescents is nutritional iron deficiency, and anemia can lower athletic performance, the Augusta team pointed out in the American Journal of Diseases of Children. A review of other articles in the literature showed that in teen athletes, the rate of iron deficiency is between 9.5% and 57%, and the rate of iron deficiency with anemia is between 6.7% and 11%,

depending on age and other factors.

Risk factors include poor socioeconomic background; following a vegetarian, weight-loss or fad diet; engaging in intense, lengthy physical activity; and a personal or family history of anemia, bleeding disorders or chronic disease, they said. Young women who have long, frequent or heavy menstrual periods are also at risk.

Oct. 13

The American Academy of Pediatrics drew fire from physicians for warning parents against putting babies to bed on their stomachs to reduce the risk of sudden infant death syndrome. Critics speaking at the academy's annual meeting in San Francisco charged that the April warning was premature. They said it causes needless anxiety for parents of healthy infants, and unnecessary anguish for parents whose babies have died of SIDS. In response to the criticism, the academy's task force on infant positioning and SIDS decided to study the issue for another year, but left the warning in place during the deliberations.

Oct. 15

Yale University researchers reported that children who

have febrile seizures are more likely to have a recurrence if the fever before the initial seizure is of short duration and low temperature. The findings may help physicians pinpoint which children are at risk of recurrent febrile seizures and get those children appropriate antiseizure medications, the researchers wrote in The New England Journal of Medicine. The study of 347 children found that 46% of those whose first fever lasted less than one hour had a recurrence by 15 months, compared with 25% whose first fever lasted up to 24 hours and 15% of those whose first fever lasted more than 24 hours. The study also found that children whose initial fever was 101 degrees Fahrenheit or less were more likely to have a recurrence.

Oct. 17

When examining children who may have been sexually abused, doctors should avoid interpreting minor abnormalities of a child's body as signs of abuse, a North Carolina pediatrician advised at the American Academy of Family Physicians annual meeting in San Diego.

The expert, who has testified in many sexual abuse cases, said that while most family physicians will be called on at some point to get involved in a child sex-

ual-abuse case, they may not have the experience to be able to distinguish the appearance of normal sex organs from abused ones.

The researcher, of East Carolina University School of Medicine in Greenville, said doctors may mistake atypical bumps or ridges as signs of damage from sexual abuse. They also should beware of mistaking straddle injury—damage from falling on a hard object that hits between the legs—for sex-abuse damage, he said.

• • •

A North Carolina physician urged physicians to donate four hours a week to providing care for poor patients. The specialist from East Carolina University School of Medicine in Greenville reported that about 25% of the 22 million American children under age six live below the poverty line, and many of these youngsters are at greater than average risk of death or malnutrition. At the annual meeting of the American Academy of Family Physicians, he said that communities and governments should provide daycare and preventive medicine programs funded from public and private sources.

Oct. 30

New York researchers advised that children not be forced to eat everything on their plates because chances are they will eat more later on to make up for the uneaten portion. Physicians at the Columbia-Presbyterian Medical Center reported in Pediatrics that children between ages three and four who ate less at one meal made up for it at a later meal.

The children in the study averaged about 1,600 calories a day. The researchers suggested that a child who skimps on dinner and is hungry later should be encouraged to have fruit, milk or graham crackers to substitute for the missed meal.

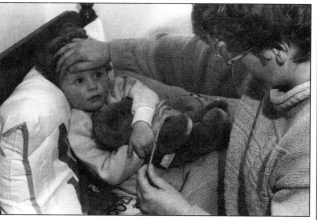

Doctors can pinpoint risk factors for recurrent febrile seizures.

Pediatrics

Nov. 1

Canadian researchers reported that infants may be quietest and most content the first 10 minutes after a feeding. The study also suggested that feeding babies more frequently than every four hours, the traditional recommendation, may make them happier and less fussy.

Researchers at McGill University in Montreal observed 53 newborns who were given bottles of water, infant formula or a solution of carbohydrates and lactose. The investigators found that the babies were awake and not crying immediately after a feeding, no matter what they were fed.

After the 10-minute honeymoon, however, babies who had been given water cried more, while babies who got lactose or formula cried less, according to the researchers' report in Pediatrics.

Nov. 5

Contrary to previous findings, hyperactivity is probably not a risk factor for injury in children, Columbia University and University of London researchers concluded. The investigators studied 702 hyperactive boys between the ages of six and eight, and compared them with a nonhyperactive control group. No relationship between hyperactivity and injuries was found, the team reported in the journal Pediatrics. The absence of an association could not be accounted for by parental protectiveness of boys designated hyperactive, the research team noted.

Nov. 7

Acetaminophen was found to be better for lowering fevers than giving warm sponge baths or removing layers of clothing, British pediatricians reported. A study of 52 children aged three months to five years found that once acetaminophen began to take effect, it worked better and longer than the other two methods. Writing in the British Medical Journal, researchers from the University of Southampton's Aldermoor Health Centre in England advised parents to offer continuous fluids in addition to acetaminophen. The findings appeared shortly after a team of Texas researchers questioned whether children's fevers need to be treated at all.

Nov. 10

Eyedrops may be the best solution for young children with amblyopia who won't wear an eye patch, physicians told the American Academy of Ophthalmology meeting in Dallas. Johns Hopkins Hospital researchers reported on 166 children, aged 2 to 12, who were treated for amblyopia for at least three weeks. Some received eyedrops containing atropine; others wore glasses with foggy lenses. Three out of four children showed improvement with either strategy. Those with the poorest eyesight at the beginning of the study improved the most, the researchers noted.

While the study did not compare the two techniques with patching, a 90% compliance rate verified that either technique is more readily accepted by children and parents. The drawback, according to the Maryland researchers, is that the foggy lens or eyedrop treatment takes longer than patching. The average treatment duration—13 months for the eyedrops and 29 months for the foggy lens treatment—is long when compared with patching, the researchers reported.

Nov. 15

A South Carolina researcher reported that rearing a child with asthma may adversely affect parents' social lives, financial well-being and overall quality of life. He told doctors at the 50th Anniversary meeting of the American College of Allergy and Immunology in Chicago that identifying the quality-of-life issues that affect these parents may help doctors improve methods of treatment of asthmatic children. If parents' concerns are addressed, it may create a more relaxed atmosphere for the child and the entire family, according to the doctor from the University of South Carolina in Columbia.

Nov. 25

Parents of asthmatic children rated home peak-flow meters useful and reassuring in a study conducted by London pediatricians. Of 50 parents surveyed, 42 were able to recall their child's best peak-flow level and the child's danger peak flow to within 10% of the correct value. Most parents said the device was very useful in judging their child's responsiveness to bronchodilators, and a smaller number of parents said they used the peak-flow meters to detect asthma when their child was asymptomatic. The researchers told Medical Tribune they were not convinced that peak-flow meters are worth the effort in apparently well children, but noted the importance of getting parents to use the device to recognize severe asthma.

Nov. 30

Ultrasound monitoring made it possible to substitute a water-based enema for barium in treating children with ileocolic intussesception, Berlin researchers found. The investigators told the Radiological Society of North America meeting in Chicago that they successfully managed 30 of 37 children using the non-radiation-requiring technique.

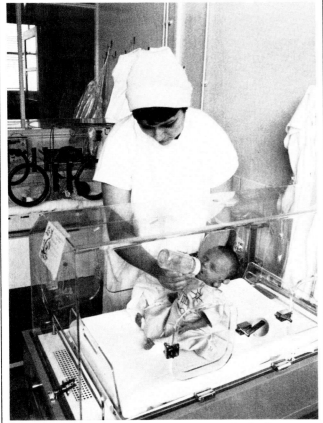

Babies most alert and content in first 10 minutes after feeding.

Pediatrics

Dec. 5

A 10-year study published in Pediatrics suggested that even when children are economically advantaged, low-level lead exposure can impair their intellectual and academic performance. The study, conducted by experts from the University of Pittsburgh and Children's Hospital in Boston, found that slightly elevated blood lead levels around the age of 24 months are associated with intellectual and academic performance deficits at the age of 10 years.

The 148 children in the study were from middle-class and upper-middle-class families; previous studies had looked at whether lead exposure was a marker of socioeconomic class rather than an independent risk. The researchers found that even blood lead levels below 10 mcg/dl, the previous lowest

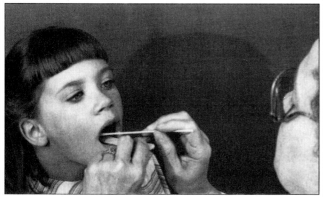

If ear pulling is sole symptom, otitis media is unlikely.

observed adverse effect level, are associated with measurable long-term cognitive deficits.

Dec. 8

Amid reports of increasing numbers of asthmatic children, a study found that these youngsters are at a modestly increased risk of experiencing academic problems. Using data from a national survey, researchers at the National Center for Health Statistics determined that 18% of children with asthma had failed a grade, compared with 15% of well children, and that 9% of asthmatic children had learning disabilities, compared with 5%

of well children. Children with asthma were absent from school an average of 7.6 days, compared with 2.5 days for well children, the researchers reported in Pediatrics.

Among children whose families earned less than $20,000 a year, those with asthma had twice the chance of being left back as well children. The researchers suggested that health professionals should be particularly alert for the risk of grade failure among asthmatic children from lower-income families.

Dec. 11

Physicians at Harvard Medical School and the Massachusetts Poison Control System found that intervention kits are only modestly effective in preventing poisonings in homes of

preschoolers. The researchers sent poisoning prevention kits to families whose preschool child had recently experienced a poisoning incident. The kit included a telephone sticker with the number of the poison control center, a $1 coupon for syrup of ipecac, a slide-style cabinet lock, a nine-step checklist for "poison-proofing" the home and information pamphlets.

While those who received the kit were twice as likely to have a telephone sticker than control families (who also had had a previous poisoning incident), and were more likely to be using at least one slide

lock, they were no more likely to have ipecac on hand, and did not indicate a higher rate of compliance with other poisoning prevention measures.

A poisoning recurrence rate of 3.7% was seen in the total sample during three months of surveillance, with no difference between the two groups, the researchers reported in Pediatrics.

Dec. 14

Contrary to the belief of many parents, ear pulling without any other signs of illness is not a sign of otitis media, concluded a Kaiser Permanente family practitioner in Bonita, Calif.

The physician studied 100 children with a chief complaint of ear pulling. Of the 20 who had no other symptoms of illness, none had otitis media, but many did have gastrointestinal complaints or behavioral complaints such as night-awakenings.

Of the 80 children with other symptoms of illness, such as fever, 12 were found to have otitis media, the physician reported in Pediatrics.

Dec. 17

Even when lab tests indicate a child is infected with relatively penicillin-resistant Streptococcus pneumoniae, pediatricians at Texas Children's Hospital found that most cases of bacteremia can still be adequately treated with penicillins or cephalosporins. Third-generation cephalosporins are generally adequate therapy for meningitis due to these resistant organisms, the investigators reported in the journal Pediatrics. Their findings were based on 19 children.

Based on this and previous small studies, the Houston physicians suggested cefuroxime (Ceftin, Allen & Hansburys), cefotaxime (Claforan, Hoechst-Roussel) or ceftriaxone (Rocephin, Roche Laboratories) as appropriate initial

treatment for children with nonmeningeal systemic infections caused by S. pneumoniae relatively resistant to penicillin.

Dec. 21

Mailing their parents flu-shot reminders can boost vaccination rates in asthmatic children 400%, announced investigators from the University of Rochester in Rochester, N.Y., and the University of Massachusetts in Worcester.

The pediatricians studied 124 parents of children with moderate or severe asthma, who were randomly assigned to receive either no flu-shot reminder or a personalized letter.

Thirty percent of those who got the letter brought their children in for a flu shot, compared with 7% of controls, the investigators reported in the journal Pediatrics. The low response rate of parents who received the letters indicates that more powerful interventions are needed to increase influenza vaccination rates further, the researchers said. In the study, high levels of parental concern about vaccine side effects were deemed to be an important variable in noncompliance.

Dec. 29

Ten years after the American Academy of Pediatrics found that its members felt deficient in their knowledge of adolescent care, learning disabilities, attention-deficit disorders, mental retardation and psychosocial and behavior problems, a new survey of 3,000 pediatricians revealed that they continue to feel inadequately trained in the same areas.

The new survey did find some encouraging news: Significantly more pediatricians identify their area of special interest or subspecialty practice as developmental or behavioral pediatrics, the researchers from Albert Einstein College of Medicine in New York and the University of California at San Francisco reported in Pediatrics.

Cold virus may deliver cystic fibrosis 'cure'

By Tom Yulsman

JAN. 9—A genetically engineered cold virus may hold the key to a treatment for cystic fibrosis.

Government researchers inserted into the adenovirus the human gene that codes for cystic fibrosis transmembrane conductance regulator protein, which is missing in the lungs of CF patients. When given to rats, the altered virus infected the lungs, sending the CFTR gene to cells lining airways. Tests showed that lung cells produced the human protein for at least six weeks. The virus was altered so it would not cause illness.

Human trials could begin in a year, according to Ronald Crystal, M.D., of the National Heart, Lung and Blood Institute.

He reported his results in Cell.

"I've no doubt that if we take the altered virus and put it in people with cystic fibrosis, it will correct the biological abnormality," he said. "The only question is whether it is safe."

Commenting on the research, Robert Dresing, president of the Cystic Fibrosis Foundation, said: "It is no longer a question of if we will have gene therapy as a cure for cystic fibrosis, it is a question of when."

Researchers found the normal CFTR gene and protein in 1989. A year later, scientists inserted the normal gene into human CF lung cells in vitro, successfully correcting a defect in salt transport that causes symptoms of the disease. But this left unsolved the problem of how to deliver the gene into the complex tree structure of the human airway.

The current rat experiments suggest that a cold virus is an effective method of delivery.

Botulinum toxin found to help relax cerebral palsy stiffness

WASHINGTON, D.C., FEB. 20—A powerful bacterial toxin may help relax the spastic muscles of children with cerebral palsy, according to Irish researchers.

Youngsters who received botulinum toxin injections were able to straighten their legs and showed improvement in muscle tone, the researchers reported at the annual meeting of the American Academy of Orthopaedic Surgeons here.

Aidan Cosgrove, M.D., of the Royal Belfast Hospital for Sick Children, injected the toxin into the spastic hamstring and calf muscles of 33 children aged two to eight with cerebral palsy. All but two showed improvement, he reported.

Relaxing the muscles also allows the limbs to grow more, reducing the need for operations to lengthen them later on, Dr. Cosgrove added.

The toxin's benefits last about six months, and some children were reinjected twice, without side effects. The injections could replace current therapies for cerebral palsy, he said.

Children with cerebral palsy are now treated with physical therapy, serial casting, and muscle weakening or lengthening surgeries to relieve muscle spasticity, said Kathy Broecker, director of physical therapy at the Richmond Cerebral Palsy Center in Richmond, Va.

For a carefully chosen group of patients, neurosurgeons perform a dorsal root rhizotomy, she said, cutting select sensory nerves in the spinal area that had been causing muscle spasticity.

Botulinum toxin injections have also been used to relax spastic muscles that keep the neck bent to one side, said Brian Younge, M.D., of the Mayo Clinic in Rochester, Minn.

"I have given it to patients who involuntarily squeeze their eyelids shut and can't open their eyes and to people who have involuntary facial twitching," he said. "The treatment works

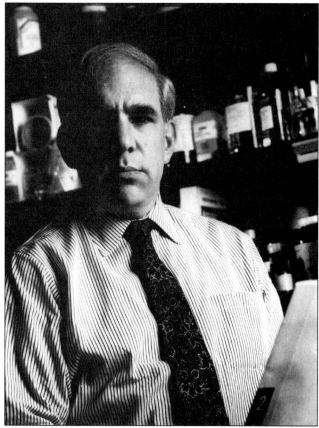

Dr. Crystal is confident in gene therapy for cystic fibrosis.

for two or three months, and then the patients have to be re-injected."

Botulinum toxin, marketed as Oculinum (Allergan, Inc.), was approved by the Food and Drug Administration in 1989 for the treatment of blepharospasm and strabismus, according to a company spokesperson.

Joseph Jankovic, M.D., of the Baylor College of Medicine in Houston, injected botulinum toxin into people who have disabling tremors of the hands, wrists and neck.

About 65% showed improvement, the investigator reported. These patients had failed to respond to other medications or surgeries.

Nationwide, resurgent TB reaching children

By Marjorie Shaffer

NEW YORK, MARCH 13—The resurgence of tuberculosis nationwide is now reaching children from the cities to the suburbs, epidemiologists report.

Although most of the cases have been reported in inner-city children plagued by homelessness, poverty and AIDS, the disease is also striking teenagers and younger children in households with adults who do not belong to any of the known high-risk groups, according to a New York City pediatrician.

"TB crosses all social lines now," said the physician, Paul Pasquariello, M.D.

Over the last 18 months, Dr. Pasquariello has treated five children, ranging in age from 5 to 15, who all come from middle-class households. In all five of the cases, he has been unable to determine the source of the infection.

"It's a mystery," he said. "No one in the family has TB. We are left with giving these kids a year of treatment, with all of the [attendant] side effects."

One child, he said, developed side effects to isoniazid and had to be switched to another antibiotic.

Nationwide, nearly 950 children under age five had active TB in 1990, an increase of 39% from 1987, according to the Centers for Disease Control. In children under age 15, the rates jumped 36% to 1,596 cases in 1990, according to the CDC.

"These cases are only the tip of the iceberg," said Jeffrey Starke, M.D., assistant professor of pediatrics at the Baylor College of Medicine, who has treated 300 children with TB over the last six years.

"We are seeing increasing numbers of children and young adults who are becoming infected but have not yet developed disease. This problem will be around for decades."

"Homelessness is contributing to the resurgence of TB in children," said Helena Aquila, M.D., a pediatrician who works at a TB clinic in Newark, N.J.

In New York City, there has been a dramatic increase in TB cases, with twice as many children affected in 1990 than in 1989. In 1991, 162 children had TB, an increase of 11% over a year earlier, according to the New York City Department of Health.

In Houston, the TB infection rate among 5,122 five- and six-year-olds tested in 1987 was 25 times higher than the previous national average of 0.2%, taken in 1970, the last year for which such tabulations were made.

In Los Angeles, as many as 35% of 10th-graders who were born outside of the United States in areas where TB is endemic tested positive on TB skin tests, according to data from 1985 and 1986.

TB in children has often been overlooked because children are not as infectious as adults, said Dr. Starke. A four-year-old with TB, for example, is not contagious, he said.

Nevertheless, some physicians are calling for aggressive TB testing in schools. But some experts say healthcare dollars would be better spent at the source of the dawning TB epidemic.

"If you want to get rid of TB in kids, you have to get rid of it in adults," Dr. Starke said. "You get the most bang for your buck by making sure sick adults are appropriately treated."

"Until you have every patient with active TB on effective treatment and completing that treatment, you have no business doing mass screening of children," said Thomas Frieden, M.D., a CDC epidemiologist assigned to the New York City Department of Health.

AAP now advocates vaccination of all infants for hepatitis B

By Andrea Kott

NEW YORK, APRIL 13—All infants and young children should be vaccinated against hepatitis B, not just those thought to be at risk of developing the disease, a leading pediatrician told a meeting of the American Academy of Pediatrics.

If all children received the vaccine, the number of hepatitis B cases would be reduced nationwide by at least 90% by the year 2015, said Saul Krugman, M.D., a professor of pediatrics at New York University Medical Center. For approximately $21, children can receive the necessary three doses of vaccine.

A baby born to a mother infected with hepatitis B has a 65% to 90% chance of becoming infected with the disease, according to Dr. Krugman.

About 30% to 40% of acute hepatitis B infections occur in people with no apparent risk factors. Of the 300,000 cases of hepatitis B estimated to strike Americans each year, as many as half are subclinical, Dr. Krugman said.

Emphasis on high-risk groups alone is not enough, according to infectious diseases expert Martha Lepow, M.D. "The cases recognized each year have been going up," explained Dr. Lepow, a professor of pediatrics at Albany Medical College in New York. "You can't predict who is high-risk now. All children today are potentially at risk," she said.

The pediatrics group recommends giving the first dose of vaccine to newborns while in the hospital, the second dose at one to two months of age and the third at six to 18 months.

Babies not vaccinated at birth should still get three doses of hepatitis B vaccine by age 18 months, the academy said.

Babies born to mothers who are infected with the virus should receive the vaccine plus one dose of hepatitis B antibodies as soon as possible after birth, the Centers for Disease Control in Atlanta advises.

A second dose of vaccine should be given at one month and a third at six months.

"Side effects of the hepatitis B vaccine are negligible," according to Dr. Krugman. The vaccine can protect babies and children for more than 10 years, he said.

The academy, following the lead of the CDC, recommended in February that all babies be immunized against hepatitis B.

The academy also considered recommending immunization against hepatitis B for teens, who are at high risk of acquiring the disease, especially if they live in areas where there is a high rate of teenage pregnancy and drug use.

A standard dose of the vaccine costs between $7 and $10, Dr. Krugman said.

Oxygen tension linked to retinopathy in preemies

By L. A. McKeown

APRIL 16—Premature infants exposed to arterial oxygen tension of 80 mm Hg or higher are at increased risk of developing retinopathy of prematurity, and the longer the exposure, the higher the risk.

Current methods of monitoring cannot prevent the condition from occurring, according to Florida researchers.

Eduardo Bancalari, M.D., of the University of Miami, reported his results in The New England Journal of Medicine.

Oxygen levels must be maintained within a very narrow range in premature infants because without sufficient oxygen the infant's brain will be damaged, but if the levels are too high, they may lead to damage in the eye, according to Dr. Bancalari. "It's a very tight rope," he said.

But factors such as the baby's weight and condition at birth

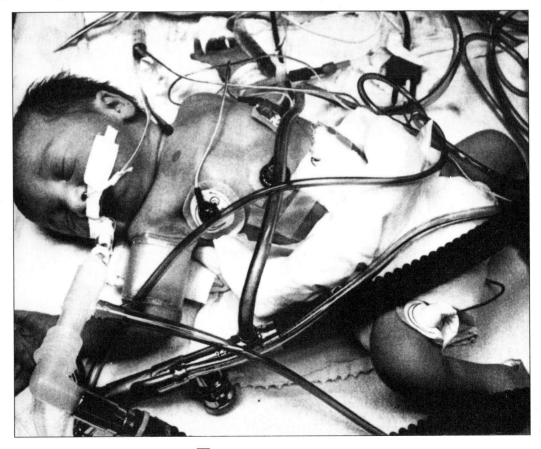

Oxygenating premature babies adequately without reaching the 80 mm Hg danger point can be difficult.

may play a bigger role in the development of retinopathy than oxygen exposure, according to the Florida investigator.

The smaller the baby is at birth, the higher the risk of ROP, said Earl A. Palmer, M.D., of the Oregon Health Sciences University in Portland.

About 6% of infants born weighing 2.7 pounds or less develop severe ROP that causes vision problems or blindness, but in infants born at 1.6 pounds or less, the rate rises to 15.5%, said the investigator.

Arterial oxygen tension in infants' blood is extremely unstable and doctors are unable to keep it constantly within the desired range with the existing equipment, he said.

The study should create the incentive for developing equipment that would allow physicians to adjust arterial oxygen tension in premature infants instantaneously, Dr. Palmer added.

In a separate study appearing in the medical journal Pediatrics, British doctors report that the amount of light that babies are exposed to in nurseries immediately after birth may account for some cases of ROP.

Babies who are always held in the same position, with their head turned to one side, may get more light exposure in one eye, since the other is usually shielded by clothing or the bottle-holder's arm, according to Alistair R. Fielder, M.D., of England's Birmingham and Midland Eye Hospital.

A study of 607 babies who were less than 3.5 pounds at birth suggested that ROP begins in areas of the retina that have had the most light exposure, according to Dr. Fielder.

If these results can be substantiated, doctors may be able to prevent ROP by adjusting light levels in nurseries, he said.

"It is still very much an open question whether light influences the development of retinopathy of prematurity," said Dr. Palmer.

Joint, limb pain in children tied to rubella vaccine

MANCHESTER, ENGLAND, APRIL 25—Children aged five and younger who are vaccinated against mumps, measles and rubella may suffer brief episodes of joint or limb pain, according to British researchers.

The rubella part of the vaccine causes the reaction, reported A. J. Silman of the University of Manchester in the British Medical Journal.

Such episodes are not as severe as the arthritis associated with rubella in adults, he added.

Vaccine expert Melvin Marks, M.D., of the University of California, Irvine, said he did not find the British results to be surprising.

"This side effect is most frequently seen in adult women who receive rubella vaccine," he said. "However, even in those cases it's extremely rare that a true case of arthritis develops."

The British researchers based their conclusions on questionnaires filled out by parents of 1,588 vaccinated children and 1,242 controls.

Among vaccinated children, 145 had some joint or limb pain during that period, compared with 73 of the non-immunized children.

Joint swelling was found to occur in 24 immunized and four nonimmunized children.

Three boys who received the vaccine required hospitalization.

The reaction is most likely to occur within six weeks of vaccination, and is more likely to affect girls than boys, according to the Manchester investigator.

According to Dr. Marks, the protective advantages associated with the vaccine far outweigh the side effects associated with it.

"Also, these side effects are not as common as the joint pain and swelling associated with the naturally occurring disease," he said.

Mothers who contract rubella while pregnant risk having babies who are born deaf or with other birth defects, Dr. Marks noted.

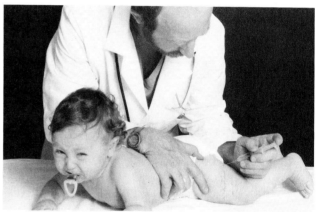

Immunization against rubella linked to transient joint pain.

Youngsters' moods not altered by theophylline

Medical World News Report

MAY 20—The asthma drug theophylline may not cause the mood changes and behavior problems that some parents have reported to their physicians, according to a study in The Journal of the American Medical Association.

University of Colorado researchers studied 31 asthmatic children aged eight to 12 whose parents had reported that theophylline caused mood alterations, learning difficulties and behavior problems in their children.

In the randomized, double-blind crossover study, the children were given the drug for a week and then a placebo for a week.

During the Colorado study, the children were tested for

attention, impulsivity, memory, activity level and mood. Parents also rated their children's behavior, using a questionnaire.

Parents could not tell which treatment their children were getting based on their behavior, the researchers wrote.

"These results are in conflict with reports of a high incidence of adverse behavioral side effects attributed to theophylline therapy," wrote Bruce Bender, Ph.D., and Henry Milgrom, M.D., of the University of Colorado Health Sciences Center and the National Jewish Center for Immunology and Respiratory Medicine in Denver.

Psychological testing showed that theophylline slightly improved memory in the children, and also improved attention span. The children also showed a mild increase in anxiety and tremor in the dominant hand while taking the drug, the study showed.

"The measured changes are typically subtle, suggesting that, for the most part, these side effects are not clinically important," the researchers wrote.

They added that the somewhat contradictory findings of improved concentration and mood disruption resemble those found with ingestion of caffeine.

James Kemp, M.D., a pediatric allergist in San Diego, said the study's conclusions seem reasonable, based on the moderate size of the study sample.

"I'm not surprised to hear the conclusions. In many children, theophylline is not a concern when it's used properly," said Dr. Kemp, who is affiliated with Children's Hospital and Health Center.

"I use theophylline extensively and feel it to be safe and effective when used properly and blood levels are monitored."

In a larger group, however, adverse effects might have surfaced, Dr. Kemp added.

"There are definitely individual patients with any drug who will respond in an adverse way, whereas the majority will not," he said.

New easier-access child vaccine rules set

By Steve Frandzel

ATLANTA, JUNE 11—Current U.S. healthcare practices fail to deliver vaccines to a large portion of the country's vulnerable preschool children, according to a panel of experts.

Members of the National Vaccine Advisory Council (NVAC) discussed the shortfall with the Centers for Disease Control's Advisory Committee on Immunization Practices.

Less than 60% of children, especially those in the inner cities, are up to date for the recommended primary immunization series, which include immunizations against diphtheria, tetanus, pertussis, poliomyelitis, measles, mumps, rubella, Hemophilus influenzae type b and hepatitis B.

A number of barriers stand in the way of efficient vaccine delivery, the council said. Many public clinics and private offices require advance appointments that involve delays. Providers often require comprehensive physical examinations as a prerequisite to vaccinations, and many opportunities to

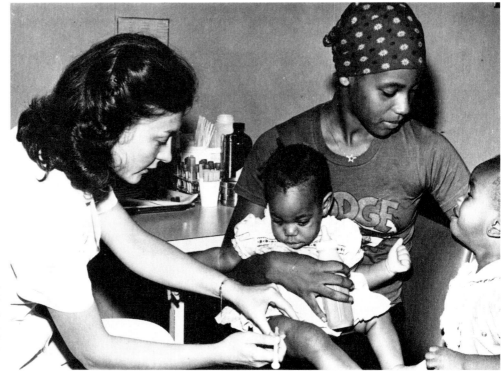

Despite vaccination programs at public health clinics, fewer than 60% of children are up to date for recommended primary immunization series.

vaccinate children who have presented for other medical services are missed.

New NVAC rules include:
• Appointment-only systems should be waived in both public and private settings, and waiting time should not exceed 30 minutes;
• In the public sector, immunizations should be free of charge;
• Each encounter with a healthcare provider should become an opportunity to screen immunization status and, if indicated, administer needed vaccines;
• Providers should administer simultaneously all vaccines for which a child is eligible at the time of each visit;
• Providers should initiate a tracking system to identify children at high risk of failing to complete the entire immunization series.

Peptide in albumin of cow's milk may trigger onset of diabetes in genetically susceptible children

New York Times/Medical Tribune News Service

JULY 29—A peptide in the albumin of cow's milk may trigger the onset of insulin-dependent diabetes mellitus in genetically susceptible infants, a Finnish-Canadian study has found.

Following a long trail of clues from epidemiologic studies and animal models, researchers performed immunoassays on 521 children and adults.

Of 142 children with recently diagnosed IDDM, all had highly elevated serum concentrations of antibodies against bovine serum albumin, most of which were specific for the ABBOS peptide. Much lower serum concentration levels for the antibodies were found in controls, with less than 3% having small amounts of ABBOS-specific antibodies.

The researchers believe that the ABBOS-specific antibodies in the diabetic children work like nearsighted pit bulls, apparently mistaking the p69 peptide on the surface of beta cells for their prey, latching on until every last beta cell is destroyed.

"The implication is that if we are right, we have a wonderful strategy to prevent the disease," said Hans-Michael Dosch, M.D., professor of pediatrics and immunology at the Hospital for Sick Children in Toronto.

"In principle, it would be a simple thing to prevent the exposure to cow's milk in the first three months of life," he said. "If we are right, it could be the beginning of the end of Type I diabetes."

But other researchers cautioned that Dr. Dosch's hypothesis, while strengthened by his study published in The New England Journal of Medicine, is far from proven.

"I hope this is really a breakthrough in diabetes," said Mark Atkinson, Ph.D., professor of pathology at the University of Florida in Gainesville and president of the International Diabetes Intervention Group.

"The potential for it to be a breakthrough is high, but now it really needs to be tested," he said.

George Eisenbarth, M.D., chief of the section of immunology and immunogenetics at the Joslin Diabetes Center in Boston, said, "If the hypothesis is true, it could be very important. The test will be to remove cow's milk from the diets of young infants who are at risk of developing diabetes, to see if the disease is prevented."

Finnish collaborators, led by Jukka Karjalainen, M.D., of the University of Oulu in Finland, began such a study recently. The results will probably not be available for five to 10 years, Dr. Dosch said.

Other researchers might attempt similar studies, said Dr. Atkinson. Or an even more practical approach might be to develop a way to short-circuit the immune system's reactivity to the bovine albumin in the first place, he said.

Both Dr. Atkinson and Dr. Eisenbarth pointed out that holes remain in the hypothesis.

Most notably, the heightened level of ABBOS-specific antibodies has not yet been conclusively demonstrated to be a marker in prediabetic children.

One-dose vaccine stops childhood hepatitis A

By Charlene Laino

AUG. 13—A study of more than 1,000 children has found that a single dose of a formalin-inactivated hepatitis A vaccine is well tolerated and highly protective against the disease.

The early protection afforded by the vaccine, which has not yet been approved by the U.S. Food and Drug Administration, should make it of special practical benefit to people at high risk, said study leader Alan Werzberger, M.D., of the Kiryas Joel Institute of Medicine in Monroe, N.Y. This includes healthy people planning to travel to areas where hepatitis A is endemic, children in daycare centers and people who live in frequently affected communities.

The immune globulin vaccine that is currently used to protect people at high risk of contracting hepatitis A provides protection for only four to six months, necessitating the inconvenience, discomfort and expense of repeated shots, Dr. Werzberger said.

To evaluate the new formalin-inactivated hepatitis A vaccine, his team studied members of a Hasidic Jewish community in upstate New York that has had recurrent outbreaks of the disease. Their findings appear in The New England Journal of Medicine.

At the beginning of a summer outbreak in 1991, 1,037 children aged two to 16 who were not infected were randomly assigned to receive either one intramuscular injection of the vaccine (Vaqta, Merck Sharp & Dohme) or placebo.

From the seventh week after the injection until the trial ended about four and a half months later, 25 cases of hepatitis A occurred in the placebo group and none in the vaccine group.

Seven cases of hepatitis A occurred in the vaccine group and three in the placebo group during the first three weeks after the injection, but these children probably had been exposed and were in the incubation phase of the disease before the trial began, he said.

All but one of the 305 initially seronegative vaccine recipients had detectable antibody one month after vaccination. No child had a serious adverse reaction, according to the researchers.

Dr. Werzberger called for widespread use of the vaccine in children. "From a public-health perspective, there can be no impact until it is universally used," he said.

William Bancroft, M.D., of the U.S. Army Medical Research and Development Council in Frederick, Md., agreed that all children should be given a hepatitis A vaccine.

In an accompanying editorial, Dr. Bancroft stated that universal hepatitis A vaccination "may prove to be the most cost-effective method of protecting large populations both nationally and universally."

A member of the American Academy of Pediatrics Committee on Infectious Diseases agreed that the vaccine will be particularly important in protecting those at high risk of hepatitis A.

But the AAP is not ready to recommend that all children receive the vaccine, said the committee member, Donald Gromisch, M.D. He said that further studies are needed to confirm the effectiveness of the vaccine.

While the NEJM trial did not study the long-term effectiveness of the new vaccine, previous studies have indicated that with a booster, the vaccine is effective for up to seven years, according to Dr. Gromisch, who is a pediatrician at the State University of New York at Stony Brook.

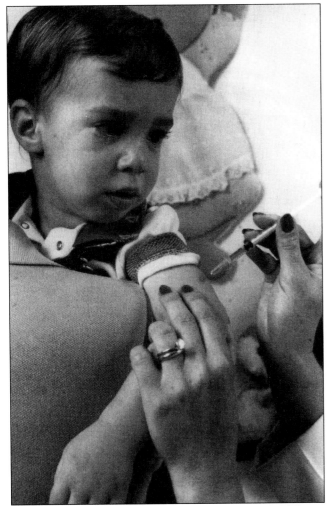

CDC was first to recommend hep B vaccine for all children.

AAFP, CDC, AAP all favor hepatitis B shots

Medical Tribune News Service

AUG. 14—The American Academy of Family Physicians has joined the Centers for Disease Control and the American Academy of Pediatrics in recommending that the hepatitis B vaccine be included in the current schedule of childhood-disease vaccines now given to infants and toddlers.

Officials at the Centers for Disease Control said the recommendation is not based on any known risk of widespread hepatitis among children, but is simply a way to ensure more people will be immunized as adults.

Adding the HBV vaccine to the existing vaccine schedule could be an important step toward the elimination of HBV, which occurs most commonly in adolescence or thereafter, according to the U.S. Public Health Service.

To be completely protected against HBV, children should be vaccinated with a series of three HBV vaccinations, said Caroline Breese Hall, M.D., chair of the AAP's Committee on Infectious Diseases.

Last December, the Centers for Disease Control first recommended that infants routinely receive immunization against HBV. In February, the American Academy of Pediatrics followed suit.

The government and the AAP recommend that newborns get their first shot before they leave the hospital or soon thereafter, the second shot at one to two months of age and the third shot at six to 18 months of age.

Older children, adolescents and adults at increased risk

also should be vaccinated against HBV, according to Dr. Hall, a professor of pediatrics and medicine at the University of Rochester School of Medicine in Rochester, N.Y.

"As resources permit, you should do universal adolescent immunization," Dr. Hall said.

The vaccine for older children should be given in a similar three-dose schedule with the first two doses about one month apart, reported Dr. Hall.

Prior to the Public Health Service's recommendation, children were vaccinated only if they were at high risk of infection with the virus. But according to Dr. Hall, this strategy was not adequate to control the spread of the disease.

Israeli study finds in-vitro fertilization babies develop as normally as naturally conceived infants

By Dan Hurley

SEPT. 1—Children conceived through in-vitro fertilization who are healthy at birth are as likely as naturally conceived children to develop normally, a new study has found.

But twins and triplets are more likely to be conceived through the procedure, and they, along with naturally conceived multiples, are at increased risk of premature birth.

The study, conducted by researchers from Haifa, Israel, is the first to assess the physical and mental growth of children conceived through in-vitro fertilization (IVF).

"The results should be very reassuring," said Barry Zuckerman, M.D., professor of pediatrics at Boston University School of Medicine. "[IVF babies] were born a little smaller, but they continued to grow on their own curve. Everything appears to be within normal limits."

Since the first successful IVF birth was reported in 1978, more than 25,000 IVF babies have been born around the world, the Israeli researchers reported in Pediatrics.

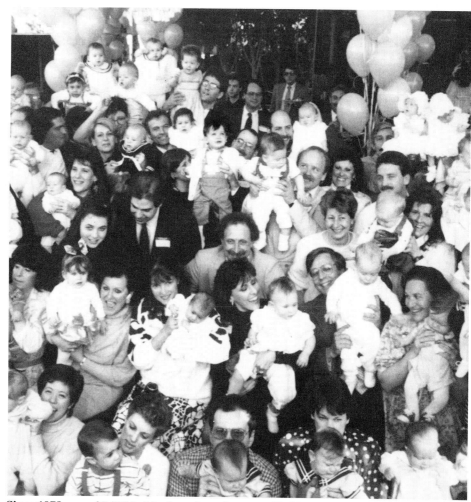

Since 1978, over 25,000 babies have been born worldwide as a result of IVF procedures.

Previous studies had found that IVF pregnancies are associated with higher rates of miscarriage, premature delivery and low birthweight. The new study is the first to determine how IVF babies who are relatively healthy at birth grow compared with naturally conceived children.

The researchers matched 66 naturally conceived singleton births with 66 IVF singletons; 19 naturally conceived pairs of twins with 19 IVF twin pairs; and four naturally conceived sets of triplets with four IVF triplet sets.

At an average of two years after birth, the children's size and weight were measured, and their physical dexterity and mental development also were measured.

The researchers concluded that when a woman gives birth to a healthy IVF baby, the infant can be expected to develop and thrive as well as a naturally conceived baby.

Earlier this year, British researchers reported that the success rate of IVF drops 8% after each attempt and that women over age 40 have a 15% chance of having a baby with the technique, compared with a 45% success rate for women age 34 and younger. A new study published in The Lancet found that IVF is successful in women up to age 52.

According to Robert Visscher, M.D., medical director of the American Fertility Society in Birmingham, Ala., the results of the new study are logical and were expected.

Every IVF cycle in which embryos are produced costs $3,000 to $8,000, he said.

One in six kids has potentially dangerous blood lead level; increased vigilance advised

By Laura Buterbaugh

SEPT. 10—Though fears that the dusty flooring of a New York elementary school was loaded with lead appear unjustified and a shutdown of the school unnecessary, lead-poisoning experts still feel that dangerous levels in many locales call for constant vigilance.

Nationwide, about one in six children—as many as 17 million—has a potentially dangerous level of lead in his or her blood, according to the Centers for Disease Control.

All children who live in older neighborhoods or attend schools painted with lead-based paint should be screened, said J. Routt Reigart, M.D., chairman of the American Academy of Pediatrics' Committee on Environmental Health.

Lead-based paint is the most common source of high-dose lead exposure for children, Dr. Reigart said.

Although lead was banned from paint in the late 1970s, it still is found in many homes and schools painted prior to that time.

Harmful lead-containing dust from renovations also can be ingested if it gets on the hands and into the mouth. "Parents shouldn't hesitate to have their children tested by their physicians," said the committee chairman.

The director of a New York lead clinic agreed. "The only way to prove children are not exposed to lead is to do a blood-lead test," said Howard Mofenson, M.D., director of the lead clinic at Nassau County Medical Center in New York, where children are tested annually.

At his clinic, the test costs $10 to $12 plus the cost of a doctor's visit. Children up to age six are considered to be at the highest risk of health problems from lead.

Parents also should check to be sure that the water supply at their child's school has been tested for lead, as required by the federal Environmental Protection Agency, Dr. Reigart said. Children also can be exposed to lead through water from old lead pipes.

Most children who suffer lead poisoning do not have symptoms, according to the CDC. Early symptoms of mild poisoning are a slight increase in nervousness or activity.

Parents should not wait until lead-poisoning symptoms appear to have their child screened, both Dr. Mofenson and Dr. Reigart said.

Recent research has found that lead levels as low as 10 micrograms per deciliter of blood—the maximum level considered safe by the government—will not produce symptoms, but can cause IQ deficiencies, growth retardation and other mental and physical problems.

Once lead levels are high enough to cause symptoms, damage is more likely to be irreversible.

Last month, the federal government instructed states to screen all children aged six months to six years who are covered by Medicaid for lead levels.

Theophylline/learning link rebutted by study

SEPT. 24—Asthmatic children given theophylline do not have more learning problems in school, on average, than their siblings without asthma, University of Iowa researchers have found.

Their results contradict earlier reports that the drug may adversely affect academic performance.

Although some parents in the new study said their asthmatic child taking theophylline was slower in school than a healthy sibling, the children's mean learning scores were not statistically different.

Scott Lindgren and colleagues studied 255 children with asthma who had taken standardized achievement tests. The national average for children taking the tests was 50 points; the Iowa children with asthma scored an average of 57 points, the researchers wrote in The New England Journal of Medicine.

Of the 255 children, the researchers identified 72 who were taking daily theophylline and compared their scores with those of their nonasthmatic siblings.

Children with asthma scored an average of 58.5 points on the tests, while their siblings scored an average of 58.4 points.

"Asthma was not associated with reduced academic performance, even when we controlled for family background by comparing children who had asthma with their [healthy] sibling," Lindgren wrote.

"It is important to recognize that the primary determinants of academic performance are factors unrelated to asthma, such as family background, intelligence, socioeconomic status, adequacy of instruction and...emotional or behavioral problems."

Many of those variables were not adequately controlled in previous studies linking theophylline to impaired cognition and school performance, said co-investigator Miles Weinberger, M.D., director of the university's pediatric allergy and pulmonary division.

One of the studies, by researchers at the University of Washington Medical School in Seattle, relied on psychiatric tests to document cognitive problems in theophylline-treated children. But the study only compared the children's test results with national norms.

"To compare local Seattle kids with some national norm is not very valid," Dr. Weinberger said. "The children might be very different; there could be many other variables that affect mood."

A 1992 study by University of Colorado researchers failed to confirm parents' accounts of their asthmatic children developing cognitive and behavioral problems following theophylline therapy. In the randomized, double-blind cross-over study, parents could not tell whether their children took the drug or a placebo, the investigators reported in The Journal of the American Medical Association.

Physicians must still be cautious, however, when prescribing theophylline, Dr. Weinberger said. "You've got to use it by the book—no ad libbing. Dosage requirements may have to change and blood levels should be monitored carefully."

High fevers, common drugs such as erythromycin, and high-dose estrogen contraceptives can all lower theophylline elimination and thus increase blood levels of the drug, he noted. "Remember that kids can be sexually active at 12 or 13 years of age; if they are on [the pill], you may have to adjust their theophylline dosage accordingly," Dr. Weinberger said.

The venerable Dr. Spock takes a jab at cow's milk

By P.J. Skerrett

BOSTON, SEPT. 29—That common dinnertime refrain, "Drink your milk," may be replaced by "Eat your tofu" if a group of physicians led by the venerable Benjamin Spock, M.D., has its way.

Once regarded as a perfect food, cow's milk is coming under increasing fire as a part of the daily diet of infants, children and even adults. "We need to leave cow's milk where it belongs—in cows," said Neal Barnard, M.D., president of the Physicians Committee for Responsible Medicine, during a press conference here.

Instead, youngsters should eat calcium-rich foods such as broccoli and tofu, the experts recommended.

It hasn't been a good year for milk. The American Academy of Pediatrics recommended that parents not give their children whole cow's milk during the first year of life, on the grounds that it causes "hidden" blood loss and possibly anemia.

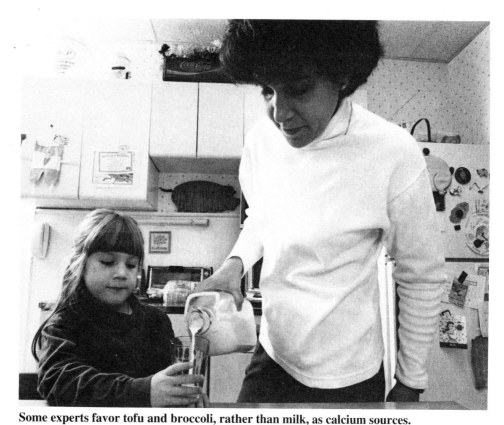

Some experts favor tofu and broccoli, rather than milk, as calcium sources.

Researchers also are increasingly finding that infants and children who are not exposed to dairy products are less likely to develop ear infections, asthma and allergies, said Russell Bunai, M.D., a Rockville, Md., pediatrician who recommends that children be kept from dairy products for at least the first two years of life.

Teens and adults also have been advised by cardiologists and nutritionists to avoid whole milk, because its fat content doesn't fit into the low-fat diet recommended to lower a person's risk of heart disease.

And a study in Canada and Finland has identified a protein fragment in cow's milk called ABBOS as a crucial trigger for juvenile-onset diabetes.

The researchers found that white blood cells in diabetes-prone infants bind to and destroy ABBOS. But a nearly identical protein sits on the surface of insulin-producing beta cells, and when mistaken for ABBOS, the beta cells in turn are attacked and destroyed.

Dr. Barnard, a Washington, D.C., psychiatrist, said that since an infant's risk of developing diabetes generally is not known, none should be given cow's milk.

Mothers who are breast-feeding their babies also should be advised to avoid dairy products, as the proteins can be transmitted through breast milk.

Parents using the bible of childrearing, "Baby and Child Care" by Dr. Spock, were encouraged to give children plenty of cow's milk. Not any more.

The 1992 edition urges mothers instead to breast-feed or use nondairy infant formulas, evaporated milk or heat-treated milk containing modified cow proteins during the first year of life.

The octogenarian author hesitated to warn parents away from milk completely. "I'm pulling my punches a little bit because I don't want to terrify 100 million parents out there," who have given their children cow's milk, Dr. Spock said.

Infants and children on no-milk diets can get adequate calcium, vitamin D and other essential nutrients from vegetables, including turnip greens, broccoli and kale, or tofu, said North Carolina dietitian Suzanne Havala.

The National Dairy Council, while supporting the pediatric academy's warning against the use of cow's milk during the first year of life, says eliminating milk from everyone's diet is going too far.

"It just isn't sound nutritional policy to make statements for teenagers and adults based on studies of infants," said nutritionist Gregory Miller, the vice president for nutrition research at the National Dairy Council.

Doctors fault warning on baby's sleeping position and SIDS; AAP to study issue for another year

SAN FRANCISCO, OCT. 13—The American Academy of Pediatrics drew fire from physicians for warning parents against putting babies to bed on their bellies.

Critics speaking at the academy's annual meeting here charged that the warning, issued in April, is premature. They said it causes needless anxiety for the parents of healthy infants and unnecessary anguish for parents whose babies have died of sudden infant death syndrome.

The warning was based on studies in New Zealand, Australia, Great Britain, the Netherlands and France that linked sleeping face down to an increased risk of SIDS.

Public health campaigns encouraging parents to put infants to bed on their backs or sides are credited with dramatic reductions in SIDS rates in some of those countries.

SIDS is the leading cause of death in babies from one week to one year of age, claiming the lives of almost two of every 1,000 babies born in the United States.

In response to criticism from doctors, the pediatric academy's task force on infant positioning and SIDS decided to continue studying the issue for another year. The warning against sleeping stomach-down will remain in place during the deliberations, said task force member John Kattwinkel, M.D.

At the time of the pediatric academy recommendations, John G. Brooks, M.D., director of pediatric pulmonology at the University of Rochester School of Medicine in Rochester, N.Y., said that changing babies' sleeping positions from tummy-down to their back or side would reduce their risk of SIDS by no more than 20%.

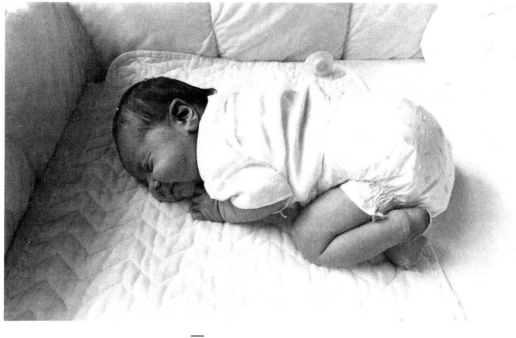

Whether putting babies to bed on their stomachs will significantly increase risk of SIDS is under debate.

COMMENTARY

Pushing for teen immunization

By Susan Baker, M.D.

IN AN INFORMAL POLL OF pediatricians in general practice and in academics, we agreed that vaccination is the biggest area of change in pediatrics.

Many of my colleagues and I concluded that before long, Hemophilus influenzae type b will be wiped out due to new vaccines. We are hopeful that hepatitis B too will become a disease of the past—but only with further change in immunization schedules.

A prototype model of the Hemophilus influenzae b vaccine was available in the early 1980s, but it was not recommended for use in children under 15 months of age. Since children are most vulnerable to the disease between the ages of three months and one year, this vaccine was limited in its usefulness.

But since the fall of 1990, when two new Hib conjugate vaccines were approved, the incidence of the disease has decreased more than 90%. The reason: The first shot is administered at two months, before the peak risk period.

Hib can be a devastating infection, manifested in several forms of invasive disease. Before the new vaccines arrived, there were estimated to be over 20,000 invasive Hib infections each year, with many resulting in meningitis, cellulitis and epiglottitis.

Of these invasive cases, there were up to 800 deaths each year. And 20% to 50% of the children who got meningitis and lived had major neurologic sequelae.

With the new vaccines, we have come to expect only about nine cases of Hib, including 3.6 cases of associated meningitis, per 100,000 children annually. Death rates due to Hib for 1991—the first year we would see the impact of the new vaccines—will not be available until early next year, according to the Centers for Disease Control and Prevention, but we expect a very low figure, or perhaps none at all.

Because Hib is the most common cause of meningitis, many pediatricians have been trained to recognize subtle signs of the infection. In the near future, when just a few pediatric patients with meningitis are seen each year in major medical centers, I believe that residents who rotate through the hospital may not see any cases.

Some of my colleagues feel this is not a problem, that training institutions will make sure that the residents all see the few cases that still occur. But those of us who are skeptical that this is possible are searching for new ways to show residents how to recognize meningitis, as well as other Hib-associated infections. Infectious-disease organizations, as well as pediatricians, are worried.

The other agent that is most important on a global basis is the hepatitis B vaccine. Hepatitis B is the third leading cause of death in the world, killing more people each year than HIV, according to the World Health Organization. Approximately 300,000 people in the United States are infected with the hepatitis B virus each year, according to the CDC, with most of the cases spread through sexual contact.

It is this method of transmission that most worries me.

Just this year, the American Academy of Pediatrics took a step toward wiping out hepatitis B by recommending that all infants—not just those at high risk—be vaccinated.

If you vaccinate children immediately at birth, you will interrupt vertical mother-to-infant transmission. With boosters at one month and six months, as recommended just this past year, the vaccine has been shown to be 98% effective as measured both by antibody levels and by the decrease in incidence among high-risk infants.

But studies have shown that antibody levels decline after five years. Adolescents who begin to engage in sexual activity, increasing their risk of the disease, will have low levels of protection.

Many of my colleagues and I therefore suggest that there should be a booster at the time of puberty; in fact, there should be a booster every five years.

I believe the AAP will eventually recommend such a schedule. The AAP does recommend adolescent immunization whenever feasible—that is, if resources are available—and has increased efforts to reach adolescents who never received the vaccine as infants.

The major impact of comprehensive immunization of infants in this country alone will not be recognized for 20 or more years. But only universal vaccination of both infants and adolescents—in all countries, not just the United States—will truly wipe out hepatitis B on a global level.

We've taken steps in the right direction. But there are still hurdles to overcome before we truly win the war against infectious disease in children.

Dr. Baker is associate professor of pediatrics at the University of Massachusetts Medical School in Worcester.

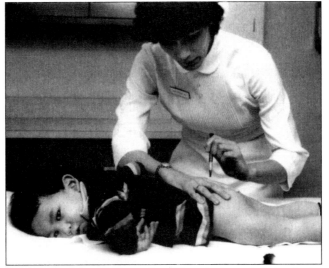

Many pediatricians believe a hep B booster is needed at puberty.

Notes

Notes

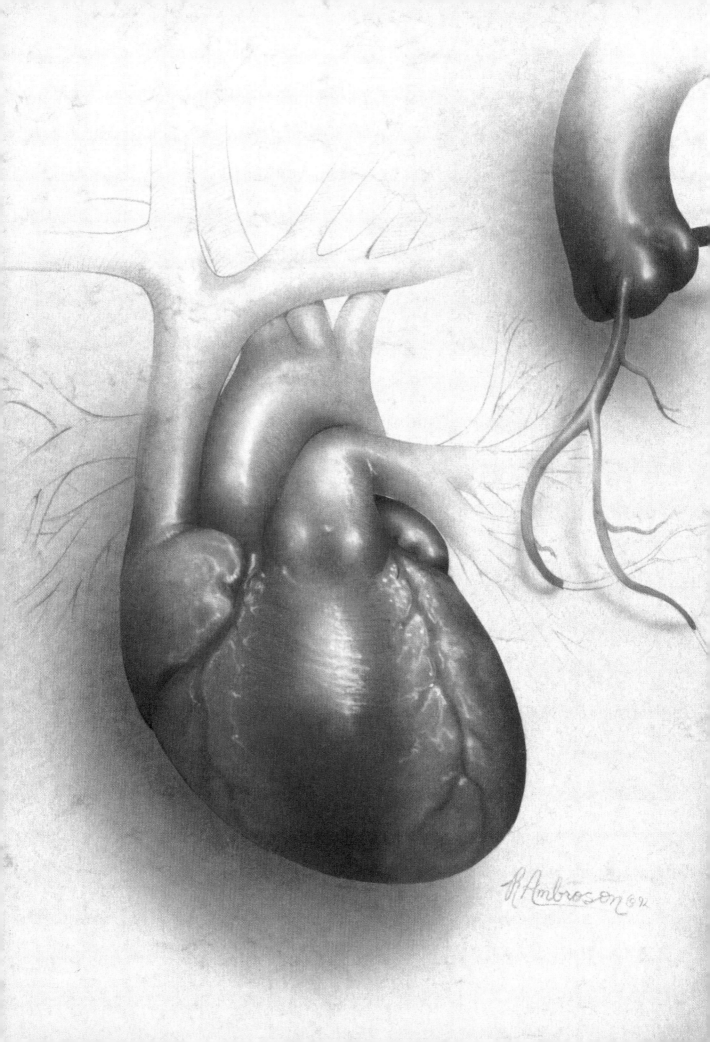

Overview 72
The year of the ACE inhibitor

Month-at-a-glance 74

Reported at the Time 86
Drugs versus angioplasty…new CPR techniques and guidelines…valvuloplasty refined…heart-disease deaths down…alcohol and CHD…updates on major trials—SAVE, SOLVD, MITI, TOMHS, VA Cooperative Study of Monotherapy in Hypertension…the latest on thrombolysis…"gender bias" in cardiac treatment…drugs augment life-style changes…apheresis update…benefits of long-term estrogen

Commentary 103
Drug trials shed light on CHD mechanisms
By John H. Laragh, M.D.

The year of the ACE inhibitor

And the discovery that endothelium-derived relaxing factor is really nitric oxide is expected to lead to important new therapeutic uses for the chemical.

In a year marked mostly by new dosage forms and broadened indications for drugs already in the armamentarium, the angiotensin-converting enzyme inhibitors stood out. The antihypertensives' ability to prevent repeat myocardial infarctions and save a substantial number of lives was documented.

The Survival and Ventricular Enlargement study (SAVE) found that the ACE inhibitor captopril (Capoten, Squibb) reduced postinfarction mortality rates, cut hospital times and lowered the risk of death from future MIs. The placebo-controlled, 2,231-patient study documented 21% fewer deaths due to cardiovascular causes among those who received captopril within three to 16 days after an MI.

Similar results were reported in the 4,228-patient Studies of Left Ventricular Dysfunction trial (SOLVD), which employed enalapril (Vasotec, Merck Sharp & Dohme). However, no survival benefit was observed in the Consensus II trial when enalapril was given within 24 hours of an MI.

Together, the studies marked an important advance in the field by showing that angiotensin-blocking action can have a beneficial effect on post-MI mortality rates, according to John H. Laragh, M.D., director of the cardiovascular center and chief of the cardiology division at the New York Hospital-Cornell Medical Center. He believes that cardiologists should begin to make ACE inhibitors part of their standard treatment for some of their post-MI patients. But he also called for a prospective trial to assess the capability of ACE inhibitors, as compared with that of calcium-channel blockers, to inhibit the angiotensin system.

Cardiologists did see a few new drugs approved this year, as well as expanded indications for agents already on the market. The FDA approved the calcium-channel blocker amlodipine (Norvasc,

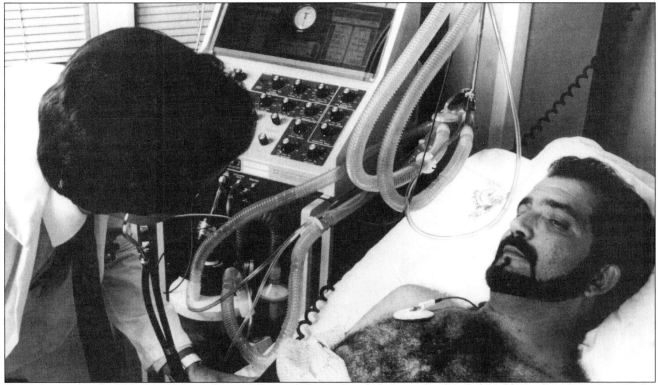

Receiving captopril within 3 to 16 days after an MI meant shorter hospital stay and reduced risk of future heart attack or death.

Pfizer) for the once-daily treatment of hypertension and angina. Diltiazem received several expanded indications: One form, Cardizem CD (Marion Merrell Dow), became available for the once-daily treatment of angina pectoris and another form, Dilacor XR (Rhone-Poulenc Rorer), was approved for the once-daily treatment of hypertension. Isosorbide mononitrate (Ismo, Wyeth-Ayerst), approved for the prevention of angina in the last days of 1991, reached the market early this year.

There were other new antihypertensives from which to choose. Injectable nicardipine HCl (Cardene, Du Pont Merck) was approved for the short-term treatment of hypertension, and prazosin HCl (Minipress XL, Pfizer) was approved for hypertension. Antihypertensives in general received a lift from the VA Cooperative Study of Monotherapy in Hypertension. The study found no increase in total cholesterol levels in mild to moderate hypertensives treated with any of the six major classes of high-blood-pressure agents.

The study was a vindication for antihypertensive agents, some of which had been thought to increase overall lipid levels. Cardiologists said that the results should alleviate fears among physicians treating hypertensives with moderately elevated lipid levels. Another boon for the pharmaceutical approach was the Treatment of Mild Hypertension Study. TOMHS found that even people with mildly elevated blood pressure benefit more from a combination of drug therapy and life-style changes than from life-style changes alone.

More questions were raised concerning possible gender discrimination in cardiac care. A Canadian study released at the meeting of the Royal College of Physicians and Surgeons found that women may be twice as likely as men to die in coronary care units. Another study comparing the cardiac treatment of men and women, which was presented at the annual meeting of the American Heart Association, found that female heart-disease patients are older and sicker when they first are seen by a doctor. The researchers theorized that women may wait longer than men before seeking treatment, and also may ignore pain and symptoms for greater periods of time.

If women do delay seeking treatment for acute myocardial infarction, another study illustrated how ill-advised that delay is. The Myocardial Infarction Triage and Intervention Trial confirmed that thrombolytic therapy is most effective when given during the first "golden" hour after the onset of symptoms.

And the discovery this year that endothelium-derived relaxing factor is really nitric oxide is expected to lead to important new therapeutic uses for the chemical, a researcher at Baylor College of Medicine in Houston told the Bristol-Myers Squibb symposium held in that city. He added that the finding means that nitric-oxide-donor drugs, such as ACE inhibitors, may actually halt or protect against the growth of atherosclerotic plaques.

Emergency cardiac treatment got a boost in 1992 with the development of a new technique that relies on a suction-cup device for CPR. Coupled with new CPR guidelines released by the AHA that advise bystanders witnessing a possible heart attack to call 911 before initiating CPR, the new device could further reduce sudden cardiac death rates, experts say.

The CDC announced this year that deaths from heart disease and stroke plummeted 24% between 1980 and 1988, an improvement attributed to better eating and exercise habits, a drop in smoking rates and improved myocardial-infarction treatments. This year's developments help guarantee that the much-awaited decline will continue.

Cardiology

Jan. 1

Researchers identified three tip-offs to help predict which atrial fibrillation patients are likely to suffer strokes.

Investigators of the Stroke Prevention in Atrial Fibrillation study found that prior stroke, high blood pressure and recent congestive heart failure identified patients at high stroke risk.

Patients with none of these factors, an estimated 40% of atrial fibrillation patients, are at low stroke risk and may not require anticoagulation therapy, the researchers reported in the Annals of Internal Medicine.

Jan. 2

Angioplasty bested drug therapy for the control of single-vessel disease, reported researchers at the Veterans Affairs Medical Centers in West Roxbury, Mass.

After six months, 64% of angioplasty patients and 46% of patients receiving antian-

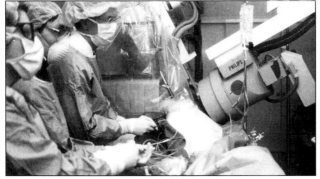

Angioplasty bested drug therapy for control of angina.

ginal drugs were free of angina, the investigators wrote in The New England Journal of Medicine. Patients receiving angioplasty were able to exercise longer on treadmill testing, but were prone to restenosis requiring additional surgery.

Jan. 4

Heart-disease patients shrank their atherosclerotic plaques using a strict regimen including a very low-fat vegetarian diet, regular yoga, exercise classes and psychotherapy, reported a physician at the Preventive Medicine Research

JANUARY

Institute at the University of California, San Francisco.

After a year in which 22 heart-disease patients limited calories from fat to less than 10% and practiced various stress-reduction measures, they lowered cholesterol levels 26% and reduced the extent of arterial stenosis 9%.

Jan. 6

Finnish researchers pinpointed a lipid profile that pegs a subset of healthy middle-aged men at high risk of heart attack.

High triglycerides and an LDL/HDL ratio greater than 5 place a man at fourfold greater risk of heart attack within the next five years, researchers from Helsinki University reported in Circulation.

Jan. 7

Older people lowered blood pressure and body fat by exercising on a cycle ergometer, reported physicians from the Medical College of Pennsylvania in Philadelphia.

After four months, healthy, sedentary people aged 60 to 86 lowered systolic blood pressure from 128.6 mm Hg to 125.3 mm Hg, and reduced body fat from 28% to 27%, the researchers reported in the Journal of the American Geriatrics Society.

During the subsequent two years, exercisers were significantly less likely to be diagnosed with cardiovascular disease than were controls.

Jan. 13

Eastern European countries topped the world in heart-attack deaths, according to statistics released by the American Heart Association at a meeting in Galveston, Texas. Japan, Switzerland and France had the lowest heart-disease rates.

Jan. 14

New Jersey investigators said they significantly improved the success rate of cardiopulmonary resuscitation via a new double-thrust resuscitation technique.

In a trial of 103 patients who experienced cardiac arrest while at St. Joseph's Hospital in Paterson, N.J., 7% of those receiving CPR with chest compression alone survived to hospital discharge, as compared with 25% of those resuscitated using alternating abdominal and chest compression.

Since all patients were treated by medical professionals, it is unclear whether bystanders can perform the abdominal maneuver, the researchers wrote in The Journal of the American Medical Association.

Jan. 16

Boston cardiologists polled by Medical Tribune called for new guidelines in managing acute myocardial infarction, including mandatory aspirin treatment and greater utilization of thrombolytics. Despite its proven efficacy, fewer than one in five eligible patients are given thrombolytic therapy after an acute MI and only one in three receives aspirin, according to physicians at Brigham and Women's Hospital, Boston, Mass.

Jan. 17

Minnesota researchers urged intensified efforts to prevent heart disease in middle-aged men. Analysis of data from the Multiple Risk Factor Intervention Trial revealed that the majority of 35- to 57-year-old men have

worrisome risk factors for heart disease. Several factors heightened the risk of death at levels lower than previously recognized, University of Minnesota researchers reported in the Archives of Internal Medicine. They said there was a graded relationship between men who smoke or who have cholesterol levels above 180 mg/dl, systolic BP over 110 mm Hg or diastolic BP over 70 mm Hg and mortality due to coronary heart disease.

Jan. 22

A new study showed that loneliness may be a heart-attack risk factor. Researchers at St. Luke's-Roosevelt Hospital Center in New York reported in The Journal of the American Medical Association that among heart-attack survivors, the risk of a second attack was almost twice as high in patients who live alone as in patients who live with others.

Jan. 23

Ulcerative plaques in the aortic arch were cited as a possible cause for an increased risk of stroke death.

Physicians at Hôpital Saint-Antoine in Paris performed autopsy examinations on patients who had died of strokes with no known cause. In 61%, they detected the ulcerated plaques, which cannot be spotted in living patients, they reported in The New England Journal of Medicine.

Jan. 30

Men were told to watch their heads as well as their cholesterol levels in assessing heart disease risk. Using data from the Framingham Heart Study, the researchers reported that men who experienced severe and rapid hair loss were twice as likely to develop coronary heart disease and three times as likely to die from it. Baldness seems to be a marker for heart disease rather than a cause of it, University of Texas researchers told the Society of General Internal Medicine meeting in New Orleans, La.

Cardiology

Feb. 1

Dobutamine (Dobutrex, Lilly) bested other pharmacologic agents for stress testing to evaluate coronary disease in patients who cannot exercise. In a comparison of dobutamine, adenosine (Adenocard, Fujisawa) and dipyridamole in stress echocardiography, dobutamine was judged most sensitive and most well-tolerated by patients, according to researchers at Brooke Army Medical Center in Fort Sam Houston, Texas. Adenosine provided the most specific test but induced more side effects, they wrote in the Annals of Internal Medicine.

Feb. 3

Epidemiologists at the University of California, San Diego, showed that middle-aged employed women had significantly lower total cholesterol and plasma glucose levels than comparable unemployed women. The results were reported in the American Journal of Public Health. The employed women, who primarily held management positions, also had lower blood pressure and lower post-challenge glucose levels.

Feb. 6

Trainees at a Buddhist temple lowered their cholesterol levels by adhering to a Zenlike diet. After one year eating a diet comprised largely of whole grains, beans and vegetables, subjects lowered their low-density-lipoprotein levels by 13% and their total cholesterol by 10%, Kyoto University researchers wrote in a letter to The New England Journal of Medicine. HDL levels also declined slightly.

• • •

California epidemiologists announced that large-vessel peripheral artery disease dramatically elevates the risk of mortality, sometimes without causing symptoms. In data from the University of California, San Diego, published in The New England Journal of Medicine, patients with severe or symptomatic large-vessel peripheral artery disease were found to carry a four- to sevenfold increase in mortality, and a 15-fold increase in mortality from cardiovascular disease.

Feb. 10

South African men discovered that their lipid levels were unrelated to the number of eggs they ate. Whether three, seven or 14 eggs a week were ingested, researchers from the South African Medical Research Council found no influence on the men's plasma cholesterol, lipids or lipoproteins. However, the researchers reported in the American Journal of Clinical Nutrition that all of the men ate a high-fat diet, gaining 40% of their calories from fat.

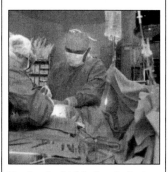

Randomized trial of angioplasty vs. endarterectomy called for.

Feb. 12

Three-cup-a-day coffee drinkers raise their levels of both plasma LDL and HDL, but so slightly that Johns Hopkins investigators determined their caffeine habit should not affect coronary heart disease risk.

In a study presented in The Journal of the American Medical Association, men drinking three cups of decaf or 1.5 cups of filtered coffee showed no change in lipid profile. Only 25% of American coffee drinkers consume three or more cups a day.

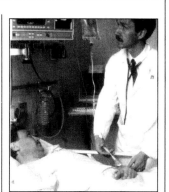

Magnesium tried in patients ineligible for thrombolysis.

Feb. 16

Endovascular experts declared that the time has come for a randomized trial of endarterectomy versus angioplasty. Impressed by successful use of brachiocephalic angioplasty to treat many proximal occlusions in the great vessels, investigators at the International Congress V: Strategies in Endovascular Interventions called for direct comparison of the surgical and nonsurgical approaches.

Feb. 17

New data challenged previous reports that moderate alcohol consumption reduces the risk of heart disease by raising levels of HDLs. Teetotalers, heavy drinkers and moderate drinkers had about the same levels of HDLs, Finnish researchers explained in the Archives of Internal Medicine.

Feb. 21

Intravenous magnesium sulfate helped save the lives of Israeli heart-attack patients who were deemed unsuitable for thrombolytic therapy. In a study of 169 such patients at the Sheba Medical Center in Tel Hashomar, 2% of those treated with magnesium died in the hospital, versus 15% of those who received a placebo.

The inexpensive and easily administered treatment may work by protecting against increased myocardial cell excitability, the investigators reported at a workshop at the University Hospitals of Geneva.

• • •

The Centers for Disease Control announced that heart disease and stroke are killing fewer Americans. From 1988 to 1989, deaths from heart disease dropped 6.3%, while those from strokes fell 5.7%. But heart disease remained the leading cause of death in the United States, followed by cancer, stroke and accidents.

Feb. 25

New guidelines for bystander response to cardiac arrest were proposed by an international panel of experts. If the guidelines are adopted, bystanders would be advised to call 911 first and then give cardiopulmonary resuscitation. For children, experts recommended clearing the airways, initiating breathing and then calling 911. The American Heart Association will consider the proposed changes early next year.

• • •

Postmenopausal women boosted their levels of estradiol and HDLs through moderate alcohol consumption. Although hormones did not reach levels achieved with estrogen replacement therapy, three drinks a week provided enough estradiol to lower the risk of coronary artery disease, University of Pittsburgh epidemiologists reported in Alcoholism: Clinical and Experimental Research. Benefits plateaued at six drinks per week.

Feb. 27

A predischarge exercise test predicted which men with unstable coronary artery disease were most likely to suffer myocardial infarction or cardiac death. Exercise-induced ST-segment depression doubled the risk for death and myocardial infarction in the postdischarge year, while the occurrence of pain without ST-depression was not of predictive value, researchers from Sweden's Linköping University reported in the American Heart Journal.

March 1

The bulk of alcohol's protective effect against coronary heart disease was attributed to its impact on high-density lipoproteins. After examining 1,768 men of Japanese ancestry who had participated in the Honolulu Heart Program, researchers from the University of California, San Diego concluded that 45% of moderate alcohol consumption's protective effect can be attributed to increased HDLs. Moderate drinking was also associated with lower LDLs (decreasing risk) and higher standing blood pressures (increasing risk), two smaller effects that were thought to negate each other, the inves-tigators wrote in Circulation.

March 4

Weight reduction and exercise most effectively reduced blood pressure in patients with high normal readings, reported the National Institutes of Health. Despite good compliance, neither stress management nor nutrition supplements reduced blood pressure significantly, the researchers stated in The Journal of the American Medical Association. In the study of 2,182 men and women with a diastolic blood pressure from 80 mm Hg through 89 mm Hg, diastolic blood pressure fell by a mean of 6.16 mm Hg in the weight reduction-exercise group versus 3.91 for controls.

March 7

London researchers stated that moderate exercise reduced the risk of stroke and heart attack among middle-aged men, even those with a history of heart disease.

By moderately exercising (regular cycling, very frequent walking or gardening, or weekly games of golf or tennis), the 7,735 men in the study halved their risk for cardiovascular events during the nine-year study period, researchers from the Royal

Free Hospital in London reported in the British Medical Journal. More vigorous exercise provided no significant advantage over moderate activity in stroke prevention, but it was associated with an increased risk of heart attack in men with symptomatic ischemic heart disease.

March 12

A University of Cincinnati team found that young and middle-aged African-Americans are more than twice as likely as whites to have an intracerebral or subarachnoid hemorrhage. Hypertension and smoking among the African-Americans probably increased their stroke risk, the researchers hypothesized in The New England Journal of Medicine. In African-Americans over age 75, the risk of intracerebral hemorrhage dropped to

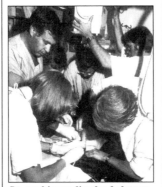

Streptokinase dissolved clots as well as pricier therapies.

one fourth that of whites, perhaps because susceptible individuals had already died, they said.

March 16

Contrary to previous reports, repeatedly losing and gaining weight does not increase the risk of heart disease, concluded a University of Minnesota researcher. In a study of 202 obese men and women, "yo-yo" dieting was not found to increase the risk of high blood pressure, blood choles-

terol, body fat or metabolic efficiency, he detailed in the American Journal of Clinical Nutrition.

March 18

A survey of all 86,463 1986 Medicare patients revealed that African-Americans are at least three times less likely to undergo coronary artery bypass grafts than are whites. Elderly African-Americans living in rural southeastern states were the least likely to undergo bypass: They received CABG six times less often than elderly whites in those states, the researchers stated in The Journal of the American Medical Association. They hypothesized that more blacks are poor and cannot afford out-of-pocket or co-pay expenses, and added that the findings have implications for such health reform schemes as national health insurance.

March 21

University of Edinburgh researchers found that people with a variation in a gene involved in fibrinogen production were twice as likely to develop peripheral atherosclerosis as healthy controls. The risk could not be attributed to differences in fibrinogen concentration. Rather, the variant gene may produce structurally variant fibrinogen with increased atherogenic potential, the team theorized in The Lancet.

March 25

The cardiovascular benefits of long-term estrogen replacement therapy for symptomatic and asymptomatic postmenopausal women outweigh the risks, agreed four experts who aired their views during a "videoconference" broadcast to 28 cities nationwide. A low oral dose of 0.625 mg of estrogen has been shown to decrease the risk of heart disease and bone loss, said an ob/gyn from the

University of Southern California, who added that he would encourage a woman with a history of cardiovascular disease and elevated serum cholesterol to start treatment even if she is asymptomatic.

There was some disagreement about the risk of breast cancer, however. While a reproductive biologist from Harvard asserted that there are no studies clearly demonstrating that estrogen increases the risk of breast cancer, the Centers for Disease Control panelist described a meta-analysis of 16 studies showing that the risk of breast cancer started to rise after about 5 years of ERT and reached a 30% additional risk after 15 years of treatment.

March 28

Streptokinase proved just as effective at dissolving blood clots as newer and more expensive therapies, concluded the third International Study of Infarct Survival. The randomized comparison of streptokinase (Steotase, Astra), tissue plasminogen activator (tPA), (duteplase, Burroughs Wellcome) and anistreplase (Eminase, SmithKline Beecham) in 41,299 patients found that there was no significant difference in death rates at 35 days or at six months among the three drugs. Fewer reinfarctions occurred up to 35 days after admission in the tPA-treated group than in those given streptokinase. But there were significantly fewer hemorrhagic strokes with streptokinase treatment than with either of the other drugs, according to the report in The Lancet.

March 30

A new nitrate became available for preventing chronic stable angina pectoris due to coronary artery disease. Patients receiving isosorbide mononitrate (Ismo, Wyeth-Ayerst) tolerated significantly longer periods of exercise on a treadmill than placebo-treated subjects.

Cardiology

April 9

Physicians told Medical Tribune that the failure rate of the Bjork-Shiley convexo-concave valve is considerably higher than previously believed. This poses a difficult clinical dilemma: Doctors must decide whether to advise recipients to undergo risky open-heart surgery or have them endure the fear that the valve might suddenly fail and kill them. According to a statement from Pfizer, the manufacturer, most clinical reports indicate that the mortality rate for reoperation is at least 5%, which is generally higher than the risk of death from valve fracture; however, a Phoenix cardiac surgeon said he decided the risk of a "re-do" operation was less than that of valve fracture in young patients in excellent health.

April 10

Valvuloplasty is much improved and offers a clear advantage over valve replacement, a Tampa surgeon told an international cardiac surgery conference. Since the mid-1980s, cardiac surgeons have refined techniques that restore the normal geometry of the mitral valve to correct prolapse and regurgitation, said the St. Joseph's Heart Institute specialist.

Because the procedure uses the patient's own tissue, clot formation is minimized, and patients can be spared a lifetime on anticoagulants, he said, estimating that 15,000 patients—about half of all mitral-valve surgery patients —are potential candidates for the procedure.

April 13

Analysis of almost 50,000 patients confirmed that women who have suffered an acute myocardial infarction are tested and treated less aggressively than men, even though they have a higher risk of death.

A researcher from the Robert Wood Johnson Medical School in Piscataway, N.J., told the American College of Cardiology meeting in Dallas that women hospitalized for a heart attack had two-thirds the chance of receiving cardiac catheterization or coronary artery bypass as men; they were less than half as likely to receive balloon angioplasty as male patients.

April 14

The case for early post-MI thrombolytic therapy was bolstered by new findings

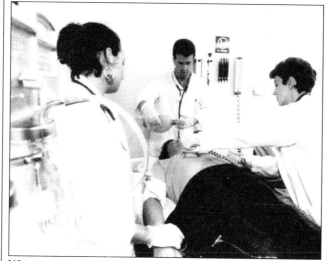

NJ team: men with MI treated aggressively, but not women.

from the Myocardial Infarction Triage and Intervention trial. When delivered within the first "golden hour" after onset of heart-attack symptoms, thrombolytic therapy cut infarct size in half and reduced mortality from 10% to 1% when compared with later treatment, researchers told the American College of Cardiology meeting.

• • •

Cocaine may boost the risk of heart attack by increasing platelet aggregation, proposed a cardiologist from the University of Southern California in Los Angeles.

To the extent that this mechanism is involved, aspirin might prove useful in lowering a cocaine user's heart-attack risk, the Ameri-can College of Cardiology meeting was told.

• • •

A Harvard researcher told cardiologists that treatment with captopril (Capoten, Squibb) can lengthen the lives of heart-attack patients. Results from the 45-center Survival and Ventricular Enlargement trial showed that patients receiving captopril after heart attack had 14% fewer repeat heart attacks and a 15% reduction in subsequent heart failure when compared with patients who received placebo instead of the ACE inhibitor. Data on 2,231 patients was presented at the American College of Cardiology meeting.

• • •

A Utah cardiologist questioned whether routine biopsies should be taken in order to rule out myocarditis in patients with congestive heart failure.

In a series of 2,224 biopsies at 23 centers, 2,015 were negative, he reported to the American College of Cardiology. Patients who were diagnosed with myocarditis gained no clear benefit from the knowledge; immunosuppressive therapy offered no advantage over standard therapy for congestive heart failure, he disclosed.

• • •

Holter monitoring proved as effective as more expensive electrophysiological tests for drug efficacy in patients with ventricular tachyarrhythmias. Using Holter monitoring, a truly effective drug was found more rapidly in about half of the cases, according to data on 486 patients presented to the American College of Cardiology by a researcher from the University of Utah.

The study also revealed that sotalol (Betapace, Bristol-Myers Squibb), a drug long available in Europe but not in the United States, reduced ventricular tachycardia by 50%, compared with five drugs on the U.S. market.

April 16

The largest study to date on congenital heart defects determined that risk factors can be identified in more than 40% of the cases. One third of 4,300 infants with heart defects came from families with a history of birth defects or genetic disorders, and 11% of the cases followed pregnancies complicated by diabetes, viral infection or exposure to medications or environmental toxins, a University of Maryland researcher told the American College of Cardiology. Previously, it was thought that only 10% of congenital heart defects could be explained by known risk factors.

April 25

Exercising at home relieved the anxiety commonly associated with recovery from heart attack, reported researchers from St. John's Hospital in Edinburgh, Scotland. Patients who exercised at home were about 50% less anxious and depressed after leaving the hospital than those who did not exercise. They were also less likely to be readmitted to the hospital with heart problems within the first six months, the researchers wrote in The Lancet.

M A Y

May 1

When healthy middle-aged men develop high blood pressure, physicians should ask them about job stress, advised investigators from New York Hospital-Cornell Medical Center. In a 1,629-man study, job strain increased systolic BP by 6.8 mm Hg and diastolic BP by 2.8 mm Hg in men aged 41 to 60—and the differential did not disappear as the men slept or unwound after work. When alcohol was added to job stress, systolic BP rose another 3.6 mm Hg and diastolic BP by 2.8 mm Hg, the researchers disclosed in the journal Hypertension. Men aged 30 to 40 were not affected.

May 4

Moderate amounts of any alcoholic beverage may help protect against heart disease, but wine appears to have an ingredient that offers better protection than beer or spirits, announced a leading epidemiologist. Citing a number of recent studies, the Boston epidemiologist told a meeting of the Wine Institute, an industry trade group, that people who drank white or red wine had lower heart disease rates and related deaths than those drinking other kinds of alcoholic beverages.

May 7

A survey of Missouri residents indicated that Americans are increasingly recognizing the importance of having their cholesterol levels measured, the Centers for Disease Control reported. The survey showed that the proportion of Missouri residents who said they never had their cholesterol checked declined from 47% in 1988 to 30% in 1991.

May 12

Future management of hypertension will focus on detecting those at risk and getting them to modify their diets, a World Health Organi-zation expert told the Fourth International Symposium on Hypertension in the Community, held in Jerusalem. To counter the adverse effects of high salt intake in many populations, the diet should be high in potassium, magnesium, fiber and amino acid-rich seafood, stated the cardiovascular specialist from Shimane Medical University in Japan. A decade-long, worldwide, multicenter study of 53 groups of people aged 50 to 54 in 22 countries confirmed that people on such a diet have lower stroke and cardiovascular disease mortality, he said.

• • •

Physicians are overlooking an effective, nonpharmacologic method of lowering their patients' blood pressure, Israeli researchers told the Fourth International Symposium on Hypertension in the Community. Biofeedback and relaxation techniques significantly reduced systolic and diastolic blood pressure and heart rate in 24 hypertensive patients, said a team from Ben Gurion University in Beer Sheva. The Israeli patients learned and practiced biofeedback techniques for two to four months and were evaluated at six months using a mental stress test.

May 18

Physio-Control of Redmond, Wash., the nation's largest maker of defibrillators, voluntarily suspended shipment of the devices after a government inspection found "numerous significant problems" in their manufacture. The Food and Drug Administration said the company made unapproved design changes and did not report all serious problems linked to the product.

May 19

Low-density lipoprotein levels dropped in patients with severe, refractory famil-ial hypercholesterolemia after they were pheresed with a device that selectively removed LDLs from their plasma. In a 30-month trial in which 20 heterozygous patients were pheresed every week or two for up to 28 months, LDL levels dropped from a mean of 287 mg/dl to 147 mg/dl, while HDL rose from 38 mg/dl to 53 mg/dl, reported researchers from the University of Saarland, Germany, at a meeting of the American Society of Artifi-

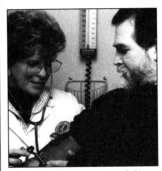

Heart problems may explain declining sexual interest.

cial Internal Organs in Nashville, Tenn.

May 22

When older men stop having sex, they might get more help from a cardiologist than from a psychiatrist, suggested new Swedish research. Men were interviewed at age 70 and again at age 75 about their sexual activity. Systemic hypertension, ischemic heart disease, congestive heart failure, diabetes or hypertriglyceridemia was present in 14 of 21 men who stopped having sex between the ages of 70 and 75, but in only three of 20 men who stayed sexually active. Moderate hypertension was the best predictor of cessation of coital activity, the University of Göteborg researchers stated in the Journal of the American Geriatrics Society.

The study found no link between psychiatric problems and a moribund sex life. How-ever, the combination of vascular disease plus a recent life stress (such as a financial setback) was present in 10 of the sexually inactive men but only one of the sexually active.

May 26

Neurologists called for randomized clinical trials of tissue plasminogen activator in the treatment of acute stroke. In open-label pilot studies, administering IV infusions of tPA within 90 minutes of stroke onset resulted in 30% of patients showing major neurological improvement within two hours after treatment. After 24 hours, 46% showed major improvement, but the effect was not dose-dependent, according to National Institutes of Health researchers.

When administered 90 to 180 minutes after stroke in a separate 20-patient study, tPA carried a 10% to 17% risk of intracranial hemorrhage. Presenting both studies in the journal Stroke, the team concluded that considerable benefit would have to be demonstrated to justify late tPA treatment.

May 28

University of Miami cardiologists cautioned that even without flow-limiting structural lesions of the coronary arteries, transient myocardial ischemia can trigger life-threatening ventricular arrhythmias. In a study of 356 survivors of out-of-hospital cardiac arrest, initial work-up revealed no identifiable etiology in 13 patients. Of these, five were found to have the combination of coronary artery spasm, silent ischemia and documented ventricular arrhythmias related to ischemia or reperfusion, the team reported in The New England Journal of Medicine. If the link holds up in future research, it would provide additional justification for intensive anti-ischemic therapy, the investigators concluded.

June 3

A new CPR technique employing a suction-cup device improved cardiopulmonary circulation during cardiac arrest, reported a researcher from North Shore University Hospital in Manhasset, N.Y. He tested the device on 10 patients with cardiac arrest who also received standard CPR. In all of the patients, the device improved the circulation of blood to the heart, and in three the device was able to restore a stable blood flow rhythm, he said. The active compression-decompression device was easy to use and inexpensive; it can be used while the patient is receiving defibrillation, making it superior to standard CPR, according to the researcher, writing in The Journal of the American Medical Association.

June 8

Two studies presented at a meeting of heart disease and stroke experts in Chicago gave contradictory answers to the question of whether daily aspirin reduces or raises the risk of stroke.

Researchers from the University of Medicine and Dentistry of New Jersey found that asymptomatic patients with greater than 50% carotid stenosis who took 650 mg of aspirin twice a day were less likely after eight years of follow-up to have had a stroke than those who did not take aspirin.

But a team from the University of Sydney in Australia told the meeting of the Society for Vascular Surgery and International Society for Cardiovascular Surgery that patients with less than a 50% stenosis were three times more likely to have a stroke if they took 162 mg of aspirin daily, about one eighth of the amount taken by the U.S. patients.

• • •

The Food and Drug Administration received a report from a Massachusetts hospital of heart attacks in five people who continued to smoke while wearing nicotine patches, and it is undertaking an investigation into the link between the two. There were three patches on the market at the time, but the FDA would not disclose which one(s) were involved.

June 10

Life-style factors, with the exception of cigarette smoking, were found to have no influence on the risk of stroke in a study conducted by researchers at the University of Oslo in Norway.

The study, published in the journal Stroke, examined 163 stroke patients and 652 control subjects from central Norway. Life-style factors often considered risks, including alcohol consumption, salt intake and level of physical activity, were not found to be associated with risk of stroke.

June 12

Preliminary results of a 15-center study suggested that antihypertensive therapy does not increase total cholesterol levels in patients with mild-to-moderate hypertension. No adverse effects on lipoprotein profiles were seen in patients treated by any of six major classes of antihypertensives used in the study, the VA Cooperative Study of Monotherapy in Hypertension. Concern about the adverse effects of diuretics on lipids and lipoproteins may have stemmed from data based on excessive dosage or methodologic flaws in some earlier trials, one of the researchers told cardiologists attending a Boston meeting on Recent Advances in Cardiovascular Therapeutics.

June 15

Levels of testosterone found in the normal adult male are capable of suppressing high-density lipoprotein concentration and may contribute to the increased risk for coronary artery disease in

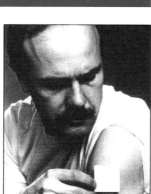

Heart attacks have been reported with nicotine-patch use.

men, announced researchers from the University of Washington and the Salk Institute. When the investigators injected healthy young men with Nal-Glu, a gonadotropin-releasing hormone antagonist, it lowered their testosterone while raising their HDLs 26%. HDLs stayed about the same in men who received placebo injections or who were injected with Nal-Glu but given enough supplementary testosterone to keep hormone levels normal, the investigators revealed in the Annals of Internal Medicine.

June 18

The Cardiovascular Health Study revealed that orthostatic hypotension can cause generalized cerebral hypoperfusion and is associated with several subclinical signs of cardiovascular disease. In a four-community study of 5,201 people over age 65, 16.2% were found to have orthostatic hypotension (defined as a drop in systolic blood pressure of at least 20 mm between the supine and standing measurements).

OH was associated with general neurological symptoms, such as frequent falls and difficulty walking, the investigators reported in the American Heart Journal. Major ECG abnormalities, the presence of carotid stenosis and isolated systolic hypertension were all significantly associated with OH, but the researchers called for further study to determine whether OH is an independent risk factor for cardiovascular or cerebrovascular events.

June 21

Body mass and gender are the most important determinants of left ventricular mass in normotensive preadolescents, researchers at the Medical College of Virginia in Richmond concluded on the basis of a study of 243 children.

Weight, supra-iliac skin-fold thickness, systolic blood pressure and heart rate accounted for 41% of the LV variation among boys, the team revealed in the journal Circulation. Weight, supra-iliac skin-fold thickness and heart rate (but not blood pressure) explained 48% of variation in girls. Fatness was found to be inversely related to LV mass.

June 27

A British study demonstrated that adding magnesium to standard thrombolytic treatment could reduce the number of heart-attack deaths by 24%. Half of 2,316 heart-attack patients were treated with intravenous magnesium upon admission to the hospital, while the other half received a saline solution as placebo. Twenty-eight days later, the death rate in the magnesium-treated group was 7.8%, while 10.3% of the placebo-treated patients had died. The magnesium-treated patients also had a 25% reduction in the risk of developing heart failure, according to the study, which appeared in The Lancet.

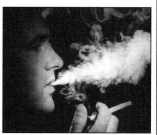

Life-style factors, except smoking, have no effect on stroke risk.

July 2

People over 75 are just as likely as younger persons to benefit from thrombolytic therapy after suspected acute myocardial infarction, a Boston team reported in The New England Journal of Medicine. After pooling data from 1,368 patients over 75 years old participating in the GISSI and ISIS-2 trials, a 14% overall reduction in mortality was found with streptokinase therapy. The Beth Israel Hospital researchers said that patients over age 75 are six times less likely than younger patients to receive the drugs.

July 8

Hypertension, diabetes, heart disease and left ventricular hypertrophy are all risk factors for postoperative cardiac events, reported University of California at San Francisco researchers. In one study of 474 men, patients with any of the risk factors were found to be at heightened risk of myocardial infarction within 48 hours of major noncardiac surgery. Patients taking digoxin also were at increased risk, according to the study in The Journal of the American Medical Association. In another analysis of the same patients, those with chronic heart disease were found to be at increased risk of MI or severe recurrent angina within two years of surgery.

July 16

Canadian researchers cautioned that the discontinuation of heparin to treat unstable angina may reactivate the disease process within hours. In research described in The New England Journal of Medicine, antithrombotics were stopped after six days in patients with unstable angina uncomplicated by a coronary event. Disease reactivation occurred in 13% of 107 patients initially treated with heparin alone, compared with 5% of 296 patients in the

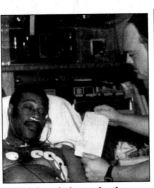
1980s' drop in heart deaths missed African-Americans.

three groups initially receiving aspirin, heparin and aspirin or placebo, said the Montreal Heart Institute team.

An accompanying editorial concluded that concomitant treatment with aspirin may markedly reduce the incidence and severity of reaction events.

July 18

Men who took 325 mg of aspirin every other day over a five-year period required less peripheral artery surgery than those who didn't take the aspirin, Harvard Medical School researchers revealed in The Lancet. In the U.S. Physicians' Health Study, 56 of 22,071 male physicians underwent surgery for arterial occlusion. Of them, 20 took aspirin, and 36 did not.

Earlier data from this study found that aspirin reduced the number of heart attacks by as much as 44% in men 50 and older.

July 21

German investigators reported that regular physical exercise and a low-fat diet can slow the progression of coronary artery disease. Using a group of 113 men with stable angina, the researchers compared the effects of 30 minutes a day of exercise and a low-fat diet with a "usual care" regimen. No lipid-lowering drugs were prescribed.

After 12 months, significant decreases in body

weight, total cholesterol and triglyceride levels were found in the intervention group, as well as significant increases in physical work capacity and myocardial oxygen consumption. Minimal progression of coronary lesion diameter was noted to have progressed in 23% of intervention patients, compared with 48% of controls, the investigators reported in Cardiology. Lesions regressed in 32% of exercisers, but in only 17% of controls.

July 23

Physicians treating heart-attack patients are strongly influenced by medical studies of cardiovascular drugs, observed a team of Boston researchers from Brigham and Women's Hospital. They analyzed the use of aspirin and calcium antagonists in 2,231 patients enrolled in the Survival and Ventricular Enlargement study.

During the 36-month study, which was reported in The New England Journal of Medicine, three clinical trials were published, all of which appeared to influence prescribing habits. For example, within two years after the second International Study of Infarct Survival found that aspirin can prevent a second MI, the number of SAVE patients given post-MI aspirin increased from 38.8% to 71.9%. Aspirin use also increased following the publication of the Physicians' Health Study, which supported the use of aspirin to prevent a first MI.

July 27

American gymnast Chris Waller became the first Olympic athlete to compete while wearing a Dacron graft to correct coarctation of the aorta. Waller's congenital heart malformation was diagnosed after his high school doctor noted that blood pressure in his arms was extreme-

ly high, while a pulse was virtually nondetectable in his lower limbs.

Since surgery to attach a graft to his ascending aorta, Waller has been normotensive, with normal left ventricular function on electrocardiography.

July 30

Physicians attending athletes at the summer Olympics worried that undetectable blood-doping techniques that boost performance may endanger the lives of athletes desperate to win. The blood-doping issue came to a head several years ago when a number of Dutch and Belgian cyclists suddenly died, allegedly of heart attacks, at the peak of their careers. Testing would require blood samples from athletes, which are currently not taken at the Olympics.

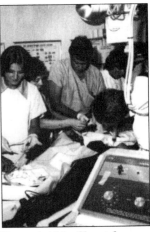
Research trials of heart drugs quickly change standard care.

July 31

The Centers for Disease Control announced that deaths from cardiovascular disease dropped 24% between 1980 and 1988. The death rate declined faster for men than for women, and faster for whites than for African-Americans, the CDC said. Government researchers attributed the improvement to better diet and exercise habits, a drop in smoking rates and improved myocardial infarction treatments.

Aug. 3

The calcium-channel blocker amlodipine besylate (Norvasc, Pfizer) received approval from the Food and Drug Administration for once-daily treatment of hypertension and angina. The medication had been available overseas for two and a half years.

Aug. 12

The death rate for stroke in the United States declined by more than 50% in the last 30 years, University of Minnesota researchers announced. They called the decreased mortality an "extraordinary public health achievement." In the report in The Journal of the American Medical Association, the team attributed the improvement to a substantial decline in the number of smokers and of people with hypertension.

Aug. 15

A team from the National Cardiovascular Center in Osaka, Japan, reported that a single moderate dose of alcohol may act to lower blood pressure in some hypertensive, habitual drinkers. Sixteen Japanese men, aged 22 to 70, with essential hypertension were randomly assigned to drink 1.0 ml/kg of vodka at dinner on a designated test day and a nonalcoholic beverage on a subsequent control day. They found that mean ambulatory systolic blood pressure fell 7 mm Hg and mean diastolic blood pressure fell 4 mm Hg after consuming an alcoholic beverage. Because the acute hypotensive effect may only be apparent during evening and late hours, ambulatory blood-pressure monitoring may be useful in habitual drinkers, the researchers wrote in the journal Hypertension.

Aug. 17

A German study showed that oral sotalol (Betapace, Bristol-Myers Squibb) was the drug of choice among 81 patients with inducible and noninducible ventricular tachycardia. At doses of between 440 and 459 mg/day, sotalol had efficacy rates of 68.4% and 82.8% for inducible and noninducible ventricular tachycardia, respectively, researchers from Westfalische Wilhelms-University in Münster revealed in the journal Circulation. The efficacy of amiodarone (Cordarone, Wyeth-Ayerst), verapamil, beta-blockers and Class Ia and Ib drugs ranged from 0% to

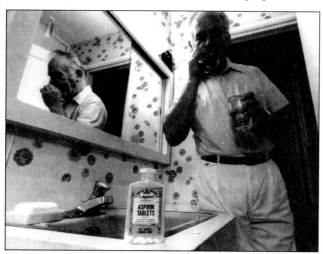

Daily low-dose aspirin reduced risk of MI and death in silent ischemia.

15.4% in the inducible group and 0% to 50% in the noninducible group. The investigators commented that verapamil and beta-blockers showed promise in a number of patients with noninducible tachycardia and may be a therapeutic alternative in this subgroup.

Aug. 19

Pfizer, Inc., announced that a Cincinnati court has approved the settlement of a worldwide class-action suit brought against it by recipients of Bjork-Shiley heart valves. The settlement is expected to cost Pfizer up to $215 million, a spokesperson said.

Pfizer will guarantee an offer between $500,000 and $2 million to each American valve recipient in the event of fracture, a spokesperson said. The company will also establish a $75-million fund for developing techniques to identify valve recipients at high risk of fracture and to pay for the replacement surgery, as well as creating a fund of up to $140 million to pay for recipients to consult cardiologists about their risk status.

About 85,000 people worldwide have had the convexo-concave valve implanted. The valves have cracked in 461 people, causing more than 300 deaths, according to Pfizer.

Aug. 23

Male smokers who quit can expect to show significantly lower levels of fibrinogen in just two days, British doctors reported in the Journal of Smoking-Related Diseases. Previous studies have found that smokers often have dangerously high levels of fibrinogen, which has been identified as an independent risk factor for heart attack or stroke. In the new study, researchers measured fibrinogen in 20 smokers before they quit and for up to two weeks afterwards. In men, levels fell by 13% within two days of quitting and remained fairly constant during two weeks' follow-up. Women's levels also dropped, but not significantly.

Aug. 29

Swedish researchers reported that daily low-dose aspirin may reduce the risk of serious cardiac events in patients with silent ischemia. In a study of 374 men—144 with silent ischemia and 230 with symptomatic ischemia with ST-segment depression—half took 75 mg of aspirin daily, and half took a placebo. All had been admitted to the hospital for unstable coronary artery disease. After three months, aspirin was found to have reduced the proportion of death and myocardial infarction by about 80% in the silent-ischemia group and by about 50% in the symptomatic ischemia group, it was reported in The Lancet. But after one year, only the silent-ischemia group continued to have a lower risk.

Aug. 31

A British researcher reported that the use of cardiac defibrillators had markedly increased. About 15,000 of the devices are implanted each year, most of them in the United States. In addition, third-generation devices are now coming into use that are able to monitor heart rhythm and can terminate dangerous arrhythmia by either pacing or electric shock, the researcher told the 14th Congress of the European Society of Cardiology in Barcelona.

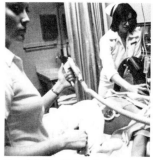

Use of defibrillators has markedly increased, says expert.

Cardiology

Sept. 1

A Stanford University research team concluded that mildly ischemic, postmyocardial infarction patients can be safely sent home sooner and with fewer tests and treatments than are commonly done. The announcement followed publication of the group's most recent finding, in the Annals of Internal Medicine, that many physicians do not distinguish between mild and severe ischemia when developing treatment plans for patients who have had a myocardial infarction.

In 1988, the group demonstrated that when mildly ischemic patients received counseling and a symptom-limited treadmill test three weeks after an uncomplicated MI, they returned to work in a median of 51 rather than 75 days, with no increase in the rate of cardiac death or recurrent infarction.

Sept. 2

Physicians at the 14th Congress of the European Society of Cardiology meeting in Barcelona were told that those who still make house calls can administer thrombolysis in patients' homes and cut mortality by 50%. In a study of 311 heart-attack patients in 27 rural practices in Scotland, about half were lysed with anistreplase (Eminase, SmithKline Beecham) at home within four hours of the onset of symptoms. The others received the drug later in a hospital. Mortality was 8% among the home-treated patients, compared with 16% in the hospital-treated patients. Median time between symptoms and injection was 105 minutes in the home-treated patients, compared with 240 minutes in the hospital-treated group.

• • •

High fibrinogen levels are more potent risk factors for myocardial infarction than high cholesterol levels, an international team reported at the 14th Congress of the European Society of Cardi-

ology in Barcelona. A study of 3,000 patients with angina compared those in the top fifth of fibrinogen levels with those in the lowest fifth. During a two-year period, the high-fibrinogen patients were three times as likely to suffer a heart attack or other cardiac problem, the researchers revealed. The coordinator of the study, from the London School of Hygiene and Tropical Medicine, suggested that fibrinogen testing be added to cholesterol screening.

Sept. 3

In a new study, an angiotensin-converting enzyme inhibitor proved useful in preventing recurrent myocardial infarctions, particularly in patients with severe left ventricular ejection damage. The Survival and Ventricular Enlargement study found 21% fewer deaths due to cardiovascular causes among patients given captopril (Capoten, Squibb) within three weeks of an MI than among those given placebo. All the 2,231 subjects in SAVE had left ejection fractions of 40% or less, the researchers stated in The New England Journal of Medicine.

• • •

Physicians at the 14th Congress of the European Society of Cardiology in Barcelona were told that thrombolytic therapy can cut cardiac mortality by 27% when given between six and 12 hours after the onset of chest pains, which suggests that the time frame for giving lytics be extended to 12 hours.

The findings come from a 247-center trial of patients (mostly men, with an average age of 63) given alteplase (Activase, Genentech), a recombinant tissue plasminogen activator. As many as 30% of heart patients in Europe and the United States may be denied thrombolytic therapy because of hospital rules against giving the drugs

more than six hours after the onset of chest pains, a researcher said at the meeting.

Sept. 14

Nova Scotia researchers reported that women may be twice as likely as men to die in coronary-care units due to less aggressive management and ill-defined cardiac symptoms. A retrospective study of 2,546 CCU admissions showed that 8.2% of women had died by the 28th day, versus 4.8% of men, investigators from Dalhousie University told the annual meeting of the Royal College of Physicians and Surgeons of Canada. Women tend to get fewer

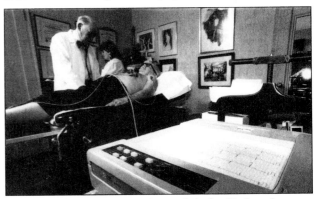

Drug trials for MI treatments often exclude the elderly and women.

antiarrhythmic agents and fewer ischemic agents when they present with chest pain, one researcher told the Ottawa gathering, adding that women are more likely than men to have nonclassical symptoms of myocardial infarction.

Sept. 16

An analysis of 214 studies found that most trials of drug therapy for myocardial infarction have excluded the elderly and have significantly underrepresented women. More than 60% of the studies excluded patients over age 75, and less than 20% of all patients were women, according to the study in The Journal of the American Medical Association. Because more than 60% of

people discharged from hospitals after MIs are over age 65, it is important to know about side effects that affect only this age group, said researchers at Brigham and Women's Hospital in Boston. Exclusion of women may be due to an unproven assumption that cardiovascular disease is similar in men and women, an accompanying editorial concluded.

Sept. 17

When faced with familial long-QT syndrome, cardiologists were cautioned not to rely solely on electrocardiogram results to determine which family members are carriers of the gene for the syndrome and at risk for recurrent syncope and life-threatening ventricular arrhythmias.

After studying 199 members of an affected family with DNA markers and electrocardiograms, researchers from the University of Utah found that if the standard electrocardiographic criteria are used (a QT interval greater than 0.44 second, corrected for heart rate), 11% of noncarrier family members will be erroneously diagnosed as having long-QT syndrome. On the other hand, if a QT interval of 0.48 second or longer is required for diagnosis, 40% of male carriers and 20% of female carriers will be missed, it was reported in The New England Journal of Medicine.

Cardiology

Oct. 1

Four-year results from the Treatment of Mild Hypertension Study indicated that drug therapy and life-style changes for mild hypertension check the disease more effectively than life-style changes alone, a University of Minnesota researcher reported.

TOMHS is comparing the effects of life-style changes alone versus combining them with one of five antihypertensive drugs in 902 middle-aged men and women with an average baseline blood pressure of 140/91 mm Hg. Life-style changes included losing weight, reducing salt and alcohol intake and exercising 150 minutes per week. The drugs were given once a day and included an angiotensin-converting enzyme inhibitor, an alpha-one inhibitor, a beta-blocker, a calcium-channel blocker and a diuretic.

At four years, there was a 32% drop in end points, including blood pressure, EKG, lipid levels and fractions, among the drug/life-style group versus those on life-style changes alone, the investigator told an American Heart Association Council for High Blood Pressure Research meeting in Cleveland.

Oct. 2

American and French researchers reported that inherited variations in the angiotensinogen gene may be the key to some familial hypertension. In a study of 379 hypertensive sibling pairs and 237 unrelated controls from the United States and France, 15 possible defects in the AGT gene were identified, they reported in the journal Cell. While normotensive people had occasional defects due to the known variability of inheritance, those with hypertension had consistent and identical variations of the AGT gene, they said. More brothers and sisters with hypertension inherited the same copy of the AGT gene from their parents than was expected by chance, said one researcher from the Howard Hughes Medical Institute in Salt Lake City.

Oct. 8

Contrary to earlier findings, two large studies of patients in cardiac arrest showed no benefit for high-dose epinephrine injections, compared with the lower doses that are more frequently used. The new studies, published in The New England Journal of Medicine, were conducted by researchers at the University of Ottawa in Toronto and Ohio State University in Columbus. The Canadian study followed 650 patients who suffered cardiac arrest in the hospital or outside. Those given up to five 7-mg units of epinephrine at five-minute intervals had no survival benefit, compared with those given up to five 1-mg injections on the same schedule. The U.S. study of 1,280 patients reported similar findings.

Oct. 10

A Johns Hopkins team found that low levels of high-density lipoproteins may predict which patients with coronary artery disease and total cholesterol levels in the normal range will have recurrent coronary events. The Baltimore researchers followed 83 men and 24 women with CAD and total cholesterol levels of less than 200 mg/dl. Over a 13-year period, 61% experienced either another myocardial infarction, death from heart disease or angina leading to cardiac surgery. Of those with HDL levels less than 34.8 mg/dl, 75% had a second cardiac problem, compared with fewer than 45% of those with levels equal to or greater than 34.8 mg/dl. Reporting in Circulation, the researchers said it remains to be seen if raising HDL can reduce cardiovascular problems in patients with desirable total cholesterol.

Oct. 15

French researchers found that a genetic mutation, called ACE deletion polymorphism, may be a new potent risk factor in middle-aged men who are considered to be at low risk for myocardial infarction. Their study of more than 1,300 patients found that those with the gene defect were three times more likely than controls to have a myocardial infarction. The researchers, from the Paris-based National Institute for Health and Medical Research, said the mutation results in an increased level of angiotensin II, a polypeptide that can damage coronary vessels and spur heart disease. If the link between the mutation and MI is confirmed, those affected would be given ACE inhibitors, the researchers reported in the journal Nature.

• • •

Marion Merrell Dow received Food and Drug Administration clearance to market diltiazem hydrochloride (Cardizem CD) for angina. The once-daily calcium-channel blocker has been available since late 1991 for the treatment of hypertension.

In one of three double-blinded, placebo-controlled trials submitted to the Food and Drug Administration, a statistically significant therapeutic difference over placebo was seen in 229 patients at doses of 180 mg, 360 mg and 540 mg.

No therapeutic difference was observed over placebo at a dose of 90 mg.

Patients should be started on 120 mg or 180 mg once daily and titrated up to a dose of 480 mg as needed, according to the company.

Oct. 24

Scottish researchers added triglycerides to the eclectic list of suspects that may trigger hostility. The University of Edinburgh team measured blood lipids and used a questionnaire to assess the personality characteristics of 1,592 men and women aged 55 to 74. They found that men in the highest quintile of triglyceride levels—85.1 mg/dl to 410.0 mg/dl—were more likely to have hostile thoughts, to be more domineering and to insult others than those in the lowest quintile—14.7 mg/dl to 37.1 mg/dl. Serum triglyceride concentrations were also positively associated with hostile acts and a domineering attitude in women, but to a lesser extent than with men (p <.05 versus p <.001), according to the report in The Lancet.

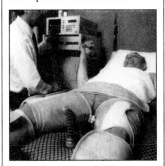

External counterpulsation: a noninvasive alternative to bypass.

Oct. 30

A noninvasive procedure that pumps blood from extremities to the heart may be an alternative for patients intolerant of bypass surgery or balloon angioplasty, said physicians at the State University of New York at Stony Brook. Twenty patients have undergone the one-hour procedure, called enhanced external counterpulsation, five days a week for seven weeks. Following treatment, all 20 said they had no pain, and many were able to decrease their cardiac medications, the researchers reported in the American Journal of Cardiology.

Nov. 5

Balloon mitral valvuloplasty resulted in immediate symptomatic improvement in 91% of patients with mitral stenosis, announced a team of researchers at the Beth Israel Hospital in Boston. Physicians were able to complete the procedure in 93% of the 146 patients they treated. Balloon mitral valvuloplasty resulted in substantial increases in the mitral-valve area and in cardiac output, the researchers revealed in The New England Journal of Medicine. The overall five-year survival rate was 76%.

Mitral-valve echocardiographic score was the strongest predictor of benefit from the procedure. Patients with multiple risk factors for restenosis were not likely to have a good long-term outcome and should be considered for mitral-valve replacement, the researchers concluded.

• • •

After this year's discovery that endothelium-derived relaxing factor is actually nitric oxide, researchers predicted that nitric oxide donor drugs will become increasingly important therapeutic tools in cardiovascular disease. The drugs have the ability to protect against the growth of atherosclerotic plaques in vascular endothelium, a Baylor College of Medicine investigator told the first annual Bristol-Myers Squibb Symposium on Cardiovascular Research in Houston, Texas. Nitric oxide drugs, such as angiotensin-converting enzyme inhibitors, could be used to produce the crucial gas in target endothelium following injury from diabetes or elevated cholesterol or blood pressure.

• • •

Researchers announced that high-cholesterol diets can damage coronary artery endothelium, thereby leading to potentially lethal constrictions well before any plaque buildup occurs.

The investigators, from Emory University School of Medicine in Atlanta, found that blood vessels from animals with extremely high serum cholesterol but no detectable plaque did not respond correctly to chemical messengers that regulate blood-vessel size.

In fact, the vessels constricted when they should have relaxed, one of the researchers said at the Bristol-Myers Squibb Symposium on Cardiovascular Research, held at the Texas Medical Center in Houston.

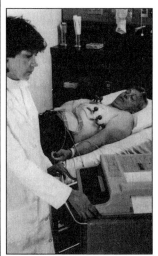

If EKG shows atrial fibrillation, warfarin may be indicated.

Nov. 6

An investigational diagnostic technique correctly identified defects in three in-situ Bjork-Shiley valves, which were then replaced, reported Michigan researchers. The technique employs computer-enhanced imaging to increase the contrast of radiographs. In initial tests, it enabled the successful detection of single-leg separations in one of the two outlet struts of three Bjork-Shiley convexo-concave mitral valves, according to preliminary findings in 70 patients in an ongoing study at William Beaumont Hospital in Royal Oak. Patients in the study have 60-degree convexo-concave mitral valves,

ranging in size from 29 to 33 mm, which are considered at high risk for fractures.

Nov. 11

The first national survey of heart attacks in Medicare patients found that approximately 26% of those who suffer an acute myocardial infarction die within a month of onset; 40% die within a year. Examining the Medicare claim forms of 218,000 patients who had suffered an infarction, Harvard Medical School investigators found that women and African-Americans are less likely than men and whites to undergo coronary angiography, bypass surgery and balloon angioplasty. The researchers suggested that although invasive procedures may not always be offered to women, patient preference may play a role in the underuse of certain procedures as well. It is also misleading to assume that more procedures are better, since the data did not indicate that patients who undergo more procedures live longer, they pointed out in The Journal of the American Medical Association.

• • •

The drug warfarin can reduce the risk of stroke by 78% in people who suffer from atrial fibrillation, a study in The New England Journal of Medicine revealed. Results of a multicenter study of the drug were so conclusive that the trial was ended so that patients on placebo could be switched to warfarin, Yale University researchers said. Elderly people stand to benefit the most from the study findings, the scientists said, because the risk of atrial fibrillation increases with age from a prevalence of four per 10,000 people in men under age 50 to nine per 10,000 people in men over 70.

Nov. 16

Several reports presented at the American Heart As-

sociation's 65th meeting in New Orleans concluded that female heart-disease patients are first seen when they are older and sicker than their male counterparts, and receive less aggressive treatment.

But researchers weren't sure whether the culprit was gender bias or a misreading of symptoms by both patients and physicians, stated an Atlanta cardiologist. An Emory University study of elective balloon angioplasty found that female patients were, on average, five years older and more likely to have hypertension and diabetes. In a Harvard study of the rate at which women with myocardial infarctions were transferred to tertiary-care units, the average time for transfer of women was 4.5 days, compared with 2.9 days for men, according to a research coordinator at the Deaconess Hospital in Boston.

Nov. 26

The survival rate of sudden-heart-attack victims could be increased from as low as 2% in many areas of the United States to 40% if communities would follow the revised cardiopulmonary resuscitation guidelines, the chairman of the American Heart Association committee that developed the guidelines told Medical Tribune.

One recommendation advised bystanders witnessing a possible heart attack to call 911 before attempting CPR. The previous version of the guidelines advised people to attempt CPR for one minute before calling 911. But many people ended up giving CPR for longer than a minute, delaying the arrival of an emergency medical team with a defibrillator.

The guidelines, agreed to earlier this year, recommended no change for helping children under age eight: One minute of CPR should be given before calling 911, said the committee chair.

Cardiology

Dec. 1

North Carolina researchers reported that enhanced magnetic resonance imaging is an effective, noninvasive method of evaluating blood flow in coronary bypass patients with grafted internal mammary arteries. The test avoids the risks and expense of angiography, the Duke University Medical Center investigators reported at the annual meeting of the Radiological Society of North America in Chicago. In a study of 15 postoperative patients, MRI was deemed very effective in differentiating between bypass-graft closure or stenosis and nonischemic causes of anginal pain.

•••

Spiral-volume computed volumetric tomography should be the screening test of choice for suspected acute thromboembolism, announced researchers from Hôpital Calmette in Nord, France, at the Radiological Society of North America meeting. The technique can detect clots in second- to fourth-division pulmonary vessels, and images were graded as good to excellent in 98% of the cases. The technique was compared with pulmonary angiography; all 23 patients with normal SVCT scans had a normal angiogram. However, in one patient asymmetry in pulmonary arterial perfusion secondary to chest trauma was misinterpreted as lobar pulmonary embolism using SVCT; the patient's pulmonary angiogram was normal.

Dec. 4

Color Doppler flow imaging won another round of kudos at the annual meeting of the Radiological Society of North America. A New Haven, Connecticut, researcher reported that the diagnostic method helps physicians effectively predict patients' responses to fibrinolytic therapy and to determine the proper time for angiography, thereby avoiding unnecessary

arteriograms. The technique may also help identify the etiology of thrombosis, the Yale investigators added.

Dec. 10

Premenopausal breast-cancer patients taking tamoxifen (Nolvadex, ICI Pharma) had a decrease in total cholesterol, low-density lipoproteins and triglycerides, as well as in their cholesterol/ high-density lipoprotein ratio, physicians reported at the 15th Annual San Antonio

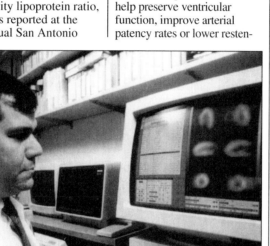

Color Doppler avoids unnecessary arteriograms, says researcher.

Breast Cancer Symposium. Similar effects were seen previously in postmenopausal women, noted researchers from the Rose Medical Center/AMC Cancer Research Center in Denver.

The study of nine premenopausal women who received adjuvant tamoxifen, 20 mg/day, found that after nine months, average total cholesterol had dropped from 182 mg/dl to 164 mg/dl; LDL had decreased from 94 mg/dl to 90 mg/dl; triglycerides had dropped from 217 mg/dl to 114 mg/dl, and the cholesterol/HDL ratio had decreased from 3.9 to 3.1.

Dec. 15

A new study concluded that an adjunctive intravenous thrombolytic agent provided no

added benefit to patients receiving percutaneous transluminal coronary angioplasty after acute myocardial infarction. Cardiologists from William Beaumont Hospital in Royal Oak, Michigan, and Moses Cone Memorial Hospital in Greensboro, N.C., randomized 122 patients with evolving MI to PTCA therapy with or without adjunctive IV streptokinase. IV streptokinase did not help preserve ventricular function, improve arterial patency rates or lower restenosis rates after PCTA, the investigators reported in the journal Circulation. Additionally, patients receiving IV streptokinase had longer, more expensive and more complicated hospital stays, according to the researchers.

Dec. 22

Mitral-valve replacement with chordal preservation preserves ejection performance in patients with chronic mitral regurgitation, concluded researchers from the University of South Carolina. The team compared postoperative left-ventricular ejection performance in seven patients who underwent mitral-valve replacement with chordal transection (MVR-CT) and eight patients who underwent MVP with

chordal preservation (MVR-CP). MVR-CT resulted in a decreased ejection performance caused in part by an increase in end-systolic stress, the investigators wrote in the journal Circulation. Conversely, MVR-CP resulted in a smaller left-ventricular size so that, although the low-impedance left atrial ejection pathway was closed, there was reduced end-systolic stress and preservation of ejection performance.

Dec. 30

Yale and Harvard researchers suggested that the implantation of a clamshell-shaped device may reduce the risk of recurrent cryptogenic stroke in patients with patent foramen ovale. In 34 patients with known right-to-left shunting and 62 instances of presumed paradoxical emboli, transcatheter closure of the patent foramen ovale was achieved via implantation of the new device. The investigators reported in the journal Circulation that complete closure was achieved in 28 patients, five were left with trivial leaks and one continued to have atrial communication. During a follow-up period of eight months, no strokes were reported, leading the team to recommend that further investigations focus on identifying the population at risk and assessing the effect of intervention.

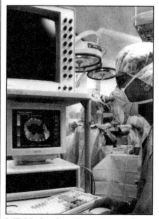

MRI helped evaluate blood flow in postoperative bypass patients.

Drugs vs. angioplasty for single-vessel disease

By Brianna Politzer

JAN. 2—A study showing that angioplasty yields better control of single-vessel disease than drug therapy highlights a therapeutic conundrum: Is the higher risk and cost of the surgery worth the increased quality of life the procedure offers?

In the study, researchers randomly assigned 105 patients with single-vessel disease to angioplasty and 107 similar patients to medical therapy with one or a combination of anti-anginal drugs, including nitroglycerin, beta-blockers and calcium-channel blockers.

After six months, 64% of the angioplasty patients were free of angina, compared with 46% of the group receiving drugs, reported Alfred Parisi, M.D., chief of cardiology at Miriam Hospital in Providence, R.I., and formerly of the Research Service at the Veterans Affairs Medical Centers in West Roxbury, Mass., where the study was conducted. Angioplasty patients also were able to exercise longer without angina on treadmill testing.

On the downside, 18 (17%) of the angioplasty patients required repeat procedures for restenosis at the six-month point. Two underwent an emergency bypass, and four had acute myocardial infarctions as a sequela of the initial procedure.

During follow-up, five more angioplasty patients required bypass surgery, and one additional patient had a myocardial infarction.

"Benefits were obtained from angioplasty in exercise test performance and freedom from symptoms, but at the expense of a small but real risk of problems and restenosis,'' said Donald Baim, M.D., associate professor of medicine at Harvard Medical School and director of invasive cardiology at Beth Israel Hospital in Boston, who wrote an accompanying editorial in The New England Journal of Medicine.

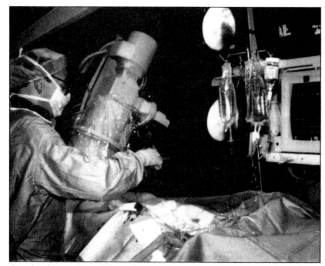

Angioplasty found best for angina, despite restenosis risk.

The expense of angioplasty, which is about $8,000-$9,000 for total hospital costs, and the rate of restenosis (between 20% and 30% after one year) make it impractical to recommend the procedure for every single-vessel disease patient, Dr. Baim said. Drug treatment costs about $1,000 a year.

"However, angioplasty might be appropriate for a patient who has angina and wants more out of life, who wants to be off medicine or who wants to be able to do more exercise," Dr. Baim said, "as long as the person understands the small risks and is willing to accept them."

Quality-of-life considerations are key, since studies suggest that surgery and medical management yield similar long-term survival rates in single-vessel disease patients.

But physicians should also take risk factors into account when deciding which therapy to employ, said William Kannel, M.D., professor of medicine and public health at Boston University and former director of the Framingham Study.

"If a patient does not quit smoking or lower their lipids, they will not derive much benefit from surgical intervention," Dr. Kannel said. "The correct approach, from the standpoint of preventing infarction, sudden death, death in general or heart failure, requires medical therapy, including lipid-lowering and blood-pressure drugs, as well as antianginal drugs and surgical therapy."

Triglycerides' role in heart attacks clarified

By Saralie Faivelson

JAN. 6—A Finnish study has finally identified the people with high triglycerides who are at high risk of heart attacks.

Healthy men aged 40 to 54 with triglyceride levels over 203 mg/dl and a low-density lipoprotein to high-density lipoprotein ratio greater than 5 at the start of the five-year study faced almost a fourfold risk of heart attacks, according to Vesa Manninen, M.D., of the Helsinki University Central Hospital.

But middle-aged men with high triglycerides and a low LDL/HDL ratio were not at high risk.

The subgroup of high-risk men experienced a 71% drop in heart attack risk after treatment with gemfibrozil (Lopid, Parke-Davis). The team reported their results in Circulation.

The study supports the contention of many international experts that aggressive treatment of hypertriglyceridemia can improve the LDL/HDL ratio by raising HDL levels. These experts also contend that lipid management guidelines in this country are inadequate.

"The current National Cholesterol Education Program guidelines, which haven't been revised in a few years, define risk in terms of LDL, but not in terms of triglycerides," said Antonio Gotto, M.D., chief of internal medicine at Methodist Hospital in Houston and chairman of medicine at the Baylor College of Medicine. "HDL is considered a risk factor only if it's under 35, but the LDL/HDL ratio isn't considered. We may revise the guidelines."

Reevaluation of data on blood fats and a reconsideration of guidelines are expected at a National Institutes of Health consensus conference next month.

"Study results will help us more efficiently identify high-risk patients and make a difference in heart disease," said Bryan Brewer, M.D., from the National Heart, Lung and Blood Institute in Bethesda.

The findings "swing the pendulum and show that high triglycerides can be a significant risk factor for some patients," agreed William Castelli, M.D., director of the Framingham Study. "The 71% drop in heart attack risk is the largest fall in heart attack rates in the history of medicine."

Abdominal maneuver during CPR evaluated

JAN. 14—Rhythmically compressing the abdomen alternately with the chest of cardiac arrest victims during cardiopulmonary resuscitation may increase chances of survival.

In a trial of 103 patients experiencing in-hospital cardiac arrest, those who received the double-thrust resuscitation technique were more likely to leave the hospital alive and functional, according to a team from St. Joseph's Hospital and Medical Center and the Seton Hall University of Graduate Medical Education, Paterson, N.J.

Interposed abdominal compression during CPR significantly improves cardiac output and blood flow to the brain and heart, reported Jeffrey Sack, M.D., of the University of California, Los Angeles, Medical Center. Dr. Sack, formerly

at St. Joseph's, reported the results in The Journal of the American Medical Association.

In the St. Joseph's trial, 25% of the patients receiving abdominal compression during CPR survived to hospital discharge, as compared with 7% of the patients who received conventional chest compression only, wrote Dr. Sack.

Abdominal compression was coordinated to coincide with the early relaxation phase of chest compression, corresponding to CPR "diastole." It was performed with hands centered over the umbilicus. All patients were intubated.

"The results are exciting and promising, and I believe the technique will eventually be incorporated into CPR guidelines for cardiac arrest," said Dr. Sack. However, "this technique

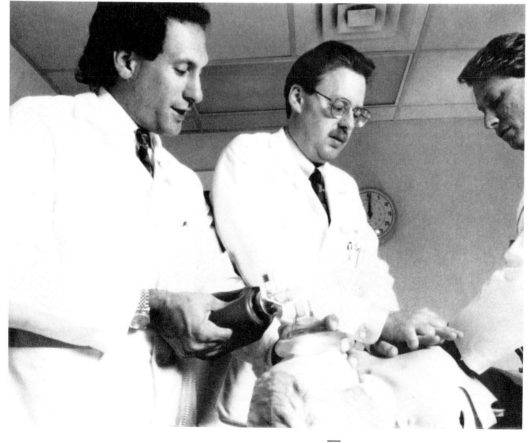

Rhythmic abdominal compression during CPR increased blood flow and survival.

was studied in a hospital, with full CPR crews, so I can't say it should be applied outside the hospital until we have studied it further."

"Intubating all the patients is a limiting factor. Obviously, bystanders could not do that," said Leonard Cobb, M.D.,

chairman of the department of cardiology at Harborview Medical Center, Seattle, Wash.

"Whether the technique will prove generally useful—in other institutions and other settings—remains to be seen, " he said.

Beginning-of-year poll: new recommendations for thrombolysis in acute MI loom for 1992

JAN. 16—New guidelines for the management of acute myocardial infarction may emerge in 1992, according to cardiologists polled by Medical Tribune.

Physicians say that despite their efficacy, thrombolytics continued to be greatly underused in the past year and they would like to see that change.

Fewer than one in five patients eligible for thrombolytic therapy receives it after an acute myocardial infarction and only one in three receives aspirin, which can reduce mortality by 25% to 30%, according to Paul Ridker, M.D., of Brigham and Women's Hospital in Boston.

Dr. Ridker said it should be mandatory for emergency room doctors to give patients aspirin after a heart attack, and that thrombolytics should be given sooner after the attack occurs.

Patients now wait an average of 81 minutes in the hospital before receiving lytic drugs, despite studies that have indicated that damage to the heart muscle can be reduced by 50% if the drugs are given within 60 minutes, according to Michael Horan, M.D., of the National Heart, Lung and Blood Institute in Bethesda.

Many other developments will take place in cardiology research in 1992. In April, for example, investigators from the SAVE study, which involves 2,200 patients in the United States and Canada, are expected to report their results at the meeting of the American College of Cardiology.

The study's goal: to see whether the ACE inhibitor captopril (Capoten, Squibb) can prevent heart failure in patients with MI and significant heart damge.

The currently ongoing ISIS-4 study, which is being conducted at 300 medical centers throughout the United States and involves up to 50,000 patients worldwide, will be completed by December 1992. Its purpose is to assess the role of IV magnesium, oral captopril and isosorbide mononitrate (Ismo, Wyeth-Ayerst) given within 24 hours of acute MI in reducing heart attack mortality.

Reports on new devices used in angioplasty will appear this year, including the use of excimer lasers. However, medical centers that have these devices continue to perform balloon angioplasties in 85% of cases, and that is unlikely to change, said John Bittl, M.D., professor of medicine at Harvard University.

Heart disease deaths down, CDC reports

FEB. 21—Heart disease and stroke are killing fewer Americans while AIDS deaths are increasing, according to the latest government figures.

From 1988 to 1989, deaths from heart disease dropped 6.3%, while deaths from strokes fell 5.7%. During that year, the latest for which figures are available, according to the Centers for Disease Control in Atlanta, AIDS-related deaths increased 33%.

Heart disease remains the leading cause of death in the United States, followed by cancer, stroke and accidents, according to a report published in an issue of the CDC's Morbidity and Mortality Weekly Report.

The AIDS mortality is only a fraction of the heart disease toll. According to the American Heart Association, 944,688 Americans died from heart disease in 1989, compared with 22,082 who died from AIDS, the CDC said.

The CDC also found that an American's overall life expectancy at birth in 1989 was 75.3 years, a new record. Life expectancy for women was 78.6 years, and 71.8 years for men.

While the gap is narrowing, women are still expected to outlive men by an average of 6.8 years, the report found.

Russell Leupker, M.D., vice chairman of the American Heart Association Council on Epidemiology and Prevention,

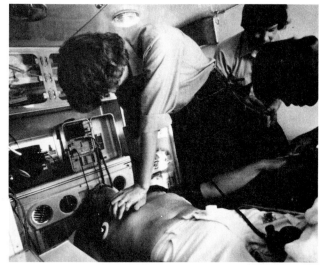

Fewer than 20% of eligible MI patients get thrombolytics.

said the decline in deaths due to heart disease and stroke is a continuation of a trend that has been seen over the last two decades.

Dr. Leupker said that by helping people control their blood pressure, lower their cholesterol and quit smoking, doctors have contributed to the decrease in deaths.

Despite this decline, however, the diseases themselves are still a big public health problem. "People are now living with the diseases and our disease rate compares very unfavorably with both Japan and most western European countries," Dr. Leupker said.

The actual number of deaths recorded in the United States in 1989 was 17,533 fewer than the number for 1988, which was a record-high year for recorded deaths.

New cardiopulmonary resuscitation guidelines

By Linda Little

DALLAS, FEB. 25—An American Heart Association committee recommended changing guidelines for bystander response to cardiac arrest. Under new guidelines, bystanders would be advised to call 911 first and then give cardiopulmonary resuscitation.

"We are dealing with the first link in the chain of survival," said William Montgomery, M.D., director of critical care units, Straub Hospital, Honolulu, Hawaii. "This could provide a dramatic improvement in shortening the interval between collapse and defibrillation."

The proposed guidelines result from research showing that defibrillation is the single most important life-saving maneuver.

More than 500 scientists and physicians attended a national conference on cardiopulmonary resuscitation and emergency cardiac care here to review guidelines set by the American Heart Association in 1985.

New guidelines emerging from the meeting will form the basis of established emergency cardiac-care techniques for the country.

The proposed guidelines for adults is to call 911 first, then initiate CPR. For children, experts recommend clearing the airways, initiating breathing and then calling 911.

The new recommendations for adults, if approved, will change the present AHA guidelines that recommend that bystanders who witness an adult collapse of heart attack determine unresponsiveness, start CPR, then call 911.

The new recommendation will delay CPR by about a minute, but will get the ambulance there quicker by having a bystander call for it first, then having the trained bystander start CPR, AHA committee members said.

Another advantage is that untrained bystanders can be talked through CPR by dispatchers, they said.

Studies from several communities have shown that survival rates decreased 3% with each minute delay of CPR. But survival rates decreased 4% with each minute of delay until defibrillation was started.

The "call first" recommendation does not apply to CPR on children, said Mary Fran Hazinski, who chairs the American Heart Association's pediatric resuscitation committee.

"If parents leave a gasping child in respiratory arrest to make a call, he or she may be unresuscitable when they return," she said.

Instead, Hazinski recommends that parents clear the airway, give the child 20 breaths, then call for an ambulance before resuming CPR. Only if a parent is untrained in CPR should he or she call first so the dispatcher can direct him or her in CPR, she said.

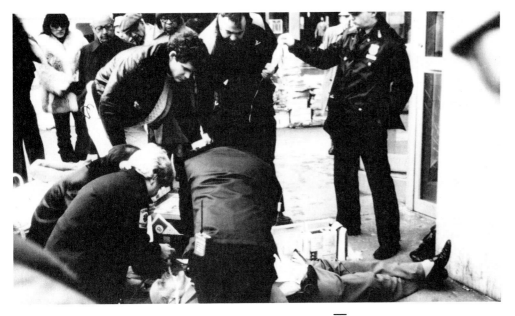

New AHA guidelines urge bystanders to call 911 before performing CPR.

Alcohol may lower coronary heart disease risk

By Andrea Kott

FEB. 25—Postmenopausal women who have at least three but no more than six alcoholic drinks a week may decrease their risk of heart disease and osteoporosis.

In a trial of 128 patients, moderate amounts of alcohol increased natural levels of estradiol by 10% to 20% of the increase that would be expected in estrogen replacement therapy, according to University of Pittsburgh researchers.

Of the 128 patients, 101 indicated during dietary recall questioning that they drank, Judith S. Gavaler, Ph.D., reported in the journal Alcoholism: Clinical and Experimental Research. Alcohol triggers the conversion of androgens into estrogens.

While ERT produces higher levels of estrogen, "the coronary heart disease risk benefit occurs at the same levels achieved in this study," said Dr. Gavaler, associate research professor of epidemiology.

Estrogen is also associated with increases in levels of high-density lipoproteins.

"The key is [that the drinking is] moderate, no more than one drink a day," Dr. Gavaler explained.

"It's important not to let ourselves fall into a thought pattern where we say, 'If a little bit of something is good, then a lot has to be better,' " she added.

"Estrogen reaches the highest level at three to six drinks per week," she added. "After that it plateaus."

The study findings do not apply to premenopausal women, Dr. Gavaler said.

"In younger women who have menstrual function and reproductive capacity, even moderate alcoholic consumption could have adverse effects, such as disruption of menstruation and infants with fetal alcohol syndrome," she said.

Having more than one drink a day, however, has been shown to increase the risk of breast cancer. Dr. Gavaler said, "The trick in this case is the lower alcoholic beverage consumption."

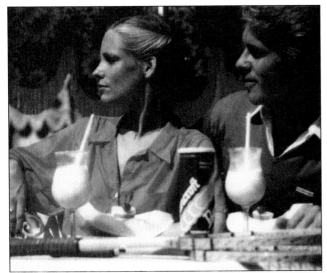

Moderate alcohol intake boosted estradiol by 10% to 20%.

Although researchers have known that estrogen therapy increases the risk of uterine cancer, there has been no consistent trend showing an increased risk of breast cancer, according to Trudy L. Bush, an epidemiologist at Johns Hopkins University in Baltimore.

Separate studies from the Boston University School of Public Health recently concluded that women who receive estrogen replacement therapy for up to 15 years do not face an increased risk of breast cancer.

"At six or seven drinks a week, studies have not been able to show statistically an increased risk of breast cancer," Dr. Gavaler said.

Long-term estrogen supported, say experts

MARCH 25—The benefits of long-term estrogen replacement therapy (ERT) for symptomatic and asymptomatic women outweigh the risks, according to four experts who aired their views during a videoconference broadcast from Atlanta to 28 cities nationwide.

The telecast was sponsored by Solvay & Cie, a Belgian company that sells Estratest, an estrogen-androgen combination replacement therapy.

"The primary prophylactic entities for which estrogen should be prescribed are osteoporosis and cardiovascular disease," said panelist Rogerio Lobo, M.D., professor of obstetrics and gynecology at the University of Southern California, Los Angeles.

Even though the Food and Drug Administration has not approved estrogen for the prevention of cardiovascular disease, "I think there is almost irrefutable evidence at this point for that benefit," he added.

A low oral dose of 0.625 mg of estrogen has been shown to prevent bone loss and heart disease, according to Dr. Lobo. He said he would not increase the oral dose to higher than 1.25 mg, and prefers the parenteral administration of estrogen if higher doses are required. Intramuscular estrogen should be avoided at all costs because of a bolus effect, he added.

"I would encourage a woman with a history of cardiovascular disease and elevated serum cholesterol to start treatment, even if she's asymptomatic" said Dr. Lobo.

While some studies have linked estrogen therapy to an increased risk of breast cancer, the panel argued that the fear of breast cancer has been overblown.

"There is not one study that clearly shows us that estrogen increases the risk of breast cancer," said Veronica Ravnikar, M.D., associate professor of obstetrics, gynecology and reproductive biology at Harvard Medical School.

The issue is not that simple, according to Karen Steinberg, Ph.D., of the Centers for Disease Control in Atlanta, the co-author of a study on estrogen use and breast cancer.

The CDC study, a meta-analysis of 16 studies, found that

the risk of breast cancer started to rise after about five years of ERT, and reached a 30% additional risk after 15 years of treatment.

The issue of treating women cured of breast cancer with estrogen therapy is becoming more urgent as more women are cured of cancer earlier in life and then face the same problems as other women who reach menopause, according to Lila Nachtigall, M.D., associate professor of obstetrics and gynecology at New York University School of Medicine.

"It is very easy to say no," she said. "The package insert says no, the FDA says no. But we have to give women some answers. Right now the patient and doctor have to weigh the risks and benefits and make that decision together."

The fourth panel member, Morrie Gelfand, M.D., professor of obstetrics and gynecology at McGill University in Montreal, discussed the efficacy of estrogen-androgen combination therapy, which he asserted has been "established beyond doubt."

"Why would one consider the use of estrogen-androgen instead of estrogen alone?" he asked. "Menopausal symptoms will be alleviated by both.

"However, in the area of quality of life the estrogen-androgen replacement therapy seems to be more positive in improving the energy, well-being and sexuality of patients," said Dr. Gelfand.

While most experts agree that estrogen therapy leads to a substantially increased risk of cancer of the uterus, progestins prescribed along with estrogen in women with an intact uterus lower the risk of endometrial cancer, said the panel.

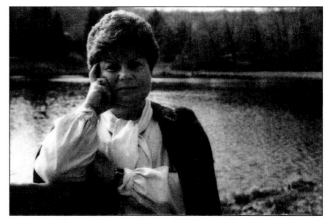

Dr. Nachtigall urges discussing ERT benefits with patients.

Valvuloplasty refined, may offer clinical benefits

Medical Tribune News Service

APRIL 10—Considering all the technological advances that have improved valvuloplasty, it could be applied more widely than it is at present, according to Dennis F. Pupello, M.D., chief of cardiac surgery at the St. Joseph's Heart Institute in Tampa, Florida.

The mitral valve procedure offers important clinical advantages to young patients who may avoid years of risky anticoagulant therapy, in the view of Dr. Pupello.

Since the mid-1980s, cardiac surgeons have refined techniques that manually restore the normal geometry of the mitral valve to correct prolapse and regurgitation, Dr. Pupello said in an interview.

He estimated that about 15,000 patients—about half of all mitral valve surgery patients—are potential candidates for valvuloplasty.

St. Joseph's Heart Institute sponsored an international cardiac surgery conference at which these advances were discussed. One important development described by Dr. Pupello is a valvuloplasty ring that restores the normal ovoid contour of the mitral valve annulus.

The ring changes the shape of the membranous fold, allowing its two leaflets to "slam shut rather than move back and forth without touching," said Dr. Pupello.

Evaluation of such repairs while the patient is still on the operating table is now feasible with the advent of trans-esophageal Doppler echocardiography, the Florida surgeon pointed out.

"We can determine whether [the repair] is satisfactory or not even before we close the chest," he said. "Five years ago, we had to fly by the seat of our pants until the patient could be subjected to other types of tests to assess the valve."

Other surgical interventions include retailoring the shape of the two valve leaflets, or altering the cords that hold each leaflet in position. "There are a number of things we can do to restore normal function of the valve," Dr. Pupello said.

Valvuloplasty is a "preferable procedure" over valve replacement because it employs the patient's own tissue, noted Mary Roman, M.D., cardiologist at New York Hospital. Patients are less likely to develop blood clots and other complications. "There is literature to suggest that the function of the left ventricle is better preserved," she said.

Avoiding the need for long-term anticoagulant therapy gives valvuloplasty a "clear-cut advantage over artificial valves," said Dr. Roman. In addition, said Dr. Pupello, valve repair is more stable than replacement, and less likely to deteriorate. The result is "improved long-term survival."

Of nearly 200 procedures performed at St. Joseph's Heart Institute, there have been only six cases that have had to be redone for "early failure" or other complications, Dr. Pupello said.

Factors that may rule against the procedure are stenosis, calcification of mitral valve leaflets or inflammation of the valve.

Dr. Roman concluded that valve repair is underutilized. "There are institutions where open-heart surgery is performed, yet surgeons aren't trained in [valvuloplasty] technique or don't feel comfortable performing it," she said.

"That's probably a real phenomenon, but it varies from institution to institution."

Heart-valve risks pose difficult clinical decisions

By Bruce Goldfarb

APRIL 9—News that the failure rate of the Bjork-Shiley convexo-concave valve is considerably higher than previously believed poses a difficult clinical dilemma: Should physicians advise recipients to undergo risky open-heart surgery to have the valve replaced, or must patients endure the fear that it might suddenly fail and kill them?

And who picks up the tab for the second operation?

The Bjork-Shiley 60-degree C-C heart valve has cracked in 461 people, causing more than 300 deaths worldwide, according to Rick Honey, spokesperson for Pfizer Hospital Products Ltd., parent company of the valve's manufacturer, Shiley Inc. The valve develops fractures in welds that attach disk-holding struts to the device's body.

A Dutch study of 2,303 recipients published in The Lancet in March found that the 60-degree Bjork-Shiley valve has a cumulative eight-year failure rate of 4.2%, five times higher than previous estimates. The large 70-degree model, in use outside the United States, has a failure rate of 17.4%. Multivariate analysis identified age under 50 years as a risk factor for strut fracture.

Pointing to the Dutch study, the Food and Drug Administration directed Pfizer to inform physicians of the new data. The agency said the rate of strut fracture was sufficiently high that some patients may elect valve removal rather than live with the prospect of potentially catastrophic consequences.

The 60-degree valve was recalled three times between 1980 and 1983 before being withdrawn from the market in 1986.

A Pfizer statement suggests that the risk of valve failure should be balanced against the risk of replacement: "Most clinical reports in the literature indicate that the mortality rate for such reoperation averages at least 5%, which is generally higher than the risk of death from valve fracture."

Phoenix cardiac surgeon Cecil Vaughn, M.D., however, has removed Bjork-Shiley valves from three patients. "My first reaction was to not do the operation, but with the information coming out, I felt that the risk of the 're-do' operation was less than the risk of these patients being subjected to a strut fracture,"

he said. "If I had it in my chest, I'm not of the temperament to walk around for the rest of my life with the thought of suddenly having an incompetent...valve."

But Dr. Vaughn believes the potential benefit of the redo operation outweighs the risk only in certain cases: young patients in excellent health.

"Somebody looking at living 30 to 35 years with this valve in place with the risk of fracture is an ideal candidate," he said.

Denton Cooley, M.D., of the Texas Heart Institute, however, contends that replacing a Bjork-Shiley valve without signs of failure is unwarranted. "There are thousands of them that are working very well," he said. "By and large, it's probably safer to leave the valve in place."

Still unresolved is the question of who pays for replacement surgery, which can cost $30,000 to $40,000. Dr. Vaughn said insurance companies have not paid for the valve replacements he has performed.

Insurance carriers will pay for a procedure if it is clearly medically indicated, a degree of certitude lacking in the case of the Bjork-Shiley valve because it is impossible to determine whether one particular valve will fail.

Some patients may soon have a pool of cash from which to pay for replacement surgery. In January, Pfizer announced that it would attempt to settle a class action lawsuit by setting aside $80 million to $130 million to pay for operations.

An expert panel would review each case to determine whether the patient should undergo the replacement procedure.

Earlier post-MI lysis bolstered by new study

By Pat Phillips

DALLAS, APRIL 14—Thrombolytic therapy delivered within the first "golden hour" after onset of symptoms of a heart attack significantly reduces morbidity and mortality, according to new findings from the Myocardial Infarction Triage and Intervention Trial.

In the study, infarct size was reduced by 50% in patients treated within an hour compared with those treated later, said W. Douglas Weaver, M.D., principal investigator for MITI, at the annual scientific session of the American College of Cardiology here.

Only 1% of patients treated early died, compared with 10% of those treated later. There was significant improvement in left ventricular ejection fraction in those treated early, according to Dr. Weaver.

Infarction was terminated in 40% of those patients treated early, and 75% were left with minimal or no damage.

Patents now wait an average of 80 minutes in the hospital before receiving thrombolysis.

"The message is that there needs to be a means to treat more patients very early in the stages of a heart attack if we want to

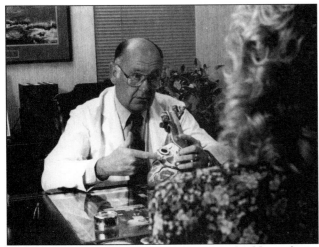

Dr. Vaughn advocates "re-dos" only in young, healthy patients.

maximize the potential benefit of these new therapies for the condition," Dr. Weaver said.

In the trial, 175 patients received thrombolysis from paramedics before arrival at the hospital, and 185 patients received treatment at the hospital.

The researchers had expected that patients receiving thrombolysis before reaching the hospital would be treated in about an hour's less time than those receiving it in the hospital. But hospital staffs participating in the trial became so motivated to initiate therapy early that there was only a 35-minute difference between the two groups. Because this time differential was small, there was no independent contribution of prehospital-initiated therapy on patient outcome, Dr. Weaver said.

Nevertheless, "prehospital initation of therapy is certainly justified, as it may be the only way to provide rapid treatment to many patients in the first golden hour," Dr. Weaver said.

Before giving therapy outside the hospital, paramedics transmitted electrocardiograms to a physician to confirm a diagnosis of MI. The paramedics also used a clinical checklist to help rule out other causes. MI was accurately diagnosed in 93% of patients, Dr. Weaver said.

ACE inhibitor benefits demonstrated in trial

DALLAS, APRIL 14—Captopril may reduce the risk of dying after a heart attack, Boston researchers reported at the American College of Cardiology meeting.

A total of 2,231 myocardial infarction patients at 45 centers in the United States and Canada were enrolled in the Survival and Ventricular Enlargement, or SAVE, trial. Half received captopril (Capoten, Squibb) and half received placebo.

The reduction in risk for death due to cardiovascular causes in the captopril group was 21%; the risk reduction for development of severe heart failure was 37%.

Patients receiving captopril also showed a 25% reduction in the risk of another heart attack, and a 22% reduction in risk of developing heart failure requiring hospitalization, said Marc Pfeffer, M.D., of Brigham and Women's Hospital.

Treatment with captopril will lengthen the lives of patients who have heart attacks, he said.

The patients enrolled in the trial were "run-of-the-mill" heart-attack patients, noted Eugene Braunwald, M.D., chairman of the steering committee of the trial. About one third had received thrombolytic therapy.

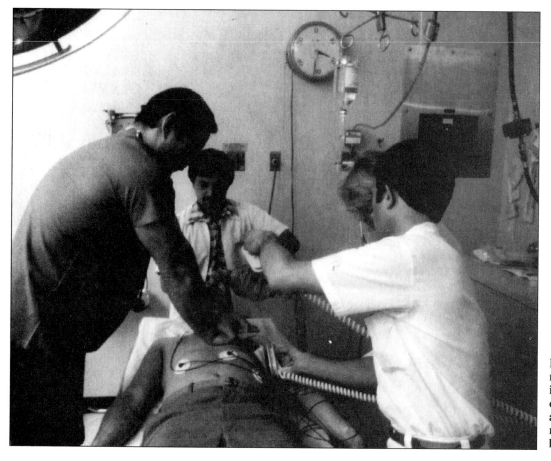

Patients with myocardial infarction given captopril had a 25% reduced risk of a repeat heart attack.

Apheresis absorbs low-density lipoprotein only

By Nathan Horwitz

NASHVILLE, MAY 19—A device that selectively removes low-density lipoprotein from plasma without significantly affecting high-density lipid levels is showing promise in the treatment of severe, refractory familial hypercholesterolemia.

"LDL-apheresis is safe and effective and appears capable of preventing the progression of atherosclerosis in some [of these] patients," said Ralph Bambauer, M.D., of the University of Saarland, Germany.

An estimated 500,000 people in the United States have the heterozygous form and about 50,000 the homozygous form of the condition, which is associated with cholesterol levels four to six times normal.

In a 30-month trial in which 20 patients with the familial disease were pheresed every week or two for up to 28 months, LDL levels dropped from a mean of 287 mg/dl to 147 mg/dl, Dr. Bambauer said at the American Society of Artificial Internal Organs meeting here. Averaging 43.5 years in age, all the patients had been unresponsive to drugs.

Mean total cholesterol declined from 436 mg/dl to 196 mg/dl, while mean HDL rose from 38 mg/dl to 53 mg/dl. Other lipid fractions associated with high atherosclerosis risk and severe stenosis were also substantially reduced. Apolipoprotein B fell from a mean of 289 mg/dl to 151 mg/dl. Lipoprotein (a), a fraction composed of LDL and apolipoproteins A and B, dropped from a mean of 64 mg/dl to 39 mg/dl.

Comparable results were achieved in a nine-center U.S. trial, reported at the American Heart Association meeting in Dallas.

During three six-week treatment phases and a four-week examining period, all 64 patients continued to take their medications—in most cases, an HMG-CoA reductase inhibitor.

In the 54 heterozygous patients, LDL was reduced from a mean 243 mg/dl at baseline to 143 mg/dl, said Bruce Gordon, M.D., associate professor of clinical medicine at New York Hospital-Cornell Medical Center. In homozygous patients, the reduction was from 447 mg/dl to 210 mg/dl. Most of the patients are continuing with the therapy, said Dr. Gordon. He cited a small British study that has reported eight-year-longer survival of homozygous patients who are pheresed than their untreated siblings.

Patented as the Liposorber LA-15 System (Kaneka American Corporation), the device used in the trials employs dextran sulfate cellulose columns to selectively adsorb lipoproteins from separated plasma. The plasma is then recombined with the patient's whole blood and returned via venous access. Thus, important plasma components such as immunoglobulins, vitamins and electrolytes, as well as HDL, are not lost as they would be during conventional therapeutic plasmapheresis.

The cost of the two-hour hospital procedure is still under review. Each treatment costs $1,500 in Japan, according to Tetsuso Agishi, M.D., of Women's Medical College, Tokyo. For once-a-week apheresis, that would annualize to $78,000. Health insurance spokespersons noted that investigational treatments like apheresis are usually not covered.

"The value of the system is that it allows you to lower LDL to almost any target you set," commented Peter Jones, M.D., associate professor of medicine at Baylor College of Medicine in Houston. "You can't do that with drugs because of dosing, side effects and patient tolerability."

Apheresis has a place in the treatment of the more severe heterozygous patients, said Basil Rifkind, M.D., chief of lipid metabolism and atherogenesis at the National Heart, Lung and Blood Institute. But in his view, the availability of pravastatin (Pravachol, Bristol-Myers Squibb) and lovastatin (Mevacor, Merck Sharp & Dohme) makes it possible to control more patients with heterozygous lipidemia pharmacologically.

New CPR technique found to spur blood flow through heart

By Peggy Peck

JUNE 3—A new technique for CPR that uses a suction-cup device is significantly more effective in restoring cardiopulmonary circulation during cardiac arrest than with standard CPR, according to a new study.

The new device, called an active compression-decompression device, is simple, easy to use and inexpensive, said researcher Todd Cohen, M.D., director of electrophysiology, Division of Cardiology, North Shore University Hospital, Manhasset, N.Y.

A more effective CPR technique is needed because most out-of-hospital heart-attack patients do not survive, Dr. Cohen noted in his study, published in The Journal of the American Medical Association.

The new device "compresses the chest just as standard CPR does, and then pulling up on the suction cup causes the natural action of the chest to suck air back into the lungs and blood back into the heart," Dr. Cohen explained.

The new device is superior to standard CPR because it can be used while the patient is receiving defibrillation, according

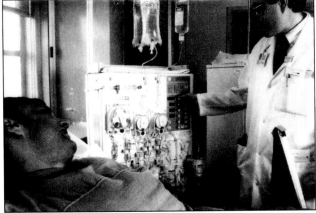

Apheresis cut LDL from a mean of 287 mg/dl to 147mg/dl.

to Dr. Cohen. "It also, I believe, will eliminate the need for mouth-to-mouth resuscitation," he said. "That advantage needs to be tested, but it can be an important improvement in the age of AIDS."

He said the device has not yet been shown to improve the long-term survival rate of heart-attack patients, but a large-scale study is now under way to test that premise.

Dr. Cohen tested the suction device on 10 patients in cardiac arrest. The patients also received standard CPR. In all 10 patients, the device improved the circulation of blood to the heart, and in three patients the device was able to restore a stable blood flow rhythm.

Dr. Cohen is coinventor of the device with Keith Lurie, M.D., a Minnesota physician who reported in JAMA in 1990 that the son of a patient had revived his father after a heart

attack by pushing and pulling on a household plunger the son had placed on the patient's chest.

The device consists of a round suction cup with a bellows on top, positioned between the nipples on the chest. The operator pushes and pulls on a handle attached to the top of the bellows. A gauge on the device can be set for a woman, a man or a large man.

In an accompanying editorial, Henry Halperin, M.D., of Johns Hopkins University Medical School in Baltimore, and Myron Weisfeldt, M.D., of Columbia University College of Physicians and Surgeons in New York, wrote that either the suction device or a pneumatic vest that they invented is likely to revolutionize cardiopulmonary resuscitation.

The vest works by alternately inflating and deflating, they pointed out.

Noninvasive blood pressure-pump may halt angina

By Fran Kritz

JUNE 11—A noninvasive procedure that pumps blood from extremities to the heart may be an alternative for patients intolerant of bypass surgery or balloon angioplasty.

Ultimately, it could be a less expensive, nearly risk-free first line of defense for people with coronary artery disease, its proponents say.

The procedure, enhanced external counterpulsation, is being tested at the Health Sciences Center at the State University of New York at Stony Brook.

Twenty patients there have undergone the one-hour procedure, administered five days a week for seven weeks. Following treatment, all 20 said they had no pain, and many were able to decrease their cardiac medications.

Counterpulsation forces blood to coronary arteries while the heart is relaxed, and therefore more receptive to receiving an increased blood flow, according to Harry Soroff, M.D., a professor of surgery at Stony Brook who helped develop the treatment.

Wide pressure cuffs are strapped around the legs, thighs and buttocks. A compressor releases air into tubes that lead to the cuffs, forcing blood to the heart.

Dr. Soroff believes the body calls tiny capillaries into play when a blockage cuts off the main arteries to the heart. When angina occurs, it sends out chemical stimuli to open these collateral channels, he said.

The counterpulsation also may stimulate the development of those channels, Dr. Soroff said.

At $5,000, the treatment is less expensive than $30,000 bypass surgery or $14,000 balloon angioplasty, he said.

The researchers used a treadmill stress test followed by a thallium scan to determine the extent of the blockage and the success of the procedure.

The researchers recently reported that of 18 patients aged 44 to 74, all said they had reduced anginal pain after counterpulsation treatment. Thallium scans showed that 12 patients regained complete heart function, and another two had significant improvement. Four did not show improvement in thallium scans.

Eight of the patients had had prior bypass surgery, and seven had previous heart attacks. No side effects were reported, although lung clots are possible.

Patients who will benefit most are likely to be those who have at least one open artery leading to the heart, as the one open vessel can transmit the increased blood flow, according to the researchers.

Lawrence Cohn, M.D., chief of cardiac surgery at Brigham and Women's Hospital in Boston, said an alternative procedure is needed for cardiac patients who cannot tolerate surgery. "But this will have to be proven many, many ways before it can be accepted," he said.

Serum lipids unaltered by most antihypertensives

Medical Tribune News Service

BOSTON, JUNE 12—Antihypertensive therapy does not appear to increase total cholesterol levels in patients with mild to moderate hypertension, according to a large, multi-center trial.

No adverse effects on lipoprotein profiles were seen in patients treated by any of six major classes of antihypertensives, according to the Veterans Administration Cooperative Study of Monotherapy in Hypertension.

Preliminary results of the 15-center study, to be published in two peer-reviewed journals later this year, suggest that concern about the adverse effects of diuretics on lipids and lipoproteins may have stemmed from data based on excessive dosage or methodologic flaws in some earlier trials, Michael Hamburger, M.D., Boston VA Medical Center, said at a meeting here on Recent Advances in Cardiovascular Therapeutics, jointly sponsored by the American College of Cardiology and Tufts University.

A total of 1,292 patients with mild to moderate hypertension (diastolic 95 to 110 mm Hg) were randomized to placebo or one of the six major classes of drugs, including a thiazide diuretic (hydrochlorothiazide); angiotensin-converting enzyme inhibitor (captopril; Capoten, Squibb); alpha-1 antagonist (prazosin); beta-adrenergic blocker (atenolol; Tenormin, ICI); central alpha-2 antagonist (clonidine); or a calcium channel blocker (diltiazem; Cardizem, Marion Merrell Dow).

Patients were titrated to a blood pressure of less than 90 mm Hg diastolic and maintained on therapy for up to two years.

Diltiazem produced the greatest drop in diastolic blood pressure, 14.4%, compared with 12.8% with clonidine. For systolic blood pressure, clonidine produced the largest percentage drop, 16.2%, with hydrochlorothiazide second, 13.8%, and diltiazem third, 13%. The investigator emphasized that these are overall data and have not been analyzed by dosage.

In an interview, Dr. Hamburger stressed the different lipid profiles seen on early- and long-term follow-up in the VA trial.

"At eight weeks, we noted that patients on diuretics demonstrated a 3 mg/dl increase in total cholesterol," Dr. Hamburger said. "But at the end of one year, there was no difference between hydrochlorothiazide and the other drugs employed in this trial."

The VA Cooperative Monotherapy trial was undertaken to test the hypothesis that most hypertensive patients can be controlled by therapy with a single drug, Dr. Hamburger explained.

"Another issue we felt it important to examine was the effect of antihypertensive drugs on lipid profiles, because of the widespread discussion of this question," he said.

Marvin Moser, M.D., clinical professor of medicine at Yale University School of Medicine, who has long contended that the lipid increases observed in diuretic therapy are short-term, said he was "delighted" by the new findings.

"If you look at any major clinical trial of antihypertensive therapy that runs two to five years, there is not one in which the cholesterol levels increase," he said.

Dr. Moser noted that the data of the Hypertension Detection and Followup Program have also shown that patients with baseline elevated cholesterol experienced decreases with thiazide diuretics, while those with low baseline levels had slight increases.

This would seem to suggest regression to the mean, rather than a specific effect of medication, he said.

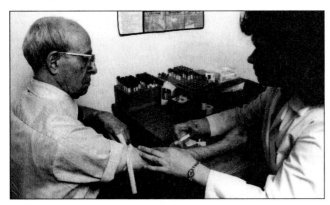

Multicenter study eased concern over diuretics raising lipids.

When the results of the VA trial were examined by subgroups, taking into account the side-effect profile, as well as the efficiency of blood-pressure reduction, diltiazem and atenolol were superior in whites under age 60, and diltiazem and prazosin in whites over age 60, Dr. Hamburger reported.

Diltiazem also scored at the top in both younger and older African-Americans, with hydrochlorothiazide also demonstrating effective blood-pressure-lowering capacity. A total of 48% of the patients were African-American.

Dr. Hamburger noted that very few investigators have followed hypertensive patients in a controlled double-blind antihypertensive study for a year or two. "Whether our data will put the discussion to rest is, however, uncertain," he said.

Franco Muller, M.D., associate professor of medicine at Cornell University in New York, said he found the lipid results of the VA trial "surprising," and wondered whether the patients had altered their diets or changed their life-styles in the course of the study.

"For one thing, we know that patients in a medical trial become health conscious. They may change their diets in the direction of fat or cholesterol reduction," he said. "Secondly, there is an immense and continuing media campaign about healthy diets as a goal in a healthy life, and the patients might have become more responsive to that kind of pressure."

Dr. Muller speculated further that the increases in cholesterol levels in the first months of the trial could have been canceled by the patients' unreported changes in diet, so that by the end of a year's treatment, there would have been no evidence of an adverse lipid effect.

He suggested that it might be interesting to analyze subgroups of patients by the dose size of diuretic or beta-blocker administered (for example, those getting 12.5 mg chlorothiazide compared with those receiving 50 mg) to see if the results were the same.

Adding magnesium to standard therapy may reduce MI mortality

Axel Springer New Service

JUNE 27—Adding magnesium to standard thrombolytic treatment could cut the number of heart-attack deaths by 24%, according to British researchers.

Previous studies have suggested that administering magnesium may be beneficial, but none of those studies were large enough to be convincing, said Kent L. Woods, M.D., of the Leicester Royal Infirmary in England.

"This study is large enough to give us clear answers," said Dr. Woods, whose study results appeared in the British medical journal The Lancet.

Dr. Woods and his colleagues studied 2,316 heart-attack patients; half received intravenous magnesium when they were brought to the hospital, the other half received a placebo solution.

"The death rate 28 days later in the magnesium group was 7.8%, while 10.3% of the placebo patients died," he said. "That's a 24% reduction in deaths."

Patients who received magnesium also had a 25% reduction in the risk of developing heart failure, according to the Leicester researcher.

Magnesium may work by enlarging the coronary blood vessels, thus increasing the blood flow through the heart, he said. "Or it could be that the increase of magnesium in the blood protects the heart muscle from the interruption of the blood supply, or reduces the damage."

"We have started using magnesium routinely because we think our evidence is good enough," Dr. Woods said. The treatment costs a few dollars per patient, he added.

Koon Teo, M.D., of the University of Alberta in Edmonton, Canada, recently conducted an analysis of studies that included 1,301 patients and found that adding magnesium to standard treatment for heart-attack patients cut the death rate by 66%.

The ISIS-4 trial, with an enrollment of 40,000 patients worldwide, is also evaluating the effect of magnesium and captopril (Capoten, Squibb) on heart-attack patients. Dr. Woods is an advisor to the Oxford-based study, and has informed Oxford investigators of his results.

The Oxford study, with 20 times more patients than the Leicester trial, will have the statistical clout to determine if magnesium saves the lives of heart-attack patients, according to cardiac experts.

Elderly patients benefit as much as younger ones from thrombolytics after myocardial infarction

JULY 2—People over age 75 are just as likely as younger people to benefit from thrombolytic therapy following a suspected acute myocardial infarction, according to a new study.

The study, published in The New England Journal of Medicine, shows a clear-cut benefit for these older patients in terms of cost savings and years of life saved.

The results are at odds with a 1990 statement by a joint task force of the American Heart Association and the American College of Cardiology, which concluded that the effectiveness of thrombolytic drugs in people aged 75 or older is "uncertain."

Harlan Krumholz, M.D., the investigator who headed the new study, said his group has clearly shown that age alone is not a reason to withhold the therapy from patients who would otherwise benefit from the drugs.

In analyzing both the GISSI and ISIS-2 trials, a team led by Dr. Krumholz of Beth Israel Hospital in Boston found that the drugs lowered the risk

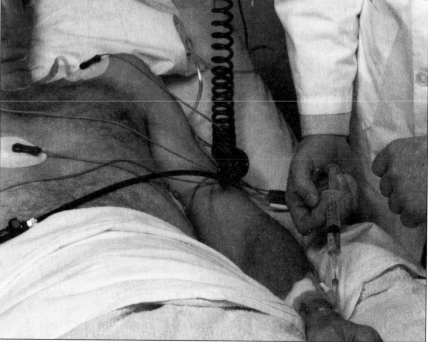

Pooling two trials, streptokinase and tPA reduced mortality in elderly patients by 14%.

of dying despite the risk of complications, including bleeding and stroke.

The overall mortality rate for the 623 patients over 75 in the GISSI study who did not receive thrombolytic therapy was 33%, while a mortality rate of 25% was seen in the 745 nonrecipient elderly patients in ISIS-2.

Pooling data from both trials, the overall reduction in mortality would have amounted to 14%, according to Dr. Krumholz. "Thrombolytic therapy with streptokinase was associated with a survival advantage even when the rate of

major complications was estimated to be as high as 4%," he added.

Accordingly, one additional life would be saved for every 33 individuals over the age of 75 treated with thrombolytic agents. This amounts to a cost savings of $22,400 per year of life saved.

Dr. Krumholz said he believes using thrombolytic therapy in older people is as cost-effective as many other ways of lowering cardiovascular risk, such as testing younger patients for moderate hypertension.

Streptokinase costs about $200 per treatment and tPA costs about $2,300.

Despite the mounting evidence that thrombolytic therapy is cost-effective and saves lives, patients over age 75 are six times less likely than younger patients to receive them, according to Eric Topol, M.D., of the Cleveland Clinic Foundation.

Dr. Topol pointed out that 14% of patients currently enrolled in the GUSTO trial to study thrombolysis after an acute MI are over age 75.

"Our experience to date suggests that American investigators have accepted the concept that elderly patients are good candidates for thrombolytic therapy, but it remains unclear whether this concept has been disseminated into standard practice," Dr. Topol said.

He said that one of the reasons that elderly patients are not given thrombolytics is that they have a worse functional status before infarction and a higher frequency of substantial coexisting illness.

Elderly patients are also more likely to present to the hospital more than six hours after symptom onset—and thus be ineligible for thrombolysis—and to have minimal or no chest discomfort at evaluation, according to Dr. Topol.

One of the complications that has been reported with the use of thrombolytic agents is an increased risk of stroke.

But in a second study appearing in NEJM, researchers from Italy found that people given either streptokinase or tPA had a relatively small risk of stroke.

However, elderly people and women were more likely than younger people and men to suffer a stroke while on the drugs.

Aldo Pietro Maggioni, M.D., one of the Italian coordinators of the GISSI-2 trial, reported that the incidence of stroke was 1.14% among 20,768 patients who received thrombolytic and antithrombotic therapy.

Mild ischemia criteria ignored by most physicians

By Dan Hurley

SEPT. 1—Ischemia, insists Robert DeBusk, M.D., is not like pregnancy. You can be a little bit ischemic.

Based on studies he has been conducting for over 20 years at Stanford University School of Medicine, Dr. DeBusk believes that patients who are only mildly ischemic following an uncomplicated myocardial infarction should be tested and treated less intensively, and sent back to work more quickly, than severely ischemic patients.

Such treatment reduces the cost of medical care and, by returning patients to work faster, increases their income, he said.

But many physicians do not make a distinction between mild and severe ischemia, according to the results of a study in the Annals of Internal Medicine on which Dr. DeBusk, a professor of medicine at Stanford, was senior researcher.

Despite guidelines on when to revascularize and how soon to let patients return to work, the study found that many physicians recommend angioplasty in equivocal cases and advise patients to take their time convalescing.

The new study comes on the heels of a 1988 trial by Dr. DeBusk's team showing that the median time a patient returned to work after an uncomplicated MI could be safely cut from 75 days to 51 days on the basis of a symptom-limited treadmill test.

In the 1988 study, half of patients were assigned to receive the standard post-MI care, and half were given an occupational work evaluation.

Patients were stratified into three groups: those who showed no signs of ischemia during a treadmill test; those with mild ischemia, consisting of either angina or 0.1 to 0.2 mV of ST-segment depression; and those with severe ischemia, above 0.2 mV of ST-segment depression.

Based on previous studies, the researchers analyzed the work-evaluation patients and predicted that the nonischemic patients had only a 5% risk of cardiac events in the next six months, and could return to work in 35 days. Mildly ischemic patients were given a 10% risk, and told to return to work at 42 days, after beginning therapy with antianginal medication.

Severe ischemics were judged to have a risk exceeding 25% and advised to undergo coronary arteriography.

As it turned out, patients who received the back-to-work advice had a rate of cardiac death and nonfatal MI of just 2%, better than the 5% rate for controls. And their quickened return to work was associated with $2,102 of additional earned salary per patient in the six months following MI.

The new study, led by Louise Pilote, M.D., also of Stanford, duplicated the older one with just one difference: This time it involved patients whose primary physicians were in a practice-based setting, rather than in a university-based setting.

The practice-based physicians followed the researchers' advice almost exactly with nonischemic patients, cutting patients' back-to-work time from a median of 65 days in the group who received standard care, to just 38 days in the group where patients were assessed and given advice by the researchers.

But in patients with ischemia, no significant difference in back-to-work time was found between treatment and control groups, who returned to work at 80 days and 76 days, respectively.

The reason: Physicians did not follow the practice guidelines used in the 1988 study, and, instead, ordered coronary angiograms for the ischemic group at a rate nearly four times higher than in the 1988 study.

They also performed coronary angioplasties at a rate more than five times higher—with no apparent improvement in cardiac events as a result.

"Doctors don't make the discrimination between mild and severe [ischemia]," Dr. DeBusk said. In the new study, "there's a lot more aggressive intervention. Who's getting that intervention? The intermediate [mildly ischemic] group."

Rolf Gunnar, M.D., chair of the American College of Cardiology-American Heart Association committee for guidelines for the treatment of acute myocardial infarction, said more information is needed about mildly ischemic patients and their outcomes.

"Should the intermediate [mildly ischemic] group be studied further? I would say there are a large number of people who feel they should be," said Dr. Gunnar, a professor emeritus at Loyola University in Maywood, Ill.

Peter Hanson, M.D., director of preventive cardiology at the University of Wisconsin at Madison, agreed. "It's not that I doubt the present study," he said, "but the overall milieu of the national cardiology scene is that a lot of tests are done. I'm not defending it, but it's a fact of life."

In the 1970s, Dr. DeBusk and Charles Dennis, M.D., a co-author on both studies and now chair of the department of cardiology at the Deborah Heart and Lung Center in Browns Mills, N.J., were the first to perform exercise stress tests three weeks post-MI.

Today, Drs. Dennis and DeBusk believe cardiologists increasingly opt to perform angiography not for scientific reasons, but for the same reason that motivates mountain climbers: because it's there.

"The evidence is there's a very low incidence of untoward events, both death and reinfarction, among miidly ischemic patients," Dr. DeBusk said.

"I have spent the best years of my life trying to convince physicians that mild ischemia is not so terrible," said Dr. DeBusk.

ACE inhibitors draw the high cards in SAVE, SOLVD trials of over 6,000 heart-attack patients

SEPT. 3—One of the best-known ACE inhibitors—captopril—may prevent subsequent heart failure in patients who have had myocardial infarctions, a new study shows.

Nineteen percent fewer deaths occurred among patients given the angiotensin-converting enzyme inhibitor captopril (Capoten, Squibb) within three weeks of having a heart attack than among patients given a placebo, according to investigators in the multicenter Survival and Ventricular Enlargement (SAVE) study.

Several large trials have been conducted over the last several years to test the benefits of ACE inhibitors, which are thought to improve survival by preventing dilatation of the left ventricle after an MI, which can lead to cardiac failure.

In a report on captopril appearing in The New England Journal of Medicine, lead researcher Marc A. Pfeffer, M.D., of Brigham and Women's Hospital in Boston reported that people on captopril survived longer, were hospitalized less and had a lower risk of death from cardiac failure than people taking a placebo.

The reduction in risk for captopril patients was 21% for death from cardiovascular causes, 37% for the development of severe heart failure, 22% for congestive heart failure requiring hospitalization and 25% for recurrent MI.

All of the 2,231 people in Dr. Pfeffer's study had left-ventricular dysfunction, with ejection fractions of 40% or less but without overt heart failure or symptoms of myocardial ischemia.

Within three to 16 days after an myocardial infarction, the patients were randomly assigned to receive double-blind treatment with either placebo or captopril. They were followed for an average of 42 months.

In another study that also appears in The New England Journal of Medicine, investigators in the Studies of Left Ventricular Dysfunction (SOLVD) of 4,228 patients found that enalapril (Vasotec, Merck Sharp & Dohme) cut the death rate by 29% among MI patients with left-ventricular dysfunction compared with a group given placebo.

Enalapril worked best at preventing heart failure in post-MI patients who had suffered the most severe left ventricle damage—those with ejection fractions of 35% or less.

However, survival was not improved among more than 3,000 people given enalapril within 24 hours of MI in a third study, the cooperative new Scandinavian Enalapril Survival Study II (CONSENSUS II). The trial, which was also reported in the same issue of The New England Journal of Medicine, was cut short when no survival benefit was shown.

In an editorial accompanying the studies, Jay N. Cohn, M.D., of the University of Minnesota said that with the exception of the European study, the data indicate that ACE inhibitors can significantly benefit patients with left-ventricular dysfunction who have already had a myocardial infarction.

Dr. Cohn suggested that physicians should be strongly encouraged to use ACE inhibitors in these patients and that further studies should be done to combine ACE inhibitors with other common treatments, such as beta-blockers, to achieve even greater benefits.

Risk of MI cut by late thrombolytic therapy

Axel Springer News Service

BARCELONA, SEPT. 3—Thrombolytic therapy given between six and 12 hours after the onset of chest pains can cut mortality by 27%, according to the results of a new international study of about 6,000 patients.

Many American heart specialists have been conservative in their use of clot busters because they are concerned the drugs are not effective if given after the six-hour cutoff.

The coordinator of the study, Robert Wilcox, M.D., estimated that as many as 30% of heart-attack patients in Europe and the United States may be denied treatment because of hospital rules against giving thrombolytic drugs when a patient comes in more than six hours after their chest pain begins.

The study, presented at the 14th Congress of the European Society of Cardiology here, analyzed the effects of tissue plasminogen activator (tPA) given more than six and less than 24 hours after chest pains begin.

The trial—called the Late Assessment of Thrombolytic Efficacy, or LATE, study—demonstrated a "highly significant benefit from treatment" in patients given tPA within six to 12 hours after heart-attack symptoms, Dr. Wilcox said.

"This significant benefit has been maintained up to one year," he said.

Half of the patients received alteplase, a recombinant form of tPA marketed by Genentech under the trade name Activase; the others received placebo.

A South American study showed that streptokinase also cut mortality when given within six to 12 hours.

The LATE study provides substantial evidence that the time frame for giving clot-busting drugs should be extended to 12 hours, said Dr. Wilcox, of the University of Nottingham in England.

The multicenter study was conducted in 247 medical centers in the United States and abroad. Most of the patients in the trial were men, with an average age of 63 years. About half had previously suffered from angina.

The investigators found that the risk of having a stroke was 2.25% in patients receiving tPA, compared with 1.1% in the placebo group.

Despite the higher risk of stroke, the study results suggest that the overall benefits of tPA outweigh the risks even when it is given up to 12 hours after chest pains begin, Dr. Wilcox said.

Women and elderly often underrepresented and less aggressively treated in cardiac trials

Medical Tribune News Service

OTTAWA, SEPT. 14—Women may be twice as likely as men to die in a coronary care unit due to less-aggressive management and less-defined cardiac symptoms, according to researchers here. Of 2,546 CCU admissions, 8.2% of women had died by the 28th day versus 4.8% of men.

"They get fewer antiarrhythmic agents and fewer ischemic agents when they present with acute chest pain," said Ronald Gregor, M.D., of Dalhousie University Medical Center in Nova Scotia. "They have fewer nuclear angiograms and fewer coronary angiograms."

In a presentation to the annual meeting of the Royal College of Physicians and Surgeons of Canada, Dr. Gregor said that in his study women also showed nonclassic symptoms of myocardial infarction more often than men. "They may present without chest pain, or with pain that's not typical. Much of the literature is based on the way males present, and treatments are also based on male study populations," he said.

A recent analysis of 214 studies showed that most trials of drug therapy for MIs have excluded the elderly and have significantly underrepresented women.

More than 60% of the studies excluded patients over 75 years old, and fewer than 20% of all patients were women, according to the results published in The Journal of the American Medical Association.

Researchers traditionally have excluded the elderly from studies of drugs because they might be suffering from other diseases that would interfere with the drug's effects, making analysis more difficult, noted the author of the new study, Jerry H. Gurwitz, M.D., of Brigham and Women's Hospital in Boston. The elderly also might experience more severe side effects with certain drugs than younger people would, he wrote.

But because more than 60% of people discharged from hospitals following heart attacks are over age 65, it is important to know about

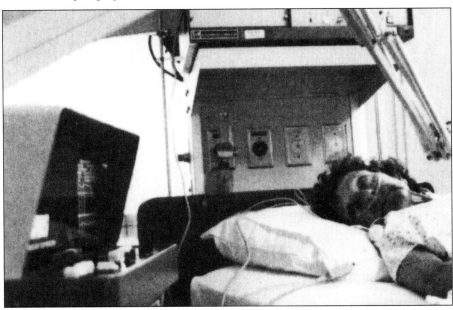

Fewer than 20% of all patients in the studies were women; figures much worse for elderly.

side effects that affect only this age group, Dr. Gurwitz concluded.

"Widespread exclusion of elderly patients from clinical trials, coupled with the tacit assumption that cardiovascular disease is comparable in women and men, has resulted in sizable gaps in our knowledge," said Nanette Wenger, M.D., of Emory University School of Medicine, in an accompanying editorial.

Dr. Wenger recently chaired a workshop on the subject involving 60 top cardiologists.

Part of the problem with including the so-called very old, those 85 and above, in drug studies has been that, until recently, they accounted for a tiny proportion of the total population.

Today people 85 years or older number 2.7 million, Dr. Wenger noted.

"They constitute the most rapidly growing subgroup among the elderly, with a projected sixfold increase by the year 2030," she added.

Recent studies have shown that patients over age 75 are as likely as younger patients to benefit from thrombolytic drugs following an MI.

The results were at odds with a 1990 statement by a joint task force of the American Heart Association and the American College of Cardiology.

Because many physicians still use the older guidelines, patients over age 75 may be six times less likely than younger patients to receive thrombolytic drugs, according to Eric Topol, M.D., of the Cleveland Clinic Foundation.

Two other studies, both published in 1991, were the first to find that elderly people between ages 70 and 84 can cut their MI and stroke risk by lowering their blood pressure.

Drugs may augment life-style in mild HBP

By Brian McCann

OCT. 1—Drug therapy and life-style changes for mild hypertension check the disease more effectively than life-style changes alone, according to the results of the Treatment of Mild Hypertension Study (TOMHS).

TOMHS, which began at four centers in 1986, is comparing the effects of life-style changes alone versus combining them with one of five antihypertensive drugs in 902 middle-aged men and women who had an average baseline blood pressure of 140/91 mm Hg. A full report on the four-year follow-up is to be given at the annual American Heart Association meeting in November. Data on lipid-lowering effects will be presented as well.

Some new data were presented at the Council for High Blood Pressure Research meeting in Cleveland by Richard Grimm, M.D., of the University of Minnesota School of Public Health.

The researchers reported that diastolic blood pressure declined 33% more in the drug/life-style group versus those on the life-style changes alone.

The drugs were given once a day and included an angiotensin-converting enzyme inhibitor, enalapril (Vasotec, Merck Sharp & Dohme); an alpha-one inhibitor, doxazosin (Cardura, Roerig); a beta-blocker, acebutolol (Sectral, Wyeth-Ayerst); a calcium-channel blocker, amlodipine (Norvasc, Pfizer); and a diuretic, chlorthalidone.

Life-style changes included a 10% reduction in body weight, at least 150 minutes a week of physical activity, reducing salt intake to 70 mmol/d and two or fewer alcoholic drinks a day.

After the first year, systolic values dropped by 18.6 mm Hg for those on drugs and life-style changes and 10.6 mm Hg in the group on life-style changes alone. Diastolic dropped by 12.8 mm Hg and 8.1 mm Hg, respectively.

"Blood-pressure lowering among mild hypertensives was linked to a decrease in four-year mortality even when diastolic blood pressure fell in the range of 70 to 80 mm Hg," said Dr. Grimm. "These findings are in contrast to other large studies that have shown higher morbidity and mortality among people who have low blood pressure."

Doctors soon may say yes to NO, says expert

NOV. 5—The discovery this year that endothelium-derived relaxing factor is actually nitric oxide is expected to lead to important new therapeutic uses for the chemical, according to cardiovascular researchers.

At the Bristol-Myers Squibb Symposium on Cardiovascular Research in Houston, researchers reported that not only is nitric oxide crucial to relaxing the vascular endothelium, it also may be a modulator of cell growth.

Paul Vanhoutte, M.D., director of the Center for Experimental Therapeutics at Baylor College of Medicine, said that nitric-oxide-donor drugs, such as angiotensin-converting enzyme inhibitors, may potentially halt or protect against the growth of atherosclerotic plaques. The injuries sustained by the endothelium render the regenerated cells incapable of producing adequate supplies of nitric oxide on demand.

According to Dr. Vanhoutte, nitric oxide drugs would target the endothelium and produce the gas when it is needed after disease or injury occurs. "I am convinced that injuries to endothelium, be they from high blood pressure, high levels of cholesterol, diabetes or any other recognized factors, set all the cardiovascular-disease processes in motion," said Dr. Vanhoutte.

Another speaker, David Harrison, M.D., of Emory University School of Medicine in Atlanta, said animal studies indicated that high-cholesterol diets cause constrictions in coronary arteries, well before plaque buildup occurs. Switching to low-cholesterol diets and lowering serum cholesterol can result in normal blood vessel relaxation, he said.

'Gender bias' in cardiac treatment debated

Medical Tribune Special Report

NEW ORLEANS, NOV. 16—Female heart-disease patients are first seen when they are older and sicker than their male counterparts, and receive less aggressive treatment, according to several reports presented here at the American Heart Association's 65th meeting.

But researchers weren't sure whether the culprit was gender bias or a misreading of symptoms by both patients and physicians. "We know that women have to get highly symptomatic before anything gets done about their heart disease," said Nanette Wenger, M.D., of Emory University in Atlanta, Ga., and co-author of three papers presented at the meeting.

"But whether that is because women don't perceive coronary artery disease as a serious health problem, or physicians equate differently the same descriptions of symptoms from men and women, is unknown."

An Emory study by Dr. Wenger and her colleagues of elective balloon angioplasty in 10,286 patients, including 2,667 women, found that the women were, on average, older than the men; 61 vs. 56 years old. Fifty-four percent of the women had hypertension, compared with 39% of the men, she said. The women also had more diabetes than the men, but less multivessel disease.

In-hospital deaths were higher among women, she added, which was partially explained by older age. The average five- and seven-year survival rates for the women were 92% and 88%, respectively, compared with 95% and 92% among the men. "What our data say is that the excess risk in women may not be female gender, but possibly that they present at an older age, they have more severe and longer-standing disease, and more severe co-morbidity," Dr. Wenger said.

In another study designed to determine whether bias played a role in determining who gets revascularized, the Emory team reviewed the records of 30,080 patients, including 6,903 women undergoing catheterization. "The decision to perform revascularization was dependent largely on severity of coronary obstructions, absence of severe left ventricular dysfunction and severity of angina, with gender playing a minor role," according to the investigators. They found no "major bias" against performing percutaneous transluminal coronary angiography or coronary artery bypass graft in women undergoing catheterization in any age group.

Another study, conducted by Daniel B. Mark, M.D., and David B. Pryor, M.D., of Duke University, concluded that the management of women, when it came to referring them for aggressive therapy, was medically appropriate.

However, a Harvard study found that the average time for transfer of women with MIs to tertiary-care units was nearly double that of men, according to Jane Sherwood, research coordinator and cardiologic nurse at the Deaconess Hospital in Boston. The average time of transfer was 2.9 days for men and 4.5 days for women, Sherwood reported.

New CPR guidelines may increase survival 20-fold

NOV. 26—The survival rate of sudden-heart-attack victims could be increased from as low as 2% in many areas of the United States to 40% if communities would follow the revised CPR guidelines, said the chair of the American Heart Association committee that developed the guidelines.

One of the new recommendations advises bystanders witnessing a possible heart attack to call 911 before attempting cardiopulmonary resuscitation.

The previous version of the guidelines advised people to attempt CPR for one minute before calling 911. But many people ended up giving CPR for longer, delaying the arrival of an emergency medical team with a defibrillator.

The guidelines, agreed to at a conference in February and announced in part at that time, recommend no change in helping children under age eight: One minute of CPR should be given before calling 911.

An effective community-wide system involving emergency medical squads, emergency rooms and a good 911 system is necessary for efforts by bystanders or family members to be effective in saving heart-attack victims, said the chair of the committee that developed the guidelines, John A. Paraskos, M.D., of the University of Massachusetts in Worcester.

He noted that although most urban and suburban communities now have 911 numbers, many still route the calls to the police, a step that can waste precious time. The guidelines recommend that 911 calls be routed to a dispatcher, who can quickly determine if CPR is necessary, and can tell the caller how to do it while an emergency medical squad is on the way.

In congested cities and sprawling rural areas, where EMS teams are routinely delayed in reaching a heart-attack victim, automatic defibrillators should be made available to security personnel and others trained to use them, said Dr. Paraskos.

The guidelines also call for all EMS teams to be equipped with a defibrillator, and for hospital emergency rooms to be prepared to offer advanced cardiac life support.

As many as 300,000 heart-attack victims die each year before reaching the hospital, according to the AHA.

An editorial accompanying the guidelines in a recent issue of The Journal of the American Medical Association noted that a Chicago study found that just 2% of cardiac-arrest victims survive. "Reports of low survival rates call into question the value of CPR and, consequently, the value of the new guidelines," wrote Carin M. Olson, M.D., a contributing editor of JAMA.

But Dr. Paraskos said that better community programs, such as the one in King County, Wash., which includes Seattle, could greatly increase survival rates. "As many as 40% of those found to be in ventricular fibrillation are able to be discharged from hospitals there with reasonable neurologic function," he said.

C O M M E N T A R Y

Drug trials shed light on CHD mechanisms

By John H. Laragh, M.D.

ONE OF THE GREAT UNSOLVED challenges in cardiology is how we can prevent the structural changes in blood vessels that lead to a myocardial infarction, stroke or kidney disease. The ultimate triumph over this problem will only emerge with a complete understanding of the factors involved in causing these structural changes.

In the absence of such information, much can be learned about causation by a careful evaluation of the differing effectiveness of antihypertensive drug types for correcting or arresting structural vascular changes and thereby preventing myocardial ischemia or infarction. In this context, agents that reduce or block plasma renin activity (i.e., beta-blockers and angiotensin-converting enzyme inhibitors) have special promise because besides reducing the cardiac burden, these agents markedly reduce plasma renin activity and angiotensin II levels. Plasma renin activity is predictive of a subsequent MI, according to both human and animal studies. On the other hand, diuretics, and to a lesser extent calcium antagonists, actually raise plasma renin value, and these treatments have so far proved less effective for cardioprevention.

A handful of trials now under way may shed more light on the question when preliminary data are released in 1993. I can think of three trials that are probably important.

The ASIST trial, or atenolol silent ischemia trial, is comparing the beta-blocker with placebo to determine if the agent can lower mortality in people with ischemia. The National Institutes of Health is sponsoring the ACIP trial, or asymptomatic cardiac ischemia pilot trial. This three-arm study will look at whether abolishing silent ischemia can affect prognosis. The 600 patients already enrolled in ACIP will receive either antianginal agents or surgery or angioplasty to revascularize. If successful, the trial is expected to expand to 6,000 patients. And the TIBET, or total ischemia burden European trial, will compare a calcium antagonist with a beta-blocker in people with ischemia.

There is no doubt that establishing whether there is a prognostic benefit to treating silent myocardial ischemia is important. It is especially important because there has never really been a study to determine if treating ischemia can affect mortality.

I also believe that 1993 will be marked by a greater interest in determining which intermediate cardiac end points can predict morbidity and mortality. As a field, we have seen fantastic advances in technology that allow us to measure many aspects of the cardiovascular system. Now we must determine which aspects are most important for predicting prognosis.

I believe efforts will likely be focused on measurements of left-ventricle mass by precise echocardiographic methods; spotting plaques down to 2 mm in carotid arteries; and the early recognition, by noninvasive methods, of changes in the arterial pressure curve and mean transit time of blood.

These are phenomenally precise and high-tech tests, and cardiologists must learn to take advantage of them. We never had these data available to us before. Now the new assignment for clinicians and researchers will be to relate these surrogate end points to the ultimate morbid events so as to establish good predictors.

Also look for big advances in the development of devices to treat coronary artery disease. I expect to see an increasing use of programmable defibrillators to prevent ventricular arrhythmias.

Antiarrhythmic drug therapy often is ineffective, leaving about 120,000 patients who could benefit from the implantable devices.

I believe we will continue to see a shift to excimer lasers for angioplasty. Admittedly, the shift from balloon angioplasty to the laser procedure has been slow, with at least three fourths of laser-equipped medical centers still performing the balloon procedure. But as more surgeons become familiar with the excimer, the shift will speed up.

Perhaps the main reason is the fact that we continue to see high restenosis rates following coronary artery bypass graft and balloon angioplasty.

While the mechanisms responsible for restenosis still have not been fully eliminated, and while we are not sure about the rates following laser angioplasty because of a lack of data, the therapy does hold the possibility of lowering restenosis rates.

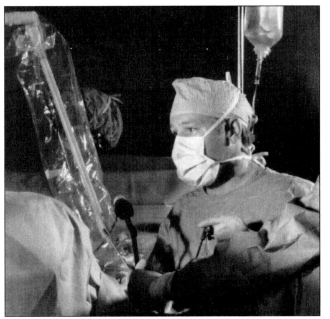

A shift to excimer lasers for angioplasty is predicted.

Dr. Laragh is director of the cardiovascular center and chief of the cardiology division at the New York Hospital-Cornell Medical Center.

Notes

Notes

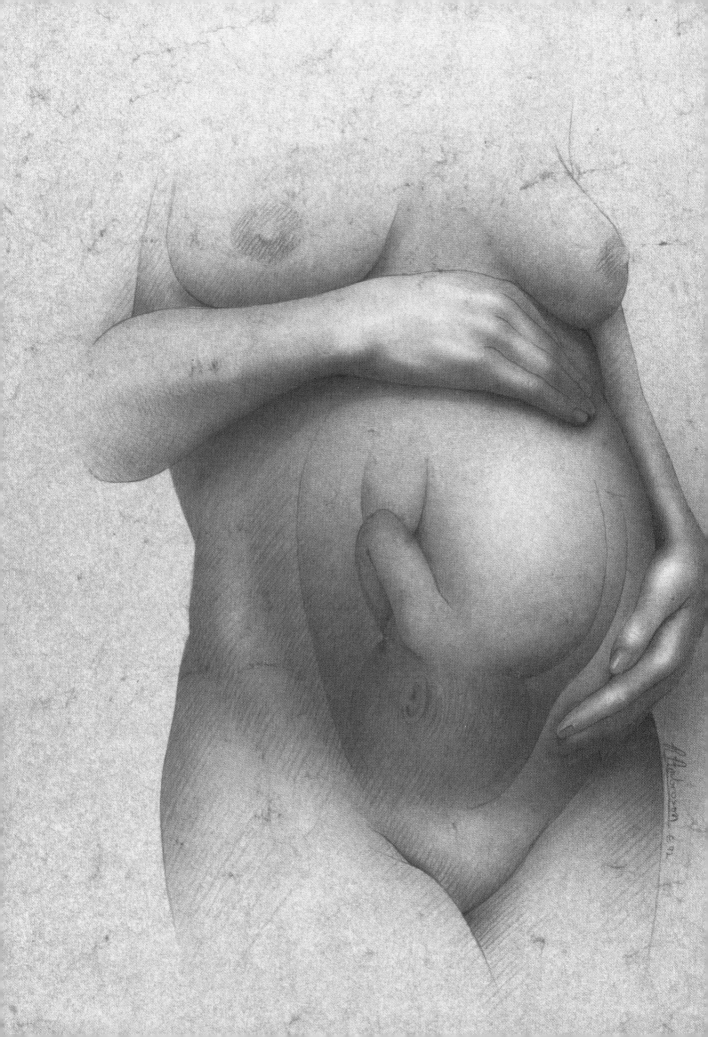

Overview 108
Obstetric advances ranged from preimplantation to postmenopause

Month-at-a-glance 110

Reported at the Time 122
Home uterine monitoring found ineffective…"baby-maker" case focuses attention on infertility standards…prenatal exercise safety debated…ACOG brief opposes abortion deterrence…ovarian-cancer screening tests termed unreliable…IVF update: success declines with age…drug news: injectable contraceptive in, ritodrine for labor criticized…the dolphin-"midwife" experiment…cystic fibrosis detected in three-day-old embryos…strep B testing for all pregnant women advised

Commentary 131
Treatment advancing, diagnosis lagging
By Luella Klein, M.D.

Obstetric advances ranged from preimplantation to postmenopause

One of the year's biggest controversies centered on silicone breast implants. After all the evidence was in, the FDA stuck by plans to restrict their use to breast-cancer patients and clinical trials.

In an age when condoms have become acceptable topics of dinner table conversation in some homes, investigators have provided a plenitude of contraceptive news.

Researchers at the University of Washington reported that people with genital herpes and their uninfected sexual partners must use condoms even between outbreaks. In the study, 70% of viral transmissions occurred at a time when the infected partner was asymptomatic. And the Centers for Disease Control and Prevention warned that women who engage in anal sex without a condom are at high risk for hepatitis B.

The Food and Drug Administration approved injectable medryoxyprogesterone (Depo-Provera, Upjohn) for use as a contraceptive. The synthetic progesterone is already approved for the treatment of inoperable, recurrent and metastatic endometrial or renal cancer, but approval as a contraceptive had been held up since the 1970s because of a paucity of long-term data and a suspected link with breast cancer.

Another controversial agent, the so-called abortion pill, RU 486, was found to be an effective postcoital contraceptive. British studies had a combined cohort of nearly 600 women, none of whom became pregnant after unprotected intercourse if they took RU 486 within 72 hours. The drug is expected to present an important policy issue to the Clinton administration.

On the diagnostic front, London researchers successfully tested a three-day-old embryo, conceived via in-vitro fertilization, for cystic fibrosis before implantation; it went on to develop into a healthy newborn girl. An important diagnostic warning was issued at the American College of Obstetricians and Gynecologists annual meeting in Las Vegas. Physicians reported that serum CA-125 and pelvic sonography should not be used

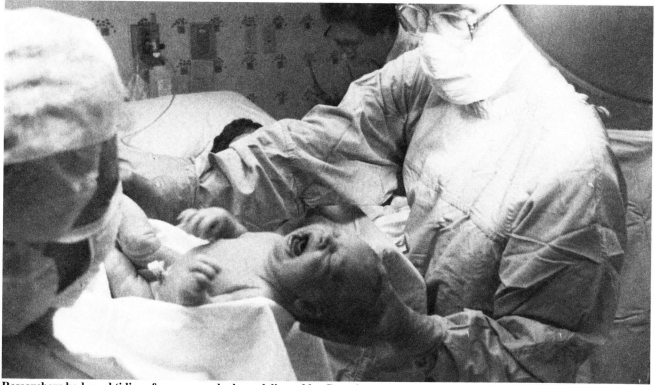

Researchers had good tidings for women who have delivered by C-section and want to go the vaginal route the next time around.

to screen for ovarian cancer in most women. The experts said the tests are not sensitive or reliable and recommended transvaginal ultrasound be used for women at high risk for malignancy.

One of the year's biggest controversies centered on silicone breast implants. First, the FDA restricted their use to breast-cancer patients and clinical trials because of doubts about the overall safety of the devices. Then, in June, a Canadian study of over 25,000 women found no evidence that implants increase the risk of breast cancer. Despite the findings, the FDA stuck with its restriction because doubts about overall safety, based on anecdotal evidence, persisted.

Another headline generator was a five-year study in which women who consumed three to six alcoholic drinks per week were found to have higher levels of estradiol than those who had fewer than three drinks per week or who abstained from alcohol. The University of Pittsburgh researchers said the findings are important considerations for women at risk of postmenopausal osteoporosis. The results stirred a call for caution in some quarters because of experimental evidence linking alcohol consumption and breast cancer.

In obstetrics, San Francisco researchers had good tidings for women who have delivered by caesarean section and want to deliver vaginally on their next birth. The study of 283 attempts at subsequent vaginal delivery showed a 63% success rate, reducing the length of hospital stays by an average of 1.3 days.

Affecting pregnancy in general, Florida investigators said this year that national guidelines for weight gain during pregnancy need to be re-evaluated. The University of Florida researchers found that women who were overweight before

pregnancy or who gained too much weight during pregnancy had unusually large infants and required caesarean sections more often than women who followed National Academy of Sciences guidelines regarding weight gain. In July, the CDC warned of the dangers of insufficient prenatal weight gain. When women gain fewer than the recommended 25 to 30 pounds during a full-term pregnancy, their risk of delivering an underweight infant increases by 75%.

The American Academy of Pediatrics also offered advice to pregnant women this year. In November, it advised that all pregnant women be tested for streptococcus B infection in the seventh month of pregnancy, in order to detect the 15% to 40% who carry strep B bacteria in their vaginal tracts.

When it comes to labor-and-delivery innovations, Medical Tribune was one of the few chroniclers of an unusual experiment in which dolphins were employed to help pregnant women relax prior to delivery. A London obstetrician arranged for 12 British women, accompanied by their husbands, to go to Israel to swim with dolphins in a closed-off bay on the Red Sea in the last weeks of pregnancy and early stages of labor. However, the Israeli Health Ministry objected to the experiment. After swimming with the dolphins for several weeks, the women ultimately gave birth in plastic minipools in a hospital.

Finally, women of "nonchildbearing age" got some rejuvenating news in September from a group of investigators at the University of Southern California. Researchers there reported that women as old as 52 were able to conceive and carry to term with the oocyte donation procedure. In November, a California grandmother did them one better by bearing twins at age 53 following IVF, using donated oocytes.

JANUARY

Jan. 2

A California ob/gyn declared that home uterine-activity monitoring is not effective in preventing preterm labor. Writing in Obstetrics and Gynecology, he criticized existing studies that claim a benefit of home uterine-monitoring saying that deficiencies in the trials may account for the small difference in outcome.

Jan. 6

Obstetricians and their patients were reassured that even when a pregnant woman contracts chicken pox during the first 13 weeks of pregnancy, the risk of severe fetal abnormalities is low. Forty women were examined by ultrasound between 16 and 20 weeks' gestation after having suffered varicella infection during the first trimester of pregnancy, according to a report in Obstetrics and Gynecology. One fetal abnormality was detected, a visceral herniation believed to be unrelated to the maternal infection, said specialists at the University of Connecticut.

Jan. 7

The National Abortion Rights Action League warned that 15 million American women are at risk of losing access to abortion. The group predicted that if the U.S. Supreme Court overturns Roe v. Wade, 13 states are likely to ban abortion immediately and another 13 will move toward stringent restrictions.

Jan. 10

French researchers determined that a hidden genetic mutation of the progesterone receptor may block the action of the progesterone analogue RU 486 in some women. The finding may explain why 1% of women do not respond to the abortifacient, researchers from Centre de Recherche Roussel-Uclaf in Romainville wrote in Science.

Jan. 11

A study of more than 2,000 eight- and nine-year-olds de-termined that women who undergo routine second-trimester ultrasonography do not increase their offspring's risk of developing learning disabilities. Testing of a subgroup of 603 children for dyslexia also showed no significant difference in incidence in those whose mothers had

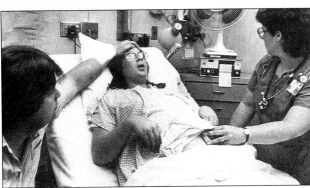
Home monitors called ineffective at preventing preterm labor.

undergo ultrasound and those whose mothers did not, Norwegian researchers reported in The Lancet.

Jan. 15

Young children with Chlamydia trachomatis were often infected at birth and not through sexual abuse, as many physicians assume, cautioned Seattle researchers. A study of 22 infants showed that those infected with chlamydia at birth can harbor the organism for as long as 28 months in the absence of antimicrobial therapy, the University of Washington team reported in The Journal of the American Medical Association.

Jan. 22

Virginia researchers announced development of a birth control vaccine that may prevent pregnancy for up to five years. The vaccine, which could be injected or given orally, would stimulate a woman's immune system to make antibodies that would bind proteins on the head of sperm and render them in-fertile, according to the Ortho Pharmaceutical Company. Because the proteins are sperm-specific, developers anticipate no problem with the vaccine's triggering an immune reaction against the woman's own tissues. Trials in baboons and humans over the next five years will clarify the vaccine's efficacy and reversibility.

• • •

Ectopic pregnancies have increased almost fivefold since 1970, but deaths are down 90%, said a specialist at the Mayo Clinic and Foundation in Rochester, Minn. Use of intra-uterine devices and fertility drugs may have contributed to the increase, he wrote in The Journal of the American Medical Association. While an ectopic pregnancy can adversely affect future fertility, he noted that tubal-conserving operations, laparoscopic approaches and treatment with drugs such as methotrexate may improve outcome.

Jan. 25

An androgenic drug diminished cyclical breast pain by 80%, German researchers announced. Women who took 2.5 mg of gestrinone (Roussel Laboratories) twice a week reported an average 80% reduction in pain, compared with 37% in women receiving a placebo. However, more than 40% of the gestrinone-treated women reported side effects, including acne, abnormal hair growth and greasy skin or hair, the Johannes Gutenberg University researchers reported in The Lancet.

Jan. 27

A Seattle physician warned that while spermicides protect against many genital infections, they can damage vaginal tissue and may actually encourage vaginal colonization with E. coli.

In-vitro tests detailed in the Journal of Infectious Diseases showed that nonoxynol-9 inhibited most strains of lactobacilli while having little or no effect on E. coli, thus allowing overgrowth of the latter microorganism.

Since nonoxynol-9 can contain high levels of toxic peroxides, damage to normal tissues is also a possibility with spermicide use, the investigator cautioned.

Jan. 31

A Food and Drug Administration advisory committee voted unanimously to recommend approval of the first condom for women, but called

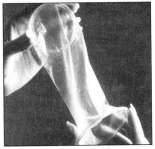
FDA called for more data on the seven-inch female condom.

for more data on the device's ability to prevent pregnancy and block the transmission of HIV and other sexually transmitted infections.

The seven-inch vaginal condom is made of lightweight, lubricated polyurethane and has two flexible rings, one that fits behind the pubic bone to cover the cervix and one that remains outside the body to cover the labia. The female condom (Reality, Wisconsin Pharmacal Co.) is twice as thick as a latex male condom.

Feb. 1

Sexual partners of persons with genital herpes were warned to use condoms even when a partner is asymptomatic. Researchers from the University of Washington evaluated 144 couples in which one partner had recurrent, symptomatic HSV. Although all couples abstained from intercourse when herpes lesions were present, 10% of the uninfected partners became infected during a one-year period. Seventy percent of the partners who transmitted the disease were asymptomatic at the time, according to data presented in the Annals of Internal Medicine. Male-to-female transmission was four times more common than men becoming infected from a female partner.

Feb. 3

A study from Boston University concluded that neither short- nor long-term estrogen replacement therapy increases a women's risk of developing breast cancer. In the study of 1,686 postmenopausal breast-cancer patients and 2,077 controls, neither short- nor long-term estrogen increased the risk, according to the report in the American Journal of Epidemiology.

Feb. 6

A new study confirmed that women who deliver their first baby by caesarean section can safely achieve vaginal deliveries in subsequent pregnancies. A review of 589 women who had had caesareans revealed that 283 attempted subsequent vaginal delivery; of these, 63% succeeded. None of the babies died or had serious injuries and no woman ruptured her uterus. Hospital stays of women who had a vaginal delivery were about 1.3 days shorter than those who had another caesarean, a San Francisco team told the meeting of the Society of Perinatal Obstetricians.

FEBRUARY

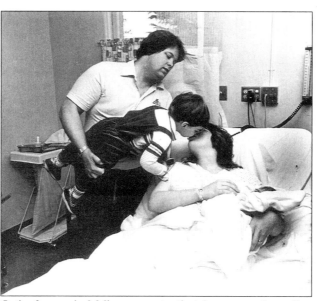

Opting for a vaginal delivery can get patients home over a day earlier.

Feb. 8

Australian researchers claimed to have achieved a 23% pregnancy rate by using microinjection of sperm to treat male infertility. The method involves ovarian stimulation, retrieving one or two eggs, placing them on a microscope slide and injecting five to 30 sperm under the zona pellucida into the perivitelline space in each oocyte.

Unlike zona drilling, another method of manipulating the gametes to aid fertilization, microinjection can succeed even when sperm have very poor motility, fertility specialists from the University of Sydney reported in The Lancet.

Feb. 10

The U.S. District Court in Virginia began hearing arguments in the case of Cecil Jacobson, M.D., an ob/gyn and self-proclaimed "baby-maker" in McLean. The charges: 53 counts of criminal fraud and perjury after allegedly using his own sperm, instead of donor sperm, to artificially inseminate as many as 75 women. Dr. Jacobson is also alleged to

have told many infertility patients that they were pregnant when they weren't, a few weeks later announcing there had been a miscarriage.

Feb. 13

Early amniotomy and use of high doses of oxytocin (Syntocinon, Sandoz) reduced the need for caesarean section in nulliparous women participating in a Northwestern University study. Women received amniotomy as soon as labor was diagnosed and were started on oxytocin at six times the normal dose if the rate of cervical dilation dropped below 1 cm per hour. Labors were shortened an average of 1.66 hours, researchers reported in The New England Journal of Medicine. The percentage of C-section deliveries in the aggressively managed labors was 10.5%, compared with 14.1% in women receiving traditional labor management.

• • •

The American Academy of Pediatrics recommended that all women of childbearing years be tested for HIV if they live in areas with a high incidence of AIDS or if they engage in high-risk behaviors.

Feb. 19

Women with atypical hyperplasia were found to be at increased risk of breast cancer, reported University of Southern California researchers. In their study of 121,700 nurses, there was a nearly fourfold increase in breast-cancer risk among women with atypical hyperplasia, as compared with women with no proliferative disease, they stated in The Journal of the American Medical Association.

Feb. 25

Both clindamycin plus cefamandole (Mandol, Lilly) and clindamycin plus doxycycline proved 100% effective in the treatment of pelvic inflammatory disease, Duke University researchers reported in the American Journal of Obstetrics and Gynecology.

The specialists also found that the specificity of clinical diagnosis was only 70%; of 33 patients who had severe PID by clinical diagnosis, only 23 cases were confirmed by laparoscopy.

Feb. 29

A multicenter study reassured women with manic-depressive illness and other affective disorders that they may safely continue lithium during pregnancy, provided that they obtain rigorous prenatal monitoring. The new study followed 138 women taking lithium (average daily dose, 927 mg) during the first trimester of pregnancy. Rates of major birth defects were no different than in 148 controls, investigators from the University of Toronto reported in The Lancet. However, one woman receiving lithium was determined to be carrying a fetus with Ebstein's anomaly, a rare cardiac malformation linked to lithium exposure in earlier case reports. The investigators suggest that pregnant women on lithium therapy should therefore receive level II ultrasound and fetal echocardiography as part of their prenatal care.

MARCH

March 1
A nine-year prospective study of more than 6,000 women found that those who smoke cigarettes may be 50% more likely than nonsmokers to develop cervical cancer or precancerous lesions. The researchers from the University of Tromsö in Norway determined that a dose-response relationship exists between smoking and risk of cancer or cervical intraepithelial neoplasia Grade III: Those who smoked 15 or more cigarettes a day, or for 10 years or more, were 80% more likely to develop the conditions. Smokers who had started before age 16 had twice the risk of nonsmokers, they stated

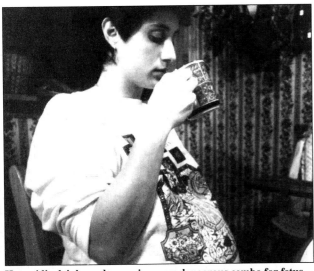

Hot acidic drinks and ceramic mugs: dangerous combo for fetus.

in the American Journal of Epidemiology.

March 3
Dutch researchers who conducted a maximal exercise test on 33 pregnant women concluded that strenuous exercise of limited duration is not harmful to the healthy mother or fetus. Exercise ECG tests revealed depression of the ST segment in 12% of the women; this incidence was unaffected by pregnancy, said the team from Erasmus University in Rotterdam. Blood pressure response to exercise was also unchanged by pregnancy. Exercise increased fetal heart

rate by an average of four beats per minute, the team stated in the American Journal of Obstetrics and Gynecology.

March 5
European researchers speculated that an immune-system gene may determine whether women with genital warts go on to develop cervical cancer. In reports in Nature, researchers found that the DQw3 version of the HLA antigen is found in increased frequency in women with cervical cancer. However, the cancer-associated version of the HLA gene is so common in the general population that it alone cannot be considered a good predictor of cancer risk.
Based on studies in rabbits, researchers from the Pasteur Institute found evidence of genetic control of wart evolution, with certain immune-system genes associated with wart regression and others with malignant transformation of virus-induced warts.

March 6
Pennsylvania's abortion law subverts informed consent and erects needless and health-threatening obstacles to abortion, the American College of Obstetricians and Gynecologists and six other medical

organizations argued in an amicus curiae brief submitted to the Supreme Court.
In a contrasting brief, the 680-member American Association of Pro-Life Obstetricians and Gynecologists asked the court to use the Pennsylvania case to abandon the Roe v. Wade decision entirely.

March 14
Extended echocardiography may be an important addition to routine screening in detecting rare fetal heart defects, said researchers from the Shaare Zedek Medical Center in Jerusalem. The standard four-chamber view revealed 11 heart defects in 5,400 fetuses, while extended ultrasound detected another seven defects, they reported in the British Medical Journal.

March 18
Home birth assisted by lay midwives proved as safe as hospital delivery and far less likely to end in caesarean section or the use of forceps or a vacuum extractor. Retrospectively comparing 1,707 deliveries at the Farm, which provides midwifery services in rural Tennessee, with a national probability sample of 14,033 physician-attended hospital deliveries, a public health physician found the rates of attended deliveries to be very low in the home birth group (2%), compared with the hospital birth group (27%). The C-section rate among the women giving birth at home was 1%, compared with 16% in the hospital, according to a report in the American Journal of Public Health. Perinatal deaths and complication rates were equivalent.

March 21
The notion that stress affects the menstrual cycle was challenged by a reproductive medicine expert at the meeting of the Society for Gynecological Investigation.

The University of California, San Francisco, physician gave metyrapone (Metopirone, Ciba Pharmaceutical) to 18 healthy women to trigger production of high levels of corticotropin-releasing factor, simulating the body's response to stress. No matter what the stage of their menstrual cycle, the drug did not affect the women's levels of luteinizing hormone, follicle-stimulating hormone or prolactin.

March 27
Four out of five American women continue to distrust the intrauterine contraceptive device, researchers told a Population Council conference. Even if it were recommended by their doctor, a mere 13% of American women would even consider using an IUD, said an official of the Alan Guttmacher Institute.

• • •

Pregnant women should be advised to avoid drinking hot beverages from lead-glazed mugs because of potential danger to their fetuses, a Food and Drug Administration official told a Senate committee. The largest single source of dietary lead is lead-glazed ceramic dishware. Hot acidic beverages, such as coffee, have a greater tendency to leach lead, said the FDA Deputy Commissioner. He also warned against storing highly acidic substances such as citrus juices in ceramic containers.

March 31
The National Center for Health Statistics revealed that pregnant women aged 35 and over are more than twice as likely to deliver via caesarean section as are teenage mothers. Statistics from 1990 presented in the journal Birth also documented that the U.S. C-section rate of 23.5% is stable, but still the third highest in the world; C-section rates in the South are significantly higher than in the West; and women with private health insurance are more likely to undergo C-section than those covered by Medicaid or paying for their own care.

APRIL

April 1

The perfect contraceptive for women at high risk for breast cancer may be a low-dose estrogen pill combined with monthly leuprolide (Lupron, Tap Pharmaceuticals) injections, a University of Southern California researcher told the annual Science Writers Seminar sponsored by the

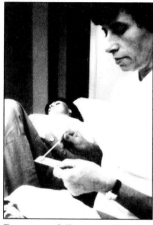

Pap smear follow-up: 60% of mild dysplasia disappeared.

American Cancer Society. The approach aims to reduce the stimulatory effect of estrogen by cutting the dose by two thirds, adding small amounts of medroxyprogesterone acetate for 13 days each month and giving leuprolide injections every 28 days, the investigator said. Results were not available on the first five women taking the combination pill.

April 4

British researchers reported that women whose Pap smears indicate mild dysplasia may not require immediate referral for colposcopy to determine if they have cervical cancer. In a study of 500 women with mildly to moderately dyskaryotic Pap smears, 300 Pap test results returned to normal and remained normal during a seven-year follow-up period, the Cambridge University team reported in The Lancet. An expert from Columbia-Presbyterian Medical Center in New York disputed their conclusion, saying that colposcopy detects cases that need rapid treatment.

April 11

Pregnant drivers were advised that a small cushion can make using a seat belt safer and more comfortable. Obstetricians from St. Helier Hospital in Surrey, England, suggested that if women tuck a small pillow under the lap belt, it will prevent the strap from riding up and pressing on the pubic bone. Women with scars from a caesarean section or other abdominal surgery may also benefit from the added cushioning, they suggested in the British Medical Journal.

April 13

A University of California obstetrician revealed that increasing numbers of medical programs are making abortion training optional or dropping it altogether. Of 225 programs responding to a survey, 12% offered compulsory or routine training in first-trimester abortions in 1991, down from 23% in 1985. He told a meeting of the National Abortion Federation in San Diego that he is concerned about access to abortion as well-trained and motivated doctors approach retirement and younger doctors fail to get the training to take their place.

April 14

The World Health Organization announced that half a million women die from complications of pregnancy and childbirth worldwide each year. In developing countries, only about 50% of births are attended by a health professional; in some countries in South Asia, the rate is 10%.

April 15

Pregnant women were warned to stay away from deli counter foods, undercooked meats and imported soft cheeses to minimize their risk of listeriosis infection. Besides killing an estimated one quarter of those infected, listeriosis during pregnancy can lead to stillbirth or cause meningitis in

the newborn. A case-control study by Centers for Disease Control investigators documented foodborne transmission of the bacteria, particularly in soft Mexican cheeses and undercooked foods.

April 18

Chilean obstetricians touted breast-feeding as a safe and effective family planning method for the postpartum months. Of 409 women who exclusively breast-fed their babies (no more than one supplemental feeding per week) and remained amenorrheic, only one became pregnant during a six-month follow-up, they reported in The Lancet. With exclusive breast-feeding, only 9% of women restarted menses by three months and 19% by 180 days, stated the researchers from Pontificia Universidad Catolica de Chile.

April 25

Danish researchers said that fish-oil supplements may be indicated for women at high risk of preterm delivery. Healthy pregnant women who took the supplements starting in the 30th week of pregnancy carried their fetuses four days longer and gave birth to infants weighing 3.7 ounces more than women given olive-oil capsules or no supplements, the researchers stated in The Lancet. A multicenter trial is under way to test their theory.

April 28

Women who are treated for precancerous cervical lesions may still develop cancer if they neglect to obtain follow-up Pap smears, cautioned physicians at the Southern California Permanente Medical Group in San Diego. Fifteen of 21 women diagnosed with cervical cancer after previous treatment had not received follow-up cytology, the physicians told the American College of Obstetricians and Gynecologists meeting in Las Vegas.

April 29

Serum CA-125 and pelvic sonography are not sensitive or reliable, and should not be used in most women for ovarian-cancer screening, a New York expert told the American College of Obstetricians and Gynecologists meeting. A researcher from the University of Kentucky said that in a study of 1,300 asymptomatic women screened with transvaginal ultrasound, 14 benign serous tumors and two primary ovarian cancers were detected. Both cancers were stage I and CA-125 and pelvic exams were normal in both cases. Experts at the Las Vegas meeting said that transvaginal ultrasound may be useful for women at high risk for malignancy.

• • •

Pregnant women who received weekly prenatal care from a nurse-midwife were less likely to give birth to a dangerously underweight infant than women who received standard prenatal care from a doctor, declared investigators from the Medical University of South Carolina. That observation emerged out of a comparison of 89 twins whose mothers had received care from a nurse-midwife at a university clinic with two other groups of twins whose mothers had been seen by residents in the high-risk obstetrics clinic. Of the twins in the midwife group, 6% were under 3.2 pounds at birth, compared with 18% and 26% in the nonmidwife groups. Speaking at the ACOG meeting, the researchers attributed the finding to better follow-up care of women in the midwife group.

• • •

Government researchers at the ACOG meeting added more data to the evidence that pregnant women who smoke can damage the placenta. For each half pack of cigarettes a pregnant woman smokes per day, the risk of placentae abruptio increases by 20%, physicians from the National Institute of Child Health and Human Development in Bethesda, Md., reported.

May 1

Postmenopausal women learned that smoking could negate the beneficial effects of estrogen. A study in the Annals of Internal Medicine described 207 women with an average age of 75 who had broken their hip. Current smoking alone did not increase the risk of a fracture, nor did current estrogen use. But women who smoked and took estrogen had the highest rate of fractures. The Brown University researchers concluded that percutaneous estrogen may be a better alternative for women who wish to continue smoking cigarettes while on estrogen replacement therapy.

May 2

Japanese researchers suggested that human papillomavirus 16 can be transmitted by sexual intercourse. In a study of 23 couples, four male partners of the 12 HPV-16-positive women harbored the same HPV type in their semen. None of the partners of HPV-negative women harbored HPV, investigators from Osaka University Medical School reported in The Lancet.

May 4

The Centers for Disease Control announced that Secretary for Health and Human Services Louis Sullivan was reviewing an educational plan aimed at increasing mammography use in minority women. The National Strategic Plan for the Early Detection and Control of Breast Cancer was drafted to work with ongoing education and screening programs run by federal and state agencies as well as public health organizations and private groups.

May 6

Overall survival at an average of 43 months' follow-up was not increased when radiation was used after lumpectomy in 837 women in a study at the Ontario Cancer Institute/ Princess Margaret Hospital. However, recurrence

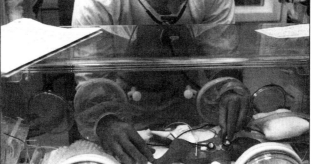
Premature births could be cut if women were treated for chlamydia.

rate was significantly different, with 26% repeat cancers in women who received only lumpectomy, compared with just 6% in women treated with lumpectomy and radiation, the Canadian researchers reported in the Journal of the National Cancer Institute.

May 9

Patients who use in-vitro fertilization to get pregnant may benefit from polymerase chain reaction testing to detect cystic fibrosis in a fertilized egg before it is put into the woman's womb, suggested a study by researchers from Brussels Free University.

PCR can be done much earlier than amniocentesis, which cannot be performed until 15 to 18 weeks into the pregnancy, according to the report in The Lancet.

May 13

A study of prostitutes became the first to implicate anal intercourse as a major risk factor in hepatitis B transmission from men to women. Among 1,368 prostitutes participating in a Centers for Disease Control study, those who did not inject drugs were most at risk for hepatitis B if they engaged in frequent anal intercourse, had syphilis or were infected with HIV. In

The Journal of the American Medical Association, the government researchers advised that women always use a barrier contraceptive.

May 20

Baylor College of Medicine researchers reported that polymerase chain reaction is a sensitive, accurate and inexpensive test for the detection of Duchenne and Becker's muscular dystrophy in fetuses. They determined that the method detects more than 80% of dystrophic gene deletions, enabling rapid diagnosis in 45% to 50% of cases. PCR requires less than one day for analysis, is easy to perform and is 99.9% accurate, noted the researchers.

May 21

Harvard researchers warned women that smoking during pregnancy can cut their newborns' lung function in half. After measuring lung capacity and airflow in 80 infants, aged two to six weeks, the investigators found that infants of smokers had smaller airways, less elastic lungs and only half the forced expiratory volume of comparably sized children of nonsmokers. In the American Review of Respiratory Disease, the physicians cautioned that poor pulmonary

function in infancy is associated with a greater incidence of asthma and other respiratory illnesses throughout childhood.

May 28

The number of premature births could be cut dramatically if all pregnant women received broad-spectrum antibiotics for chlamydial infections, University of Maryland researchers said at the American Society for Microbiology meeting in New Orleans.

Giving all pregnant women antibiotics would also be more cost-effective than screening and treating only those with the infections, they said. The pediatric team estimated that giving antibiotics to all pregnant women would save $2,728 per pregnant woman, while treating only those who tested positive for chlamydia would save $228 per pregnant woman. Their theoretical model proposed that the women receive erythromycin and their partners receive doxycycline for seven days, at a total cost of $19.

• • •

University of Mississippi researchers claimed that pregnant women who already have a child may be as adept as physicians at predicting the weight of their babies. The physicians asked 93 women in labor to predict the weight of their babies. Almost half estimated within 5% of the actual birthweight and 66% guessed within 10%, according to a report in The New England Journal of Medicine.

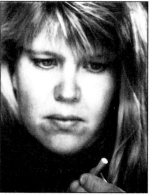
Babies born to smokers are more likely to have poor lung function.

June 1

Ob/gyns are hit with the lion's share of lawsuits for failure to diagnose breast cancer, warned attorneys who specialize in malpractice. Most cases are settled outside of court for between $500,000 and $2 million, a New York attorney told a symposium on breast-cancer malpractice. Recipes for defendant failure include using "so-what" arguments that early diagnosis would not have helped, relying solely on negative mammogram results (an estimated 20% are false negatives) and any defense in which a physician altered office records, the attorneys cautioned.

•••

A woman who exercises regularly can reduce the discomforts of pregnancy without harming her fetus, reported physicians from Kaiser Permanente in Oakland, Calif., at the American College of Sports Medicine meeting in Dallas.

A prospective study of 388 women from 15.5 weeks' gestation through delivery found that those who exercised the most reported the fewest symptoms, such as nausea and bloating. The exercise had no effect on the infant's birthweight, the study found.

June 6

Conception and live birth rates achieved with in-vitro fertilization decline with age, with women over age 40 having a 15% chance of having a baby after five IVF attempts, reported researchers at the King's College of Medicine in London. In contrast, more than half of women between 20 and 34 conceived after five cycles, and 45% had babies, they reported in The Lancet.

Based on one IVF unit's experience with 5,055 consecutive IVF cycles in 2,735 women and 518 live births, they found that the success rate drops by about 8% after each attempt and is greatly reduced when the male is infertile or the female has multiple infertility problems.

June 11

Geneticists warned that a new fluorescence in-situ hybridization test for prenatal diagnosis of aneuploidy is inadequate and should not be used as an alternative to karyotyping. They reported the case of a 40-year-old woman at 19 weeks' gestation who was told, based on a FISH analysis of amniotic-fluid cells, that her fetus was female and had Turner's syndrome. But an ultrasound exam at the time of amniocentesis showed that the woman was carrying a male fetus and a subsequent karyotype showed the fetus was

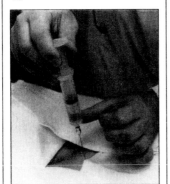

Amniocentesis is relatively safe for fetus if done before 12 weeks.

normal, the geneticists wrote in a letter to The New England Journal of Medicine. The woman gave birth to a normal baby boy.

Integrated Genetics, which makes the InSight Rapid Chromosome Analysis FISH test, replied in the journal that the test has a high accuracy rate, and should be used in combination with, not as a substitute for, standard chromosome tests.

•••

A Canadian study of 3,407 women revealed that artificially inducing labor in women who were more than two weeks past their expected delivery date lowered the rate of caesarean sections and fetal distress. The study did not find statistically significant differences in the rate of infant death or illness between women

whose pregnancies were artificially induced and those who were simply monitored. However, when combined with previous studies, the results showed that artificial inducement was slightly safer than monitoring and should be the method of choice, the researchers concluded in The New England Journal of Medicine.

June 13

Women with mild dyskaryosis can safely be followed with a series of repeat Pap smears, concluded British gynecologists. When women received repeat Pap smears at six, 12 and 24 months after mild cytological abnormalities were detected, only one third eventually required colposcopy and 4% developed more serious precancerous conditions (small cervical intraepithelial neoplasia Grade 3 lesions), the multicenter team reported in The Lancet.

•••

Researchers from Taiwan reminded gynecologists that the presence of genital human papillomavirus does not necessarily indicate sexual contact. When the polymerase chain reaction was used to detect HPV in vulvar swabs from 118 women undergoing premarital physical examinations, women who reported no sexual experience were infected about as frequently as women who reported having had sexual experience (15% vs. 12%). Writing in The Lancet, the team theorized that the virus may have been transmitted via nonsexual contact, or the women might have become infected at birth.

June 18

The silicone breast implant debate was fueled by a Canadian study of more than 25,000 women that found no evidence that implants increase a woman's risk of breast cancer.

Researchers from the Alberta Cancer Board searched the

medical data registries of 11,676 women who underwent cosmetic augmentation from 1973 to 1986 and 13,557 women diagnosed with primary breast cancer. In the cohort that underwent silicone implantation, 86.2 cases of breast cancer were expected and 41 cases were observed, the researchers reported in The New England Journal of Medicine.

Despite the findings, the Food and Drug Administration stuck with its restrictions on the use of the implants because of doubts about the overall safety of the devices, according to a report by the FDA commissioner.

June 19

An FDA advisory committee recommended approval of the injectable contraceptive medroxyprogesterone (Depo-Provera, Upjohn).

The synthetic progesterone is already approved in the United States for the treatment of inoperable, recurrent and metastatic endometrial or renal cancer and in 90 other countries as a contraceptive.

The depot contraceptive was denied approval in 1978 after some studies indicated it could increase the risk of breast cancer. A recent nine-year World Health Organization study found that the drug does not increase the overall risk of breast cancer, although that risk does increase slightly within the first four years of taking the drug, mainly in women under 35.

June 25

Amniocentesis, traditionally done 16 to 18 weeks into pregnancy, was found to be relatively safe for the fetus when done at less than 12 weeks, reported University of California, Davis, researchers. The miscarriage rate for 936 women who had the procedure at 12 weeks or less was 3.4%, compared with 0.3% to 2.8% when done at 15 to 18 weeks, according to the study, published in the American Journal of Obstetrics and Gynecology.

July 1

Mayo Clinic researchers reported that estrogen patches can prevent fractures and even rebuild bone mass in women with established osteoporosis.

They gave 39 women a combination patch containing estrogen and progesterone, and 39 a placebo. During a one-year period, seven women in the treatment group suffered eight new fractures, compared with 20 fractures in 12 women in the placebo group. Spinal bone density also increased 5% in the women who used the patch, the investigators stated in the Annals of Internal Medicine.

• • •

Canadian researchers alerted obstetricians that episiotomies often lead to tearing of the rectal sphincter and rectum and may delay the resumption of intercourse after childbirth.

Obstetricians for more than 1,000 women in the McGill University study were randomly instructed to attempt to either "avoid a tear" or "avoid an episiotomy." Of the 47 severe tears that entered the rectal sphincter or rectum, 46 occurred in patients who had received an episiotomy, it was reported in the Online Journal of Current Clinical Trials. Women who had not undergone an episiotomy resumed intercourse a week earlier than those who had the surgery. Urinary problems occurred in 20% to 30% of the women, regardless of whether they had had an episiotomy.

July 7

National Institutes of Health scientists reported that the controversial abortion pill RU 486 may be effective as a contraceptive.

Their research showed that RU 486 (Roussel-Uclaf) retarded endometrial maturation in six of nine women and reduced peak levels of a placental protein in all nine. Participants in the study, which appeared in the

American Journal of Obstetrics and Gynecology, took 1 mg of the medication a day, as compared with the 600-mg dose used as an abortifacient. Previous research had demonstrated that daily RU 486 prevented pregnancy in guinea pigs.

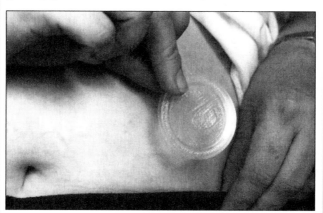

Estrogen patch may rebuild bone mass in women with osteoporosis.

July 15

Federal researchers revealed that the number of multiple live births has more than doubled during the past two decades.

Multiple births rose 152% for white women aged 30-34, and 165% for white women aged 35-39, according to researchers from the National Center for Health Statistics. There was a 22% increase in multiple births among African-Americans, they reported in the American Journal of Diseases of Children. The rise was attributed to increasing use of fertility drugs as women get older.

July 23

University of Pittsburgh researchers found that three to six alcoholic drinks a week may lower the risk of postmenopausal osteoporosis by increasing estradiol levels. Their five-year study of 128 women determined that estradiol levels increased in a stepwise progression, starting with three drinks a week and leveling

off at six drinks a week. Women who abstained from alcohol had the lowest levels of estradiol, the investigators told Medical Tribune. Given some experimental evidence linking alcohol consumption with breast cancer, it was advised that the results be interpreted with caution.

July 26

German researchers reported that infants of mothers who smoke are more likely to have bronchial hyperresponsiveness upon exercise by the time they reach elementary school than infants of nonsmokers. Maternal smoking during pregnancy or after infancy does not seem to cause the condition, according to the report in the Journal of Pediatrics.

The University Children's Hospital in Freiburg research project involved 1,461 first-grade children in southern Germany. Nine percent of children whose mothers smoked during their infancy had bronchial hyperresponsiveness, compared with about 6% of children whose mothers did not smoke during their infancy.

July 30

The Canadian Preterm Labor Investigators Group revealed that use of the beta-adrenergic agonist ritodrine

may hurt pregnant women more than it helps their infants. In a randomized comparison of intravenous ritodrine (Yutopar, Astra) and placebo, 708 women at six hospitals were treated for preterm labor. Ritodrine delayed delivery by 24 to 48 hours, but there was no difference in perinatal outcome: Rates of death, low birthweight, respiratory distress and other complications were similar. However, more side effects were reported among women receiving ritodrine than those on placebo, chiefly chest pain and cardiac arrhythmias, the team reported in The New England Journal of Medicine. One woman taking ritodrine developed pulmonary edema.

July 31

Scientists from the Centers for Disease Control warned that many women still gain insufficient weight during pregnancy, thereby increasing their chance of delivering a low-birthweight infant. After reviewing almost four million birth certificates, the CDC investigators found that approximately 17% of white mothers and 27% of African-American mothers who carried their pregnancies at least 40 weeks gained 20 pounds or less, compared with the recommended 25 to 35 pounds. Failing to gain sufficient weight during pregnancy increases the risk of having an underweight infant by an estimated 75%.

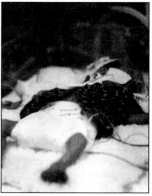

Scanty weight gain in pregnancy boosts low-birthweight risk 75%.

AUGUST

Aug. 1

Researchers at the University of Florida in Gainesville called for a re-evaluation of national guidelines recommending substantial weight gain during pregnancy. They found that women who gain too much weight during pregnancy, or who are overweight before they become pregnant, are at higher risk of having unusually large babies and needing emergency caesarean sections.

In a study of 3,191 women of varying weight, published in the American Journal of Obstetrics and Gynecology, 12% had babies weighing more than nine pounds. These women were more likely to have been overweight before becoming pregnant, or to have gained substantial weight during pregnancy.

Using multiple logistic regression, the team showed that if weight gain were limited in all cases to the maximum National Academy of Sciences recommendation, the predicted unscheduled C-section rate would be 9.7%; if all weight gain were limited to the lowest NAS recommendation, it would fall to 8.1%. The investigators did not, however, offer specific new weight-gain guidelines.

Aug. 7

Medical Tribune reported on an unusual experiment in which pregnant women would spend time swimming with dolphins as an aid to relaxing prior to delivery. Greater relaxation should lead to less pain and fewer complications during delivery, explained the London obstetrician who initiated the project.

A group of 12 British women and their husbands were scheduled to travel to Israel, accompanied by five physicians, volunteer midwives and massage therapists, said the obstetrician from Whipps Cross Hospital. Each day during the last weeks of pregnancy and the early stages of labor, the women were to

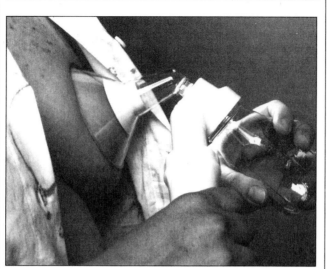

Mothers who use breast pumps likely to breast-feed longer.

swim in a closed-off bay on the Red Sea with six adult dolphins and one baby dolphin. They would then give birth in the bay or, if the water were found to be contaminated, in a separate shallow pool.

Aug. 8

Fluoxetine may relieve the symptoms of severe premenstrual syndrome, researchers at Otago Medical School in Dunedin, New Zealand, reported in the British Medical Journal.

Fifteen of 21 women with PMS who were given fluoxetine (Prozac, Dista) for three months showed a good or very good response, the investigators said. When the women were switched to placebo for three months, only three showed improvement, as compared with baseline. The drug enhances serotonin levels in the brain, which are thought to be blunted premenstrually, the researchers said.

Aug. 15

University of Iowa pediatricians reported that new mothers who are sent home from the hospital with manual breast pumps are likely to breast-feed longer than those who receive samples of infant formula. An eight-week study of 146 women found that

"the breast pump facilitated the feeding process" and kept the mothers breast-feeding about 1.5 weeks longer than those using infant formula alone.

The breast pump also had a significant impact on the subgroup of women who believed that bottle-feeding made night-time feeding easier. Thirty percent of these women breast-fed their babies during the study period, compared with 8% of mothers given formula samples, the physicians wrote in Pediatrics.

Aug. 19

Pregnant women should be advised to forgo hot tubs and saunas in the first trimester. That was the message from a study of 23,491 pregnant women that looked at whether heat is a teratogen.

Women exposed to heat from hot tubs or saunas in the first trimester had more than twice the risk of having an infant with a neural-tube defect than women who were not exposed, reported Boston University researchers in The Journal of the American Medical Association. Exposure to heat from a fever in early pregnancy almost doubled the risk, but heat from an electric blanket did not substantially increase risk, they found.

Aug. 20

Pregnant women who have light snacks just before delivery may have shorter labor and stronger babies, an Irish study found. Researchers at the Jubilee Hospital in Belfast studied 90 women, half of whom drank only clear fluids during labor, and half of whom ate scrambled eggs, toast, jelly or ice cream until they were in advanced labor. Those who ate during labor required fewer labor-inducing drugs and painkillers, the researchers told Medical Tribune. Their babies also had stronger heartbeats and better muscle tone. A heavy meal, however, was not recommended, in case a caesarean section is needed that requires general anesthesia.

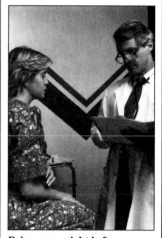

Being overweight before pregnancy may lead to C-sections.

Aug. 27

The combination of alpha-fetoprotein, estriol and chorionic gonadotropin is more effective than alpha-fetoprotein alone when screening for Down's syndrome, researchers reported in The New England Journal of Medicine. In a study of 1,661 women, the combo screen detected 58% of Down's cases, compared with 35% using alpha-fetoprotein alone.

In an accompanying editorial, a California obstetrician said that screening for all three markers "could reduce the number of women who undergo amniocentesis" to confirm the diagnosis.

SEPTEMBER

Sept. 1

University of California researchers found that an ultrasound-guided biopsy may be used to detect Duchenne muscular dystrophy prenatally. The procedure, performed around the 20th week of pregnancy, uses an ultrasound-guided needle inserted into the abdomen to extract a fetal muscle biopsy from the gluteal region. Fluorescent antibody molecules that attach only to normal dystrophin are used as markers to detect the presence or absence of the protein, the San Francisco researchers explained in the German journal Human Genetics. The procedure may be of added benefit in dystrophy detection when the results of DNA testing with amniocentesis or chorionic villus sampling are inconclusive, said the investigators.

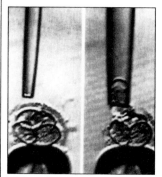

Eight-cell embryos can be checked for cystic fibrosis gene.

Sept. 7

In a nine-month follow-up of 91 women with abnormal squamous cells detected on Pap smear, most returned to normal without treatment, announced University of California, Los Angeles, gynecologists. Of 203 women with original Pap readings of low-grade squamous intraepithelial lesions, 78% resolved with no treatment, the UCLA team revealed in Obstetrics and Gynecology.

The investigators recommended repeat Pap smears every three months, as well as an initial colposcopic examination, as an alternative to immediate treatment for women with low-grade lesions.

Sept. 9

University of Southern California researchers demonstrated that oocyte donation can help women up to age 52 successfully conceive and carry their pregnancies to term. The doctors studied three groups of women: two groups, 65 postmenopausal women aged 40 or older and 35 women below age 40, were implanted with fertilized, donated oocytes. The third group of 57 women over age 40 underwent standard in-vitro fertilization with their own eggs. The researchers reported in The Journal of the American Medical Association that just over one third of the over-40 women using donated eggs, including a 51-year-old and a 52-year-old, gave birth to healthy babies. That rate was as good as that for women under 40 receiving donated eggs, and considerably better than the 9% rate for the women over 40 who had attempted IVF with their own eggs, said the investigators.

Sept. 11

Transvaginal alcohol sclerosis was used to treat postmenopausal women with ovarian cysts with a low risk of malignancy, McGill University physicians reported. In a preliminary study, the researchers tested the technique on seven patients with recurrent ovarian cysts. After aspirating the cyst contents, approximately two thirds of the aspirated fluid was replaced with 100% alcohol that was left in place for 20 minutes and then reaspirated. Four cysts had not recurred at follow-up exams performed 2, 5, 7 and 12 months, respectively, after sclerosis, the Montreal team reported in Radiology.

Sept. 16

A group of pregnant British women who flew to Israel to give birth right after swimming with dolphins in the Red Sea were told by the Israeli Health

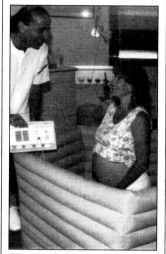

Women who hoped to give birth with dolphins landed in minipools.

Ministry to make alternative birthing plans. The government said births are forbidden in unlicensed locations, so the women decided to give birth in plastic minipools at a hospital. The idea behind the dolphin project was to create an enjoyable and relaxed environment for the expectant women and their babies, possibly reducing the pain, trauma and risk of complications associated with delivery.

Sept. 24

British and Texas researchers announced the birth of a girl who had passed preimplantation testing for cystic fibrosis. The method, which relies on a variant of polymerase chain reaction to amplify shards of genetic material, may be used to screen for other genetic diseases, such as hemophilia, Tay-Sachs disease and muscular dystrophy, said the investigators.

After in-vitro fertilization, the researchers pierced the zona pellucida with an acid and siphoned off one cell from each of the eight-cell embryos. They then used what they called nested PCR, in which primers were used to amplify the trinucleotide deletion on the cystic fibrosis transmembrane regulator gene. The technique, reported in The New England Journal of Medicine, could persuade many couples not to abort, but would require even fertile women to undergo costly IVF.

Sept. 26

British physicians advised that pregnant women be counseled about the risks of vaginal delivery of a breech baby, after finding that breech fetuses delivered by caesarean section are more likely to have a good outcome.

Researchers at St. Mary's Hospital in London studied 3,447 breech births over three years, 42% of which were delivered by a planned C-section, 30% by emergency C-section and 28% vaginally. Excluding stillbirth and death from unrelated birth defects, eight infants who were delivered vaginally died during or just after birth, while one infant died after C-section delivery, the team reported in the British Medical Journal. In addition, the numbers of low Apgar scores and neonatal intubation were doubled in babies born vaginally or by emergency C-section compared with those delivered by an elective operation.

• • •

Levels of relaxin secreted during pregnancy were found to be above normal in diabetic women, even when they maintained tight control of their diabetes, said a researcher from the University of Newcastle upon Tyne in England. As described in The Lancet, serum relaxin levels were found to be significantly higher in each trimester in 23 insulin-dependent diabetic women than in nine healthy non-diabetic controls. The researcher noted that the physiological importance of the higher levels of relaxin in diabetics—including whether they contribute to the higher incidence of major anomalies in the fetuses of diabetic mothers—is yet to be determined.

Obstetrics/Gynecology

Oct. 8

Scottish researchers found that RU 486 is a highly effective postcoital contraceptive. The University of Edinburgh team found that none of over 400 women given RU 486 (Roussel-Uclaf) within 72 hours after unprotected sexual intercouse became pregnant, compared with four of about 400 women who received the standard therapy of high-dose estrogen and progestogen. Nausea and vomiting were reported by signficantly fewer women given RU 486 than women on the standard therapy, although RU 486 did delay onset of the next menstrual period more frequently, they stated in The New England Journal of Medicine.

Oct. 10

Results from an Australian study indicated that women who undergo amniocentesis are less likely to suffer a miscarriage than women who undergo prenatal testing via chorionic villus sampling.

Researchers at the Murdoch Institute for Research into Birth Defects in Parkville, Australia, studied 150 hospitals with maternity facilities and over 300 obstetric practices, and reported in The Lancet that 1.3% of women miscarried after amniocentesis and 2.9% miscarried after CVS.

Two previous studies had shown that the two prenatal tests were equally safe. Those studies found that women simply are more likely to abort spontaneously earlier in their pregnancies, coincidentally the time when CVS is performed.

Oct. 12

Pregnant women with asthma were advised to continue taking their medication. Most asthma drugs pose no known risks to the unborn and can improve the supply of oxygen to the fetus, the chairman of the group of experts that prepared the report told the First National Conference on Asthma Management in Arlington, Va. Studies have shown that women whose asthma is left untreated during pregnancy tend to have more low-birthweight babies and a higher incidence of miscarriages and stillbirths than women without asthma or women whose asthma is controlled, the specialist from Rush-Presbyterian-St. Luke's Medical Center in Chicago said. He added that these women should monitor their lung function daily with a peak-flow meter to ensure that the fetus is getting enough oxygen. Women on theophylline should have their blood levels monitored because the drug can produce a stimulating effect on the fetus in high doses, he said.

Oct. 14

A new oral contraceptive containing the first new progestin marketed in the United States in more than 20 years was introduced by the Ortho-Pharmaceutical Corporation of Raritan, N.J. Norgestimate/ethinyl estradiol (Ortho-Cyclen) contains 0.25 mg of norgestimate combined with 35 mcg of ethinyl estradiol. Norgestimate has been widely used in Europe for six years, according to a company spokesperson.

Oct. 16

All women should undergo estrogen replacement therapy unless they have a family history of cancer, a Georgia physician told the annual meeting of the American Academy of Family Physicians in San Diego. While some studies have shown an increased risk of breast and uterine cancer in women taking estrogen, just as many studies have shown no increased risk, said the doctor from the Medical College of Georgia in Augusta. He said studies that have shown an increased risk pinpointed subgroups of women, such as those who had had hysterectomies, and not the general population.

Oct. 17

British investigators found that the abortion pill RU 486 is an effective "morning-after" pill, in a study that confirms research published earlier this month. None of almost 195 women given a single oral dose of RU 486 within 72 hours of unprotected intercourse became pregnant, compared with five pregnancies in 191 women given the standard therapy of high-dose estrogen and progestogen. And significantly fewer women given RU 486 had unwanted side effects (chiefly nausea and vomiting) than women given standard therapy, the University of Manchester team reported in the British Medical Journal.

Oct. 24

Boston researchers found that mammograms are an effective way of detecting early breast cancer in women under age 50, contradicting the findings of an unpublished Canadian study that was widely publicized earlier this year, which reportedly found no benefit in screening younger women.

Researchers at Massachusetts General Hospital studied 117 women under age 50 diagnosed with breast cancer through a mammogram between 1978 and 1991, and 928 women whose cancer was detected through a physical exam. Some 50% of women whose cancer was caught through a mammogram had early-stage cancer, compared with 30% of women in the physical-exam group. The survival rate after five years for women whose cancer had been found through a mammogram was 95%, while survival in women whose cancer had been detected through manual examination was 74%, they reported in The Lancet.

Oct. 29

New York State Psychiatric Institute researchers reported that women are likely to become depressed after a miscarriage regardless of the length of gestation or their attitude toward the pregnancy. Childless women are particularly prone to depression after a miscarriage, the researchers wrote in the American Journal of Public Health.

They interviewed 232 women within four weeks of miscarriage, 283 pregnant women and 318 women who had not recently become pregnant. Among women who had miscarried, the proportion who were highly symptomatic on the Center for Epidemiologic Studies Depression Scale was 3.4 times that of pregnant women and 4.3 times that of community women. Among childless women, the proportion of women who had miscarried and who were highly symptomatic was 5.7 times that of pregnant women and 11.0 times that of community women, the researchers found.

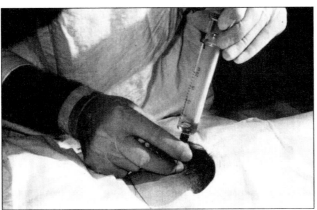

Women who undergo amniocentesis found less likely to miscarry.

Nov. 2

Attendees at the American Fertility Society meeting in New Orleans were told that a new technique for viewing the narrowest passageways of a woman's fallopian tubes may improve nonsurgical diagnosis and treatment of infertility-causing tubal diseases. In the technique, a lighted instrument called a falloscope is inserted through the vagina and into the narrow first portion of the fallopian tube. The falloscope looks for blockages and lesions that can render a woman infertile, and can also spot ectopic pregnancies, said the researcher from Flinders Medical Center in Adelaide, Australia.

He presented results of an international study that included 19 infertile women. A total of 20 abnormal lesions were found in 32 fallopian tubes. In 13 of the women, the new technique spotted problems unseen by traditional diagnostic techniques, resulting in an alteration of treatment.

Nov. 4

Omaha researchers reported that even women in their 20s can build bone mass by consuming more calcium and exercising a few times a week. The study, published in The Journal of the American Medical Association, also found that women who take oral contraceptives gain more bone mass than those who do not.

The Creighton University researchers followed 156 college-aged women for five years and found that those who consumed on average no more than 220 mg of calcium a day lost over 1% of their bone mass. Women who consumed 700 mg of calcium daily gained more than 3% bone mass, compared with a gain of more than 6% at an intake of 1,000 mg a day; a nearly 10% at 1,400 mg; and more than 16% at 2,100 mg.

In a separate analysis, sedentary women gained only about a quarter of a percent of spinal bone mass during the five-year period, while those who exercised regularly gained over 8%.

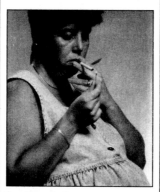

Smoking during pregnancy may put infants at risk of strabismus.

Nov. 5

Philadelphia physicians reported on an often-overlooked cause of pelvic infections: cat scratches.

A patient presented with a two-day history of crampy, intermittent right lower-quadrant pain radiating to the back and epigastrium. Diagnostic laparoscopy revealed a yellow, purulent exudate throughout the pelvis. Cultures of the pelvic fluid for gonorrhea and chlamydia proved negative, but on the fourth postoperative day they grew Pasteurella multocida. At that point, her physicians at the Hospital of the University of Pennsylvania learned she had been scratched several times on the legs by her cat. An ultrasound of her pelvis found a large infected mass that required the removal of her right ovary, they wrote in The New England Journal of Medicine. The Pennsylvania doctors said that at least three other researchers have reported cases of women who were infected by animals and had evidence of the same bacteria—P. multocida—in their cervical secretions.

• • •

The American Academy of Pediatrics issued guidelines advising that all pregnant women be tested for streptococcus B infections when they are seven months' pregnant, in order to reduce the risk of passing it on to their newborns during delivery.

The AAP recommendations include screening all pregnant women for strep B between weeks 26 and 28 of gestation; certain positive patients may require treatment with intravenous antibiotics during labor. Pregnant women admitted to the hospital for conditions such as premature labor or premature rupture of membranes should be tested immediately if it has not already been done, according to the AAP.

Nov. 7

An international team of researchers reported that women who take estrogen or calcium after menopause can significantly decrease their risk of suffering a hip fracture as they get older. The Mediterranean osteoporosis study compared 2,086 women who had suffered a hip fracture and 3,532 healthy women with no fractures. The relative risk of hip fracture was 0.55 in women taking estrogen, 0.75 in women taking calcium and 0.69 in women taking calcitonin, the investigators reported in the British Medical Journal. Medications containing vitamin D, fluorides or anabolic steroids conferred no fracture protection, according to the study.

Nov. 10

A 53-year-old woman gave birth to premature twin girls who were conceived by in-vitro fertilization using donated eggs fertilized with her 32-year-old husband's sperm, announced spokespersons from Martin Luther Hospital in Anaheim, Calif. The grandmother and former bodybuilder became the oldest postmenopausal women to deliver an IVF baby in the United States.

During the IVF process, four embryos were transferred and two survived. The pregnancy was supported with exogenous hormones during the first trimester of pregnancy. The successful pregnancy bore out recent research that suggested that infertility problems in older women are principally due to their ova, not to any inability of an aging uterus to carry a pregnancy.

Nov. 14

At its annual meeting in San Francisco, the American Medical Women's Association asked President-elect Bill Clinton to make RU 486 (Roussel-Uclaf) available for large-scale research trials in the United States.

Nov. 16

Colorado researchers reported that women with breast implants may be at increased risk of developing autoimmune disease. In the study by doctors at the University of Colorado in Denver, 30% of women with breast implants tested positive for antinuclear antibodies, compared with 5% of women without the implants. These antibodies may lead to autoimmune diseases such as scleroderma, lupus and rheumatoid arthritis, although no research has isolated breast implants as a cause of these diseases, the scientists reported at the 50th Anniversary meeting of the American College of Allergy and Immunology in Chicago.

Nov. 24

Women who smoke during pregnancy may be putting their children at risk of strabismus, suggested researchers from the Wilmer Eye Institute in Baltimore. In a case-control study of 377 babies with strabismus, women who smoked throughout pregnancy had almost twice the risk of having a baby with esotropia than women who did not, the investigators reported in the Archives of Ophthalmology. Smoking was not associated with an increased risk of exotropia, however.

DECEMBER

Dec. 6

Delegates to the American Medical Association interim meeting debated whether it would be cost-effective to insist that family planning services be reimbursed by health insurers. Paying for contraceptives would be costly, but far less so than reimbursing patients for prenatal care or abortion services following unintended pregnancy, proponents told the physicians' meeting in Nashville.

Dec. 9

The March of Dimes Birth Defects Foundation recommended a six-pronged evaluation for women who have suffered two or more unexplained miscarriages. At a symposium in New York, obstetricians suggested that a multiple-miscarriage workup include genetic counseling to detect the estimated one in 20 couples in which a balanced chromosomal translocation can explain multiple miscarriages; a gynecologic exam to detect an incompetent cervix or abnormalities of uterine shape; laboratory testing of the woman, including endometrial biopsy to detect luteal phase defects, as well as blood or tissue cultures to detect asymptomatic infections linked to miscarriage (particularly mycoplasma and chlamydia); a full physical focused on detecting immune system disturbances such as antiphospholipid syndrome; HLA testing of parents to detect overcompatibility syndrome; and an evaluation of possible toxic exposures in both parents.

• • •

Young breast-cancer patients do not have to forgo menstrual regularity if they undergo chemotherapy, doctors at Rush-Presbyterian-St. Luke's Medical Center in Chicago reported.

The researchers evaluated 43 node-negative, estrogen-receptor-negative women under age 50 who were still menstruating prior to receiving adjuvant therapy with methotrexate, 5-fluorouracil and leucovorin. Of 30 patients who received the three-agent combination alone, 26 maintained menstrual regularity through and after treatment. Of 13 women who received tamoxifen as well as the three-drug regimen, 12 maintained menstrual regularity. The remaining women reported regular periods before, amenorrhea during and irregular periods since treatment.

Four women in the study attempted to become pregnant; three succeeded. The researchers, speaking at the 15th Annual San Antonio

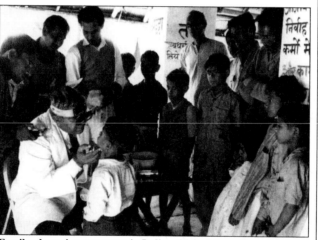

Family plannning programs in India criticized by policy analyst.

Breast Cancer Symposium, concluded that the trio of chemotherapeutic agents has minimal impact on menstrual regularity, making it an attractive alternative for node-negative, ER-negative women seeking to preserve ovarian function.

• • •

Breast self-examination proficiency is poor among women with a family history of breast cancer, Johns Hopkins University oncologists told fellow physicians at the 15th Annual San Antonio Breast Cancer Symposium.

The researchers assessed mastery of BSE in 101 first-degree relatives of breast-cancer patients. At baseline, women's proficiency was poor, but after they were randomized to one of two training techniques (MammaCare or concentric circle), their ability improved. The doctors concluded that these two commonly used BSE teaching techniques can enhance proficiency.

Dec. 11

Obstetricians were advised to encourage both their pregnant patients and their patients' families to stop smoking. Sudden infant death syndrome, which has been associated in past studies with maternal smoking during pregnancy, was linked with passive tobacco exposure after birth by researchers at the National Center for Health Statistics. Analyzing data from a national sample of 10,000 births and 6,000 infant deaths, the researchers found that compared with infants not exposed to tobacco smoke, normal-birth-weight infants were twice as likely to die of SIDS if they were exposed to passive smoke after birth. Infants exposed both pre- and postnatally were three times as likely to die of SIDS, the government researchers reported in the journal Pediatrics.

Dec. 21

After 40 years of national family planning programs, a policy analyst has concluded that population control measures in India have failed to improve the health of the country's citizens. Despite population control measures ranging from forced sterilization, instituted under Indira Gandhi's government, to a variety of noncoercive family planning services, indices of general health have not changed, the investigator wrote in Issues in Reproductive and Genetic Engineering. Infant and maternal mortality rates in India remain extremely high, the analyst added.

Dec. 29

Women who undergo in-vitro fertilization or other modern reproductive technologies to become "nongenetic" mothers feel forced to maintain secrecy about the origins of their pregnancies, an Australian researcher from the Royal Melbourne Institute of Technology reported in Issues in Reproductive and Genetic Engineering. Interviews with Melbourne women who had become pregnant through IVF using donor ova revealed that they had often felt coerced into trying every available technology. The women predicted that they would never escape the need to keep their ordeal a secret from most friends and family members.

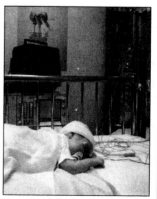

Parents advised to stop smoking to reduce babies' SIDS risk.

Studies indicate gauging uterine activity at home may be ineffective in preventing preterm labor

JAN. 2—Home uterine-activity monitoring is not effective in preventing preterm labor in women at risk, according to a review of randomized controlled trials.

The goal of the home monitoring technique is to detect preterm labor early enough so that drug therapy to prevent labor can be effective.

But five studies of the technique, although they were published in peer-reviewed journals, did not meet accepted standards of scientific rigor, according to David Grimes, M.D., of the University of Southern California School of Medicine, Los Angeles.

When Dr. Grimes combined the relative-risk calculations from the five published studies, he found that women who used the home uterine-activity monitoring devices were only 10% less likely to deliver preterm than women who did not use the devices.

Writing in Obstetrics and Gynecology, Dr. Grimes pointed out that the small improvement in outcome could easily have resulted from a number of methodological shortcomings.

Deficiencies in the trials included failure by the authors to explicitly state the differences in rates among treatment groups, mixing of the effects of frequent nursing contact and home monitoring of uterine activity, analysis of findings before the intended sample size and power had been reached and inappropriate randomization, he reported.

Daily nursing attention during pregnancy did seem to help prevent premature birth among women at risk, but the additional information provided by home uterine monitoring did not confer additional benefit, Dr. Grimes said.

Dr. Grimes is not alone in his opposition to clinical use of the home uterine monitoring technique.

"Home uterine-activity monitoring is a high-cost, ineffective approach to the all-important problem of prematurity," wrote Benjamin Sachs, M.D., in a New England Journal of Medicine column last November. "If we are to make progress with the multifaceted problem of prematurity, we must first provide basic preventive health care for all pregnant women."

The technique can cost more than $5,000 per patient, according to Dr. Sachs, chief of obstetrics and gynecology at Beth Israel Hospital in Boston.

In 1989, the American College of Obstetricians and Gynecologists Committee on Obstetrics stated that the technique should remain investigational and recommended against clinical use.

Despite the lack of evidence of efficacy, the Food and Drug Administration has approved a monitoring system, called the Genesis Home Uterine-Activity Monitor, for early detection of preterm labor in women who have had a previous preterm delivery.

'Baby-maker' case focuses attention on infertility standards

FEB. 10—Treating infertility is largely unregulated, as the trial of Cecil Jacobson, M.D., self-proclaimed "baby-maker," is likely to show.

But legislation introduced recently in Congress would set minimum standards that might help physicians make informed choices when referring patients to fertility specialists.

On Feb. 10, the U.S. District Court in Alexandria, Virginia, began hearing arguments in the Jacobson case. The physician is accused of using his own sperm, instead of donor sperm, to artificially inseminate as many as 75 women. He faces 53 counts of criminal fraud and perjury, which carry a maximum sentence of 285 years in prison and $500,000 in fines.

According to a 1988 study by the Congressional Office of Technology Assessment, artificial insemination is at least a $150-million-a-year industry, with 11,000 private physicians, 400 sperm banks and well over 200 fertility centers responsible for the birth of 30,000 babies annually.

Artificial insemination is largely unregulated. Many states do not even require anonymous donors to be tested for STDs.

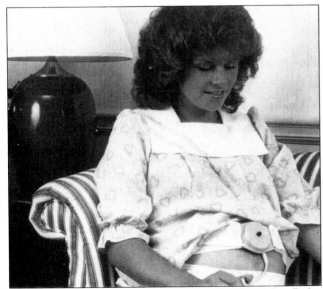
Home uterine monitoring may be of little benefit, review finds.

But studies have shown that large fertility clinics generally do a good job of testing donors and assuring quality control. Abuses like the ones of which Dr. Jacobson is accused are most likely to occur in private practices.

"I would recommend that a woman or a couple seeking treatment for a fertility problem go to a center that's associated with a hospital or a medical school," said fertility specialist Hanna Lisbona, M.D., assistant professor of medicine at Case Western Reserve University School of Medicine in Cleveland. Such centers are subject to institutional review, and physicians are subject to peer review by hospital medical staff.

The American Fertility Society has about 240 clinics in its registry, said a spokesperson. But the AFS is not a certifying agency.

Member clinics are asked to abide by minimum, non-binding standards adopted by the Society for Assisted Reproductive Technology. The minimum standards cover personnel and procedures.

Resolve, a national organization headquartered in Somerville, Mass., that helps persons seeking treatment for infertility, maintains a list of 800 recommended fertility specialists. To be listed, a physician must be board certified in obstetrics and gynecology, endocrinology or urology, and 30% of the physician's practice must involve infertility

treatment. Physicians who lack board certification can make the list if they have special training in reproductive medicine and if 50% of their practice is devoted to infertility.

When it comes to in-vitro fertilization and other procedures at the cutting edge of assisted reproductive technology, even board-certified physicians and a hospital-affiliated fertility center may not offer a patient good odds of success.

According to David Schulke, chief health policy adviser to Rep. Ron Wyden (D-Ore.), IVF centers can be judged in a general way by their "take-home baby rate": the percentage of egg retrieval procedures that result in the birth of a baby. At the best centers, the success rate is about 20%, according to fertility experts. However, a center that specializes in complicated cases may have a lower overall rate. Thus, it is also important that patients and their primary-care physicians look at a clinic's success rate in treating the particular problem a couple is experiencing.

Wyden has introduced legislation in the House that would require Health and Human Services to establish a model program that would "set basic standards for these clinics in terms of facilities, personnel and procedures," Schulke said. States would be encouraged to adopt the nonmandatory model.

Schulke, however, predicts that if the bill passes—and he expects it will because it is not opposed by the Bush administration—most states will adopt the model.

Experts differ on the safety of prenatal exercise

MARCH 3— Dutch researchers who conducted a maximal exercise test on 33 pregnant women concluded that strenuous exercise of limited duration is not harmful to the healthy mother and fetus. But an expert on maternal fetal medicine said that such a broad interpretation is unjustified.

"The conclusion should be that a maximal exercise test is not harmful to the mother or fetus," said Neil Mandsager, M.D., who has studied maternal exercise at the University of Cincinnati School of Medicine. "From a research point of view, that's an important piece of information to know. But to then say that strenuous exercise of limited duration is all right, to me that's a different ballgame, and I would be cautious about making that kind of statement."

Researchers at Erasmus University in Rotterdam led by Marieke B. van Doorn, M.D., studied 33 women at 16, 25 and 35 weeks' gestation and again at seven weeks after delivery. They found that exercise ECG tests revealed depression of the ST segment in 12% of women in the absence of clinical signs of ischemia.

"The incidence of these changes was unaffected by pregnancy," the researchers wrote in the American Journal of Obstetrics and Gynecology.

Blood pressure response to exercise at 75% of maximal heart rate was virtually unaffected by pregnancy, they found. Fetal heart rate was increased by an average of four beats per minute, without a change in pattern, and a transient increase in uterine activity after maximal exercise was found in 6% of the tests.

Robert McMurray of the University of North Carolina at

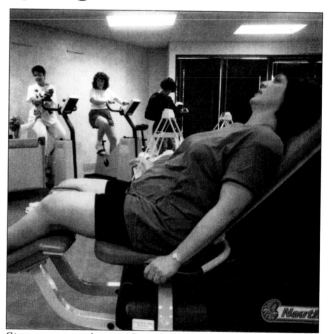

Strenuous exercise may be safe in some pregnant women.

Chapel Hill agreed with the Dutch researchers. "We have been finding that women can exercise safely at levels higher than the guidelines set by the American College of Obstetricians and Gynecologists with no harmful effects to pregnancy outcome or the mothers," he said.

Guidelines by the obstetricians' group state that maternal heart rate should not exceed 140 beats per minute, and that women should not exercise strenuously for more than 15 minutes.

"Women who exercised before pregnancy could certainly exercise for more than 15 minutes during pregnancy," said Janet Walberg-Rankin, associate professor of physical education at Virginia Polytechnic Institute and State University in Blacksburg.

Walberg-Rankin, a first-time mother of twins at age 36, swam for a half-hour two or three times a week during her pregnancy.

Guidelines from the American College of Obstetricians and Gynecologists on exercise during pregnancy are being reviewed, said Dr. Mandsager. New guidelines may be issued in two years extending the limit for moderate exercise to 20 minutes.

ACOG brief opposes abortion deterrence laws

By Susan Ince

MARCH 6—Pennsylvania's abortion law subverts informed consent and intrudes on the marriage relationship, the American College of Obstetricians and Gynecologists argued in an amicus curiae brief submitted to the Supreme Court, which heard widely publicized oral pro and con arguments on the law's restrictions last month.

The eventual High Court ruling in the case of Planned Parenthood v. Robert Casey may set a precedent for further state restrictions on abortion and could undermine the 1973 Roe v. Wade ruling that established abortion as a constitutional right.

A federal appeals court upheld provisions of the Pennsylvania law requiring that women wait 24 hours for an abortion and receive specified counseling from physicians on alternatives, but struck down a requirement that married women notify their husbands of their intention.

In oral arguments, attorneys representing Pennsylvania maintained that what a physican tells a patient can be legally restricted because it is "commercial speech."

But "far from promoting true informed consent, [the counseling requirement] will interfere with constructive consultation between physicians and their patients and will undermine patients' health," according to the ACOG brief.

Together, the "obstacles placed in the path of a woman seeking abortion—notification, consent, waiting periods and public disclosure," constitute "an effort to deter [her] from making a decision that, with her physician, is hers to make," said the ACOG brief, in which six other medical organizations joined.

And by requiring in-person parental consent, the Pennsylvania law "ensures that minors will face needless and health-threatening delay," the ACOG brief stated.

In a contrasting amicus curiae brief, the 680-member American Association of Pro-Life Obstetricians and Gynecologists and the Association of Pro-Life Pediatricians urged that the Pennsylvania case be used to abandon the Roe v. Wade decision entirely.

Legalized abortion in general violates the medical precept of "do no harm" and "uniformly places the socioeconomic concerns of the mother...above the life of the unborn child," the pro-life medical groups argued.

Matthew J. Bulfin, M.D., the Fort Lauderdale, Fla., ob/gyn who heads AAPLOG, said he is not concerned that scripted informed consent procedures might interfere with the doctor-patient relationship.

"Our freedom to practice medicine has already been greatly curtailed by restrictions placed [on it] by insurance companies, Medicare and Medicaid," said Dr. Bulfin. "The restrictions in this case shouldn't be such a shock to our nervous systems."

U.S. women's fears of IUDs contradicted by international study

MARCH 27—Monogamous women properly fitted with modern, copper-releasing IUDs face little if any risk of developing pelvic inflammatory disease, according to a major international study.

Even so, four out of five women in the United States continue to distrust the device, researchers reported at a conference in New York last month sponsored by the Population Council.

The study of PID, published in The Lancet, found that the overall rate of the disease for 22,908 IUD insertions in 23 countries was 1.6 cases per 1,000 woman-years of use.

PID risk was more than six times higher during the first 20 days after insertion than during later times, according to the study. The risk remained low and constant for up to eight years of follow-up.

"These are safe devices for monogamous women," said co-author Michael J. Rosenberg, M.D., of Health Decisions, a private research group in Chapel Hill, N.C.

An editorial accompanying the study concluded, "It is essential that all patients should be adequately assessed before the fitting of an IUD, and that it should be fitted under strict aseptic control. To reduce the risk associated with insertion, the devices should be left in place as long as possible."

The researchers acknowledged that their recommendation to keep the intrauterine devices in place as long as possible contradicted the recommendations several groups had previously made that the devices be replaced at regular intervals irrespective of need.

The researchers also found that PID rates were lower among women who had their IUDs inserted more recently, which the authors said could be attributed to doctors' growing awareness of sexually transmitted disease risk as a contra-indication to IUD use.

Although 84 million women worldwide were using IUDs by 1987, the number of American women using the devices dropped from 2.2 million in 1982 to just 700,000 by 1988, according to the World Health Organization.

In large part, the dropoff was due to widespread publicity surrounding a 1981 study that pointed to a higher incidence of pelvic inflammatory disease among women using IUDs, including the Dalkon Shield.

The results of that study, although since put in doubt by a reevaluation published last April by the Journal of Clinical Epidemiology, sparked millions of dollars in lawsuits against Dalkon Shield's manufacturer, A.H. Robins, and led to Robins's withdrawal from the market.

Only 13% of American women would even consider using an IUD if it was recommended by their doctor, according to Jacqueline Darroch Forrest, vice president for research at the Alan Guttmacher Institute in New York.

In contrast, women who currently use IUDs are very happy with the choice, ranking their satisfaction higher than users of any other method, said Daniel Mishell, Jr., M.D., of the University of Southern California School of Medicine in Los Angeles.

Women's fears should be allayed by the new research, Dr. Mishell added.

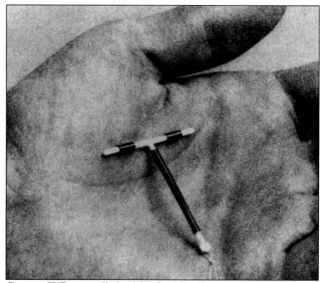

Copper IUDs pose little risk of pelvic disease, experts suggest.

One in 200 women using an IUD becomes pregnant each year, according to Patrick Rowe, M.D., of WHO. A woman using an IUD for nine years has about a one-in-50 chance of accidental pregnancy during that time, he said.

Women who want an IUD may have a hard time finding a doctor experienced in inserting one, according to a study by Carolyn Westhoff, M.D., of Columbia-Presbyterian Medical Center in New York. "We have young doctors who don't know how to insert IUDs, and older doctors who know how, but are afraid of being sued," she said.

Ovarian cancer-screening tests termed unreliable; ultrasound is probably best option, expert says

By Celia Slom

LAS VEGAS, APRIL 29—Screening tests for ovarian cancer are often unreliable, signaling cancer when none is present and leading to unnecessary surgery, according to a cancer expert at the annual meeting of the American College of Obstetricians and Gynecologists.

But of all the available methods, transvaginal ultrasound appears to be the most promising, and could be offered to women at high risk for the malignancy, said William Hoskins, M.D., of the Memorial Sloan-Kettering Cancer Center in New York City.

Because serum CA-125 and pelvic sonography are not sensitive or reliable, most women should not bother having the tests, according to Dr. Hoskins.

"We can't recommend screening now. There's no clear-cut evidence it's effective," said the New York researcher.

Pelvic exams alone do not increase the early diagnosis of cancer, and have not been shown to decrease the death rate, Dr. Hoskins said.

In a pioneering study conducted last year, Jack van Nagell, M.D., of the University of Kentucky in Lexington, screened 1,300 asymptomatic women with transvaginal ultrasound.

He found 14 benign serous tumors and two primary ovarian cancers. Both were stage I. CA-125 and pelvic exams were normal in both cases.

The five-year survival rate is 95% for stage I, 20% for stage III and 5% for stage IV.

Only about 23% of all cancers are detected in the early stage, according to the American Cancer Society.

Although he would not advocate screening women at high risk—those with a family history of the disease, women with no children and those who started menstruating by age 12—tests should be provided to those who request them, said Dr. Hoskins.

But Steven Piver, M.D., director of the Gilda Radner Familial Ovarian Cancer Registry at the Roswell Park Cancer Institute in Buffalo, N.Y., thinks women at high risk (in his view, those with two first-degree relatives with the disease) have a 50% chance of developing ovarian cancer and should get triple screening twice a year—pelvic exam coupled with ultrasound and a serum CA-125.

Several studies have suggested that oral contraceptives, which reduce the frequency of ovulation, protect against ovarian cancer.

Early age of first pregnancy and early menopause also seem to reduce the risk.

The National Cancer Institute is planning to test various methods of ovarian cancer-screening on 37,000 women aged 60 to 74.

In-vitro fertilization success declines with age

JUNE 6—Rates of conception and live births achieved with in-vitro fertilization decline with age, with women over age 40 having a 15% chance of having a baby after five IVF attempts.

In contrast, more than 50% of women between the ages of 20 and 34 conceive after five IVF cycles, and 45% succeed in having babies, according to Seang Lin Tan, M.D., of the King's College School of Medicine in London.

He reported the results of a study of 5,055 consecutive in-vitro fertilization cycles in 2,735 women and 518 live births in The Lancet.

The success rate of in-vitro fertilization drops by about 8% after each attempt, and is greatly reduced when the male is infertile or the female has multiple infertility problems, the study found.

"Our findings suggest that infertile women over 30 years who are considering IVF should avoid unnecessary delay before they start treatment," the British infertility researchers wrote.

All the women were seen at the Hallam Medical Center in London, a clinic that has been in operation since 1984 and is considered to have success rates comparable to those of other top centers in the United States and Europe, Dr. Tan said.

He said that the study is the largest ever done in a single center.

Among women aged 35 to 39, the conception rate was 38.7%, while the live-birth rate was 28.9%, according to the London researchers.

Among women aged 40 or above, the conception rate was 20.2%, while the live-birth rate was 14.4%.

Conception and live-birth rates were similar for women of the same age who conceive naturally, according to the researchers.

"There's no question that age has an impact on success rates for any reproductive treatment," said Robert D. Visscher, M.D., medical director of the American Fertility Society in Birmingham, Ala.

He said that the dropoff in success rates after repeated IVF attempts has also been suspected for a long time. "There's certainly a law of diminishing returns," he said.

According to the American Fertility Society, approximately 240 centers across the United States offered some form of assisted reproductive technology in 1990.

The standard technique is IVF, which results in 2,000 births in the United States annually, according to the society.

Rep. Ron Wyden (D-Ore.) proposed a bill in February that would require fertility clinics to report their success rates in a uniform manner, and would set standards for laboratory personnel and quality control.

One reason for the low overall success rates of most in-vitro fertilization programs is the high proportion of older women who seek treatment, said Dr. Tan.

Thirty-seven percent of the women at the London clinic were over the age of 34, he said.

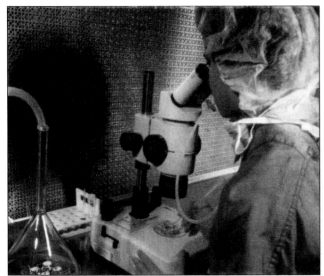

IVF results in about 2,000 births in the U.S. every year.

FDA committee now recommends approving injectable contraceptive

By Laura Buterbaugh

JUNE 19—More than a decade after the Food and Drug Administration denied approval for medroxyprogesterone (Depo-Provera, Upjohn) amid concerns that the injectable contraceptive increased the risk of breast cancer, an advisory committee of the FDA recommended approval of the drug.

The final decision on whether to approve the drug now is up to FDA Commissioner David Kessler, M.D., who is not bound by advisory committee recommendations.

The synthetic progesterone already is approved in the United

States to treat inoperable, recurrent and metastatic endometrial or renal cancer and in 90 other countries as a contraceptive.

Upjohn estimated that due to off-label prescribing, about 10,000 U.S. women have received the drug as a contraceptive. The drug would be delivered intramuscularly every three months to suppress ovulation.

The depot contraceptive was denied FDA approval in 1978, after some studies suggested it could increase the risk of breast cancer.

A recent nine-year World Health Organization study found that the drug does not increase the overall risk of cervical, liver, ovarian, endometrial or breast cancer. The study did find that the risk of breast cancer increased slightly within the first four years of using the drug, mainly in women under 35.

A 1991 study suggested that medroxyprogesterone may lower women's bone density.

James Jones, M.D., an assistant professor of obstetrics and gynecology at the University of Florida Health Science Center in Jacksonville, said initial studies that showed an increased breast-cancer risk were done on beagles, and cannot be extrapolated to humans.

Depot medroxyprogesterone may be an attractive contraceptive because it is cheaper than the birth-control pill and may only have to be taken every three months. It also has a 99% success rate, comparable to those of the pill and the recently released levonorgestrel implant (Norplant, Wyeth-Ayerst).

Both the levonorgestrel implant and depot medroxyprogesterone can cause heavy irregular bleeding in some women. The latter also can cause weight gain.

"You can use progesterones in women [who are not candidates for the pill]: heavy smokers over 35, patients with sickle-cell disease, patients who are breast-feeding and insulin-dependent diabetics," Dr. Jones explained.

In Jacksonville, depot medroxyprogesterone is about $28 for a three-month supply, compared with about $45 for a three-month supply of the pill, he said.

Other methods still being developed include contraceptive vaginal rings that release steroids through the vagina, and monthly injections for men of testosterone to block sperm production. A new IUD called the Flexigard has been shown in early studies to be highly effective, but has not been approved by the FDA.

The first female condom recently was recommended for approval by an FDA advisory committee.

Little benefit, many risks seen with drug for labor

By Charlene Laino

JULY 30—The only drug approved in the United States for the treatment of preterm labor did not significantly reduce infant mortality and increased maternal morbidity in a Canadian study of more than 700 women.

Ritodrine (Yutopar, Astra) delayed delivery for one to two days, but the delay did not translate into better clinical outcome, according to the Canadian Preterm Labor Investigators Group.

"Ritodrine should no longer be approved for premature labor," said Kenneth Leveno, M.D., professor of obstetrics and gynecology at the University of Texas Southwestern Medical School, Dallas.

He said that previous studies have shown that between 3% and 9% of women treated with ritodrine develop pulmonary edema, while there has been no evidence to show that the drug helps fetuses.

In the new study, 708 women in preterm labor were randomly assigned to receive intravenous ritodrine at a maximum rate of 0.35 mg per minute until the cessation of uterine activity or placebo.

Of 771 infants born, 23 deaths occurred in the ritodrine group and 25 deaths occurred in the placebo group, the Canadian researchers reported in The New England Journal of Medicine.

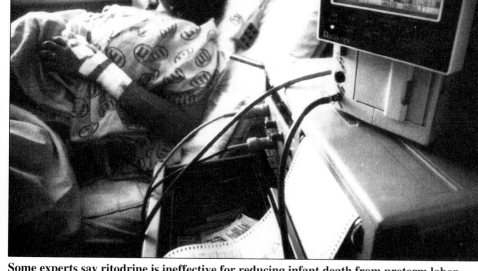

Some experts say ritodrine is ineffective for reducing infant death from preterm labor.

There was no difference between the groups in the incidence of premature deliveries or the proportion of infants weighing less than 2,500 g.

More side effects were reported in the ritodrine group, chiefly chest pain and cardiac arrhythmias, than in those on placebo. One woman taking ritodrine developed pulmonary edema.

The Food and Drug Administration issued a statement saying that the study raises few new issues regarding the use of ritodrine, noting that the risks associated with the drug are clearly marked on the label. The agency will, however, reassess the maternal risks and neonatal benefits of the drug.

"The drug did exactly what it was supposed to do—delay delivery by 24 to 48 hours," said Nigel Rulewski, M.D., vice president of medical affairs at Astra. The delay gives the physician time to administer corticosteroid therapy, which has been shown to enhance lung maturation and reduce the incidence of respiratory distress syndrome, he said. The delay also gives the pregnant woman time to be moved to a specialized care center for delivery.

"It's up to the physician to do something useful with that time," he said.

The FDA approved ritodrine in 1980 after smaller studies indicated it effectively delayed delivery. Within a few months of the approval, the agency was criticized for its decision because of concerns over efficacy and safety, Dr. Leveno stated in an accompanying editorial.

Dolphins to be tested as 'midwives' in Israel; U.S. obstetrician/gynecologist urges caution

By Luba Vikhanski

AUG. 7—A group of pregnant volunteers is scheduled to take part in an unusual experiment in which they will spend time every day swimming with dolphins in Israel before giving birth.

Twelve British women and their husbands are planning to make the trip, which is expected to cost from $2,000 to $5,000 per couple.

They will be accompanied by five physicians, as well as volunteer midwives and massage therapists, according to Gowri Motha, M.D., of Whipps Cross Hospital in London.

The women will give birth in the Israeli resort of Eilat after swimming with dolphins in the Dolphin Reef sanctuary on the Red Sea.

The idea is to create an enjoyable and relaxed environment for the mothers and their babies, reducing the pain and risk of complications associated with delivery, said Dr. Motha, an obstetrician who initiated the project.

"It's a fun project," she said. "If children are born into a fun environment, then hopefully the world will become a more fun place for us to live in than at the moment."

Three pregnant Israeli women are expected to join the group, she said.

The expectant mothers can spend time every day swimming in the sanctuary—a closed-off expanse of the bay that is home to six adult dolphins and one baby dolphin—during the last weeks of pregnancy and until the early stages of labor. They would then give birth in the bay.

Dr. Motha and her colleagues will study samples of the seawater for the presence of infectious organisms every day. If it is found to be contaminated, the women can give birth in a separate shallow pool, she said.

In the event of complications, the women will be rushed to a nearby hospital.

But an ob/gyn from the University of Southern California in Los Angeles said that pregnant women should enter the study with a great deal of caution.

Keith Russell, M.D., said that while some ob/gyns in the United States and England recommend keeping a woman immersed in water during early labor to alleviate pain, act/ually delivering the baby under water is risky and the benefits of interacting with dolphins at childbirth are "purely theoretical."

Neural-tube defects linked to pregnancy overheating: study

AUG. 19—Increases in the body temperature of pregnant women caused by hot tubs, saunas or fevers during the first three months of pregnancy can more than double the risk of having an infant born with a neural-tube defect.

Aubrey Milunsky, M.D., director of the Center for Human Genetics at Boston University, surveyed 23,491 pregnant women in New England. Overall, 1,254 reported using a hot tub, 367 a sauna and 2,883 electric blankets during the first two months of pregnancy.

An additional 1,865 pregnant women reported having a fever over 100 degrees in the first trimester.

The study appeared in The Journal of the American Medical Association.

Use of a hot tub yielded a relative risk of 2.8 for neural-tube defects, compared with 1.8 for saunas, 1.2 for electric blankets and 1.8 for fevers.

Using an electric blanket was not found to significantly increase the risk of neural-tube defects.

In all, 49 of the pregnancies resulted in a birth defect.

Dr. Milunsky said that given the findings, it would be prudent for women to avoid taking very hot baths in the first trimester of their pregnancies.

The March of Dimes Birth Defects Foundation recommends that women who are in their first trimester of pregnancy or who are considering pregnancy avoid hot tubs and saunas.

However, another researcher, Sterling Clarren, M.D., of the University of Washington in Seattle, said that women who have already used hot tubs or saunas during their pregnancy should not be unduly alarmed by the study results.

"Hot tubbing and sauna bathing do not necessarily raise body temperature if you get in and get out quickly," said Dr. Clarren.

He cited previous research by himself and others showing that before damage to the fetus occurs, the body temperature of the mother must rise to at least 102 degrees—a point at which the woman would begin to feel light-headed and nauseous.

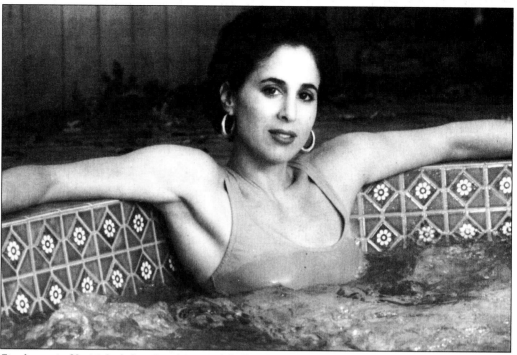

Staying out of hot tubs is best bet, but a quick dip of the lower body is okay, says Dr. Clarren.

"If you keep your arms, your head and your chest out of the water in a hot tub, your core temperature will never go up," Dr. Clarren said.

"For most people who use a hot tub or sauna correctly, there should be no harm," he said.

Cystic fibrosis identified in three-day-old embryos

By Dan Hurley

SEPT. 24—Using a technique that could be described as polymerase chain reaction squared, researchers have siphoned off a single cell from a three-day-old embryo conceived through in-vitro fertilization and successfully tested it for the presence of cystic fibrosis genes. One woman gave birth to an apparently unaffected child after a select embryo was implanted.

The advance, which could obviate the perceived need for abortion, could also be used in couples who are carriers of other genetic diseases such as hemophilia, sickle-cell anemia, Tay-Sachs disease and muscular dystrophy, said the researchers at Hammersmith Hospital in London and the Institute for Molecular Genetics and Center for Reproductive Medicine and Surgery at Baylor College of Medicine in Houston.

In 1990, the same London researchers reported on the grandfather of the technique, in which couples at risk for conceiving a child heterozygous for hemophilia underwent the genetic screening procedure.

Without the sophisticated polymerase chain reaction test, however, only sex could be screened for, resulting in the elimination of all male embryos for couples who wanted to rule out the possibility of having a child with the blood disorder.

By taking an additional genetic step, finding and amplifying single genes, researchers have taken reproductive medicine into a new ethical morass, according to Arthur Caplan, M.D., director of the Center for Bioethics at the University of Minnesota.

"We should not be confused that this technique is limited to a few couples," Dr. Caplan said. "One can envision a future in which couples—fertile or otherwise—will sit down and pick from an array of embryos."

But at $7,000 to $10,000 per in-vitro fertilization attempt, plus the additional $2,000 for the new technique, the procedure is off limits to those without insurance or their own financial means.

And the live-baby success rate of in-vitro fertilization, which the American Fertility Society puts at about 15%, may turn away other fertile couples.

Even so, Jerome H. Check, M.D., head of the department of endocrinology and infertility at the Robert Wood Johnson Medical School in Camden, N.J., said, "I think it's very exciting, very interesting, and will definitely have application to a minority of potential parents. It's very practical for people at high risk of having a child with a genetic defect."

In the study, published in The New England Journal of Medicine, three sets of fertile parents who had previously given birth to children with cystic fibrosis went through standard in-vitro fertilization. After three days, when the developing embryo had reached the eight-cell stage, researchers used a micropipette to aspirate one cell from each embryo after having pierced the zona pellucida with an acidified medium (pH 2.4).

The new PCR technique, dubbed nested PCR by the researchers, was then employed. Traditional PCR is unable to amplify DNA from a single cell.

In nested PCR, primers to amplify DNA fragments containing the sequence CTT (cytosine, thymine, thymine) first were used. CTT is the trinucleotide deletion which, when it occurs on the cystic fibrosis transmembrane regulator gene on chromosome 7, is thought to be responsible for the disease, according to a report in 1990.

After the first CTT-primer PCR pass, researchers used traditional PCR to amplify the already amplified gene sections.

In the study, one set of parents had five embryos, two of which were heterozygous for cystic fibrosis, two homozy-

gous and one free of the gene deletion. The unaffected embryo and one homozygous embryo were implanted, but no pregnancy occurred.

The second couple had two embryos. Analysis was unsuccessful on one; the other was heterozygous. Neither was implanted.

The third couple had six embryos: Two were heterozygous, two unaffected, one homozygous and in one, genetic screening was unsuccessful. The woman had an unaffected and homozygous embryo implanted and gave birth to a girl with no copy of the mutated gene.

Amniocentesis and chorionic villus sampling both carry their own risk of birth defects. And if either method found that the fetus had the genetic defect and the parents wished to terminate the pregnancy, an abortion would be required.

Mark R. Hughes, M.D., an assistant professor at Baylor and director of the prenatal genetics program at Methodist Hospital in Houston, said testing the eight-cell embryo through IVF involves a group of cells no bigger than a grain of sand. "It's postconception, but pre-pregnancy," he said. He said some couples may find the technique less ethically troubling than abortion.

Pediatric group now recommends strep B testing for pregnant women to reduce infant infections

Medical Tribune News Service Report

Nov. 5—All pregnant women should be tested for streptococcus B infection when they are seven months' pregnant, to reduce the risk of passing the bacterium to their newborns during delivery, according to new guidelines issued by the American Academy of Pediatrics.

Streptococcus B—serologically classified as Lancefield group B Streptococcus agalactiae—is one of the major causes of sickness and death in newborns, especially those born prematurely.

It can lead to pneumonia or meningitis in infants, and in pregnant women can cause infections of the urinary tract and the amniotic sac surrounding the fetus, as well as inflammation of the uterine lining.

Between 15% and 40% of women carry strep B bacteria in their vagina during pregnancy, the academy estimated. About 12,000 newborns each year come into contact with the coccus in the birth canal and develop a potentially fatal strep B infection, according to the organization.

Illness and death resulting from strep B infection "make prevention strategies imperative," academy members wrote in an article accompanying the proposed guidelines in the journal Pediatrics.

The new guidelines recommend that
• All pregnant women should be screened for strep B between weeks 26 and 28 of gestation, to determine if they should be treated with antibiotics.
• Pregnant women who test positive for the germ but do not

have symptoms of infection should not be treated, unless they have the bacteria in their urine.
• Pregnant women admitted to the hospital for conditions such as premature labor or premature rupture of the amniotic sac who have not been tested for strep B should be tested immediately.
• Women who test positive for strep B and have certain risk factors should be treated with intravenous antibiotics during labor. Those risk factors include premature labor, rupture of the amniotic sac, fever during labor and multiple births.
• Women who have previously given birth to an infant with strep B-caused disease should be treated with antibiotics during the birth of all future children.

These guidelines "represent the best approach currently available," said Jeffrey Greenspoon, M.D., director of perinatal intensive care at Cedars-Sinai Medical Center in Los Angeles.

"Many private physicians have already been doing this," Dr. Greenspoon said. "Others have been waiting for recommendations, because they weren't assured it was cost-effective. But studies have shown that it is."

Intravenous antibiotic treatment is extremely effective for treating strep B infection when given during labor, when the baby is exposed to the bacteria, Dr. Greenspoon said. It is not as effective when given earlier in the pregnancy, because it only wipes out the bacteria temporarily, he said.

Effective antibiotics for treating maternal strep B infections include intrapartum intravenous ampicillin or penicillin G, or, for penicillin-allergic women, clindamycin or erythromycin intravenously.

COMMENTARY

Treatment advancing, diagnosis lagging

By Luella Klein, M.D.

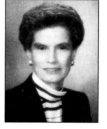

IN 1993 AND BEYOND, THERE are a number of areas in which both specialists and physicians as a whole will see change.

One exciting advance that I think will be of tremendous importance in the long run is the recommendation from the Centers for Disease Control and Prevention that all women of childbearing age start taking 0.4 mg per day of folic acid to reduce the risk of having a baby with neural-tube defects; this is especially important for women who have already had a baby with a neural-tube defect. The CDC recommends that women take the vitamin prior to conception and throughout the pregnancy. Folic acid is a cheap vitamin that can go a long way toward ensuring healthy outcomes.

An area that I think physicians are not paying enough attention to is the heterosexual transmission of HIV infection. Women are becoming infected at an alarming rate, and we simply are not sufficiently and thoroughly counseling and testing women, especially pregnant women, who might be at risk.

Another big issue that I see gaining in importance is Norplant. This product has turned out to be a fairly popular long-term contraceptive. The biggest problem is the cost (approximately $350 plus a fee to have the implants inserted), but Norplant lasts at least five years and is cheaper than five years' worth of birth control pills. I would recommend Norplant for any woman who knows that she doesn't want to have a baby for several years.

The National Cancer Institute and the American Cancer Society have said that one woman in nine will get breast cancer in her lifetime. That statistic underlines the importance of ensuring that women receive mammograms on the recommended schedule. We know that only about one third of women who are eligible for screening are getting them on a regular basis. This is just too low. Unfortunately, many of us are part of the problem because we just don't talk to our patients enough about the importance of screening. Given that there will be approximately 180,000 new cases of breast cancer in the United States this year and about 46,000 deaths, I think we need to talk to our patients, we need to get the cost of mammography lowered and we must get third-party payment for mammograms.

From a technological viewpoint, I think that laparoscopy is becoming an increasingly important part of our field. Gynecologists are using laparoscopy for ovarian, tubal and pelvic procedures, and even to assist vaginal hysterectomies. As the light sources, equipment and visualization improve, I think the number of endoscopic procedures is very likely to increase. One of the biggest problems with laparoscopy, however, is that many physicians are not sufficiently trained. To ensure that the physician is proficient at the procedure, hospitals now require a certain number of supervised procedures before doctors can perform one on their own. Only physicians who complete a full training program should attempt the procedure.

Two artificial surfactants have proved in clinical trials to reduce deaths in nurseries by about 40% in the first 28 days of life; this should be reassuring to expectant mothers. Exosurf, a synthetic product, and Survanta, a bovine product, are already on the market. Both have helped physicians in neonatal centers achieve a significant reduction in the death rates of small infants.

The safety of silicone-gel breast implants was a topic that raised much controversy in 1992 but was never really resolved. Most surgeons are offering only saline implants, and companies still making the silicone implants are stymied because they are awaiting some direction from the Food and Drug Administration.

Another thing that continues to touch every physician is healthcare reform. If there is healthcare reform—and I think there will be—it will affect women and infants first. Of course, there are so many different proposals, I don't see how anyone can make any definitive statement about what direction it will take. I guess the best thing we can do is wait it out, because judging by President-elect Bill Clinton's proposal in The New England Journal of Medicine, it isn't very clear what he intends to do.

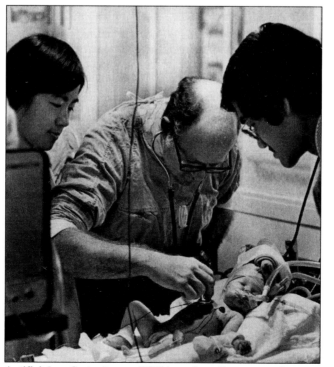

Artificial surfactants ease RDS to reduce time on respirators.

Dr. Klein is professor and chair of the department of gynecology and obstetrics at Emory University School of Medicine, Atlanta.

Notes

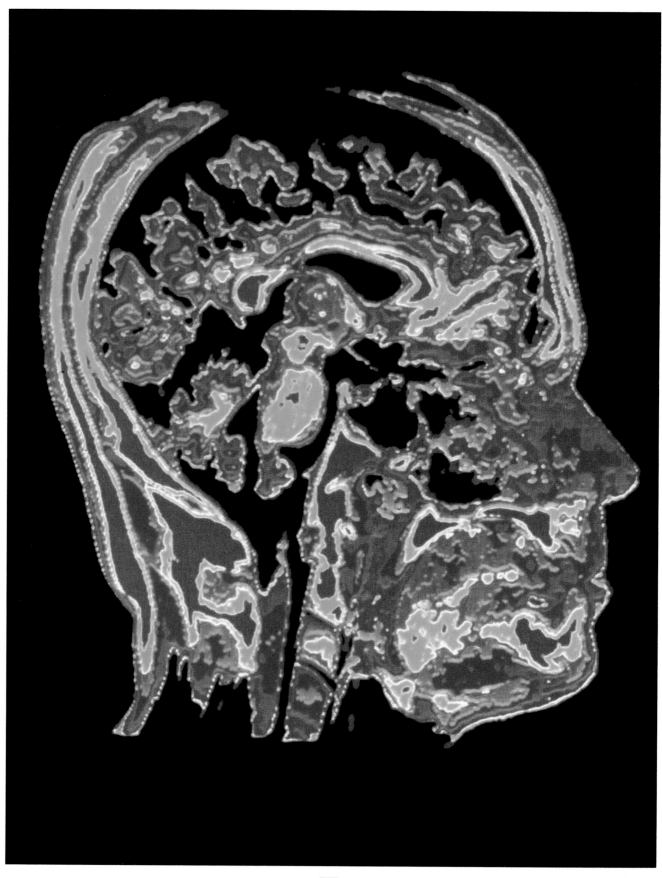

Jan. 4

Headache experts at London's Charing Cross Hospital found that weekend migraines are more common in men than in women. They collected data from questionnaires from 11 male and 22 female patients with migraine or tension-type headaches that occurred on the weekends. All 11 males suffered from migraines, while only 17 of the 22 women had migraines. Although migraines affect three times as many women as men, men are more likely to suffer weekend attacks, the London team wrote in a letter to The Lancet. Friday-night drinking, changes in stress levels, skipped

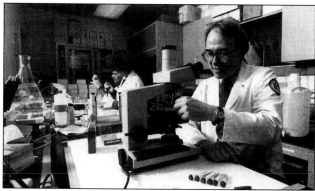

PCR betters traditional antibody tests for spirochete detection.

breakfasts, reduced caffeine consumption and changes in sleep patterns have been considered as triggers for the weekend headache pattern.

Jan. 7

Charlottesville researchers speculated that clozapine (Clozaril, Sandoz) may be useful in the treatment of anorexia nervosa, after finding that schizophrenics gained up to 45 pounds during their first 16 weeks on therapy with the serotonin antagonist. Of 21 hospitalized patients placed on clozapine for the treatment of schizophrenia or schizoaffective disorder, eight increased their body weight by more than 10% and another six gained between 5% and 10% of their baseline weight, according to psychiatrists at the University of Virginia School of Medi-

1992 HIGHLIGHTS

cine. Those gaining the most weight also showed the most improvement in psychiatric symptoms, they reported in the American Journal of Psychiatry.

Feb. 3

Omaha researchers suggested that the antianxiety drug buspirone (Buspar, Mead Johnson) may help smokers quit the habit. The Creighton University team found that buspirone blunted nicotine withdrawal symptoms in long-term smokers. In a four-week study, 40 people who smoked at least a pack a day were asked to cease smoking in three weeks. Half received buspirone three times a day, in the weeks prior to quitting; others received a placebo. In the withdrawal week, 79% of the buspirone group completely abstained from smoking, compared with 50% of smokers given a placebo. Placebo-treated patients had significantly higher ratings for craving, anxiety, irritability, restlessness and sadness during tobacco withdrawal, according to data published in the Archives of Internal Medicine.

Feb. 5

Aluminum may play an active role in the neurodegenerative process in Alzheimer's patients, an international team reported. Aluminum appears to trigger the biochemical se-

quence that leads to the progressive aggregation of the cerebral neurofibrillary tangles that are pathognomonic of the disease, they wrote in the Journal of Molecular Biology. Their conclusion is based on the finding that beta-pleated protein sheets characteristic of the tangles are formed in vitro when aluminum is added to the key protein fragment of the neurofilament. It has yet to be shown that ingested or exogenous aluminum crosses the blood-brain barrier.

Feb. 7

Case Western Reserve University researchers found that beta-amyloid, the protein that accumulates in the brains of Alzheimer's patients, is also present in smaller quantities in the brains of normal people. Until now, it was thought that the protein was unique to Alzheimer's patients, the Cleveland team said. The discovery led to speculation that scientists may be able to slow down beta-amyloid production when too much is being generated, they hypothesized in Science.

Feb. 14

Short-term psychotherapy may benefit patients suffering from specific problems due to drug addiction or grief as much as long-term psychological counseling, determined University of Pennsylvania researchers. They reached that conclusion after comparing findings from 12 studies that examined treatment of people suffering from depression, drug addiction, personality disorders, posttraumatic stress disorder or grief. The analysis, in the American Journal of Psychiatry, encompassed various types of psychotherapy, such as hypnotherapy, self-help groups and cognitive or dynamic therapy lasting 12 to 40 sessions.

Patients found most likely to benefit from short-term therapy included those with specific problems relating to

substance abuse, rape or other physical injury, property loss or death.

Feb. 15

Patients who suffer from migraines may need a second injection of sumatriptan (Imitrex, Glaxo) to prevent headache recurrence, declared researchers from the Gothenburg Migraine Clinic in Gothenburg, Sweden. Despite initial relief, 26 of 48 migraine patients who self-injected sumatriptan had another headache an average of 13 hours later, it was reported in The Lancet. When the 26 patients administered a second shot within 24 hours of the migraine, only one sufferer had a recurrence.

March 11

The cerebrospinal fluid of patients with negative CSF laboratory tests was found to contain Lyme disease spirochetes. Using polymerase chain reaction technology, researchers from the State University of New York at Stony Brook detected Borrelia burgdorferi spirochetes in eight of 10 Lyme disease patients, only two of whom had CNS infection detectable with traditional antibody tests.

High doses of amoxicillin, doxycycline or ceftriaxone (Rocephin, Roche) may be indicated for all people with early Lyme disease to prevent the spirochetes from remaining in a CNS "sanctuary," and then emerging periodically to cause recurrent arthritis and other problems, the investigators suggested in The Journal of the American Medical Association.

April 1

Failure to consider confounding variables may have resulted in overestimating the link between beta-blockers and depression, said Philadelphia geriatric specialists who found that the drugs do not appear to cause depression. In a case-control study of 4,302 Medicaid recipients, the Presbyterian Medical Center team found that depressed patients

Central Nervous System

were about 45% more likely to have taken beta-blockers in the year prior to diagnosis. But after controlling for such variables as benzodiazepine use, frequent outpatient visits and frequent use of other medications, there was no difference in use of beta-blockers between depressed patients and controls, according to The Journal of the American Medical Association report.

April 9

The antidepressant fluoxetine (Prozac, Dista) was found to relieve chronic headaches, a Chicago investigator told Medical Tribune. More than 65% of 52 patients with recurrent, severe headaches reported pain reduction after taking fluoxetine for two weeks to a few months, said the neurologist. Fluoxetine is associated with fewer side effects than other drugs used to treat severe headaches, he added.

May 5

Some bulimic patients were found to benefit from daily light therapy. At a meeting in Washington, D.C., of the American Psychiatric Association, University of British Columbia researchers said a half-hour each day in front of 10,000 lux white fluorescent light reduced the number of bulimic episodes by 43%, while exposure to a red light for the same period reduced the episodes by 12%. The therapy, which has been used in seasonal affective disorder, may be most helpful to bulimics who experience some seasonal variation in their symptoms, said the Canadian team.

• • •

Wider access to the schizophrenia drug clozapine (Clozaril, Sandoz) has more than doubled the number of Americans receiving the drug since last year, the drug's manufacturer reported at the meeting of the American Psychiatric Association.

About 25,000 patients are receiving clozapine, up from 10,000 a year ago, when the Health Care Financing Ad-

1992 HIGHLIGHTS

ministration ordered state Medicaid programs to pay for the drug, said the director of scientific affairs for Sandoz.

But tens of thousands of patients who could benefit from the drug are still not receiving it, he said. He estimated that the drug, which costs $7,500 a year, could benefit about 10% of the country's 2.5 million schizophrenics: the 250,000 who are resistant to standard antipsychotic drugs.

May 6

North Carolina researchers told a session at the American Academy of Neurology meeting in San Diego that positron emission tomography can spot brain abnormalities several years before the diagnosis of Alzheimer's disease. Researchers from Duke University evaluated 54 Alzheimer's patients three years after a PET scan and found that 28 with worsening symptoms had telltale signs in the temporal and parietal lobes in the original scan.

• • •

Physicians at the American Academy of Neurology meeting were told that patients who suffer head injuries may develop memory loss or epilepsy if cells in the hippocampus are damaged. The theory was based on experiments on rats with surgically induced concussions. If substantiated, the findings could lead to the development of drugs that would protect the hippocampus cells in head-injured patients, a neurologist from the University of California at San Francisco said.

• • •

A survey of over 5,000 physicians revealed that doctors have a pattern of prescribing tranquilizers or pain relievers for themselves that could increase their chances of drug abuse or addiction. One of every nine doctors had prescribed his or her own tranquilizers in the past year,

and one in six had self-prescribed pain medicine in the past year without supervision from another doctor, according to the study from the University of South Florida in Tampa. Physicians were more likely to use prescription tranquilizers or pain relievers than the general population, according to the study in The Journal of the American Medical Association.

May 18

A Food and Drug Administration advisory committee announced that the widely used sleeping pill triazolam (Halcion, Upjohn) is safe and effective. Critics had claimed that the drug induced anxiety, depression and short-term memory loss. The committee recommended that the drug be kept on the market and called for warnings on labels to be strengthened and simplified.

May 28

Neurologic and respiratory problems were linked to indoor ice-skating rinks, warned the Centers for Disease Control.

At least 60 of 130 Wisconsin students who attended an ice hockey tournament reported headaches, nausea, dizziness, vomiting or coughing spells within a day or two of the games.

Health officials attributed the illnesses to toxic doses of nitrogen dioxide and carbon monoxide released by the Zamboni ice-cleaning machine, and by the heaters used to heat the stands.

June 1

A sleep-disorder consultant asserted that patients who take one lesson in a technique called imagery rehearsal can get rid of their nightmares.

When patients have a bad dream, have them write it down and then change it or imagine that it has a different ending, he told the American Sleep Disorders Association meeting in Phoenix. The University of New Mexico re-

searcher presented the results of a study showing that four of 10 people who reported nightmares had complete relief after a single session of imagery rehearsal, and the average number of nightmares per month dropped from seven to two for the entire group.

June 2

Physicians were told that a new, more convenient form of light therapy may be as effective in the treatment of seasonal affective disorder as conventional light treatment. The new treatment is a low-intensity light that simulates the dawn by gradually increasing in intensity while the person is asleep, a University of Washington psychiatrist reported at the Association of Professional Sleep Societies meeting.

In a preliminary study, 13 SAD patients who received two hours of the gradual light treatment between 4 a.m. and 6 a.m. showed a significant improvement in their symptoms.

June 6

A newly identified defect on the p450 gene, coupled with years of exposure to common environmental pollutants, may lead to Parkinson's disease, reported researchers from the Imperial Cancer Research Fund in Edinburgh, Scotland.

The flaws may inhibit the body's ability to flush out environmental toxins, they theorized in The Lancet. Defects in the p450 gene were found to be twice as frequent in 229 Parkinson's patients as in 720 controls.

June 11

Radiologists at Brigham and Women's Hospital in Boston found that impaired blood flow through affected areas in cocaine users' brains improved when use of the drug was stopped. Previously, researchers had thought the drug permanently reduced the brain's blood flow by constricting blood vessels.

In a small study of 10 drug

addicts who were evaluated with high-resolution SPECT and MRI, impaired blood flow increased by 11% after one week without the drug and by 23% after 17 to 29 days, the radiologists told a meeting of the Society of Nuclear Medicine in Los Angeles.

June 24

Attendees at a headache conference in Toronto were told that intramuscular injection of a drug normally used intravenously for migraine headaches could relieve moderate to severe headaches within an hour. Forty-six percent of 311 patients reported either no pain or only mild pain 30 minutes after an injection of dihydroergotamine (D.H.E. 45, Sandoz), said a Florida investigator. At the end of an hour, 72% felt no pain or only mild pain. Although half the patients were given an antiemetic along with the D.H.E. 45 injection, the slower intramuscular absorption of the drug appeared to obviate the need for routine antiemetic use, said the codirector of the Palm Beach Headache Center in West Palm Beach.

• • •

New York and Baltimore researchers found that physicians often fail to diagnose migraine headaches; their patients may therefore fail to benefit from the latest treatments, they suggested. Their survey of 20,468 people aged 12 to 80 found that migraines were only diagnosed in 41% of female and 29% of male sufferers. Older, high-income migraine patients are more likely to be diagnosed and treated than younger, poorer ones, the researchers stated in the Archives of Internal Medicine.

July 13

Boston University investigators reassured the siblings and children of Alzheimer's disease patients that although they are at increased risk of developing the disease, it will likely occur late in life. In an evaluation of the relatives of

1992 HIGHLIGHTS

198 Dutch Alzheimer's patients, 10% developed the disease by age 65 and 13% by age 75. Overall, the risk of developing Alzheimer's was estimated at 39% by the age of 90, the team told the Third International Conference on Alzheimer's Disease in Padua, Italy.

July 14

Tacrine hydrochloride (Cognex, Warner-Lambert) was found to produce at least a short-term gain in cognitive function in Alzheimer's patients. At the Third International Conference on Alzheimer's Disease in Padua, Italy, the Warner-Lambert researchers said that more than 50% of 468 patients who received tacrine showed a four-point improvement on the Alzheimer's cognitive function scale at 12 weeks. Also, 23% of those treated with tacrine scored an eight-point gain on the cognition scale—the equivalent of avoiding about one year of cognitive decline. Elevations of transaminase resulted in the withdrawal of 25% of the tacrine patients from the study. Side effects such as nausea, vomiting and diarrhea forced another 10% to withdraw from treatment with the cholinergic compound.

• • •

The first guidelines for the nursing-home care of Alzheimer's patients were released by the Alzheimer's Association. The guidelines, issued at the annual meeting of the Alzheimer's Disease and Related Disorders Association in Chicago, called for ongoing training of staff; preadmission examination to assess care requirements; and re-evaluation of care as the disease progresses.

July 23

Some canned soft drinks were found to have a high aluminum content, which may pose a risk for Alzheimer's

disease if a link between Alzheimer's diease and aluminum intake is ever confirmed, said Australian researchers. The team from John Hunter Hospital in Newcastle investigated 52 beverages and found the aluminum content of noncola drinks was almost six times higher in cans than in bottles. The aluminum content of cola drinks was nearly three times higher in cans than in bottles, they told Medical Tribune. The difference did not hold for beers, they said. A Brandeis University researcher has hypothesized that aluminum may trigger a biochemical sequence that leads to the progressive aggregation of neurofibrillary tangles in the brain, but ingested aluminum has never been shown to cross the blood-brain barrier.

• • •

Investigators began testing what they hope will be the first drug to slow the course of amyotrophic lateral sclerosis. The new agent, Human Ciliary Neurotrophic Factor (Regeneron Pharmaceuticals) is a genetically engineered version of a protein found in small quantities in human nerve and muscle cells, the company told Medical Tribune.

In preliminary testing of 12 patients injected with the drug over a four-month period, none experienced toxicity, said a researcher at the Cleveland Clinic, one of four institutions where Phase I trials are under way.

July 31

The Food and Drug Administration approved an expanded indication for the anti-anxiety drug buspirone (Buspar, Mead Johnson), to include treatment of anxiety even in the presence of depressive symptoms. Buspirone already was approved for the management of anxiety disorders, or for short-term relief of the symptoms of anxiety.

Aug. 1

University of Pittsburgh researchers found that elevated levels of autoantibodies may be linked to cerebrovascular disorders in people with dementia. They studied 40 age-matched patients: 10 with probable Alzheimer's disease, 10 with possible Alzheimer's and cerebrovascular disease, 10 with vascular dementia and 10 nondemented controls. Autoantibodies were found in all patients with possible Alzheimer's/cerebrovascular disease, 80% of those with vascular dementia, 40% of those with probable Alzheimer's and 30% of the controls. The highest levels of autoantibodies were found in patients with vascular dementia and possible Alzheimer's/cerebrovascular disease, although no autoantibody could differentiate Alzheimer's from cerebrovascular disorders, the Pittsburgh team reported in Stroke.

Aug. 18

A new study added evidence to the theory that a genetic predisposition may trigger the onset of Alzheimer's disease. As reported in the American Journal of Psychiatry, the study revealed that patients with a family history of Alzheimer's had a faster course of dementia. Evaluating 462 Alzheimer's patients, a team of psychiatrists from the University of Chicago, University of Miami and University of Wisconsin-Milwaukee found that 76.7% of patients with a familial history of dementia showed a rapid deterioration in neurological symptoms, compared with 56% among those who did not have a positive family history.

The patients who degenerated rapidly were also more likely to have a family history of psychiatric disorders (18.6% vs 7.2%), as reported by caregivers.

Aug. 27

Postmortem magnetic resonance imaging examinations revealed a striking reduc-

1992 HIGHLIGHTS

tion in gray matter of the left temporal lobe in men with schizophrenia, reported Harvard researchers.

Using new MRI neuro-imaging techniques to derive volume measurements and three-dimensional reconstructions of temporal lobe structures, they examined 15 right-handed schizophrenics and 15 controls.

As compared with the controls, the volume of gray matter in the left anterior hippocampus-amygdala of schizophrenics was reduced by 19%, the left parahippocampal

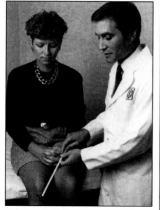

TCE-polluted well water linked to neurologic symptoms.

gyrus by 13% and the left superior temporal gyrus by 15%. In the 13 schizophrenic patients who had been evaluated on a thought disorder index, there was a high correlation between the extent of thought disorder and the reduction in volume of the left superior temporal gyrus, the team reported in The New England Journal of Medicine.

Sept. 10

Yale University researchers found that the efficacy of antiepileptic drugs in controlling symptoms depends on seizure type. The study of 480 adults with symptomatic epilepsy indicated that valproate (Depakote, Abbott) was as effective as carbamazepine (Tegretol, Ciba-Geigy) for the treatment of grand mal seizures. However, carbamazepine provided better control of partial seizures than valproate

and had fewer long-term adverse effects, the neurologists reported in The New England Journal of Medicine. In previous studies, the same team had found carbamazepine to be as effective as phenytoin (Dilantin, Parke-Davis) for partial seizures.

Since most adult epileptics have both kinds of seizures, the study suggested that carbamazepine and phenytoin be used first, but if they prove toxic or ineffective, valproate may be tried, according to the chief investigator.

Sept. 15

A small trial revealed that treating elderly depressed people with fluoxetine (Prozac, Dista) can result in significant weight loss, nausea and anorexia. Seven of 15 patients who were over 75 years old lost more than 5% of their body weight during four months of fluoxetine therapy, the California team revealed in the Journal of the American Geriatrics Society. In contrast, only two of 20 fluoxetine-treated patients between ages 60 and 71 lost more than 5% of their body weight, said the physicians from Palo Alto Veteran's Affairs Hospital. Twenty patients over 75 years of age achieved an average weight gain of nearly half a pound during treatment with tricyclics.

Oct. 2

For the second time in two weeks, Alzheimer's researchers announced findings that broadened the understanding of the brain-wasting disease. In a report in Science, a team from Case Western Reserve University in Cleveland confirmed two reports that had appeared in the previous week's issue of Nature: All three teams found that beta-amyloid protein, which aggregates and forms neurofibrils in the brains of Alzheimer's patients, is also secreted by normal cells in healthy people.

Harvard researchers also reported in last week's Nature that the protein can be measured in blood and cerebrospinal fluid, and researchers at Athena Neurosciences said they had begun the testing of drugs to lower beta-amyloid production. But the Case Western Reserve team said that there is not a one-to-one correlation between high levels of the protein and a predisposition to the disease, which points to an as-yet-unidentified factor that leads to precipitation of the amyloid and formation of the fibrils in Alzheimer's patients.

Oct. 8

A Chicago neurologist cautioned that exposure to trichloroethylene, a chemical solvent used in a variety of industries and found in numerous water supplies, may be a cause of severe, chronic headaches. He told the American Academy of Pain Management convention in Albuquerque that of 106 Illinois residents whose wells were polluted with TCE, 62% had severe or frequent headaches. After excluding migraines, the Rush-Presbyterian-St. Luke's Hospital researcher attributed 57 unexplained headaches to TCE pollution.

Oct. 23

Seattle scientists said that a defective gene on chromosome 14 appears to cause some cases of early-onset Alzheimer's disease, bringing the total number of chromosomes found to be involved in Alzheimer's to three. The University of Washington researchers collected blood samples and compared the genetic material from members of nine families with the disease with samples of genetic material taken from people in nonaffected families. Markers on chromosome 14 appeared to be close to one possible Alzheimer's gene, according to the report in Science.

Oct. 29

A new study of the investigational Alzheimer's drug tacrine (Cognex, Warner-Lambert) found that it improved mental functioning, but not to the extent that the patients' doctors noticed the change. Nonetheless, the head of the National Institute on Aging said that the study proves for the first time that Alzheimer's disease can be altered with drug therapy, and noted that other studies are under way to test whether tacrine might be more effective at higher doses.

As described in The New England Journal of Medicine, 215 patients were given either 40 mg or 80 mg of tacrine for six weeks, or placebo. Patients taking tacrine had a slight, statistically significant improvement on the Mini-Mental State Examination, and a significantly smaller decline in the activities of daily living than those on placebo. The study found that 42% of the patients taking tacrine showed dangerous changes in liver function. The liver function in all patients returned to normal after discontinuing the drug.

Nov. 5

British researchers suggested that studies dating back to 1965 linking aluminum deposits in the brain to Alzheimer's disease may be wrong.

Aluminum in microscopic dust particles might have contaminated the dyes that scientists used to compare the brain tissue of Alzheimer's patients with brain tissue of people who had died of other causes, the researchers wrote in the journal Nature.

Aluminum clings to certain proteins present in large amounts in the diseased brain tissue of Alzheimer's patients. Thus the aluminum may have accumulated in the brain tissue during the staining process in the lab, instead of originating from the brain tissue itself, the researchers said.

If high aluminum content poses Alzheimer's risk, beer in cans appears safer than some soft drinks

By Chris Gerrans

NEWCASTLE, AUSTRALIA, JULY 23—Some canned soft drinks have a high aluminum content, which may pose a risk for Alzheimer's disease if a link between aluminum intake and Alzheimer's ever is established.

Australian researchers investigating 52 beverages found the aluminum content of noncola drinks was almost six times higher in drinks packaged in cans than in bottles. The aluminum content of cola drinks was nearly three times higher in cans than in bottles. The difference did not hold for beers.

Overall, the highest aluminum content was found in noncola drinks and the lowest in beers.

Soft drinks are more acidic than beers and therefore allow aluminum to dissolve more easily into the drinks, said John Duggan, M.D., from the department of gastroenterology at John Hunter Hospital.

He suggested that imperfections in the protective lacquering on the walls of cans allow the acidic contents to slowly dissolve the aluminum.

Although the 106 cans and bottles investigated were obtained from different parts of Australia and from New Zealand and Thailand, Dr. Duggan could not confirm whether aluminum cans in other countries would reveal similar results. "I could only think that they must be very similar," he said.

A review that appeared in The Lancet in March attempted to establish a link between aluminum intake and Alzheimer's disease, but failed to provide a definite answer, Dr. Duggan said. "The jury is out."

The normal aluminum intake among Western Europeans is less than 10 mg/day, but some researchers recommend a maximum daily intake of less than 3 mg/day. Soft drinks were found to contain up to 3.9 mg per can, he said.

The World Health Organization and European Economic Community recommend a maximal aluminum concentration of 7.4 mcM/l in drinking water. The concentrations of aluminum in bottled cola drinks (8.9 mcM/l), cola drinks in cans (24.4 mcM/l) and noncola drinks (33.4 mcM/l) all exceeded this recommendation.

Dr. Duggan said that there is no cause for concern, but further research is required to identify other possible sources of dietary aluminum and verify its passage accross the blood-brain barrier.

Gerald Fasman, Ph.D., of Brandeis University in Waltham, Mass., has hypothesized that aluminum may trigger a biochemical sequence that leads to the progressive aggregation of neurofibrillary tangles in the brain.

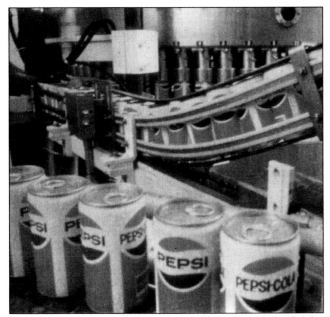

Acid in soda allows aluminum to dissolve easily into the drinks.

Antiepileptics' efficacy depends on seizure type and patient tolerance

SEPT. 10—In one of the largest studies of antiepileptic drugs ever completed, researchers have found that the efficacy of drugs in controlling symptoms of epilepsy depends on seizure type.

The findings are very significant and provide "important new information for the practicing clinician," according to Timothy A. Pedley, M.D., director of the Comprehensive Epilepsy Center at Columbia-Presbyterian Medical Center in New York. He said the majority of patients with seizures can be adequately cared for by primary-care doctors, sometimes in consultation with a neurologist.

The study was conducted over five years and involved 480 adults with symptomatic epilepsy, the most common type of the disease caused by brain injury. It compared two antiepileptic medications, carbamazepine (Tegretol, Ciba-Geigy and valproate (Depakote, Abbott).

Valproate, the newer drug, was as effective as carbamazepine for the treatment of grand mal seizures, according to Richard Mattson, M.D., professor of neurology at Yale University School of Medicine in New Haven, Conn.

Dr. Mattson was lead author of the study, which was part of a larger trial of antiepileptic drugs that involved more than 1,100 patients at 12 Veterans Affairs Medical Centers throughout the country and spanned nearly 15 years. The current report appeared in The New England Journal of Medicine.

The findings "mean that we now have five drugs that are effective and can control symptoms in more than two thirds of people with seizures," Dr. Mattson said.

However, carbamazepine provided better control of partial seizures than valproate and had fewer long-term adverse effects. In Dr. Mattson's previous studies, carbamazepine had been shown to be as effective as phenytoin (Dilantin, Parke-Davis).

When all five major antiepileptics are considered, "the big conclusion for the primary-care physician is that carbamazepine and phenytoin have a slight edge in efficacy over the other three drugs [valproate, phenobarbital and primidone (Mysoline, Wyeth-Ayerst)] for partial seizures," Dr. Mattson said.

According to him, the differences in efficacy had failed to emerge from earlier trials because they are rather minor and only became apparent in a larger study.

Since most adult epileptics have both types of seizures, the new study suggests that carbamazepine and phenytoin may be used first, but if they prove toxic or ineffective, valproate may be tried, he said.

However, no antiepileptic medication can be viewed as the drug of choice, according to Dr. Mattson.

While some of these medications appear equally effective in a large population, "for any given individual one medication may work when another has failed to control seizures," he said.

Moreover, there may be significant differences in side effects between the five medications.

In the study, valproate was more frequently associated with weight gain, hair loss and tremor, while carbamazepine more often caused an allergic reaction.

Overall, both drugs were very well tolerated and produced no clinically serious effects on liver function or white blood cell count, according to Dr. Mattson.

He stressed that the choice of antiepileptic drugs must be individualized on the basis of efficacy, side effects and cost.

Physicians should try one drug at a time and resort to a combination only after two or three drugs have failed, he said.

Epilepsy, which affects about two million Americans, is the third most common neurological disorder in the United States.

A beta-amyloid screening test for Alzheimer's?

By Charlene Laino

OCT. 2—Three new studies independently confirmed that beta-amyloid protein, which aggregates and forms debilitating fibrils in the brains of Alzheimer's patients, is also secreted by normal cells in healthy people.

One of the research teams also showed that the protein can be measured in samples of blood and cerebrospinal fluid.

Another of the studies showed that there is not a one-to-one correlation between high levels of beta-amyloid and a predisposition to Alzheimer's disease, making it unclear whether drugs that reduce beta-amyloid production would be beneficial.

"It is not yet clear whether high levels of beta-amyloid correlate with the development of Alzheimer's disease," commented Sam Gandy, M.D., Ph.D., assistant professor of molecular cell biology at Cornell University Medical School in New York.

Until such time as that is known, measurement of beta-amyloid levels should be done on a research basis only, he emphasized.

Current research points to an as yet unidentified factor that leads to precipitation of the amyloid and formation of the fibrils in Alzheimer's patients, he said.

Steven Younkin, M.D., professor of pathology at Case Western Reserve University School of Medicine in Cleveland and colleagues Mikio Shoji, M.D., and Todd Golde, M.D., reported their findings in Science. Dennis Selkoe, M.D., and his team at Brigham and Women's Hospital in Boston and a team from Athena Neurosciences Inc. in San Francisco reported their findings in Nature.

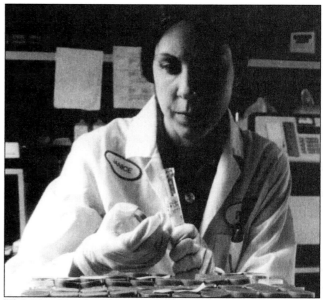

High blood levels of beta-amyloid do not necessarily correlate with development of Alzheimer's disease, said Dr. Gandy.

There are three major implications to the new studies, said Dr. Selkoe, professor of neurology at Harvard Medical School.

"First, it will make it much easier to study the protein because normal cells make it all the time," he said. Second, it could help to develop diagnostic tests for excess levels of the protein in the blood and spinal fluid.

Even if excess beta-amyloid protein in the blood does not directly cause Alzheimer's, it appears to be a risk factor for the disease, just as high blood cholesterol is for heart disease. Unlike Dr. Gandy, Dr. Selkoe does foresee beta-amyloid screening.

Third, it allows for the testing of drugs to lower beta amyloid protein, he said. Researchers at Athena Neurosciences in San Francisco have already begun such testing.

The studies also leave unanswered why, at autopsy, the fibroid plaques have been found in the brains of some healthy elderly people.

"It could be that these people were just at a very early stage of Alzheimer's; it's just another unknown about this disease," said Neil Kowall, M.D., assistant professor of neurology at Harvard Medical School.

One third of patients improve on tacrine

Medical Tribune News Service

Nov. 11—About one third of people suffering from mild to moderate Alzheimer's disease who take the experimental drug tacrine (Cognex, Warner-Lambert) regain about six months worth of the mental functioning they had lost to the disease's progression, a new study has found.

The study's findings, involving 486 patients at 23 medical centers in the United States and Canada, are only slightly more hopeful than conclusions of another major study on tacrine released two weeks ago. That study found that the drug did not benefit patients to the extent that examining doctors could detect the improvement.

The new study found that both the patients' doctors and the patients' daily caregivers were able to see improvements.

"These patients actually got better," said the lead author of the study, Martin Farlow, M.D., associate professor of neurology at Indiana University Medical Center in Indianapolis. "It's the equivalent of rolling back the clock symptomatically by six months or so."

An editorial accompanying the article in today's Journal of the American Medical Association described the drug's effects as modest, but clinically meaningful.

Even that cautious assessment, however, was more positive than the one in an editorial two weeks ago in The New England Journal of Medicine that accompanied the publication of the first major study of tacrine.

John H. Growdon, M.D., an associate professor of neurology at Harvard Medical School in Boston, called the drug's effects trivial and said that research on tacrine and other drugs that work like it should be abandoned.

"I stand by my position," said Dr. Growdon, in response to the new study's slightly better results. "The new study confirms that tacrine has some beneficial effects in a small number of patients, that the benefit is still quite small and that there is a high rate of side effects. So I don't see any surprises here."

No drugs have been approved by the Food and Drug Administration to treat Alzheimer's, except those involved in experimental studies.

A researcher who was on the FDA advisory committee that permitted expanded testing of the drug last year said that the new study showed only marginally better results than the one published two weeks ago. "I haven't changed my personal opinion that it's not a clinically meaningful benefit," said Steven H. Ferris, Ph.D., executive director of the aging and dementia research center at New York University.

The new study involved 468 people, all at least 50 years old, with mild or moderate Alzheimer's disease and no other significant medical conditions. For the first six weeks of the study, patients took placebo, 20 mg of tacrine or 40 mg of tacrine. In the next six weeks, half the patients were given stronger doses than they had been receiving, and half were given the same.

Of those who did not have to drop out of the study due to side effects or for other reasons, 51% of patients taking 80 mg of tacrine in the second six-week phase had at least a four-point gain on a test of mental functioning—the Alzheimer's Disease Assessment Scale.

But about 18% of patients taking the inactive placebo showed an equal gain, a fact that the researchers attributed to random fluctuations in the course of the disease. So, they explained, the four-point gain can be attributed to the effects of the drug for only about one third of the patients taking tacrine.

The mental functioning scale ranges from zero to 70, with 70 being the worst impairment. On average, Alzheimer's patients decline by about eight points per year. The four-point gain is therefore considered equal to reversing about six months' worth of average decline.

Researchers do not yet know what effects the drug might have beyond 12 weeks.

In the new study, one fourth of the patients given tacrine showed dangerous elevations in liver function tests and had to stop taking the drug. The liver function in all patients returned to normal after discontinuing the drug. Because of the possible liver damage, any patient taking the drug must be tested for changes in liver chemistry once a week and must stop taking tacrine if harmful changes are found.

In the multicenter study published two weeks ago, the researchers offered tacrine to 632 Alzheimer's patients. Since prior research had suggested that many patients probably would not benefit at all from the drug, the researchers eliminated 417 patients who did not respond to treatment in a preliminary test.

With the remaining 215 patients, the researchers gave half of them either 40 mg or 80 mg of tacrine every day for six weeks, and gave the other half a placebo drug.

After six weeks, patients on tacrine had gained an average of 2.4 points, a change that was not noticeable by the patients' doctors. The study also found that 42% of the patients taking tacrine showed dangerous changes in liver function. Slightly more than one fifth of the patients had to stop taking the drug because the changes were so severe. Liver function in all patients returned to normal after discontinuing the drug.

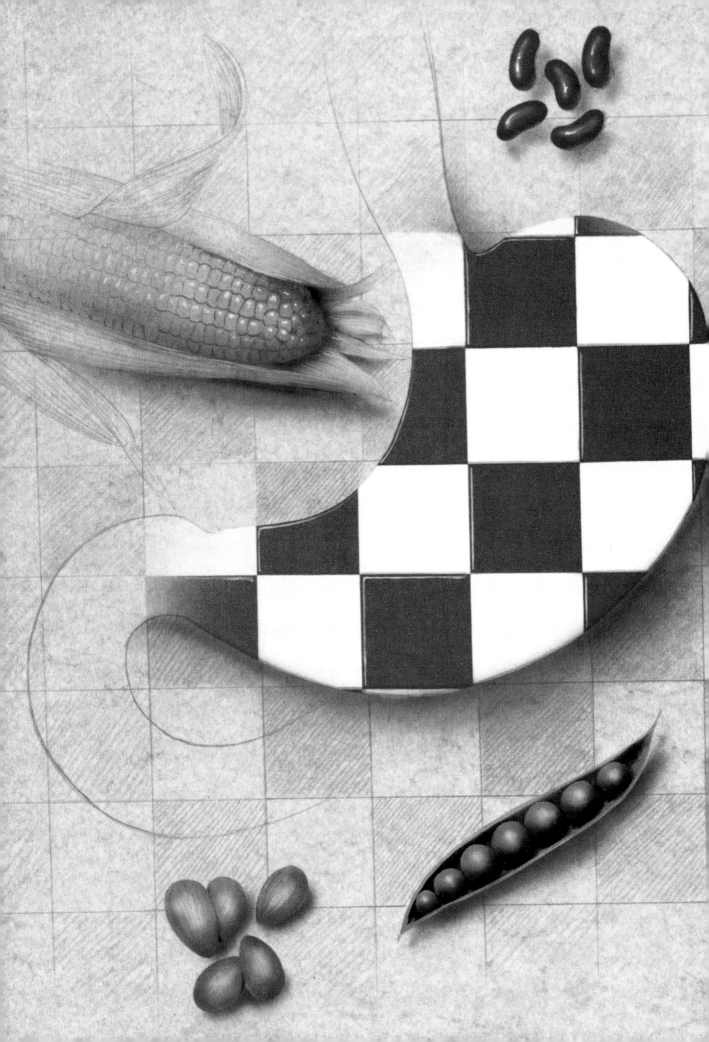

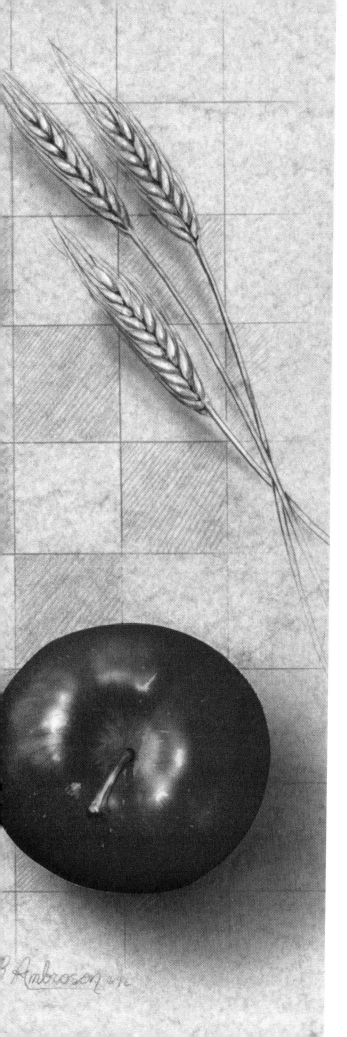

Overview 144
Despite insights on nutrient-disease links, advice the same: less fat, more veggies

Month-at-a-glance 146

Reported at the Time 158
Fast food and sugar linked to Crohn's disease…low folic acid and HPV increase cervical-cancer risk, CDC recommends folic acid for women…Institute of Medicine, USDA publish diet guidelines…sailors demonstate ACS diet is practical…modified citrus pectin slows tumor-cell growth…FASEB meeting news: saccharin only a rodent carcinogen, zinc counteracts harmful chemical by-product of exercise, eat garlic raw to reap benefits…wide variation in vitamin D quantities in milk discovered…diets for autoimmune disease, cardiac patients, nursing mothers, postop patients…meta-analysis confirms anticancer role of fruits and veggies, but Nurses' Health Study finds fat, fiber don't affect breast-cancer risk

Commentary 171
Dietary research is bearing fruit
By Johanna Dwyer, D.Sc.

OVERVIEW

Despite insights on nutrient-disease links, advice the same: less fat, more veggies

The four basic food groups are out, replaced by a pyramid that downplays milk and meat and prods Americans to consume more grains, fruits and vegetables.

In 1992, a year in which scientists came closer to understanding nutrition's role in cancer, heart disease, birth defects, allergies and other areas of health, the overall dietary message for physicians and patients stayed the same: lower fat intake and increase consumption of fruits, vegetables and grains.

The evidence that diet plays a role in some types of cancer continued to accumulate. Researchers at the University of California, Berkeley, reviewed 156 studies on the role of fruits and vegetables in cancer prevention; 128 concluded there was a protective effect. The review found that for most types of cancer, the 25% of the world's population with the highest intake of fruits and vegetables had roughly half as many cancers as the 25% with the lowest intake.

And a study of more than 7,000 men conducted at the Harvard School of Public Health found that eating a high-fat, low-fiber diet increased the risk of developing colorectal adenomas.

But the long-held assumption that a high-fat, low-fiber diet also increases breast-cancer risk was cast into doubt by a report on almost 90,000 women who are part of the Nurses' Health Study. Researchers found that a high-fat diet did not increase women's breast-cancer risk, nor did a high-fiber diet lower the risk. But the researchers were quick to point out that high-fiber, low-fat diets are still desirable since they reduce the risk of colon cancer.

In the area of weight loss, there was some discouraging news and a few rays of hope. A National Institutes of Health consensus panel broke no new ground when it concluded that to lose weight, people must diet and exercise. Up to 95% of dieters regain almost all their lost weight within one to three years, the panel noted.

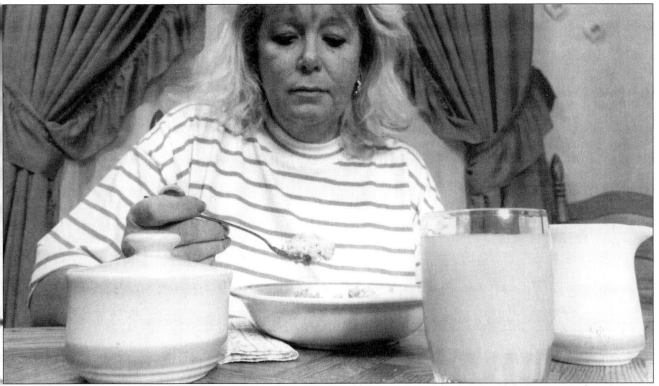

Eating breakfast helped reduce impulsive snacking and fat consumption, and contributed to weight loss, study found.

Still, a few new trials seemed to help some dieting patients. Boston nutritionists reported at the American Dietetic Association annual meeting in October that women who used artificial sweeteners in their desserts and coffee lost significantly more weight and were more likely to keep it off, compared with women who used sugar.

In a study from Vanderbilt University in Nashville, eating breakfast helped reduce impulsive snacking and fat consumption. Over a three-month period, women who ate three meals a day, including breakfast, lost about 18 pounds, compared with an average 13-pound loss for those eating only two meals a day.

The government made several changes in nutrition policy in 1992. The Centers for Disease Control recommended in September that all women of childbearing age consume 0.4 mg of folic acid daily to reduce the risk of birth defects. Folic acid can reduce the risk of neural-tube defects if it is taken starting at least a month before a woman becomes pregnant and continuing through the first trimester of pregnancy.

The U.S. Department of Agriculture replaced its old food chart, which had promoted the basic four food groups, with a new food guide pyramid. The pyramid de-emphasizes meats and dairy products and recommends that people use fats, oils and sweets "sparingly." Instead, the new guide encourages people to eat plenty of grains, such as bread, cereal, rice and pasta, along with fruits and vegetables.

For patients concerned with lowering their cholesterol levels and risk of coronary artery disease, several studies suggested strategies that go beyond a low-fat diet. A team from the University of California, San Diego, found that

eating four meals a day may result in lower average cholesterol levels than eating meals less frequently, even when more calories, fat and cholesterol are consumed.

Eating raw garlic can lower both cholesterol and hypertension, Tulane University School of Medicine researchers reported at the Federation of American Societies for Experimental Biology meeting. And eating fish was found to be more effective than taking fish-oil supplements in lowering cholesterol, according to Australian researchers. A team from the University of Western Australia in Perth studied men aged 30 to 60 and found that those who ate fish every day for 12 weeks showed a 20% reduction in total cholesterol, compared with a 14% drop in those who took fish-oil supplements.

A number of provocative studies on nutrition and health suggested directions in which future research may go. Several studies suggested that vegetarian diets may have a role to play in the treatment of various autoimmune diseases, including lupus. Finnish researchers found that the hot flashes of menopause may be eased by soy-based foods such as miso soup and tofu. Soy products are rich in isoflavonoids, which bind to estrogen receptors, they hypothesized. Soy sauce, as well as garlic and cauliflower, also contains diallyl sulfide, which researchers found prevented cancer in rodents.

And a compound in broccoli, sulforaphane, seems to bolster the activities of enzymes known to detoxify carcinogens, Johns Hopkins researchers reported.

In sum, 1992 findings move physicians closer to a time when they may be able to prescribe diets to prevent or treat an ever-larger number of diseases.

Nutrition

Jan. 2

Harvard pediatricians warned that infants may be subject to lead poisoning as a result of contaminated water-based formula. About one fourth of 41 cases of lead intoxication were traced to the water used to prepare formula. Although the labels on powdered and concentrated infant formulas recommend boiling for five minutes for sterilization, excessive boiling increases the lead concentration of the water, the researchers pointed out in Pediatrics.

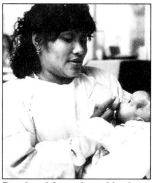

Powdered formula and lead-heavy water: poisonous combo.

Jan. 7

A fast-food diet is risky for the gut as well as the heart, asserted Swedish researchers. People who regularly eat at fast-food restaurants, consuming an overall diet high in sugar and fat, are at increased risk of Crohn's disease and ulcerative colitis, according to researchers from the Karolinska Institute. The risk of either disease was lowered in people eating a high-fiber diet, according to a 602-person, case-control study reported in Epidemiology.

Jan. 9

Homemade beer with a high iron content was linked to a syndrome often misdiagnosed as chronic liver disease in sub-Saharan Africans. A study of 236 people in Zimbabwe revealed that those with a genetic predisposition to hemochromatosis are susceptible to iron overload when they routinely drink beer mixed in steel drums that leach iron, according to researchers from the Metro-Health Medical Center in Cleveland. In The New England Journal of Medicine, they cautioned that beer-related iron overload can result in symptoms of bronze skin color, diabetes, heart disturbances, abdominal pain and loss of sex drive, which should not be attributed to liver damage.

Jan. 13

The Food and Drug Administration announced that the advocacy group Public Voice is developing new, voluntary food labels designed to teach children how to tell if a product's ingredients are nutritious. The labels, which will be bold and simple with an emphasis on graphics, are intended to augment the detailed nutritional labeling mandated by the FDA by 1993.

Jan. 15

Male patients who consume diets high in saturated fat and low in fiber were shown to face an increased risk of colorectal adenoma. Among

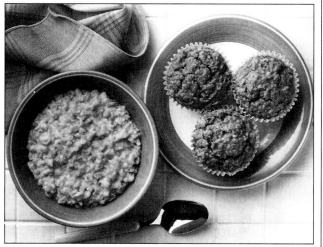

Low-fat, high-fiber diet may decrease colorectal adenoma risk.

7,284 men studied, those on a high-saturated-fat, low-fiber diet had 3.7 times the risk of developing the precancerous growths compared with those on low-saturated-fat, high-fiber diets. The data support recommendations to substitute chicken and fish for red meat and to increase consumption of vegetables, fruits and grains, Harvard School of Public Health researchers concluded in the Journal of the National Cancer Institute.

Jan. 22

A new study suggested that HPV-16, the strain of human papillomavirus most closely linked with development of cervical cancer, does most of its damage in women with inadequate stores of folic acid. In a case-control study of 464 young women presented in The Journal of the American Medical Association, the presence of HPV-16 alone raised the risk of cervical dysplasia by one tenth, but the risk increased 500% in those infected with HPV-16 and with red-blood-cell folate levels at or below 600 nmol/l. With HPV exposure estimated to affect 30% of sexually active women in their twenties, University of Alabama researchers concluded that increasing folic acid in the diet may prevent the initial cervical epithelial changes that are caused by HPV.

Jan. 23

Researchers in Zaire found that a single dose of iodine can shrink goiters and correct severe iodine deficiency for an entire year.

When 75 people with visible goiter were given a single oral dose of iodine (either 47 mg or 118 mg), goiters shrank 36% in three months. At one year, goiter size was reduced 44% in persons on low-dose iodine and 52% in those on the higher dose, according to Belgian and Zairean researchers writing in The New England Journal of Medicine. Meanwhile, people who received a noniodized dose of vegetable oil showed a 9% increase in goiter size.

Jan. 25

Public health experts announced that one large dose of vitamin A reduces the risk of death among malnourished toddlers.

In a study of more than 3,700 children in Nepal and India, the risk of death was 26% less among those who received vitamin A supplementation (50,000 to 200,000 IU each) than among those who did not, they reported in the British Medical Journal.

Each death was prevented for just $11 extra in health-care costs, according to the International Center for the Prevention and Treatment of Major Childhood Diseases.

Jan. 31

Government researchers warned that consumption of an unripe tropical fruit can cause fatal toxic hypoglycemia. Six people died and another 22 suffered the hypoglycemic syndrome after eating unripe ackee, the national fruit of Jamaica, according to the Centers for Disease Control.

Unripe ackee fruit contains a liver toxin that induces hypoglycemia by inhibiting oxidation of fatty acids. Ackee is found in the Antilles, Central America and southern Florida, as well as Jamaica.

Nutrition

Feb. 1

Infant formula of the future may include two breast-milk components known to be vital building blocks of brain and nervous tissue, predicted researchers from Cambridge University. After a seven-year follow-up study showed an 8.3-point boost in IQ scores for premature infants receiving breast milk over formula, formula manufacturers got a nudge toward adding the two complex lipids, docosahexanoic acid and arachidonic acid. Previously, formula makers assumed that infants could make enough of the substances themselves from other, less complex fats included in formula. The additives, already recommended by a European nutrition committee, are likely to be included first in formulas specifically for premature infants, the researchers reported in Medical Tribune .

•••

The World Health Organization recommended that a rice-based oral rehydration formula be used in treating diarrhea caused by cholera. In a meta-analysis of 13 studies involving 1,367 patients, published in The Lancet, rice-based oral rehydration solution proved 36% more effective in adults and 32% more effective in children than the standard glucose-based mixture.

Rice-based formula was also 18% more effective in treating noncholera diarrhea in children, but the WHO stopped short of recommending its widespread use in these cases because the mixture is three times as expensive. Other studies have shown that the rice formula speeds healing and leads to quicker weight gain in infants.

Feb. 3

Obese patients may lose weight on an 800-calorie, high-protein diet, but the pounds shed are likely to be gained back, warned a Pittsburgh psychologist. Long-term weight loss is

more likely when the very-low-calorie diet is accompanied by psychological therapy, the psychologist wrote in Diabetes Care. On average, people on very-low-calorie diets lose 44 pounds in three months, she said.

Feb. 5

Vitamin C may be of use in delaying or preventing the chronic complications of diabetes, speculated researchers from Whittington Hospital in London. Whether it is useful depends on the vitamin's ability to inhibit glycosylation of proteins when

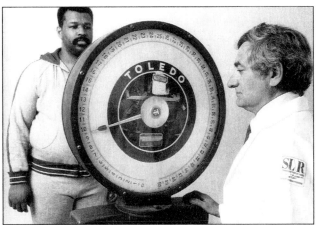

Exercise and 10%-fat diet cut weight, triglycerides and BP.

administered at doses unlikely to cause deleterious effects, they explained in Diabetes. In a study of 12 healthy, nondiabetic volunteers, 1 g of vitamin C daily for three months inhibited the glycosylation of the short-lived proteins albumin and hemoglobin.

Feb. 7

Sixty-nine of 72 overweight, hypertensive patients with normal total serum cholesterol were able to lose weight and reduce high blood pressure, high triglycerides and high insulin levels by exercising and reducing fat intake to 10% of total calories for 26 days, California researchers associated with the Pritikin Longevity Center

reported in the American Journal of Cardiology.

Feb. 13

After an epidemiological study linking low levels of folic acid to cervical damage from human papillomavirus, an Alabama nutrition professor suggested that the recommended daily allowance of folic acid be returned to 400 mcg/day. In 1989, the National Academy of Sciences lowered its RDA to 180 mcg/day for women and 200 mcg/day for men. Although there is no evidence that folic acid can prevent

cancer, increasing the amount of the vitamin in the diet may prevent the initial cervical epithelial changes that are caused by HPV, the University of Alabama researcher told Medical Tribune.

Feb. 19

To lower the risk of most common chronic diseases, the Institute of Medicine recommended limiting total fat intake to 30% or less of daily calories and eating five or more servings a day of fruits and vegetables. In its nutrition report, "Eat for Life,'' the institute further advised people to get moderate, regular exercise; limit salt intake to slightly more than one teaspoon per day; maintain adequate calcium intake by

consuming low-fat or nonfat milk products and dark-green vegetables; maintain an optimal level of fluoride in the diet; avoid taking vitamin and mineral supplements in excess of the U.S. RDA; eat no more than six ounces a day of protein; and limit alcohol intake to no more than two drinks a day.

•••

Sailors who traded their traditional fare of meat and potatoes for the American Cancer Society's low-fat, high-fiber diet lost weight and lowered their cholesterol levels, according to an unpublished ACS study. During a six-month deployment, sailors who ate the ACS diet lost an average of 12 pounds and trimmed their waistlines by 2 inches; 44% lowered their cholesterol levels. Shipmates on the standard Navy diet gained seven pounds and 1.5 inches around the waist.

Feb. 25

Three out of five Americans surveyed said they would buy a food labeled "healthy," rather than a similar food without the label, reported the National Consumers League. Nearly four out of five people would expect a product labeled "healthy" to be low in sodium, cholesterol and fat; 72% believed it would be a good source of fiber; and two out of three shoppers thought it would have all these attributes. Yet the foods do not have to meet these high standards under current labeling regulations, said the consumer group.

Feb. 26

Three years after the first media reports linking Alar-treated apples to an increased risk of cancer, and the subsequent voluntary removal of the chemical from the market, scientists from the chemical-industry-funded American Council on Science and Health released a report saying the chemical never posed a cancer risk to adults or children.

March 1

Candidal colonization and infection was reduced in women who ate an eight-ounce cup of yogurt with active cultures every day for six months. In a crossover trial of 13 patients, vulvo-vaginal candidal infections were decreased threefold when subjects consumed the "live yogurt" containing Lactobacillus acidophilus, said a team from Long Island Jewish Medical Center. However, tests showed that some products touting their live cultures did not contain the gram-positive, fermentative bacteria, the researchers cautioned in the Annals of Internal Medicine.

March 4

Stanford University researchers said microwaving breast milk markedly decreased the effectiveness of two substances in the milk that defend against infectious organisms. The new study, published in Pediatrics, found

Microwaving may zap infection fighters in breast milk.

that microwaving breast milk decreased activity of lysozymes and IgA antibodies.

The researchers studied microwaved milk in an intensive-care nursery, where mothers' breast milk is given to their infection-susceptible premature infants.

March 6

Eating breakfast may help people lose weight by reducing impulsive snacking

---

and reducing dietary fat, said researchers from Vanderbilt University. A three-month study of 52 women who were 30% to 60% above ideal body weight revealed that those who ate three meals a day, including breakfast, lost about 18 pounds, while those who ate two meals daily lost about 13 pounds. All the women consumed 1,200 calories a day and participated in a 12-week behavior-modification program consisting of weekly 90-minute group meetings, the researchers stated in the American Journal of Clinical Nutrition.

March 9

Saying bottle-feeding leads to more than one million infant deaths each year, UNICEF and the World Health Organization kicked off a campaign to promote breast-feeding in developing countries. Many of the deaths are the result of chronic diarrhea, caused by bacteria that can be transmitted in unsterilized bottles or milk diluted with unclean water, UNICEF officials said. Breast milk supplies an infant's total nutrient requirements for the first four to six months of life, and provides nourishment through the second birthday, the agency said.

WHO promotes breast-feeding to cut infant diarrhea deaths.

March 13

Eating four meals a day may result in lower average cholesterol levels than eating meals less frequently, suggested a University of California at San Diego team. A study of 2,034 whites aged 50 to 89 found that those who ate four or more meals a day had total cholesterol levels that were about 2.5% lower than those of people who ate once or twice a day, even though the people who ate more frequently consumed more calories, fat and cholesterol. Low-density lipoprotein cholesterol was an average of 6.0 mg/dl lower in people eating four or more meals a day, they stated in the American Journal of Clinical Nutrition.

March 15

A compound in broccoli, sulforaphane, seems to bolster the activities of enzymes known to detoxify carcinogens, reported researchers from Johns Hopkins University. Sulforaphane appears to block tumor formation in animals, and it will presumably do the same in humans, they predicted in the Proceedings of the National Academy of Sciences.

• • •

A modified form of citrus pectin appears to interfere with the way in which cancer cells cluster together and form secondary tumors, said researchers from the Michigan Cancer Foundation.

Injections of citrus pectin led to a threefold increase in tumor-cell colonization compared with controls, while the modified form reduced the number and size of tumor cell clusters in mice. If these findings are confirmed, modified pectin could be given intravenously before and after surgery, when cancer cells are likely to metastasize, they predicted in the Journal of the National Cancer Institute.

March 24

Although rapid weight loss has been associated with gallstone formation, Harvard researchers found that obesity carries an even greater risk. Analyzing 2,122 cases of cholecystectomy and 488 other cases of symptomatic gallstones among women participating in the Nurses' Health Study, they found that women of average height who weighed more than 269 pounds had the highest risk of developing symptomatic gallstones, about 2% per year. Substantial or extreme weight loss also increased the risk of gallstones, but the risk was less than that associated with obesity. Sustained weight loss may reduce the incidence of gallstone formation, they concluded in the American Journal of Clinical Nutrition.

March 28

British researchers suggested that a man's chances of dying of heart disease may depend in part on how he was fed as an infant. A study of 5,741 men revealed that those who were exclusively breast-fed or bottle-fed but not weaned at one year had higher cholesterol levels and died from heart disease about 20% more often than men who received both types of milk as infants. The exclusive breast- or bottle-feeders died of heart disease about 10% more often than those on breast milk who were weaned at one year, the University of Southampton team reported in the British Medical Journal.

Nutrition

APRIL

April 1

Older Americans may have cut their fat consumption, but they are still not getting enough fiber in their daily diet, said University of North Carolina researchers. The team compared the dietary practices of people over 65 who were part of both the 1977-1978 and 1987-1988 Nationwide Food Consumption Surveys. The comparison revealed that the elderly have not increased their consumption of fruits, vegetables and high-fiber cereals, while they have decreased their consumption of high-fat beef and pork, the researchers reported in the American Journal of Clinical Nutrition.

• • •

A National Institutes of Health consensus development panel reached what might seem an obvious conclusion: To lose weight, people must diet and exercise. Dieters need to set modest goals based on realistic ideals, said the panel, which did not specify which types of diet and exercise are best. More than one third of women and almost one fourth of men are trying to lose weight at any given time, noted the panel. Up to 95% of dieters regain almost all their lost weight within one to three years.

April 2

A study of nearly 129,000 people found that three to five alcoholic drinks a day reduces the chance of premature death by 20% compared with not drinking at all, reported a team from the Kaiser Permanente Medical Center. In contrast, six or more drinks a day carried a 30% higher correlative risk, the Oakland, Calif., researchers told the Alcoholic Beverage Medical Research Foundation conference. They noted that such factors as not smoking, exercise and attention to high lipids and blood pressure are more important than moderate drinking in avoiding premature death.

April 8

Zinc supplements may prevent cell-damaging superoxides from building up in the bloodstream during strenuous activity, announced a researcher from the Uniformed Services University in Bethesda, Md. When five runners took either a placebo or two 25-mg zinc pills a day for four days prior to exercise, those receiving zinc developed fewer superoxides after two hours running on a treadmill, the researcher reported.

Superoxides, produced by white blood cells during exercise, can suppress the immune system and increase the risk of infections, he explained at the Federation of American Societies for Experimental Biology meeting in Anaheim, Calif.

• • •

The artificial sweetener saccharin may not be harmful to humans, a University of Nebraska Medical Center researcher announced at the same meeting. The sweetener has carried a label for 15 years in the United States warning that it may cause cancer in laboratory animals. However, the researcher said that humans lack a protein (alpha-2-u-globulin) that binds to saccharin in rats, creating a toxic substance that irritates the lining of the bladder, and it is the combination of saccharin and the protein that causes cancer.

April 9

Garlic can lower cholesterol and hypertension, but only if eaten raw, Tulane University School of Medicine researchers reported. The healthy effects of garlic depend on the amount of allicin, the ingredient that gives the herb its odor, the researchers told a meeting of the Federation of American Societies for Experimental Biology.

The amount of allicin in about two cloves of garlic was able to lower blood pressure in rats and reduce cholesterol levels by 11% in patients with high cholesterol, the researchers said.

Cooking the herb deactivates allicin, the chemical that holds the key to garlic's beneficial effect, the researchers added.

April 15

Adding to the evidence that nutrition plays a role in preventing colon cancer, a 41-patient case-control study at the University Hospital of Linkoping, Sweden, revealed that high dietary intake of fiber, phosphorous and calcium each had a protective effect against adenocarcinoma of the colon or rectum. The study, presented in the journal Cancer, also showed that high alcohol consumption increased cancer risk.

April 18

Indian researchers reported that if heart-attack patients switch to a low-fat diet rich in

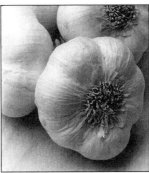

Use garlic raw to reap benefit of blood-pressure-lowering allicin.

fiber and vitamins, they will significantly reduce their risk of death or a second heart attack. In a one-year follow-up study of 406 heart-attack survivors, 75% of those who increased their daily intake of fruit, vegetables, nuts and grains and reduced their consumption of meat, butter and eggs went for a year without experiencing a second heart attack, they reported in the British Medical Journal. By comparison, 60% of patients who lowered their fat without increasing fiber and vitamin intake went for a year without a second heart attack, reported the team from the Medical Hospital and Research Center in Moradabad.

April 25

World Health Organization officials warned that supplementing the diet of breast-fed infants with tea, juice or water increases the risk of diarrhea. In Peru and the Philippines, studies have found that infants younger than six months whose diets were supplemented with other fluids had at least twice the risk of diarrhea that infants did who were exclusively breast-fed, the officials stated in the British Medical Journal.

April 28

The U.S. Department of Agriculture replaced its old food chart, which had promoted the basic four food groups, with a new food guide pyramid.

The pyramid, which lists grains such as bread, cereal, rice and pasta, along with fruits and vegetables, as the base for good nutrition, de-emphasizes meats and dairy products and recommends that people use fats, oils and sweets "sparingly." It recommends six to 11 small servings daily of grains, three to five of vegetables, two to four of fruits and two to three of both dairy products and meats.

April 30

Milk and infant-formula preparations rarely contain the amount of vitamin D stated on the label, and may be either over- or underfortified, stated a team of Boston researchers after diagnosing hypervitaminosis D in eight patients. Only a third of the milk tested was within 20% of the amount of vitamin D on the label. Seven of 10 samples of formula had more than twice the stated amount, the researchers said in The New England Journal of Medicine.

Nutrition

May 5

In a three-month attempt to lower children's low-density lipoproteins with diet, success hinged on how much the youngsters reduced the amount of saturated fat in their diet, said Mayo Clinic researchers. Thirty-two children, each with LDLs above 110 mg/dl, were placed on a diet in which no more than 30% of calories came from fat (with no more than 10% saturated fat and 10% polyunsaturated fat). Overall, the average decrease in LDLs was 10.4%, according to the Mayo researchers. Only the change in number of grams of saturated fat eaten correlated with LDL response (not total fat, cholesterol, polyunsaturated fat or the percentage of any type of fat in proportion to calories), they reported in Pediatrics.

May 6

A protein in breast milk protects infants against diarrhea, which causes 200,000 hospitalizations and 500 infant deaths in the United States each year, a Johns Hopkins infectious-disease expert told a meeting of the Society for Pediatric Research in Baltimore. The protein, called mucin, protects against diarrhea-causing rotavirus by inhibiting its reproduction in the intestine, the researcher said. While it has long been known that breast milk protects babies against diarrhea, it was not known that a protein in the milk was the key factor.

May 7

A Finnish study suggested that supplementary inositol, a B-complex vitamin abundant in breast milk, may improve survival and reduce complications in premature infants with respiratory distress syndrome. Out of 114 RDS infants given inositol, 11% died and 71% survived the first 28 days without developing bronchopulmonary dysplasia. Of 107 RDS babies on placebo, 24% died

and 51% survived the first 28 days without BPD, the University of Helsinki team reported in The New England Journal of Medicine.

Infants on placebo were also twice as likely (26% vs 13%) to develop retinopathy of prematurity, or retrolental fibroplasia.

May 9

Two reports in The Lancet prompted researchers to suggest that vegetarian diets may have a role to play in the treatment of various autoimmune diseases.

Physicians at Tottori University in Yonago, Japan, reported that a 16-year-old girl with systemic lupus erythematosus clinically improved and her antibody titers dropped to normal and were maintained for five years on a vegetarian diet. Another group of researchers, at the San Carlo Hospital in Milan, reported that 20 people with nephrotic syndrome improved after eating a vegetarian soy-based diet for eight weeks.

May 11

The effectiveness of milk-digestion aids varies widely, a Baylor University physician told the Digestive Disease Week meeting in San Francisco.

When compared with placebo in seven patients diagnosed with lactase deficiency, Lactrase proved 100% effective in relieving symptoms, Lactaid Tablets 86% effective and Dairy Ease 57% effective, he said.

May 16

Miso soup, tofu and other dishes derived from soybeans may ease the hot flashes brought on by menopause, suggested Finnish researchers. Soy-based foods are rich in isoflavonoids, said the University of Helsinki team in The Lancet. Isoflavonoids are known to bind to estrogen receptors and themselves have

weak estrogenic activity, which the researchers suggested as a plausible explanation for the women's lack of menopausal symptoms.

May 19

Hungarian researchers predicted that if pregnant women took daily supplements of folic acid (0.4 mg is recommended), 75% of all neural-tube defects would be prevented. In a 5,000-woman clinical trial in Hungary, six women receiving placebo delivered infants with NTDs. There were no NTDs in infants born to women who

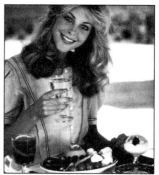

Vegetarian diet may help treat some autoimmune diseases.

received the B vitamin starting one month before conception and through the second month of pregnancy.

While folic acid supplements are currently recommended in the United States only for women who have already delivered a child with the abnormality, investigators from the National Institute of Hygiene in Budapest told a New York Academy of Sciences symposium in San Diego that all women should receive the supplements, since only 5% of NTDs are recurrences.

May 21

Eating fish was found to be more effective than taking fish-oil supplements in lowering cholesterol.

In a study of 120 men aged 30 to 60, those who ate fish every day for 12 weeks

showed a 20% reduction in total cholesterol, whereas those who took fish-oil supplements showed a 14% reduction, reported researchers from the University of Western Australia, Perth, writing in the Medical Journal of Australia. Their investigation was the first cholesterol study to control for both the fat and fish content in diets.

• • •

A compound derived from a food preservative used in dairy products may be effective in ridding the upper GI tract of Helicobacter pylori, a bacterium implicated in peptic ulcer disease, researchers told Medical Tribune. The antibacterial peptide nisin, a pure form of the preservative nisaplin, kills the ulcer-related bacteria in the laboratory, said the research director of Applied Microbiology Inc. of Brooklyn. The company plans to file applications with the Food and Drug Administration next year to start clinical trials of its nisin product in the treatment of ulcers and dental plaque.

May 25

A retrospective case-control study comparing children with juvenile diabetes and those without revealed that among blacks, exposure to any breast-milk substitute (whether based on cow's milk or not) before three months of age poses a threefold increase in the risk of developing insulin-dependent diabetes before the age of 17. The relationship with early feeding was not seen in white diabetic patients, the University of Pittsburgh investigators reported in Diabetes Care.

May 28

Government officials reminded salad lovers that the dressing for Caesar salad, which is made with raw eggs, can cause salmonella poisoning. Researchers at the Centers for Disease Control reported several cases of salmonella poisoning in Georgia among Caesar salad eaters.

JUNE

June 1

Mothers who vigorously exercise were advised to breast-feed their infants before a workout. In research at Indiana University in Bloomington, 26 two- to six-month-old infants were less likely to accept breast milk taken from their mothers 10 to 30 minutes after they exercised, compared with milk expressed prior to exercise. The reason: Concentrations of sour-tasting lactic acid increase significantly after exercise and remain elevated for at least 90 minutes, the investigators reported in Pediatrics.

June 3

Obese people who have insomnia or who sleepwalk may be likely to make after-midnight raids on the refrigerator, reported a researcher at the annual meeting of the Association of Professional Sleep Societies in Phoenix.

The investigator from St. Luke's-Roosevelt Hospital Center in New York City presented anecdotal reports supporting her theory, and said that nighttime binge eating is common among her patients.

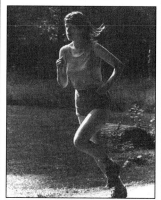

Mothers who breast-feed should do so before strenuous exercise to avoid sour-tasting milk.

She advised patients to eat satisfying meals during the day, and to seek help through a nutritionist or a sleep disorder clinic if necessary.

June 5

Attendees at a pediatric conference in Philadelphia were told that their index of suspicion should be raised when parents switch their infant from one formula to another because it doesn't agree with their baby. For example, if parents switch because they think a formula is causing diarrhea or constipation, a urinary-tract infection or stomach virus may be overlooked and the source not identified, said a Temple University pediatrician and nutritionist.

She also noted that infants who are fed formula should not receive cow's milk formula until after their first birthday to avoid the risk of iron-deficiency anemia.

June 12

A new case-control study linked a diet high in fruits and vegetables with a lower risk of breast cancer. In a comparison of 310 women with breast cancer and 316 women without the disease, researchers at the State University of New York at Buffalo found that cancer-free women consumed more fruits and vegetables. Total intake of folic acid, carotenoids, vitamin C and fiber may contribute to the observed cancer protection, the investigators told the Society for Epidemiologic Research meeting in Minneapolis. At least in adulthood, such nutritional protective factors may be of greater importance than the amount of fat in the diet, the researchers said.

June 17

University of Alabama researchers blamed foiled attempts to keep cholesterol levels down on poor patient compliance with low-fat diets. Forty-two of 73 patients who followed a cholesterol-lowering diet with 30% or less of total calories derived from fat had lowered their cholesterol levels by at least 10% after four weeks. But after six months, only 22 of them continued to have a 10% or greater reduction in cholesterol levels, the team reported in the Archives of Internal Medicine.

June 20

French researchers speculated that wine generates its heart-protective effect by inhibiting platelet aggregation. The researchers from the Nutrition and Vascular Physiopathology Research Unit in Bron, France, examined the habits of residents in Toulouse, France, where consumption of bread, wine and cheese is high, but heart-disease mortality is low. Wine's protection could not be attributed to increased levels of high-density lipoproteins, they stated in The Lancet.

• • •

A British woman who suffered signs of severe dyserythropoiesis and autoimmune thrombocytopenia was the victim of arsenic poisoning from kelp supplements, physicians at Royal London Hospital concluded in The Lancet.

After taking three 550-mg kelp tablets each day for six weeks, the British woman suffered abnormal bleeding, bruises all over her body and tiny subcutaneous hematomas. Kelp is known to concentrate heavy metals, and the researchers found that a daily dose of this woman's kelp pills contained 2.2 mcg of arsenic.

Kelp supplements, available at most health-food stores, are a source of iodine and are used by some people who have iodine deficiency or thyroid problems.

• • •

Putting a breast-feeding mother and her child on a strict diet devoid of known food allergens may prevent the child from developing future allergies, asthma and eczema, claimed researchers at St. Mary's Hospital on the Isle of Wight, England.

The British team studied 120 breast-feeding mothers and babies with a family history of allergies. About half were put on a diet excluding cow's milk, eggs,

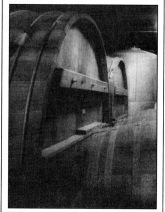

Wine may protect heart by inhibiting platelet aggregation.

fish, nuts, soy, wheat and oranges, and their homes were treated with products to control dust mites.

After one year, 13% of babies in the special diet group had allergies, compared with 40% of controls, according to a report in The Lancet. And just 7% of the treatment group developed asthma, compared with 19% of controls, they found. Likewise, 7% of the diet group developed eczema, compared with 19% of controls.

June 29

Thermogenic beta-3 agonists may overcome the body's tendency to slow its metabolism when given fewer calories, a University of London physiologist reported. The drugs increase the metabolic rate above the normal set point, preventing the body's metabolism from going below normal when dieting, the physiologist told a meeting of the Association for the Study of Obesity, a British medical group. A study has shown that obese patients who were on a diet and taking beta-3 agonists lost 54% more weight after 18 weeks than those on a diet alone. Several pharmaceutical companies are testing the agonists.

JULY

July 1

Recovering abdominal-surgery patients who received a fortified liquid diet were found to have a lower rate of infection and better immunologic function than those on a typical postoperative diet. In a randomized study of 85 patients, those who were given formula supplemented with arginine, omega-3 fatty acids and RNA had 70% fewer nosocomial infections than those on a standard diet, University of Pennsylvania researchers reported in the journal Surgery. The patients on

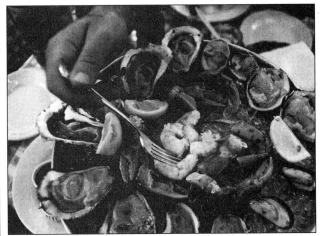

CDC advice: Keep cocktails strong when eating raw oysters.

the fortified diet also were discharged from the hospital an average of four days earlier, said the Philadelphia team.

July 4

A new study in the journal Epidemiology provided further support for current recommendations to increase consumption of fruits and vegetables in order to reduce lung-cancer risk.

An analysis of data compiled over 24 years on 1,960 middle-aged men showed that those who rarely or never consumed foods rich in beta-carotene had a 48% increased risk of developing lung cancer, according to University of Texas researchers. The men whose diet provided at least 5,000 IU of beta-carotene daily were found to have the lowest risk of lung cancer, they reported.

July 7

University of Hawaii researchers warned that heavy consumption of foods high in animal fats boosts the risk of lung cancer. After studying 326 lung-cancer patients and 865 controls, the epidemiologists found a dose-response relationship between the amount of dietary animal fat and the risk of lung cancer. Bacon, sausage, lunch meats, whole milk, ice cream, eggs, custard and cream pies were among the studied foods most commonly associated with the cancer, they disclosed in the journal Epidemiology.

The investigation also revealed an upward trend in risk with increasing consumption of cured meats containing nitrates and dimethylnitrosamines.

July 10

Government scientists said better nutrition may be a factor in the drop in spina bifida cases in the United States. The rate decreased by almost half in the last few years, from 59 per 100,000 births in 1984 to 32 per 100,000 in 1990, the Centers for Disease Control reported. In recent years, there has been increasing attention given to the importance of consuming adequate folic acid during early pregnancy to protect against spina bifida, they noted. Another factor in the decrease may be advances in prenatal testing, allowing women whose fetuses are found to be affected to terminate the pregnancy, the researchers said.

July 13

The fat substitute olestra can lower fat intake without making people hungry later, although it may not significantly reduce calorie count, Johns Hopkins University researchers reported. They studied 24 men randomized to receive for three days biscuits made with either 36 g or 20 g of olestra, or biscuits made with regular fat. Men who ate the olestra biscuits derived 35% of their total calories from fat, compared with 41% for men who ate the other biscuits, according to the report in the American Journal of Clinical Nutrition. Total daily calories and degree of satiety did not differ significantly between the two groups.

July 19

Centers for Disease Control researchers reported that drinks with more than 10% alcohol concentration (wine or whiskey) may protect against hepatitis A infection. Following an oyster-borne outbreak of the virus in Florida, the investigators found that people who drank alcohol while eating the oysters were less likely to become ill than those who ate oysters but did not drink alcohol. The study, which appeared in the journal Epidemiology, speculated that stronger alcohol may block or reduce transmission of the virus into the circulatory system.

July 22

Even when smokers eat plenty of vitamin A, the nutrient may fail to reach vital tissues, claimed a University of Missouri researcher. When rats were fed normal amounts of vitamin A along with benzopyrene, a chemical thought to be the major carcinogen in cigarette smoke, blood levels of vitamin A were normal but levels in the lungs, intestines and liver were abnormally low, the internist told Medical Tribune.

However, when rats were fed beta-carotene, the animals maintained normal tissue vitamin A levels despite benzopyrene exposure, he said.

July 26

Lecithin was suggested as a possible treatment for anosmia. Daily therapy with a pungent licorice-flavored syrup preparation of phosphatidylcholine (PhosChol, Advanced Nutritional Technology) was tested against a similarly flavored placebo in 20 patients unable to smell the concoction. The Chicago neurologist who conducted the study told the International Cholinergic Symposium in Toronto that seven people in the PhosChol group dropped

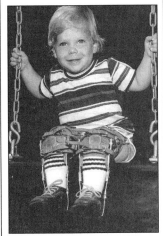

Better nutrition partly credited with reducing spina bifida.

out of the study after two and a half months, complaining of the syrup's taste and smell. No placebo patients reported gains in taste or smell. The PhosChol dropouts were not asked if they could smell or taste other foods, said the researcher, who plans a larger trial with 100 patients.

AUGUST

Aug. 1

Women who take daily supplements of vitamin D may reduce their risk of osteoporosis, Cambridge University researchers reported, confirming previous findings that the supplement leads to less bone loss in women. Based on a study of 138 women, the researchers estimated that increasing daily vitamin D intake to 400 IU or exposing the face and lower arms and legs to sunlight for 30 minutes a day would increase bone density by 5% to 10%. The researchers predicted in the British Medical Journal that a 5% increase in bone density could reduce the incidence of fractures by 20%.

Aug. 3

A panel of health experts convened by the Center for Science in the Public Interest, a nonprofit consumer advocacy group, released nutritional standards for processed foods commonly eaten by children. The panel found only a handful of children's processed foods—but not a single cookie, frozen dessert, granola bar, hot dog or luncheon meat—that met the panel's guidelines. All were too high in fat, salt or sugar, the center said.

Aug. 5

The General Accounting Office warned that the Food and Drug Administration and individual states are failing to protect the public from dangerous drug residues found in the nation's milk supply.

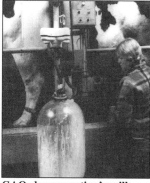

GAO charges nation's milk supply is not adequately tested.

States routinely test milk for only four of the 82 drugs used in dairy cows, the new report stated. The residues have been linked to cancer and other health problems, it said.

The FDA and dairy-producing states should create a plan to develop and implement new tests, the report advised. But FDA officials maintained that the agency and states have already made progress in ensuring the safety of the milk supply.

Aug. 8

Boston researchers announced that women who eat large amounts of vegetables rich in vitamin A and take vitamin C supplements for years can greatly reduce their risk of developing cataracts. The data linking the antioxidant micronutrients and a decrease in cataracts were collected from 50,828 women enrolled in the Nurses' Health Study. Writing in the British Medical Journal, the Brigham and Women's Hospital investigators speculated that the high intake of antioxidant-rich vegetables, such as spinach, sweet potatoes and squash, protects the eyes by preventing oxidation of proteins in the lens that lead to the formation of cataracts.

• • •

Physicians learned that cat and dog foods in developed countries are more nutritious than the food doled out to refugees throughout the Third World.

In a letter to The Lancet, an Oxford University scientist pointed out that most pet foods have "an excellent micronutrient composition." For example, most pet foods are fortified with more vitamin A, iron and niacin than a typical ration of wheat flour, kidney beans, vegetable oil, sugar and tea given to refugees. The refugees' rations contain virtually no vitamin A or C, placing the recipients at risk of internal hemor-

rhaging and blindness, he wrote. Riboflavin, niacin and iron levels are also dangerously low in these rations, the investigator added.

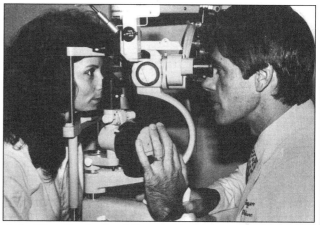

Antioxidant vitamins A and C may protect women against cataracts.

Aug. 10

A University of South Carolina psychiatrist found that the national obsession with weight loss and body image has reached the schoolyard: More than 40% of youngsters in grades 5 through 8 said that they feel fat and want to lose weight, according to the first survey of eating disorders among grade-school children ever conducted.

Speaking at the annual meeting of the National Mental Health Association in Charleston, S.C., the physician reported on the 3,100 children surveyed: 55% of the girls and 29% of the boys wanted to lose weight; 43% of girls and 20% of boys had gone on diets; 11% of girls and 6% of boys had fasted; and 4% of girls and 1% of boys had taken diet pills.

The physician warned that an "eating disorder could be a sign of depression, anxiety, sexual abuse or other problems."

Aug. 25

Compounds found in garlic, cauliflower and soy sauce prevented cancer in rodents, several teams of researchers

reported at the American Chemical Society meeting in Washington, D.C. Investigators found that diallyl sulfide in garlic prevented colon-cancer tumors in rats injected with a carcinogen; it also reduced lung cancer in mice exposed to a cigarette carcinogen. Other studies found that a naturally occurring chemical in cauliflower, brussels sprouts and cabbage prevented about 80% of colon tumors, and that a flavoring compound in soy sauce reduced the risk of esophageal cancer in mice.

Aug. 26

A survey of 12 health and bodybuilding magazines revealed that they contained ads for more than 300 types of pills touted as nutritional supplements. The pills often contained doses of vitamins far higher than those recommended by medical groups, Centers for Disease Control researchers reported in The Journal of the American Medical Association.

In all, 235 ingredients were discovered, including some the CDC had never heard of, such as conch grass and muira puama. Many doctors never learn that their patients are taking these supplements because patients are embarrassed or may not consider them drugs that they need to inform their physician about, the CDC investigators noted.

Nutrition

Sept. 1

A nutrition expert said that obese patients who go on eating binges may benefit from behavior modification and psychotherapy. Studies show that 50% to 70% of these people can abstain from overeating at the end of treatment, which takes about 16 to 20 weeks, the Rutgers University nutritionist told the annual meeting of the North American Association for the Study of Obesity in Atlanta.

Another speaker, from the University of Pennsylvania, cautioned physicians that behavioral strategies alone generally fail to work in patients with a predisposition to weight gain. He urged patient education to emphasize the benefits of exercise and a balanced diet.

Sept. 2

Confronting an emerging body of evidence that yo-yo dieting can cause serious health problems, a government obesity expert said middle-aged patients can still gain moderate amounts of weight—12 to 17 pounds— and retain healthy lives. Speaking at a meeting of the North American Association for the Study of Obesity, he said that putting on a little weight as you get older actually seems to be beneficial.

At the Atlanta meeting, a Michigan State University psychologist suggested that moderately overweight people learn to accept their figures instead of feeding the nation's $33-billion weight-loss industry.

Sept. 8

Pennsylvania State University researchers found that microwaving infant formula in plastic bottles can be safe if certain precautions are taken. In addition, they found that microwave heating will not decrease the amount of vitamin C or riboflavin. In the journal Pediatrics, the researchers recommended using only plastic bottles,

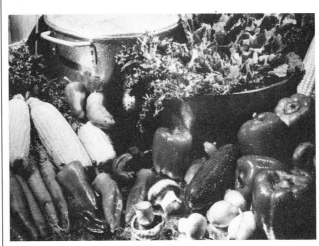

People who eat large quantities of fruits and vegetables have half as many cancers, reported team from University of California, Berkeley.

heated without the nipple or cap. Using at least four ounces of refrigerated formula at a time, the milk should be microwaved for no more than 30 seconds for a four-ounce bottle or 45 seconds for an eight-ounce bottle. Once heated, the bottle should be gently shaken 10 times and tested on the tongue, not the inside of the wrist.

Sept. 11

Women who learn how to shop for and prepare low-fat meals for themselves often end up reducing the fat content of their husbands' diets as well, Seattle researchers reported in the American Journal of Public Health. A team from the Fred Hutchinson Cancer Research Center followed 188 women enrolled in a program that taught them to prepare low-fat meals, rather than eat special diet foods, and compared them with 180 women not enrolled in the program. After one year, the husbands of the women in the program were receiving an average of 32.9% of their calories from fat, compared with 36.9% among the husbands of wives not participating in the program.

Sept. 14

The Centers for Disease Control recommended that all women of childbearing age consume 0.4 mg of folic acid daily to reduce the risk of birth defects. The researchers noted that folic acid can reduce the risk of neural-tube defects if it is taken starting at least a month before a woman becomes pregnant and continuing through the first trimester of pregnancy. The CDC cautioned that women should not take more than 1 mg of folic acid per day, unless a greater dose is recommended by a physician, since the effects of high levels of the nutrient have not been established.

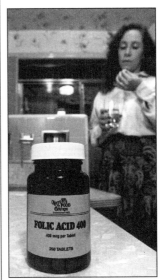

Folic acid supplements help reduce the risk of birth defects.

Sept. 15

A Missouri researcher reported that cigarette smokers may have low levels of vitamin A in their lungs and other organs, despite consuming recommended amounts of vitamin A-containing foods. The main carcinogen in cigarette smoke, benzopyrene, seems to prevent vitamin A from reaching the tissue where it is needed most, the researcher told a conference on tobacco smoking and nutrition at the University of Kentucky in Lexington. Rather than taking potentially dangerous megadoses of the vitamin, the University of Missouri at Columbia researcher advised smokers to quit or, if they can't, to eat foods rich in beta-carotene, which the body converts into vitamin A.

Sept. 21

A review of 156 studies on the role of fruits and vegetables in cancer prevention revealed a protective effect in 128 of them. The review showed that for most types of cancer, the 25% of the world's population with the highest intake of fruits and vegetables had roughly half as many cancers as the 25% with the lowest intake, the University of California at Berkeley researchers stated in Nutrition and Cancer.

Sept. 29

Harvard researchers reported that patients with type-I glycogen storage disease can maintain normal blood glucose concentrations during the day if they are fed uncooked cornstarch at three-to four-hour intervals. A daytime feeding regimen consisting of mixed meals that provide all the nutrients required for normal growth and development, supplemented by uncooked cornstarch with the meals and three hours later, can achieve blood glucose concentrations that eliminate symptoms of hypoglycemia, they stated in the American Journal of Clinical Nutrition.

OCTOBER

Oct. 1

Experts reported in the Archives of Internal Medicine that eating local fish in tropical locales can result in a unique type of poisoning that is known to worsen with sexual activity. The experts, from the Johns Hopkins University School of Medicine and elsewhere, linked 23 cases of ciguatera poisoning to barracuda eaten while in a tropical area or imported from a tropical area. Diarrhea, abdominal pain, nausea and vomiting started about six hours after eating the fish and lasted for days or weeks. The researchers said barracuda should never be eaten, and travelers should exercise caution when eating grouper, red snapper and amberjack.

Oct. 5

Australian researchers reported that reduction of both weight and alcohol consumption is a simple, non-pharmacologic way to cut risk factors for coronary artery disease. For 18 weeks, scientists from Royal Perth Hospital in Perth, Australia, studied 73 overweight men

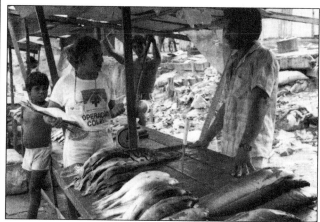

Ciguatera poisoning was linked to barracuda consumption.

who were moderate drinkers. All the men who ate a restricted diet and drank less alcohol achieved normal blood pressure, compared with 80% of those who dieted only and 75% who only drank less alcohol. Fifty-seven percent of men who did not alter their alcohol or food intake achieved normal

blood pressure. Men who restricted both their diet and alcohol also had the most improved cholesterol and triglyceride levels, the researchers wrote in Hypertension.

Oct. 12

A Brooklyn pediatrician told colleagues that he was at odds with the American Academy of Pediatrics' recommendation that children over age two should limit their fat intake to 30% of daily calories. The Maimonides Medical Center physician said that children over the age of two have just stopped breast-feeding, from which they were getting 50% of calories from fat. To switch them suddenly to a diet that's only 30% fat makes no sense, he said at the American College of Nutrition meeting in San Diego.

Oct. 15

Johns Hopkins researchers reported that people who stop drinking as little as two cups of coffee or cola a day may experience the symptoms

associated with caffeine withdrawal. The study of 44 women and 18 men who drank about two strong cups of coffee a day found that abstaining from caffeine for two days caused about one half to have moderate to severe headaches and about one tenth to experience fatigue,

moodiness, depression and anxiety. Caffeine withdrawal also was associated with some loss of coordination, the Baltimore team reported in The New England Journal of Medicine.

Oct. 19

Boston nutritionists reported that using artificial sweetener instead of sugar helped people lose weight and keep it off. In a study of 420 men and women, people lost weight regardless of whether they followed a fat-restricted diet or used Slimfast shakes and snacks with artificial sweeteners. At the American Dietetic Association annual meeting in Washington, D.C., researchers from Deaconess Hospital said women who used artificial sweeteners in their desserts and coffee lost significantly more weight and were more likely to keep it off than were women who used sugar.

Oct. 20

Physicians were told to advise parents not to ban sugary cereals from the breakfast table. At the annual meeting of the American Dietetic Association in Washington, D.C., a Tulane University specialist said that most types of cereal provide children with important nutrients.

Sugary cereals are better than some popular alternatives among children these days—skipping breakfast altogether, or eating cakes, cookies and dessert for the morning meal—said the New Orleans researcher. Based on findings from the Bogalusa Heart Study, which has been following the diet of about 1,400 youngsters since 1973, she said that children who eat any type of cereal have a higher vitamin and mineral intake than kids who don't.

Oct. 21

Contrary to previous reports, a high-fat, low-fiber

diet does not appear to increase a woman's chance of getting breast cancer, a study of almost 90,000 women concluded. But such a diet does increase the risk of colon cancer and heart disease,

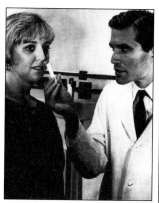

Aromatherapy with corn chip odor may aid weight loss.

researchers from Brigham and Women's Hospital in Boston reported in The Journal of the American Medical Association.

For eight years, the researchers followed 89,494 women enrolled in the Nurses' Health Study. They identified 1,439 cases of breast cancer, including 774 in postmenopausal women. After adjusting for age, risk factors and calories consumed, researchers found that a high-fat diet did not increase breast-cancer risk, nor did a high-fiber diet lower the risk.

Oct. 31

A Chicago study suggested that aromatherapy with a scent akin to that of Fritos may suppress the urge to eat in some people. Overweight people who inhaled and liked a chemical that smelled like the corn chip lost an average of 4.17 pounds in two weeks, and those who didn't even like the Frito odor lost an average of 3.79 pounds, doctors at Rush-Presbyterian-St. Luke's Medical Center reported at the American Society of Bariatric Physicians annual symposium in Chicago. Those who inhaled a different-smelling placebo lost 1.59 pounds.

Nov. 5

Boston researchers found that men who had been overweight as teenagers were twice as likely to die prematurely as those who had been lean adolescents. Women who were overweight during their teen years die no earlier, but they are at elevated risk of heart disease and arthritis, according to a study in The New England Journal of Medicine.

Researchers at Tufts University studied 508 people who had participated between 1922 and 1935 in the Harvard Growth Study of children and teens. Both men and women who had been overweight as teens were seven times more likely to develop atherosclerosis, the study reported. Men were nine times more likely to die of colorectal cancer if they had been overweight as teens, but the number of deaths was small. Women who had been overweight as teens were about one and a half times more likely to develop arthritis, according to the study.

• • •

An Italian study suggested that a serotonin precursor believed to have an inhibitory influence on eating behavior may help overweight people lose weight.

Researchers from the University of Rome studied 20 people with an average weight of 200 pounds, half of whom received the drug 5-hydroxy-tryptophan(5-HTP) and the other half of whom received placebo. For six weeks, both groups were told to eat normally, and then for six more weeks, to follow a diet.

Those in the group taking a placebo lost less than two pounds during the entire 12-week period. But members of the group taking 5-HTP lost about four pounds even while they were allowed to eat what they wanted, and lost seven more pounds during the six-week diet phase, achieving a total loss of 11 pounds.

The only side effect was slight nausea that tended to diminish with extended use of the drug, the researchers reported in the American Journal of Clinical Nutrition.

• • •

A survey of more than 30,000 men found that those who frequently ate fruit and other high-fiber foods were less likely to develop hypertension than those who rarely ate even small amounts of fiber-rich foods, reported researchers at the Harvard School of Public Health. The survey also concluded that calcium was not likely to be protective against hypertension, and sodium showed no significant effect, the researchers reported in Circulation. Magnesium was found to decrease hypertension risk. The researchers cautioned against taking fiber supplements instead of eating fruits, noting that it may be the global effect of eating fruits that is protective, not just their chemical components. The Boston investigators suggested that if all Americans were to increase their fiber intake to 24 g a day, the rate of hypertension in the United States would be cut by 11%.

Nov. 7

Canadian researchers reported that people over age 65 could increase their ability to fight infections, and cut their number of sick days in half, by taking vitamin supplements. Researchers at the Memorial University of Newfoundland in St. John's studied 96 healthy, elderly Canadians who took either vitamin pills or inactive placebos. They found that those taking the vitamins had increased levels of certain T-cell subsets, as well as increased interleukin-2 production, and higher antibody response and natural killer-cell activity. Those in the placebo group were sick due to infections 48 days during the year, whereas the number of sick days was 23 a year for those receiving vitamins.

The 11-vitamin, seven-mineral supplements contained the recommended dietary allowance of most of the standard vitamins and trace minerals. Beta-carotene and vitamin E were included at levels about four times higher than those usually obtained through diet, according to the report in The Lancet.

Nov. 8

The Secretary of Agriculture blocked the publication of new food-labeling regulations due to be released November 9, opening up the possibility of protracted court battles and reopened public hearings that could delay clearer nutritional labels by months.

The block reflected a failure of representatives from the Department of Agriculture and the Department of Health and Human Services to compromise on regulations. Labeling regarding the fat content of food is a particularly sensitive issue to the Department of Agriculture, which fears that proposed labeling on fat—including a maximum number of desired grams per day—will discourage consumers from eating meat and dairy products.

Nov. 11

Beringer Vineyards halted formerly government-approved plans to hang tags from the necks of its wine bottles that tout the potential health benefits of wine, after it learned that the government had switched its position on the labels. U.S. Surgeon General Antonia Novello, M.D., reportedly felt the tags did not contain enough information about the dangers of alcohol along with evidence that moderate wine consumption reduces the risk of heart disease.

Nov. 17

Women taking vitamin E supplements lowered their heart-disease risk by 46%, reported Harvard researchers. In men, vitamin E supplementation reduced the risk by 26%, the investigators told the American Heart Association scientific sessions in New Orleans. The researchers, who presented data compiled from the Nurses' Health Study and a Harvard study following 45,720 middle-aged men since 1986, considered people with no history of cardiovascular problems who had taken 100 IU or more of vitamin E per day for at least two years. The RDA for the vitamin is 30 IU.

Nov. 18

Doctors caring for elderly patients should be on the lookout for a weight loss of 10% or more, announced Ohio researchers at the annual meeting of the Gerontological Society of America. Nursing-home patients who lost 10% of their weight were at increased risk of dying within two years, they reported.

A precipitous drop in cholesterol may also be a marker for mortality in the elderly, cautioned doctors at the University of Illinois in Chicago. Twenty-percent drops in cholesterol levels were seen in 47% of study patients who died, but in only 13% of the survivors, they said.

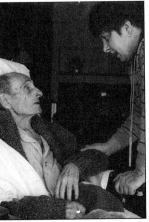

Weight loss of 10% or more in elderly is warning signal.

Nutrition

Dec. 2

Dietary guar gum, a fiber known to improve glucose tolerance, may be useful in slowing the progression of diabetic nephropathy, a Minnesota researcher reported. Rats with established diabetes were fed a modified diet or a diet of 5% guar gum. The guar-gum diet resulted in smaller kidney weight and lower urinary albumin excretion after eight weeks.

Glycated hemoglobin was 12.4% in the guar-gum group, compared with 14.4% in the modified-diet group, investigators from the University of Minnesota in St. Paul reported in the Journal of Nutrition.

The findings indicated that guar gum warrants further study to determine whether it is useful in slowing the progression of renal complications of diabetes, stated the researchers.

Dec. 5

Breast-feeding women who smoke cigarettes were found to have decreased milk production, with lower fat concentrations in their milk. The study of 11 smoking women and 29 controls, all of whom had had preterm infants, found that at two weeks postpartum, 24-hour milk volumes averaged 406 ml for mothers who smoked and 514 ml for controls.

Between two and four weeks postpartum, the mean 24-hour milk volume of control subjects increased, while milk volume of smoking mothers remained unchanged, the researchers from the U.S. Department of Agriculture, Baylor College of Medicine in Houston and Cornell University in Ithaca, N.Y., reported in Pediatrics. They also found that milk fat concentration was 19% lower in the milk of mothers who smoked.

Dec. 6

States should not hesitate to impose tougher and more specific regulations on dietary supplements than does the federal Food and Drug Administration, asserted the

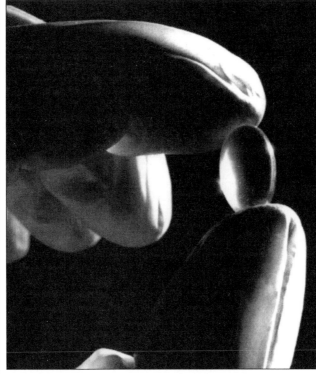

Stiffer labeling rules on dietary supplements are advocated.

head of the Division of Food of the Texas Department of Health.

The regulator called for cooperation between state attorney generals in confronting fraudulent or unsubstantiated claims regarding nutritional supplements.

Depending on claims in promotion and labeling, the products fall under various Texas regulations involving foods, food additives or drugs, the official explained in the Food and Drug Law Journal.

Dec. 10

Three garlic compounds slowed proliferation of human breast-carcinoma cells in a study presented at the 15th Annual San Antonio Breast Cancer Symposium. Forty-eight hours after the com-

pounds, aged garlic extract and two of its components, S-allyl cysteine (SAC) and S-allyl mercaptocysteine (SAMC), were added to the carcinoma cells, the researchers noted an increasing antiproliferative effect.

The researchers from New York's Memorial Sloan-Kettering Cancer Center concluded that certain constituents of aged garlic extract may be able to inhibit growth of the breast-carcinoma cells.

Dec. 14

The Center for Science in the Public Interest announced that it will soon release an enhanced version of the government's food pyramid. While the U.S. Department of Agriculture's pyramid rates categories of foods (emphasizing fruits and vegetables and recommending less meat consumption), a three-

dimensional pyramid was created by CSPI as an educational tool to help consumers make food selections within groups. For example, within the meat and protein group, consumers will be guided to emphasize beans and eat red meats more sparingly, a CSPI spokesperson explained.

Dec. 16

If Americans increased their dietary fiber intake by 70%, or about 13 g a day, there could be 50,000 fewer cases of colon cancer a year, declared an international team of researchers. In a combined analysis of 13 case-control studies from various countries, rates of colon cancer fell as dietary fiber increased, the investigators reported in the Journal of the National Cancer Institute. After adjusting for fiber intake, vitamin C and beta-carotene had only a weak inverse relationship to colorectal-cancer risk, according to the research team led by epidemiologists from the University of Toronto.

Dec. 22

A new study suggested that fiber consumption can have a big influence on whether increased fat intake translates into increased levels of low-density-lipoprotein cholesterol.

University of Arizona nutrition researchers fed guinea pigs diets that included 15% lard.

One group's food included fiber in the form of cellulose; the other ate food that had dietary pectin isolated from prickly pear as part of its fiber content.

Plasma LDL cholesterol levels in the prickly pear pectin group were lowered by 33%, the investigators reported in the Journal of Nutrition. Plasma very-low-density- and high-density-lipoprotein cholesterol concentrations were unchanged.

Fast food and sugar linked to Crohn's disease

JAN. 7—People who regularly eat at fast-food restaurants and who eat too much sugar may increase their risk of developing Crohn's disease or ulcerative colitis, according to a study by Swedish researchers.

But an American expert disagreed with the findings, saying that scientists have not identified any particular foods that may cause either disease.

Researchers from the Karolinska Institute in Stockholm interviewed 152 people with Crohn's disease, 145 with ulcerative colitis and 305 healthy people about their eating habits in the five previous years.

Those who ate fast food at least two times a week were 3.4 times more likely to develop Crohn's disease and 3.9 times more likely to develop ulcerative colitis, reported Per-Gunnar Persson in Epidemiology.

Fast food in the Swedish study consisted of a hamburger or hot dog with mustard and ketchup plus french-fried or creamed potatoes and a soft drink.

In addition, people who ate more than 55 g of sugar per day were found to be 2.6 times more likely to develop Crohn's disease.

Stephen Hanauer, M.D., associate professor of gastroenterology of the University of Chicago Medical Center, however, disagreed with the Swedish findings.

"There's a major problem with this type of recall study," Dr. Hanauer said. "People can't remember what they ate last week; how can they recall accurately what they ate five years ago?"

People in the Swedish study probably started eating certain foods in response to their symptoms, not the other way around, according to Dr. Hanauer.

"They probably started eating high-sugar, high-calorie food to gain weight, and foods low in fiber to reduce their diarrhea," he said.

"No study has identified any dietary factor that may increase the risk of these diseases," Dr. Hanauer added.

The Swedish study found that eating whole-grain bread or Muesli cereal prevented people from developing Crohn's disease, as did drinking coffee regularly. The coffee finding has been reported before, but Persson wrote that more research is needed to determine a clearly beneficial effect.

Low folic acid levels and HPV may increase cervical-cancer risk

JAN. 22—Women infected with the human papillomavirus may be able to reduce their risk of developing cervical cancer by increasing their daily intake of folic acid.

In a study of 464 women, those with low levels of folic acid who were infected with HPV were over five times more likely to develop precancerous changes of the cervix than infected women with adequate amounts of the vitamin, University of Alabama researchers reported in The Journal of the American Medical Association.

"It's sort of a double whammy," said Charles Butterworth, Jr., M.D. The new findings may warrant changes in the recommended dietary allowance of the vitamin, according to Dr. Butterworth.

In 1989, the National Academy of Sciences lowered its recommended allowance of folic acid from 400 mcg/day to 180 mcg/day for women and 200 mcg/day for men. Dr. Butterworth recommends going back to the 400 mcg/day allowance.

A typical serving of liver has 383 mcg, pinto or navy beans about 84 mcg, spinach about 70 mcg, broccoli 53 mcg and orange juice 43 mcg.

Although there is no evidence that folic acid can prevent

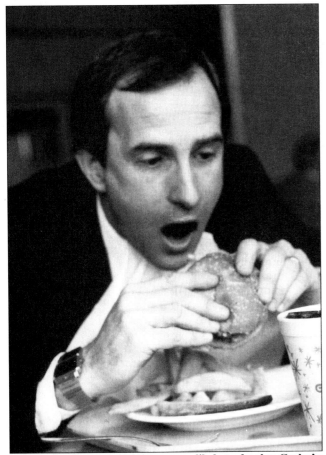

Fast-food eaters were 3.4 times more likely to develop Crohn's.

cancer, increasing the amount of the vitamin in the diet may prevent the initial cervical epithelial changes that are caused by HPV, Dr. Butterworth explained.

Up to 90% of women with such changes have evidence of the virus, said Mark Schiffman, M.D., of the National Cancer Institute in Bethesda, Md.

Up to 30% of sexually active women in their 20s have been exposed to HPV, but only a few will develop the type of changes that lead to cancer, Dr. Schiffman said.

Deficiencies of other nutrients also may play a role in the development of cervical cancer, said Nancy Potischman, Ph.D., of NCI.

Pritikin researcher: exercise and diet reduce 'deadly quartet' of heart-disease risk factors

FEB. 7—People with a "deadly quartet" of noncholesterol CHD risk factors can reduce their risk through a rigorous diet and exercise program, a researcher affiliated with the Pritikin Longevity Center has reported.

According to R. James Barnard, M.D., who also is vice chair of the department of kinesiology at the University of California, Los Angeles, the deadly quartet is obesity, hypertension, high triglyceride levels and hyperinsulinemia.

In a study, 69 of 72 overweight, hypertensive patients with normal cholesterol, were able to lose weight, reduce high blood pressure, high triglycerides and high insulin levels by reducing fat intake to 10% of total calories and exercising for 26 days, according to University of California doctors.

Dr. Barnard reported on the study in the American Journal of Cardiology.

The exercise program consisted of 30 minutes of brisk walking four to five times a week, along with walks of 45 minutes at a slower pace once a week.

The patients also attended exercise classes, consisting of 10 to 20 minutes of stretching exercises followed by 40 to 50 minutes of aerobic exercise five times a week.

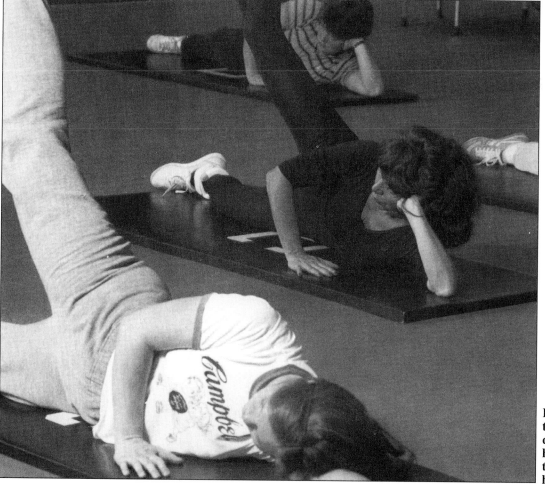

Regimen reduced the "deadly quartet" of obesity, hypertension, high triglycerides and hyperinsulinemia.

Institute of Medicine publishes diet guidelines

Medical Tribune News Service Report

FEB. 19—United States Government scientists have boiled down nutrition recommendations to nine simple guidelines.

Following the rules, such as limiting total fat intake to 30% or less of daily calories and eating five or more servings of vegetables and fruits, will help prevent heart disease, cancer and other chronic diseases, said Paul Thomas, co-editor of "Eat for Life," the nutrition report published by the Food and Nutrition Board of the Institute of Medicine.

"Americans labor under a big misimpression that nutrition is complex and controversial, and no two nutritionists will agree on anything," Thomas said.

"But there is a remarkable degree of consensus on what constitutes good eating," he added.

To lower the risk of the most common chronic diseases, health experts across the board endorse a diet that includes whole grains, legumes, fruits and vegetables, with smaller amounts of dairy, meat and poultry products, he said.

The six other dietary guidelines advise people to
• Get moderate, regular exercise.
• Limit the amount of salt to slightly more than one teaspoon per day.
• Maintain adequate calcium intake by consuming low-fat or nonfat milk or milk products and dark-green vegetables, which are rich in calcium.
• Maintain an optimal level of fluoride in the diet through the water supply or through a fluoride supplement.
• Avoid taking vitamin and mineral supplements in excess of the U.S. Recommended Daily Allowances, in any one day.
• Eat a moderate amount of protein, no more than six ounces a day.

"Eat for Life" also advises against drinking alcohol altogether, but for those who won't follow that recommendation, it calls for limiting drinks to no more than one or two a day.

Sailor crew demonstrates ACS diet is practical

FEB. 19—Switching from meat and potatoes to a low-fat, high-fiber diet helped a crew of U.S. sailors lose weight and lower their cholesterol levels, an unpublished American Cancer Society study has found.

During a six-month deployment in the Mediterranean, the crew aboard the guided-missile destroyer USS Scott ate meals prepared according to ACS guidelines, which emphasize low-fat and high-fiber foods.

The typical American high-fat, low-fiber diet has been associated with an increased risk of cancer, heart disease and other chronic disorders, said Walter Lawrence Jr., M.D., the ACS president.

Sailors who ate the ACS diet were compared with crew members on another ship, who ate a standard U.S. Navy diet. The society found that:
• Crew members on the USS Scott lost an average of 12 pounds each, whereas those on the other ship gained an average of seven pounds.

• Of the USS Scott crew members who weighed 200 pounds or more at the beginning of the six months, 74% lost weight. Only 26% of the other sailors over 200 pounds lost weight.
• About 44% of the crew in "low-stress" jobs showed a decline in cholesterol levels; 35% showed no change, and 20% showed an increase. (Cholesterol testing of serum samples from sailors on the other ship has not been completed.)

"It's one thing to set out guidelines, but it doesn't mean anything if they aren't used," Dr. Lawrence said. "This study proves that our guidelines are easily implemented and that people don't miss the other diet. A good number of the sailors, who are accustomed to a meat and potatoes diet, like eating according to the ACS guidelines."

Modified citrus pectin slows tumor-cell growth

By L.A. McKeown

MARCH 15—A modified form of citrus pectin appears to interfere with the way in which cancer cells cluster together and form secondary tumors, according to Michigan researchers.

In a study published in the Journal of the National Cancer Institute, the researchers found that injections of citrus pectin led to a threefold increase in tumor-cell colonization compared

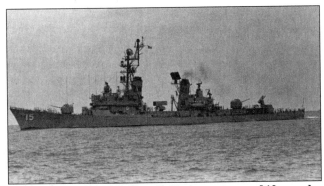

Sailors on low-fat, high-fiber diet lost an average of 12 pounds.

with controls, while the modified form reduced the number and size of tumor cell clusters in the lungs of mice.

Lead researcher Avraham Raz, M.D., of the Michigan Cancer Foundation in Detroit, said that if future studies confirm the findings, the modified pectin could be given intravenously before and after surgery, when cancer cells are likely to metastasize.

"This is a natural, cheap product that's abundant and commonly available," said Dr. Raz, director of the Metastasis Research Program. "It could be the first natural, nontoxic treatment regimen of its kind."

In the study, tumor cells of female mice were injected with either citrus pectin or the modified version with added galactose.

One researcher who has worked with pectin stressed caution in interpreting the results.

"I would say that what these researchers need to do is find out more about the mechanism in which pectin acts on the body," according to Michael Parisa, M.D., director of the Food Research Institute at the University of Wisconsin in Madison.

According to Dr. Parisa, this is the first study he has heard of in which pectin is administered intravenously.

Last year, researchers at the University of Texas Health Science Center in San Antonio reported that dietary pectin can significantly reduce cholesterol levels and may play a role in preventing colon cancer.

Saccharin may be only a rodent carcinogen

By John Carpi

ANAHEIM, CALIF., APRIL 8— The artificial sweetener saccharin, which has carried a label for 15 years in the United States warning it may cause cancer in laboratory animals, may not be harmful in humans.

Saccharin may lead to bladder cancer only in rats, Samuel Cohen, M.D., of the University of Nebraska Medical Center in Omaha reported at the Federation for American Societies of Experimental Biology meeting here.

"People, and in fact most other animals, do not respond to saccharin the way rats do," he said.

A spokesperson for Kraft Inc. in Northfield, Ill., manufacturer of Sweet 'N Low saccharin sweetener, said that the company has always held that the product is safe for humans.

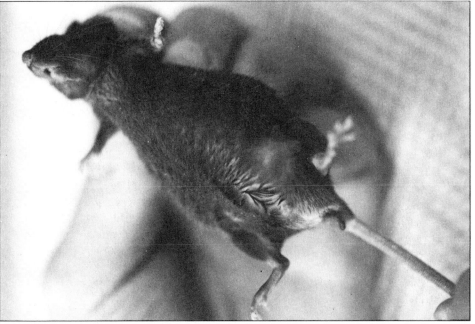

While some toxicologists maintain that saccharin only causes cancer in lab animals, one consumer advocate group said it is too early to give the sweetener a clean bill of health.

The consumer watchdog group Center for Science in the Public Interest said it still was too early to tell if the sweetener should get a clean bill of health.

"Saccharin-containing products carry a warning label mandated by the federal government, and until enough evidence accumulates to reverse that label, there is no reason not to heed it," said a spokesperson for the Washington-based group. "People don't have to avoid saccharin-containing products but they shouldn't go overboard with them either."

Dr. Cohen found that saccharin can only lead to cancer if it combines with a certain protein in rats called alpha-2-u-globulin to create a toxic substance that irritates the lining of the bladder.

"It's not the saccharin itself that causes the cancer, but saccharin combined with alpha-2-u-globulin," he said.

Humans do not have alpha-2-u-globulin, and they have a related saccharin-binding protein in a concentration only one-thousandth of that in rats, Dr. Cohen said.

Even if people had enough of the protein needed to combine with saccharin, a 180-pound man would have to consume about 1,000 packets of Sweet 'N Low a day to get cancer, he said.

After tests in the 1970s showed that rats who had received the equivalent of 1,000 cans of saccharin-sweetened diet soda every day for life developed bladder cancer, the U.S. Food and Drug Administration approved a ban on the sweetener in 1977.

A tremendous public outcry led to a Congressional exemption from the Delaney Act, which automatically bans carcinogenic foodstuffs.

Congress settled on the warning label. In 1990, the congressional exemption was extended for another five years.

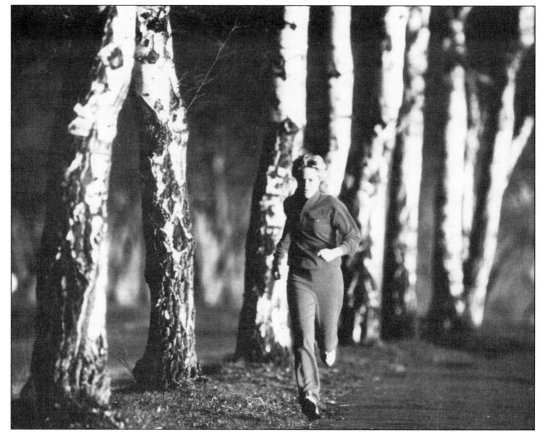

Supplements may inhibit superoxides, which have been linked to increased rates of respiratory infections in marathon runners.

FASEB meeting news: zinc counteracts harmful chemical by-product of strenuous exercise

ANAHEIM, CALIF., APRIL 8—Zinc supplements may prevent cell-damaging superoxides from building up in the blood during strenuous exercise.

Superoxides, produced by white blood cells during physical exertion, can increase the risk of infections, reported Patricia Duester of the Uniformed Services University in Bethesda, Md., at the Federation of American Societies for Experimental Biology meeting here.

"We've known for years that these chemicals build up after exercise, and their accumulation may explain why runners are prone to upper-respiratory infections after a marathon," said Ms. Duester, who is director of the university's human performance laboratory.

Ms. Duester studied five runners who ranged in age from 24 to 42. They took either two 25-mg zinc pills a day or a placebo for four days.

On the fourth day the runners ran for about two hours on treadmills. Ms. Duester found that runners who had taken the zinc had less of the damaging chemicals in their blood, compared with those on placebo.

She also found that runners who took placebo instead of the zinc had suppressed immune systems.

"It seems as though zinc can block that suppression," she said. Ms. Duester said it was too soon to advise joggers to take zinc supplements. She did say that in the doses given in the study, zinc probably is harmless, and that people who exercise on a regular basis generally have lower zinc levels in their blood than experts advise for the maintenance of good health.

Garlic's effects depend on eating it raw

ANAHEIM, CALIF., APRIL 9—Garlic can lower cholesterol levels and high blood pressure, although patients' friends and family may soon wish they were taking conventional medication.

The garlic cloves must be crushed and eaten raw in order to exert their beneficial effects on lipid levels and blood pressure, according to Dennis McNamara, Ph.D., professor of pharmacology at Tulane University School of Medicine in New Orleans.

Dr. McNamara presented his findings here at the Federation of American Societies for Experimental Biology meeting.

Cooking garlic deactivates allicin, the chemical that gives the herb its odor and holds the key to garlic's beneficial effect, Dr. McNamara said. He and his colleagues found that the amount of allicin in about two cloves of garlic lowered blood pressure in rats.

Another study, conducted by Gilbert McMahon, M.D., also of Tulane, found that the same amount of allicin lowered cholesterol by about 11% in patients with average cholesterol levels of 235 mg/dL.

Better diet helps cardiac patients avoid 2nd attack

MORADABAD, INDIA, APRIL 18—By replacing meat, butter and eggs in the diet with foods high in fiber and beneficial vitamins, patients can significantly reduce their risk of a second heart attack, researchers in India have found.

Seventy-five percent of heart-attack survivors who increased their daily intake of fruit, vegetables, nuts and grains, and reduced their consumption of meat, butter and eggs, went for a year without experiencing a second heart attack, the researchers here reported in the British Medical Journal.

By comparison, 60% of patients who reduced their consumption of meat, butter and eggs without increasing fiber and vitamin intake went for a year without a heart attack, according to Ram B. Singh, M.D., from the Medical Hospital and Research Center.

The fiber- and vitamin-rich diet also reduced patients' risk of dying from any cause, the study

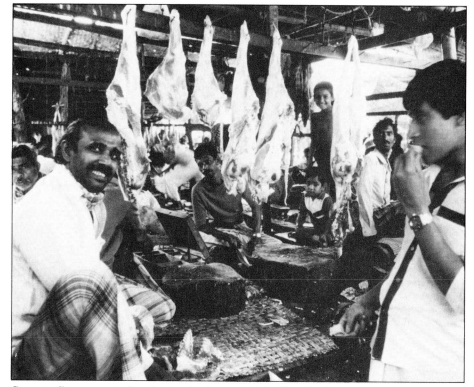

Seventy-five percent of patients who favored high-fiber foods over meat, butter and eggs went a year without a second heart attack, versus 60% of those who cut only fat.

showed. About 10% of patients on the diet died within a year, compared with 19% of patients not on the diet, the study of 406 patients found.

The diets were begun within 24 to 48 hours of the first heart attack.

Drugs used in therapy included propranolol, verapamil, nitrates, furosemide and aspirin.

In the study, patients also received counseling from dietitians every one to 12 weeks.

Those on the fiber and vitamin diet were encouraged to eat a variety of fruits, vegetables, nuts and grains, including guava, onion, garlic, bitter gourd, soybeans, peanuts and almonds. The goal was consumption of at least 400 g/day of fruits and vegetables.

In the study, cholesterol dropped by an average of 29 mg/dL in those on the fiber and vitamin diet, compared with 12 mg/dL among the other patients.

In addition, patients on the fiber and vitamin diet lost an average of 14 pounds, compared with five pounds in those not on the diet, the researchers reported.

Patients on the fiber and vitamin diet also had better compliance.

USDA issues new food guide pyramid

WASHINGTON, D.C., APRIL 28—After 20 years of promoting the basic four food groups as the key to nutrition, the U.S. Department of Agriculture has replaced its old chart with a new food guide pyramid.

The pyramid, which lists grains such as bread, cereal,

rice and pasta, along with fruits and vegetables, as the basis for good nutrition, deemphasizes meats and dairy products and recommends that people use fats, oils and sweets "sparingly."

"It's a big improvement over the 'basic four,'" which listed meat, dairy, bread and fruits/vegetables as the main food groups, said Felicia Busch, a registered dietitian and nutrition consultant in St. Paul, Minn.

The food guide pyramid recommends six to 11 servings daily of grains, three to five of vegetables, two to four of fruits and two to three servings of both dairy products and meats.

Busch cautioned that the serving sizes on which the pyramid is based are small.

Pat Harper, a dietitian and nutrition consultant in Pitts-

burgh, said the new pyramid should be easy for patients to understand.

"The old recommendations just did not reflect the current research and trends. It's going to be a useful tool both for the medical and nutrition communities," she said.

The American Dietetic Association has endorsed the new food pyramid.

The USDA planned to release the guide last year, but put it on hold after concerns arose that some lower-income and less educated people might not understand it.

At the time, some criticized the agency for bowing under to complaints from the meat and dairy industries. The USDA has produced pamphlets explaining the new food guide pyramid. To order copies, call (301) 436-8617.

Wide variation in vitamin D levels discovered in milk and infant formula; monitoring suggested

By Peggy Peck

APRIL 30—Eight cases of hypervitaminosis D highlight the need for a national program to monitor vitamin D supplementation of whole milk, according to two groups of Massachusetts researchers.

Spurred by the report of eight patients who became ill, a team of researchers evaluated 13 brands of milk and five brands of infant formula. Only a third of the milk brands and none of the infant formulas contained 80% to 120% of the amount of vitamin D stated on the label, reported Michael F. Holick, Ph.D., of the Boston University School of Medicine.

Both reports of mislabeling appear in The New England Journal of Medicine.

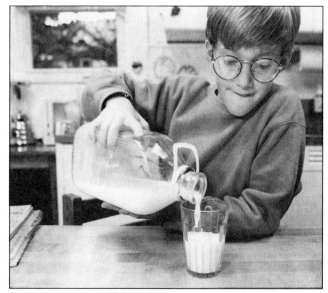

Amount of vitamin D in milk often misstated on label.

Seven adults and one child suffered weakness, fatigue and weight loss after drinking milk that contained 580 times the amount of vitamin D recommended by the U.S. Food and Drug Administration, according to Ellen W. Seely, M.D., of Brigham and Women's Hospital in Boston. All the milk came from the same dairy.

Boston University School of Medicine researchers then tested 42 containers of milk and 10 cans of infant formula purchased in Massachusetts, New Hampshire, New Jersey, Vermont and Virginia, according to Dr. Holick.

Twelve of the 42 containers of milk had within 80% and 120% of the label amount of vitamin D, 26 had less than 80%, and four had more than 120%, reported the Boston researcher.

Of the 10 samples of infant formula, which were made by five different manufacturers, seven had more than 200% above the label concentration of vitamin D.

"We have no knowledge of any such mislabeling," said a spokesperson for the Food and Drug Administration. "I'm not a lawyer and I cannot say if that would violate FDA regulations."

The spokesperson did say that FDA testing has also turned up some variation in vitamin D concentrations, but insisted that they did not constitute a health risk.

Infant formula manufacturers probably add higher concentrations of the vitamin, figuring that the product will sit on the shelf for a while and by the time it is used some of the vitamin may have dissipated, according to Dr. Holick.

Infant formula is not overfortified, according to the Infant Formula Council in Atlanta. "Infant formula is the most intensely regulated food product in the U.S.," according to a prepared statement by the manufacturer's trade group. The group questioned the methods used in the study to determine the vitamin D levels.

The FDA leaves the testing of milk to individual states, which sample it every six months. "I think that testing should be done at the least once a month, and once a week would be better," Dr. Holick said.

The FDA spokesperson said that it would be premature for the agency to make any such changes in testing policy.

"The labels on the packages usually do not match the content of the food," said Dr. Holick. "Milk is also supposed to be fortified with vitamin A. When we tested it we found that it doesn't contain vitamin A. This is potentially a problem that has wide-ranging ramifications because of the potential toxicity of various vitamins."

The lack of vitamin D in milk can have serious consequences in both children and elderly people, who depend on milk for their vitamin D requirement, according to Dr. Holick.

Several U.S. studies have suggested that 30% to 40% of patients with hip fractures have vitamin D deficiencies, he added.

Several European countries stopped fortifying milk in the mid-1950s when 204 cases of hypercalcemia were reported. However, Dr. Holick said he is opposed to halting fortification.

If milk was not fortified, most Americans would not suffer a vitamin D deficiency, according to John G. Haddad, M.D., of the University of Pennsylvania School of Medicine in Philadelphia, in an accompanying editorial.

But pregnant women, infants, disabled persons and those with little sunlight exposure would be at risk for a deficiency, he added.

Vegetarian diet may improve autoimmune disease

New York Times/Medical Tribune News Service

MAY 9—Vegetarian diets may have a role to play in the treatment of various autoimmune diseases, according to two reports that appeared in The Lancet.

Physicians at Tottori University in Yonago, Japan, reported that a 16-year-old girl with systemic lupus erythematosus clinically improved and her antibody titers dropped to normal and were maintained on a vegetarian diet during five years of follow-up.

"A vegetarian diet may be of benefit to someone with lupus because it is so low in calories," according to Richard S. Rivlin, M.D., program director of the clinical nutrition research department at New York Hospital-Cornell University Medical College.

"Malnutrition affects the ability of the body to mount an immune response, and also decreases inflammation," he said.

Dr. Rivlin cautioned patients with lupus against starting a starvation diet in an effort to improve symptoms. "They should not make any drastic changes in their diets without consulting their doctor. It's still too early to tell if this report is significant."

The Japanese girl's improvement could have been caused not by any dietary changes but by a spontaneous remission, added Dr. Rivlin.

In another report, a group of Italian researchers at the San Carlo Hospital in Milan reported that 20 people with nephrotic syndrome improved after eating a vegetarian soy diet for eight weeks.

The diet consisted of 28% of calories from fat, was low in protein, cholesterol free and rich in monounsaturated and polyunsaturated fatty acids. The patients consumed 40 g of fiber a day.

"During the soy-diet period, there were significant falls in serum cholesterol and apolipoproteins A and B, but serum triglyceride concentrations did not change," wrote Giuseppe D'Amico, M.D. Urinary protein excretion fell significantly, he added.

"Diets such as ours, low in protein and phosphate, seem to slow progression of renal damage in chronic glomerular disease, and are not harmful to patients with severe proteinuria," he wrote.

"'This might be useful, although only a small number of patients were studied," said William Mitch, M.D., of the Emory University School of Medicine in Atlanta. "Even though we treat nephrotic syndrome with prednisone, we really don't have a good treatment."

"This diet wouldn't be my first line of treatment," added Dr. Mitch. "But if a patient of mine didn't respond to drugs, I would try this diet."

In a Lancet study published last year, rheumatoid arthritis patients who ate a vegetarian diet had less pain, joint swelling and stiffness than sufferers who ate a regular diet, according to Norwegian researchers.

But the American College of Rheumatology issued a position statement last year cautioning that "until more data are available, patients should continue to follow balanced and healthy diets, be skeptical of 'miraculous' claims, and avoid elimination diets and fad nutritional practices."

Wine found to guard the French from CHD

BRON, FRANCE, JUNE 20—Liberal wine consumption may protect the French from cardiovascular disease, despite a national predilection for foods rich in saturated fat, according to researchers here.

The French regularly consume about 20 to 30 g of alcohol every day, wrote S. Renaud, M.D., in The Lancet. That amount can reduce the risk of heart disease by at least 40%, he reported.

A can of beer has about 13 g of alcohol, a glass of wine about 11 g, and a shot of whiskey about 15 g.

Calling it the "French paradox," Dr. Renaud noted that study participants in Toulouse, France, have one of the lowest rates of heart disease in the study, despite a high intake of saturated fat. "This paradox may be attributable in part to high wine consumption."

Because studies have shown that alcohol increases HDL cholesterol and that HDL is inversely related to cardiovascular disease, alcohol was thought to be cardioprotective via changes in HDL levels.

But HDL levels in the French study were not above average. Instead, alcohol may prevent cardiovascular disease by inhibiting platelet aggregation and preventing blood clotting and myocardial infarction, the scientist reported.

"Thus, alcohol taken in moderation may be one of the most efficient drugs for protection from coronary heart disease," Dr. Renaud wrote.

Other cardiovascular disease risk factors that could skew the results, such as blood pressure, body-mass index and cigarette smoking, are no lower in France than in other industrialized countries, he wrote.

Dr. Renaud and colleagues at the Nutrition and Vascular Physiopathology Research Unit in Bron based their findings on the World Health Organization's MONICA cardiovascular disease study.

The 10-year study, started in 1985, is gathering information from people enrolled in 39 medical centers in 26 countries, according to Ivan Gyarfaf, M.D., chief of the cardiovascular disease unit at WHO headquarters in Geneva.

An American expert thinks the study may be an over-simplification. "I think they're going too far by concentrating only on alcohol," said Eric Rimm, Ph.D., of the Harvard School of Public Health.

"There are many life-style factors, like stress and exercise and other parts of the diet, like processed foods, that differ from country to country and have not been looked at," Dr. Rimm said.

Dr. Gyarfaf believes the French are protected partly because they follow the so-called Mediterranean diet: small quantities of butter and a lot of bread, vegetables, fruit, cheese, vegetable fat and wine, which is known to protect the heart.

"Even in different parts of France, the closer you get to the Mediterranean Sea, the lower the death rates from heart disease," he said.

The MONICA study shows that the death rate from heart disease in Strasbourg, in northeastern France, is 102 per 100,000 men, while the death rate in Toulouse, near the southern border and closer to the sea, is 78 per 100,000 men.

In contrast, already high death rates in Eastern Europe are rising, Dr. Gyarfaf said.

"Their diet is full of animal fat, they have a very high alcohol intake, they smoke a lot and have low levels of physical activity," he said.

The MONICA study found that Japanese men have the lowest death rates from heart disease—33 per 100,000 men—while in the United States the rate is 182 per 100,000 men. In Glasgow, Scotland, the rate is 380 per 100,000 men.

Allergen-free diet while nursing protects babies

Medical Tribune Report

JUNE 20—Putting a breast-feeding mother and her child on a strict diet devoid of known food allergens may prevent the child from developing future allergies, a new British study has found.

Controlling the level of dust mites in the home also may limit allergies in high-risk children, according to the study, led by researchers at St. Mary's Hospital in Newport on the Isle of Wight. They reported their findings in The Lancet.

In the study, 58 breast-feeding mothers and babies from families with a history of allergies spent one year on diets that excluded known allergens, including cow's milk, eggs, fish and nuts.

The infants' diets also were free of soy products, wheat or orange, and their homes were treated with products to control dust mites.

After one year, the rate of allergies in infants on the restrictive diet was less than one third that of a control group of 62 babies on a normal diet whose houses were not treated for mites. Whereas 25 (40%) of the control infants developed allergies, eight (13%) in the dieting group did.

Infants on the diet also were less likely to develop asthma or eczema, the study found. Twelve infants (19%) in the control group and four (7%) in the diet group developed asthma. The numbers were identical for eczema.

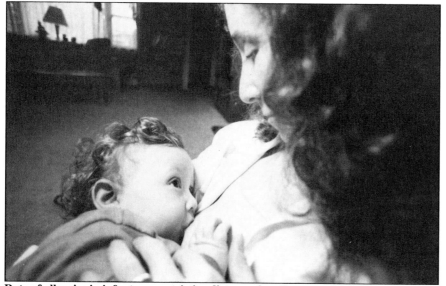

Rate of allergies in infants on restrictive diets was less than one-third that of controls.

The new study supports the findings of other research that has found that restricting the diets of nursing mothers can lower the rate of allergies among at-risk infants, the British researchers wrote.

The researchers also found that parental smoking was a significant risk factor for increasing the possibility of childhood allergies.

According to the American Academy of Allergy and Immunology, a child has a 25% chance of developing allergies if one parent has them, and a 66% chance of developing allergies if both parents have them.

The Lancet researchers, led by Syed H. Arshad, M.D., said follow-up studies are needed to determine if the lower allergy rates will continue as the children grow.

"If the benefit shown in this study is maintained, it is likely to outweigh the costs of dietary supervision, hypoallergenic formulas and anti-dust-mite measures," the researchers wrote."

"This is very exciting because it confirms other studies that I and other researchers have previously done," said Robert N. Hamburger, M.D., director of the allergy-immunology laboratory and professor of pediatrics emeritus at the University of California in San Diego.

Beginning in the 1970s, Dr. Hamburger was one of the first researchers to show that allergies develop not only because of a genetic predisposition, but also because of environmental triggers.

Howard J. Schwartz, M.D., clinical professor of medicine at Case Western Reserve University in Cleveland, said the new study points up the importance of reducing the concentration of house dust mites to avoid allergies.

Liquid diet aids recovery from abdominal surgery

Medical World News Report

JULY 1—A supplemented liquid diet can reduce infection in patients recovering from abdominal surgery and help them leave the hospital sooner than a typical postoperative diet, according to Pennsylvania researchers.

The cohort of 85 patients was randomized to receive either a standard enteral diet or a supplemental version following surgery for upper gastrointestinal malignancies.

The supplemented formula contained the amino acid arginine, omega-3 fatty acids and RNA.

According to John M. Daly, M.D., of the University of Pennsylvania School of Medicine in Philadelphia, patients on the supplemented diet had 70% fewer nosocomial infections and left the hospital an average of four days earlier than patients on the standard diet.

"The new formula significantly lowered the rate of infections and wound complications," Dr. Daly said. Fewer of the surgical wounds reopened among patients receiving the new formula, and fewer patients developed pneumonia, he reported in Surgery.

In addition, patients on the supplemented diet had a return to preoperative levels of immunologic function that were noticeable within seven days.

The percentage of patients who were still hospitalized by day 21 was 16% for the supplemental group and 30% for the standard group.

Diarrhea was slightly more common in the supplemented group."It's a very significant study," said Elie Hamaoui, M.D., chief of nutrition at the Veterans Administration Medical Center in Brooklyn, N.Y. "We knew these substances improve immune function in patients, but is it really good to beef up the immune system in these patients? It may be too much of a stimulus and harm the patient."

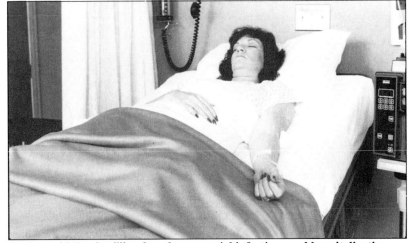

Amino acid "cocktail" reduced nosocomial infections and hospitalization.

Dr. Hamaoui said that now that the supplemental diet is known to improve outcome, it is clear that it would be helpful to patients after surgery.

Nutrient supplements raise new worries

By Saralie Faivelson

AUG. 26—Government researchers would like to deflate the pumped-up claims of some pills promoted as nutritional supplements in health and bodybuilding magazines.

The supplements often contain doses of vitamins far higher than those recommended by national medical groups, or list mysterious substances, Rossanne M. Philen, M.D., of the

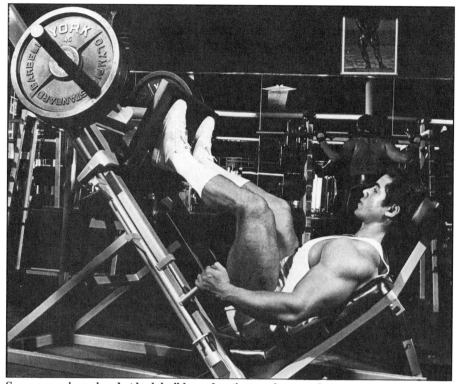

Some magazines aimed at bodybuilders advertise supplements that may pose toxicity risk.

Centers for Disease Control, wrote in The Journal of the American Medical Association.

Dr. Philen and colleagues at the CDC conducted a survey of 12 health and bodybuilding magazines, and found that they contained ads for more than 300 types of pills promoted as nutritional supplements. "I was surprised to see the vast number of different ingredients, and how little we knew about what they were," she said.

The researchers discovered 235 ingredients, including some they had never heard of, such as conch grass, muira puama and uva ursi, she said.

Amino acids were the most frequently mentioned ingredient. The most frequently used claim: muscle and strength development.

"My greatest concern is that since we have no information about these products, we don't know what kinds of side effects they produce," Dr. Philen said.

People who take supplements often take more than one, increasing the chance of side effects, Dr. Philen said. "Then they go to their doctor, who has no way of knowing what caused the symptoms because they don't know the ingredients in the supplements."

Many doctors never find out their patients are taking the supplements because patients may not consider them drugs they must tell their doctors about, or are embarrassed to tell the doctor they are taking health pills, she said.

If more than one type of pill is taken at the same time, patients can get symptoms of vitamin overdose. Some of the pills contain large doses of vitamin A, which could lead to headaches, blurred vision, diarrhea, joint and bone pain, dry skin, and loss of hair and vision, according to Liz Marr Diemand, a spokesperson for the American Dietetic

Association. Others have large amounts of vitamin D, possibly causing kidney damage, high blood pressure and high blood cholesterol, she added.

To highlight the possible dangers of taking food supplements, Dr. Philen pointed to cases of eosinophilia-myalgia syndrome (EMS), some of which resulted in death, among people who took pills from contaminated batches of L-tryptophan supplements.

As of August, the CDC had received reports of 38 deaths and 1,512 cases of EMS linked to contaminants in L-tryptophan, said Chuck Fallis, a CDC spokesperson.

L-tryptophan was sold in drug-stores and health-food stores across the country as a treatment for premenstrual syndrome, stress, depression and insomnia.

"The real issue with these supplements is what kind of claim are they making and are they supporting it," said Michael Taylor, deputy commissioner for policy at the Food and Drug Administration. "If they don't, it's plain old-fashioned health fraud. And if they are promising health benefits, then these substances should be considered drugs, and submitted to the FDA for the standard approval process."

CDC recommends folic acid for women

SEPT. 14—All women of childbearing age should consume 0.4 mg of folic acid daily to reduce the risk of having a baby with birth defects, the government recommended.

Folic acid, a B vitamin, can reduce the risk of having a baby with neural-tube defects if it is taken starting at least a month before a woman becomes pregnant. About 2,500 U.S. infants are born each year with neural-tube defects, the most common of which are spina bifida and anencephaly.

The folic acid recommendation was presented to experts at a meeting of the Centers for Disease Control this summer. Until now, folic acid supplements have been advocated only for pregnant women who already have given birth to a baby with a neural-tube defect.

Folic acid can be found in leafy, dark green vegetables, citrus fruits and juices, bread and beans and fortified breakfast cereals. Women also can take folic acid supplements or daily multivitamins containing 0.4 mg of the nutrient, which fosters cell growth and reproduction.

James Mason, M.D., head of the U.S. Public Health Service, said, "It seems possible that we can reduce the number of serious neural-tube defects through a good diet and/or supplements. If we can do this, we will have produced a major reduction in the disability that today impacts many families and communities."

The newly released government recommendations state that women should not take more than 1 mg of folic acid per day unless a greater dose is recommended by their doctor, since the effects of high levels of the nutrient are not well understood.

Anticancer role of dietary fruits and vegetables confirmed by meta-analysis of 156 studies

By Luba Vikhanski

SEPT. 21—People who eat a lot of fruits and vegetables have about half the risk of developing most cancers compared with people who rarely include these foods in their diet.

The finding comes from a review of 156 studies on fruits, vegetables and cancer risk, which appeared in the journal Nutrition and Cancer. In 128 of the 156 studies, fruits and vegetables were found to have a protective effect against cancer.

"This is the most consistent evidence of a relationship between diet and cancer that we have ever found," said lead author Gladys Block, Ph.D., professor of public health at the University of California at Berkeley.

The review lends further support to the National Cancer Institute's new "5 A Day" program launched in July, in which Americans have been encouraged to eat five servings or more of fruits and vegetables a day, according to Regina Ziegler, an epidemiologist at the NCI.

Generalists are encouraged to advise their patients to follow the NCI guidelines, in which a serving is defined as one-half cup of fresh fruits or one cup of leafy vegetables.

While evidence of the protective effect of fruits and vegetables against cancer has been accumulating over the past 10 years, the consistency with which the link has emerged from the new report is impressive, Ziegler said.

The review showed that for most types of cancer, the 25% of the world's population with the highest intake of fruits

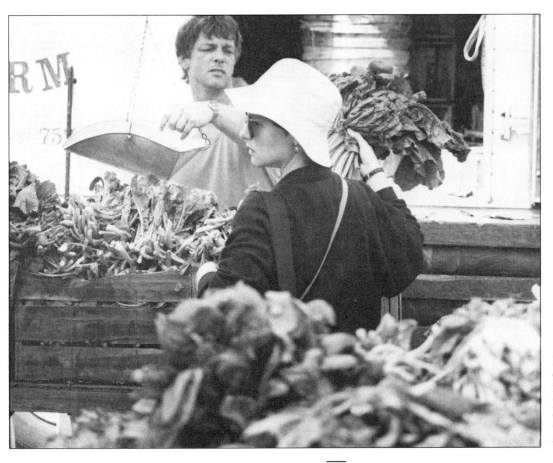

Review of over 150 studies reaffirms the protective effect of fruits and vegetables against cancer.

and vegetables had roughly half as many cancers as the 25% with the lowest intake.

A diet rich in fruits and vegetables significantly reduced the risk of cancers of the lung, larynx, mouth, esophagus, stomach, colon, rectum, bladder, pancreas, cervix, ovary and endometrium, according to the report.

The protective effect may be due to a combination of nutrients, or because people who consume many fruits and vegetables tend to eat a diet low in fat and meat, according to Ziegler.

"As a scientist, I am concerned when doses of beta-carotene and vitamin C in pill form are touted as a way to reduce the risk of cancer because of this fruit-and-vegetable effect," she said. "They may not be the mechanism."

The effect of fruits and vegetables on cancer risk has been overlooked because people have been trying to find a single protective nutrient, or "magic bullet," like beta-carotene or vitamin C, Dr. Block said.

"I don't for a minute believe it's one thing. There are some cancers for which one nutrient is more important than another. But then the opposite is true for another cancer. Nature packaged them all together in fruits and vegetables," she said.

While eating five servings a day may sound like a lot, Dr. Block said that it is not so difficult if you remember to have a vegetable with every meal and a fruit for a snack.

Because different foods contain different nutrients, it is important to eat a variety, said Amy Subar, an NCI nutritionist and coauthor of the new report.

"Someone eating five apples every day isn't doing what we are telling them to do," she said.

It is difficult to know exactly how many fruits and vegetables people consume per day, but on the whole, Americans are thought to fall far short of the goal set by the NCI.

According to one recent survey, only 10% of the United States population eats the recommended amounts of fruits and vegetables, Dr. Block said.

Study: Fat, fiber don't affect breast cancer risk; NCI stands by its low-fat recommendations

By Charlene Laino

OCT. 21—Contrary to previous reports, a high-fat, low-fiber diet does not increase a woman's chance of getting breast cancer, according to a study of almost 90,000 women.

But such a diet does increase the risk of colon cancer and heart disease, said researchers from Brigham and Women's Hospital in Boston.

Even before the study was published in The Journal of the American Medical Association, a government breast-cancer prevention expert rushed to issue a statement cautioning women against interpreting the study to mean they can smother extra butter on their toast without consequences.

The National Cancer Institute continues to recommend that all Americans consume 30% or fewer of their total calories from fat, said Peter Greenwald, M.D., director of the Division of Cancer Prevention and Control at the National Cancer Institute.

The study looked at women with an intake of dietary fat ranging from about 27% to 50% of their total calories. "Therefore, the data can only be interpreted for women who eat within that range," Dr. Greenwald said.

In a typical woman's 1,800-calorie-a-day diet, 27% of calories from fat would translate into 54 g of fat; 50% of calories from fat would mean 100 g of fat.

Therefore, any woman on an 1,800-calorie diet consuming fewer than 54 g of fat a day actually may be protecting herself against breast cancer; that was not looked at in this study, Dr. Greenwald said.

He added that the results of the Boston study make the National Institutes of Health's long-term trial, the Women's Health Initiative—which is examining the health effects of

consuming just 20% of total calories from fat—that much more important.

Recommendations to decrease fat consumption are justified even though the link between fat and breast cancer may not be very strong, according to Geoffrey Howe, Ph.D., of the National Cancer Institute of Canada Epidemiology Unit at the University of Toronto.

"Even a weak association can be of major importance in public health terms," he wrote in an editorial accompanying the new study. "A reduction in risk of 10% would reduce the number of breast-cancer cases occurring in the United States each year by about 18,000."

In the new study, the researchers reported on 89,494 women who are part of the Nurses' Health Study. The women, aged 34 through 59 in 1980, were followed for eight years, during which time they periodically filled out questionnaires about diet and breast cancer.

Some 1,439 cases of breast cancer were identified, including 774 in postmenopausal women.

After adjusting for age, established risk factors such as family history of the disease and total calories consumed, no link was found between total fat intake and risk of breast cancer, said Walter Willett, M.D., of the department of medicine, Brigham and Women's Hospital.

A similar absence of any positive association was observed without adjustment for energy intake; for tumors less than 2 cm in diameter as well as 2 cm or greater in diameter; for saturated, monounsaturated and polyunsaturated fat, and after excluding the first four years of follow-up, he said.

In addition, the researchers found that a high-fiber diet did not significantly reduce a woman's risk of breast cancer.

COMMENTARY

Dietary research is bearing fruit

By Johanna Dwyer, D.Sc.

DURING THE NEXT FEW YEARS, as research answers more of our questions about diet's role in health and disease, we also must address the questions of how nutrition fits into the day-to-day practice of medicine and how nutritional services can reach those who most need them.

Here are some areas in which we are particularly likely to make research advances or where we most need to do so:

• We must define the role of nutrition in patients' ability to function and in quality of life. We don't have very many good ways to assess subtle changes in patients' daily functioning, which is particularly a problem as people age. Research end points should include functional outcomes rather than morbidity as estimated by mortality rates or changes in biochemical measures.

• Randomized clinical trials of promising dietary interventions should yield important information on nutritional strategies and therapies. Particularly interesting are trials of diet-related adjuncts to various medical treatments and studies, such as the National Cancer Institute's Designer Foods Program, that look at the biological effects of nutrients and nonnutrients.

• Women have been in the quiet corner of the clinical trial business; a study of dietary manipulations in middle-aged and older women is long overdue to help reduce major diet-related disease incidence.

• Advances in clinical nutrition will continue in newer methods of feeding, such as total parenteral nutrition and special enteral therapies, for example. We are learning more about specific nutrient requirements of specialized cells, such as colonocytes in the gut that have special fatty-acid requirements or enterocytes that need glutamine as a conditionally essential amino acid.

• We must pay more attention to how we integrate concerns about nutrition across the entire spectrum of disease—not just in prevention but also in amelioration and palliation, such as with terminal disease. We need to realize that dietary recommendations for primary prevention aren't necessarily sufficient or appropriate for disease treatment, and to apply appropriate measures for each condition and stage of disease.

• We will try to learn more about food composition, especially in terms of non-nutrient substances that have biological significance.

• We are gaining more understanding of nutrition's role in preventing chronic degenerative disease. In terms of immunology, we're just beginning to understand the relationship between diet and immune response. Scientists are looking into nutrition and AIDS, food allergies and a lot of other diseases that we don't think of as immune related, but that might be.

In nutrition policy, I am concerned about resource allocation in several areas:

• We must make sure that as medical care dollars continue to be limited and as we devise new systems for payment, nutrition doesn't get overlooked. When services are bundled together or cut, clinical nutrition usually is not at the top of decision makers' priority lists, even though it often should be.

• Physicians will begin identifying older patients who are having problems with nutrition or general health. One program that is helping them do this is the Nutrition Screening Initiative, sponsored by medical groups, including the American Academy of Family Physicians, the American Dietetic Association and the National Council on Aging, with a steering committee of 30 other health professional groups. The program's materials, available for all health professionals, help ensure that patients having nutritional problems get help earlier.

• As biotechnology advances, we must make sure that the fruits of that technology are translated quickly and safely into health applications. As we have seen with fat substitutes, there are difficult regulatory issues that must be addressed.

• We should continue to fund the government's program surveillance and monitoring system of the nation's nutritional status, and to strengthen the National Center for Health Statistics and other data-collection systems. We need to make sure we fund monitoring of national representative samples and have long-term follow-up. We also must evaluate nutrition programs that are in place and integrate them with other health services.

• Nutrition education needs to be more sophisticated. We should equip patients to be good consumers and to be advocates on their own behalf with respect to nutrition.

Johanna Dwyer, D.Sc., is professor of nutrition at Tufts University School of Medicine and the Tufts School of Nutrition, and director of the Frances Stern Nutrition Center at the New England Medical Center Hospital in Boston.

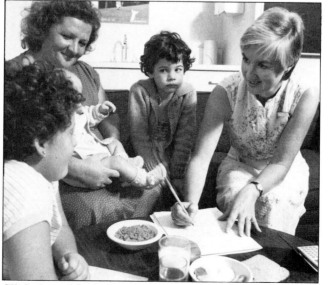

Clinical nutritionist suggests better eating strategies.

Urology

1992 HIGHLIGHTS

PSA screening said to be useful in distinguishing between benign and cancerous growths only when prostate size is known.

Feb. 5

Infectious-disease experts warned that electing not to circumcise a son may place him at increased risk for urinary-tract infections as an adult. After reviewing records from a sexually transmitted disease clinic in Seattle, University of Washington researchers found that 31% of men diagnosed with UTIs were uncircumcised, versus only 12% of men attending the clinic who did not have a UTI diagnosis. Infections with urovirulent strains of E. coli that produce urethritis as well as UTIs were particularly common in uncircumcised men, the team reported in The Journal of the American Medical Association.

Earlier studies by the same investigators had demonstrated a higher incidence of UTIs among uncircumcised newborns.

March 11

Men over 40 should be rejected as semen donors, the director of the American Fertility Society announced at an American Medical Association meeting. He cited evidence that the incidence of serious genetic mutations in sperm from men over 40 was four times higher than the rate among men under 35.

Previously, the cutoff age for semen donors was 50.

March 12

Duke University researchers detected human papillomavirus 16 in tumor specimens from eight out of 29 patients with squamous-cell carcinoma of the penis.

The HPV may be responsible for more than one quarter of penile cancers, the investigators concluded. HPV was also detected in the metastatic lesions of three out of six patients with more advanced disease, the team reported in the International Journal of Cancer.

March 19

Male infertility may be linked to a defective protein on the head of sperm, announced San Francisco researchers.

In laboratory experiments the protein, PH-30, proved necessary in order for sperm to recognize, fuse with and penetrate an egg, the University of California team reported in Nature. In the future, it may be possible to design a male contraceptive that prevents fertilization by interfering with PH-30, the researchers predicted.

March 21

Urologists can reassure their patients that having a vasectomy will not increase their risk of testicular or prostate cancer, British researchers announced. Oxford University investigators compared 13,246 men aged 25 to 49 years who had undergone a vasectomy with 22,196 controls. There was no significant difference in cancer rates between the two groups, the team reported in the British Medical Journal.

March 30

The prostate-specific antigen test can help distinguish between prostate cancer and benign enlargement of the gland, but works well only if prostate size is known, said Ann Arbor, Mich., researchers. For example, if a man's level of serum PSA is 10 ng/ml and the prostate volume is over 105 cc (as measured by ultrasound), it may be normal, but if the gland volume is only 25 cc, he almost certainly has cancer, radiologists from St. Joseph Mercy Hospital told an American Cancer Society seminar.

April 9

The active ingredient in

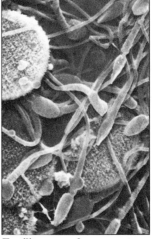

Fertility researcher suggests men over 40 not donate sperm.

marijuana may inhibit the ability of the sperm to fertilize eggs, announced a researcher from the State University of New York at Buffalo. By treating sea urchin sperm with tetrahydrocannabinol, the euphoriant in marijuana, the sperm's ability to penetrate the egg was reduced by 93%, the researcher reported at the Federation of American Societies for Experimental Biology meeting in Anaheim, Calif. He said the sea urchin may prove useful as a model in studying a range of marijuana effects.

May 2

Japanese researchers cautioned that they have detected human papillomavirus 16 in semen from the sexual partners of infected women, confirming that the cancer-linked virus can be sexually transmitted. In a study of 23 couples, four male partners of the 12 HPV-16-positive women harbored the same HPV type in their semen. None of the partners of HPV-negative women harbored HPV, investigators from Osaka University Medical School reported in The Lancet.

May 10

To detect prostate cancer early, while it is still curable, the digital rectal exam should be supplemented by the prostate-specific antigen test, a specialist told the American Urological Association meeting in Washington, D.C. In two studies of more than 17,000 men, only 27% of patients screened with PSA and digital rectal exams were diagnosed after their cancers had become advanced, compared with 67% of those tested with only the rectal exam, reported the Washington University School of Medicine urologist. But many other urologists questioned the value

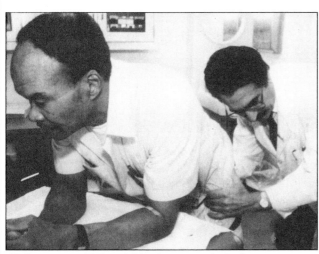

CDC reports a 30% and 8% rise, respectively, in prostate cancer among white and African-American men.

1992 HIGHLIGHTS

of mass screening in men over 50 with the PSA test because it is unable to distinguish between cancers that are likely to spread and those that will remain indolent.

May 11

Silent prostate cancer is relatively common, even in younger men, reported researchers from Wayne State University in Detroit. Of 144 males aged 10 to 49 who had died of causes other than prostate cancer, autopsy revealed that 41% of those aged 40 to 49 had precancerous lesions of the prostate, as did 22% of those aged 30 to 39, they told the American Urological Association meeting in Washington, D.C.

May 12

Two drugs could replace surgery as the treatment of choice for benign prostatic hyperplasia, said researchers at the American Urological Association meeting in Washington, D.C.

Finasteride (Proscar, Merck Sharp & Dohme) was tested in two independent trials in which patients received either 5 mg of the drug or placebo. At the conclusion of the trial, all patients were allowed to continue on finasteride. Among 850 patients treated

for two years on the drug, prostate size decreased by 25% and urine flow increased by 2.3 ml/sec, said the executive director of clinical research at Merck.

In an 18-month study, terazosin (Hytrin, Abbott Laboratories) eased urethral constriction by about 50% in 484 patients, said a Medical College of Wisconsin researcher. Urine flow improved by 32%.

Hytrin is approved for the treatment of hypertension.

May 13

University of Wisconsin Medical School researchers predicted that within a few years a vaccine against urinary-tract infections will be available in the United States. The vaccine, which is introduced as a liquid into the vagina, is already available in Europe.

During a five-month follow-up of 22 women prone to UTIs, nine women had fewer than expected infections after receiving the vaccine, the investigators told the American Urological Association meeting in Washington, D.C.

May 21

Along with generally reassuring news about the long-term safety of vasectomy, Harvard researchers reported an unexplained link between lung cancer and vasectomy.

In a retrospective study of over 14,000 men, vasectomy did not increase the overall risk of dying from heart disease or cancer, the investigators reported in The New England Journal of Medicine. However, men who had had the procedure more than 20 years ago were 44% more likely to die from cancer, particularly lung cancer, said the Harvard researchers. They had no explanation for this increased risk and recommended further study.

June 11

A high-fat, high-cholesterol diet may lead to

erectile dysfunction by promoting plaque buildup in penile arteries, a prominent urologist suggested. In a study of 31 New Zealand male rabbits, the Boston University School of Medicine researcher found that 93% of those fed a high-fat, high-cholesterol diet developed erectile dysfunction. Angioplasty restored penile function to the rabbits, the researcher reported in the Journal of Urology.

In man, studies have shown that atherosclerotic stenosis of penile arteries can cause erectile dysfunction. Once penile arteries become occluded, starting a patient on a low-fat diet may not reverse the condition, according to the urologist.

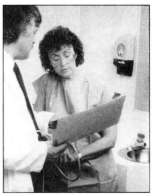

Follow-up of vaccine trial demonstrated fewer UTIs.

June 12

The Centers for Disease Control reported that the rate of prostate cancer in American men has increased steadily, especially among white men, although African-Americans are twice as likely to die from the disease. From 1980 to 1988, the rate of the disease increased 30% among white men and 8% among African-Americans. During those years, death rates increased 2.5% in whites and 5.9% in African-Americans.

The rising rate of diagnosis may be due in part to greater availability of screening tests, said a CDC epidemiologist. He said the higher death rate in blacks may be due to postponement of therapy or less access to medical care.

June 30

After a 14-month review, the Food and Drug Administration approved finasteride (Proscar, Merck Sharp & Dohme) for the treatment of benign prostatic hyperplasia.

July 17

Nitric oxide enzymes concentrated in penile neurons may be responsible for causing erections, suggested Johns Hopkins University researchers. Their studies of rats, reported in the journal Science, showed that when these enzymes were inhibited with injections of L-nitroarginine, electrically stimulated erections either decreased or disappeared. The findings have potential application in the therapeutic treatment of priapism, the researchers stated, noting that nearly 40% of sickle-cell anemia patients suffer from priapism and could possibly benefit from injections of L-nitroarginine.

Aug. 10

Traffic cops who hold radar guns on their laps may be at increased risk of testicular cancer, scientists told the Senate Subcommittee on Consumer and Environmental Affairs. Police officers requested the hearing because of concerns that the guns may cause or promote testicular cancer as well as cervical, eye and brain cancers.

Scientists told the committee there is not enough evidence to conclude that the radar guns do in fact cause cancer, but said more scrutiny is needed. Officers testified that they often hold the guns in their laps, or rest them over their shoulders, thus exposing themselves to unshielded radiation.

Aug. 15

Prostate-cancer support groups are emerging throughout the country, the American Urological Association reported. The groups offer newly

diagnosed patients and those who have just begun to undergo treatment a chance to obtain information about different treatment options, prognosis and posttreatment follow-up in a relaxed atmosphere, according to a New York urologist who started one of the nation's first support groups.

Sept. 2

Radical prostatectomy via the perineal route may be the best choice for men with adenocarcinoma of the prostate, a Philadelphia urologist told Medical Tribune. The Jefferson Medical College urologist said he believes that the perineal procedure is superior to a retropubic approach because it is less invasive, resulting in significantly less blood loss and less postoperative impotence.

Sept. 12

Men's sperm counts plummeted by more than half over the last 50 years, and Danish researchers blamed chemical pollution for the damage to male fertility. After reviewing more than 60 studies, investigators from the University of Copenhagen found that both ejaculate volume and sperm concentration had declined. Neither laboratory errors nor life-style factors (such as smoking and an increase in sexually transmitted diseases) account for the dramatic changes, the researchers, who aimed their scrutiny on exposures to environmental toxins, stated in the British Medical Journal.

Sept. 14

Penile injections of a genetically engineered prostaglandin prior to intercourse can help men achieve an erection quickly and more comfortably than implants, an Australian urologist told the International Society for Impotence Research meeting in Milan. When injected into the base of the penis, the prostaglandin produces an erection within

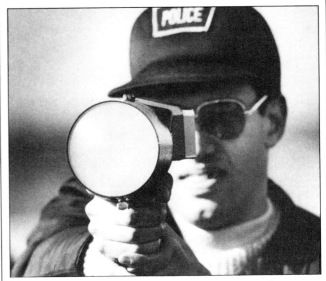

Traffic cops who hold radar guns on their laps may be at increased risk of testicular cancer, say scientists.

two minutes that lasts about half an hour, reported the Sydney urologist. Priapism is not a problem, he said.

Sept. 24

Patients with a chlamydial infection of the urethra can be successfully treated with a single oral dose of azithromycin (Zithromax, Pfizer), investigators from Louisiana State University reported. They studied 141 patients given azithromycin (1 g once orally) and 125 given doxycycline (100 mg orally twice daily for seven days) for treatment of urethral or endocervical chlamydial infection. Of the patients evaluated 21 to 35 days after treatment, none of 112 repeat bacterial cultures were positive in the azithromycin group compared with one of 102 in the doxycycline group, the New Orleans team reported in The New England Journal of Medicine.

Oct. 22

In a multicenter study reported in The New England Journal of Medicine, finasteride (Proscar, Merck Sharp & Dohme) modestly but significantly decreased the volume of enlarged prostates and diminished symptoms of obstruction. Thirty-one percent of the men taking finasteride had an increase of at least 3 ml/sec in their maximal urinary-flow rate, which the researchers considered significant; 17% of men receiving placebo had an equal improvement.

Finasteride may interfere with doctors' ability to detect prostate cancer, cautioned some scientists. For now, the drug should only be used among men who have moderate to severe symptoms of an enlarged prostate and who do not wish to undergo the quicker and more reliable minor surgery that is the standard treatment, according to an editorial accompanying the study.

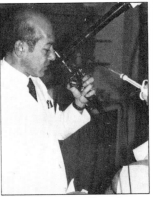

Finasteride significantly reduced prostate volume.

Research points way to contraceptive for men, and may also help to explain male infertility

MARCH 19—Scientists have determined the structure of a protein needed for sperm to penetrate an egg, pointing the way to a male contraceptive that would knock out the protein to prevent fertilization.

The protein, PH-30, is found on the heads of sperm and may help them recognize and fuse with an egg, University of California, San Francisco, researchers reported in Nature.

In an accompanying editorial, a Scottish fertility expert said the research also may help explain male infertility.

The PH-30 protein anchors the sperm to the surface of an egg, and then it fuses the egg and the sperm. Each action is carried out by different units of the protein.

"The long-range implication for contraception is that we may be able to interfere with the binding protein or make an antibody against that part of the protein," said coauthor Judith White, M.D., associate professor of pharmacology at the California university.

The research follows reports that scientists have deciphered the composition of other proteins found on the surface of sperm and eggs. It is still unclear which proteins will prove the most important for an eventual male contraceptive.

"It is possible now to start thinking of a male contraceptive," said William Byrd, M.D., of the University of Texas Southwestern Medical Center in Dallas. "It might work. But you would have to make sure it is...reversible."

John Altken, M.D., of the Center for Reproductive Biology in Edinburgh, Scotland, who wrote the Nature editorial, believes that researchers can begin to look at fusion proteins on sperm to see if they are defective. The research "carries implications for the diagnosis and treatment of male infertility," he wrote.

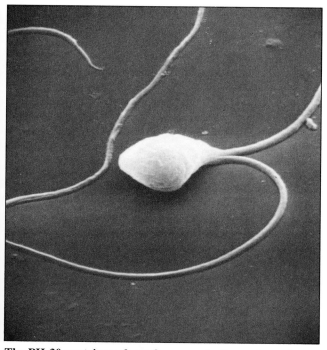

The PH-30 protein anchors the sperm to the surface of an egg, and then it fuses the egg and the sperm.

AUA meeting news: 2-way screen detects prostate cancer early

WASHINGTON, D.C., MAY 10—A new study has confirmed that the prostate-specific antigen (PSA) test combined with a digital rectal exam can detect most cases of prostate cancer early, while they are still curable, according to William Catalona, M.D., chief of urology at the Washington University School of Medicine in St. Louis.

But urologists question the value of screening all men over 50 with the PSA test because it is unable to distinguish between cancers that are likely to remain indolent and those that will spread.

In two studies of more than 17,000 men, patients screened with PSA and digital rectal exams (DRE) had less than half the number of advanced cancers as those tested only with DRE, reported Dr. Catalona at the American Urological Association meeting here.

The study is the first evidence that PSA screening detects more localized prostate cancers than the standard digital rectal exam alone, he noted.

According to Dr. Catalona, 67% of men in the new studies who were given only DRE had advanced prostate cancer, compared with 35% screened via PSA and 27% given both PSA and DRE.

The findings offer more support for his recommendations that the PSA blood test, together with DRE, be used in men the way that mammograms are used for women, Dr. Catalona told the meeting.

But many urologists are not yet swayed.

"PSA could also stand for 'priority seems awry,'" said William Fair, M.D., chief of urology at Memorial Sloan-

Kettering Cancer Center in New York City. "We don't have any evidence that early detection leads to increased survival [and] we don't have the faintest clue of how to distinguish indolent from more aggressive [prostate cancer]."

This means that physicians may treat patients with prostate cancer who could suffer morbidity or mortality from biopsy or treatment, but may never have progressed to life-threatening cancer, he noted.

Even if Medicare would offer reimbursement, as Sen. Robert Dole (R-Kan.) has proposed, the test's price is still prohibitive, Dr. Fair said. "The cost of the test can be as high as $85, so screening the 28 million American men over 50 could cost $2.4 billion. That's $400 million more than the National Cancer Institute's entire budget."

Urologists will have more information on the PSA test's impact on survival when results from the National Cancer Institute's multicenter 16-year study of screening tests and mortality rates for prostate, lung and colorectal cancers in high-risk men between the ages of 60 and 74 begin to come in. The study is scheduled to begin in late 1992 or early 1993.

"We expect to find out answers before the 16 years are up," said Barnett Kramer, M.D., associate director of the NCI's early detection and community oncology program.

He suspects that the study will find subsets of men, such as blacks, who are at higher risk for prostate cancer than whites, who will benefit more from screening. "The reason we're studying [the PSA test] is that we think it may well save lives, though it could still cause a net harm," said Dr. Kramer.

Vaccine found to prevent urinary-tract infections

WASHINGTON, D.C., MAY 13— A vaccine already available in Europe may be on the market within a few years in the United States to prevent urinary-tract infections in women who are prone to them.

Researchers at the University of Wisconsin Medical Center in Madison said the vaccine was found safe in older women and shows promise in reducing the number of repeat infections.

In the study, reported at the American Urological Association meeting here, 22 women between ages 45 and 70 who suffered from recurrent UTIs were given the vaccine, which is introduced as a liquid into the vagina.

After five months of follow-up, the only effect noted was minimal vaginal irritation that required no treatment, said David Uehling, M.D.

Nine of the women had one or no infections during the time

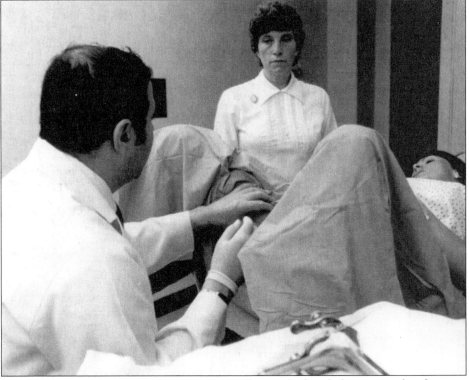

Agent shows promise in reducing recurrences. Research already has proven it safe.

they were followed. Dr. Uehling said that these women normally would have had two or three infections during that time.

The other women continued to have two or more infections. No placebo group was studied.

Standard treatment is oral antibiotics, but they can cause yeast infections and allergic reactions.

"It would be better to completely prevent the infection than treat the symptoms," said Perry Nadig, M.D., clinical professor of urology at the University of Texas Health Science Center in San Antonio.

It is likely to be at least several years before the vaccine is

approved in the United States, according to the investigators who reported their findings.

An injectable form of the vaccine already is approved in Europe. The European version, called Urovac, is made by Solco of Basel, Switzerland, and is given as an injection in the arm.

Although it has been proven effective, it also caused mild to moderate side effects, including pain at the injection site and fever in 47% of women surveyed, said Dr. Uehling. He is currently waiting for Food and Drug Administration approval for a second phase of vaccine testing that will compare the U.S. version with a placebo.

After 14-month review, new drug is approved for the treatment of benign prostatic hyperplasia

By Fran Kritz

JUNE 30—After a brief 14-month review, the Food and Drug Administration has approved finasteride (Proscar, Merck Sharp & Dohme) for the treatment of benign prostatic hyperplasia.

In studies of 1,600 patients at 76 centers worldwide, finasteride produced a 24% median reduction in prostate size over two years in 50% of men taking 5 mg per day. It also increased urine flow by 2.3 ml/sec.

The drug's effect may not be evident for at least six months after treatment begins. The medication must be taken for the remainder of the patient's life at a cost of about $1.75 a day. Corrective surgery can cost $7,000 to $8,000.

The most frequent side effects: impotence (3.7%), decreased libido (3.3%) and decreased volume of ejaculate (2.8%).

Another potential problem: By decreasing the amount of prostate tissue, prostate-specific antigen levels also are reduced, possibly masking malignancy. Merck maintains that the drug did not alter cancer detection rates in controlled trials.

William Catalona, M.D., head of urology at the Washington University School of Medicine in St. Louis, who studied the PSA test, said he does not think the issue is resolved.

Patrick Walsh, M.D., chairman of the urology department at Johns Hopkins University in Baltimore, said finasteride should not be used for mild symptoms that may need no treatment, or for severe symptoms such as urinary retention or incomplete voiding that may require surgery.

Dr. Walsh said he believes most urologists have been conservative about surgery and will welcome finasteride as a pharmacological alternative.

It is the first of the 5-alpha reductase inhibitors, which inhibit the enzyme that converts testosterone to dihydrotestosterone.

Terazosin (Hytrin, Abbott Laboratories), approved for hypertension, has been shown to ease urethral constriction by up to 50% in men with BPH. Studies are under way to test terazosin with finasteride in men with prostate enlargement and urethral constriction.

Finasteride study sparks debate on efficacy

By Dan Hurley

OCT. 22—A new study concluding that the first drug approved in the United States to treat enlarged prostates is beneficial has sparked a debate among experts, some of whom say the drug is only minimally effective in a small group of men.

But a coauthor of the new study, Patrick Walsh, M.D., chairman of the urology department at Johns Hopkins University in Baltimore, is more optimistic about the drug's usefulness.

Finasteride (Proscar, Merck Sharp & Dohme) "provides significant improvement in symptoms in about a third of patients. It's effective in low doses taken once a day, and has very few side effects, " Dr. Walsh said.

"I've been taking care of men with enlarged prostates for a long time, and I've never had any medical therapy to offer them until now," he said.

The new study of 895 men with symptoms of enlarged prostate glands was carried out for a year, with half taking finasteride and half taking placebo.

The men taking 5 mg of finasteride each day had an average 22% increase in the maximal urinary-flow rate, and a 19% decrease in the size of their prostate gland. According to the report, 31% of the men had an increase of at least 3 ml/sec in their maximal urinary-flow rate, which was considered significant; 17% of the men in the placebo group had an equal improvement.

The main side effects of the drug—impotence, decreased sex drive and difficulty ejaculating—affected about 3% of men, and generally abated after the drug was discontinued, the investigators reported in The New England Journal of Medicine.

Finasteride should only be used among men who have moderate to severe symptoms of an enlarged prostate, such as difficulty urinating, and who do not wish to undergo the quicker and more reliable surgery that is the standard treatment, according to an accompanying editorial.

Even then, doctors must check the patient for prostate cancer periodically, since the drug may interfere with prostate-specific antigen (PSA) tests, and discontinue the drug if it has no effect, wrote Paul H. Lange, M.D., chairman of the urology department at the University of Washington in Seattle.

Doctors at Merck Sharp & Dohme said that studies are currently under way to learn more about finasteride's effects on prostate-specific antigen levels.

A coauthor of the study, John McConnell, M.D., of the University of Texas Southwestern Medical Center in Dallas, also sees limited use of the drug for patients with mild symptoms. Dr. McConnell is chairman of a panel jointly sponsored by the American Urological Association and the Agency for Healthcare Policy. The panel will release standards in the spring of next year indicating that "watchful waiting" is the only appropriate treatment for men with mild symptoms, he said.

Notes

Notes

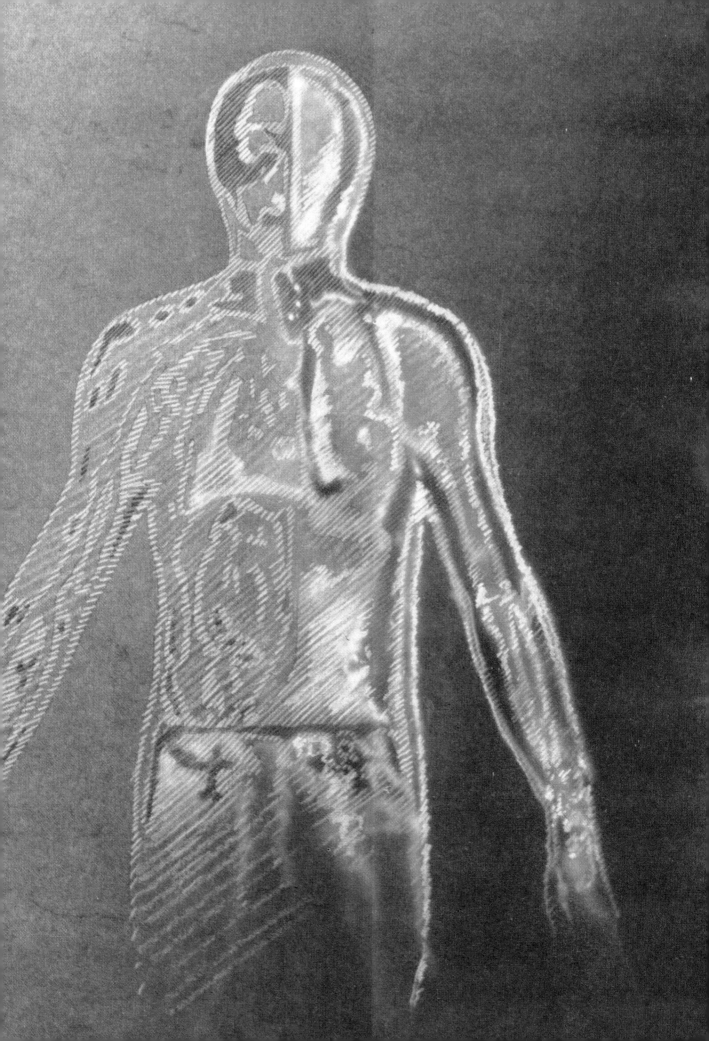

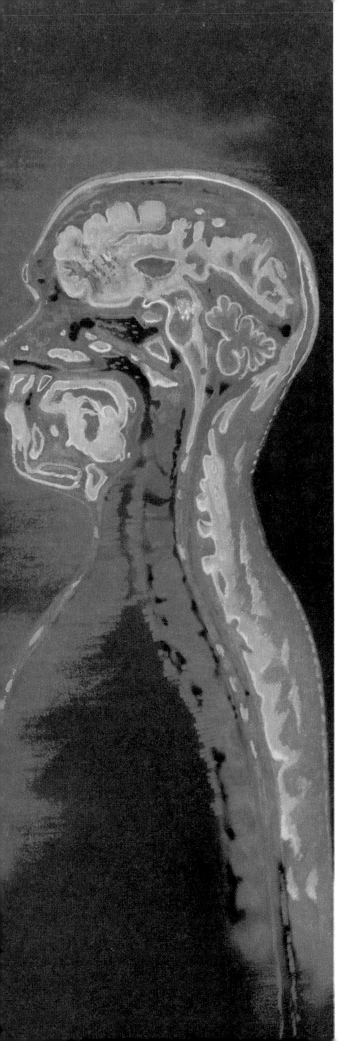

Clinical Medicine

Overview 182
Drug resistance, some infectious diseases on the rise in 1992

Month-at-a-glance 184

Reported at the Time 196
Steroid slows alcoholic hepatitis...self-administered heparin for deep-vein thrombosis...Bushes' double thyroid trouble coincidental...enzyme eases breathing in cystic fibrosis...TB update: step-care proposed, hospital workers at high risk...sustained estrogen for osteoporosis...alcohol may protect heart, but heavy drinking poses health hazard...diabetes news: exercise for prevention, aspirin to reduce complications...tacrine shows promise for Alzheimer's...new chronic fatigue test...Gulf vets suffer mystery ills...pig-liver transplant sparks ethics debate...oral cholera vaccine

Commentary 211
Building bone with drugs and diet
By Theodore Fields, M.D.

Drug resistance, some infectious diseases on the rise in 1992

"Without immediate and massive efforts to address the threat of tuberculosis, this country faces the possibility of an epidemic of TB that is resistant to all available treatments."

The year 1992 saw a resurgence of tuberculosis and measles, along with a wave of drug resistance to bacterial infections. The specter of emerging infectious-disease epidemics arose after disease surveillance efforts were stymied by years of severe cuts in public health budgets.

However, a team of French and British researchers reported the first evidence of a genetic basis for TB-drug resistance. By identifying a gene missing in clinical isolates from patients with isoniazid-resistant TB, the researchers raised the hope of a molecular-genetics approach to treatment.

On the diagnostic front there was also some good news. Pathologists reported at the meeting of the American Society of Microbiology that a newly developed test can diagnose TB in 24 hours or less, compared with the three to 12 weeks needed for conventional tests.

In the medical trenches, however, the onslaught of multi-drug-resistant TB strains took a steady toll on already over-burdened inner-city hospitals. Nonresistant TB can be cured with a six-month course of antibiotics, but the multidrug-resistant strains require 18 months of therapy and are often fatal–some 50% of patients with them die.

Inner-city hospitals, shelters and drug clinics scrambled during the year to deal with the rising number of both uncomplicated and drug-resistant tuberculosis cases, but often found that they lacked the resources to deal with the emergency.

At Chicago's Cook County Hospital, one in 100 cases of TB was reported to be resistant to at least isoniazid and rifampin. In New York City, the epicenter of multidrug-resistant TB strains in 1992, at least 7% of cases were

Clinical Medicine

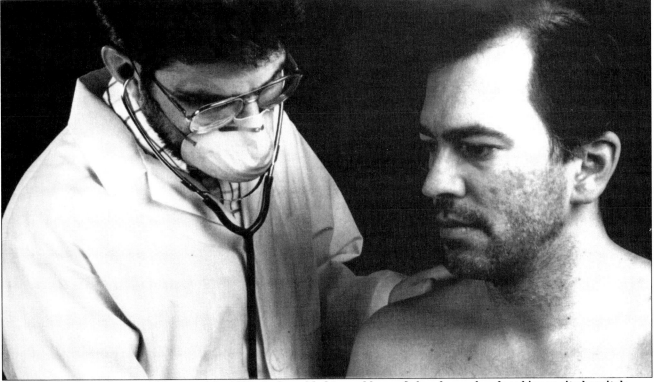

In the medical trenches, multidrug-resistant TB strains added to problems of already overburdened inner-city hospitals.

estimated to be resistant to at least these drugs. Overall, over one third of all TB cases in New York City in 1992 were estimated to be resistant to one or more drugs.

Sounding the alarm, Allan Bloch, M.D., of the Centers for Disease Control and Prevention, told a House subcommittee that "without immediate and massive efforts to address the threat of tuberculosis, this country faces the possibility of an epidemic of TB that is resistant to all available treatments."

The disease has made an alarming comeback following nearly two decades of severe cuts in public health programs and amid the AIDS epidemic and significant increases in homelessness and drug abuse. In the United States, the number of TB cases has been increasing since 1985, and in 1991 cases rose 9.4% to nearly 26,000. No state was TB-free.

Tuberculosis was not the only disease in which drug resistance posed a threat in 1992. Many other bacterial diseases were found to be unresponsive to at least one antibiotic, according to a series of reports in the journal Science that underscored the growing crisis in drug resistance. Staphylococcus, Streptococcus, pneumonia, dysentery, gonorrhea, meningitis and malaria were among the infections already resistant to the commonly used antibiotics. "It is an ongoing battle," said Harold Neu, M.D., an antibiotics expert at Columbia University and an author of one of the Science articles. "The bugs want to survive, just like we do," he said.

As the battle against drug-resistant bacterial infections continued throughout the year, some relief in the viral arena arrived when the Food and Drug Administration approved alfa interferon for the treatment of hepatitis B. The Department of Health and Human Services reported that recombinant interferon alfa-2b, administered in doses of 5 to 10 million IU subcutaneously three times a week for four months, led to a loss of hepatitis B serum markers in about 40% of study group subjects.

In the battle against hepatitis C, there was some encouraging news in 1992 from a group of Johns Hopkins University researchers who reported that the incidence of the infection from blood transfusions had decreased dramatically since the introduction in 1990 of an ELISA screening test that detects HCV antibodies. And in March, 1992, the FDA licensed an even more sensitive ELISA test that screens antibodies to three viral antigens, replacing the single antigen test.

Another widespread affliction, at least in the industrialized world, received a flurry of attention in 1992. A number of new reports reaffirmed the role of Helicobacter pylori in the pathogenesis of duodenal ulcers. In one study of 109 patients, David Graham, M.D., chief of digestive diseases at the Veterans Administration Medical Center in Houston, found ulcers recurred in 12% of patients taking ranitidine plus antibiotics, while ulcers returned in 95% of those taking only ranitidine.

However, other physicians cautioned that it was too early to make any blanket statements about whether H. pylori was the cause of the most common ulcers. They said only large, double-blind, long-term studies could confirm the relationship between the bacterium and the ulcers.

Overall in clinical medicine, 1992 was a year marked by solid progress in the battle against some well-entrenched diseases. But, unfortunately, the year also brought many sobering reminders that infectious diseases that once could be prevented have emerged with new, more deadly defenses.

Clinical Medicine

Jan. 1

Some ulcer drugs may boost blood alcohol levels, reported researchers at the Veterans Affairs Medical Center in New York. After a standard dose of alcohol, men treated with cimetidine (Tagamet, SmithKline Beecham) had peak blood alcohol levels 92% higher than those achieved with the same amount of alcohol prior to H_2-receptor antagonist treatment. Ranitidine (Zantac, Glaxo) raised blood alcohol 34%, but famotidine (Pepcid, Merck Sharp & Dohme) did not significantly increase blood alcohol levels, the researchers stated in The Journal of the American Medical Association.

Jan. 4

Norwegian researchers found that careful control of blood glucose levels in diabetic patients can slow the progression of retinopathy. A seven-year study of 45 insulin-dependent diabetics

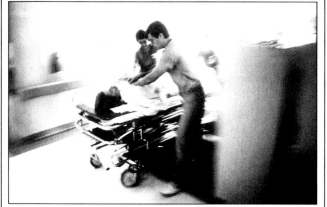

Will heart-attack patient survive? Poverty may lessen the chance.

showed that intensified insulin treatment and home blood glucose monitoring improved glycated hemoglobin concentrations, thus diminishing progession of retinopathy, Trondheim University specialists reported in the British Medical Journal.

Jan. 7

Schizophrenics gained up to 45 pounds during their first 16 weeks on clozapine (Clozaril, Sandoz) therapy, leading researchers to speculate that the serotonin antagonist may be useful in treating anorexia nervosa. After 21 hospitalized patients were placed on clozapine for treatment of schizophrenia or schizo-affective disorder, eight increased their body weight by more than 10%, and another six gained between 5% and 10% of their baseline weight, according to psychiatrists at the University of Virginia School of Medicine. Those gaining the most weight also showed the most improvement in psychiatric symptoms, they reported in the American Journal of Psychiatry.

Jan. 9

Harvard University researchers suggested that polymerase chain reaction testing may be useful for detecting Lyme disease. The method correctly identified Borrelia burgdorferi in 45 of 55 patients with Lyme disease, while producing no false-positive results in any of 106 healthy individuals tested. In addition, PCR correctly predicted clinical outcome in eight patients from whom cerebrospinal fluid was obtained before and after antimicrobial therapy, the team stated in Neurology.

Jan. 15

Researchers at the University of Texas Southwestern Medical Center at Dallas took the first step toward creation of a genetically engineered artificial beta-cell that could be used in the treatment of diabetes. Further development of the artificial cell could offer an alternative to human islet-cell transplantation, they stated in the Proceedings of the National Academy of Sciences. The cells have not yet been tested in humans or animals.

Jan. 18

Stroke-wary people learned that they are at high risk in the morning. In a study of 578 patients, the hours between 8 a.m. and 10 a.m. were found to be the peak time for strokes to occur, specialists at London's National Hospital for Neurology and Neurosurgery reported in the British Medical Journal. The cause of the circadian variation requires further study, they noted.

Jan. 22

Poverty emerged as an important factor influencing long-term survival following heart attacks. During a five-year follow-up of 1,965 patients, those with annual incomes under $10,000 died at almost twice the rate of heart attack survivors with a household income of $40,000 or more, Duke University researchers reported in The Journal of the American Medical Association.

Jan. 25

A Dutch physician warned that patients with fair complexions who sunbathe may be at increased risk of developing gallstones as well as skin cancer. The researcher from University Hospital Leiden conducted a case-control study of 206 fair-skinned people. Those who liked to sunbathe had twice the risk of cholelithiasis of those who did not, he wrote in a letter to The Lancet.

•••

Analysis of a decade of research in Europe and Australia confirmed that a low-protein diet delays the progress of end-stage renal disease. Regardless of the type of kidney disease, patients on a diet at least 0.2 g protein/kg/day lower than controls stayed off dialysis longer and suffered fewer renal deaths than those on more liberal protein diets, French nephrologists reported in the British Medical Journal.

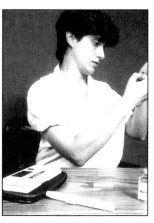

Home glucose monitoring found to cut diabetic retinopathy risk.

Jan. 27

An official of the American Academy of Family Physicians warned that benzodiazepines—often prescribed for the nearly one third of American adults who have trouble sleeping—can cause depression and rebound anxiety and insomnia.

Jan. 30

A Boston internist called for global surveillance of antibiotic resistance in response to an alarming Finnish report that erythromycin-resistant group A streptococci had increased sixfold between 1988 and 1990. Medical decision makers need to know whether they are dealing with isolated clusters or a growing trend in resistance to a particular antibiotic, he explained in The New England Journal of Medicine.

Clinical Medicine

Feb. 1

A study of more than 9,000 male twins suggested that the risk of having a stroke is strongly influenced by genetics. Men with a homozygous twin brother who had suffered a stroke had a more than fourfold greater risk of having a stroke than men with a heterozygous twin brother who had had a stroke, the Yale researchers explained in the journal Stroke.

Feb. 5

An 11-year study revealed that alcoholics who abstain have the same life expectancy as nonalcoholic men, while relapsed alcoholics are almost five times as likely to die prematurely. Of 199 men who had been heavy drinkers for at least five years, 101 resumed drinking and 98 remained sober. There were 19 deaths among the relapsed alcoholics over a period from one to 11 years; statistically, 3.83 were expected. Among abstinent alcoholics, there were four deaths, the University of California at San Diego researchers reported in The Journal of the American Medical Association.

Feb. 6

Scientists announced that they had detected a genetic defect specific to individuals with myotonic dystrophy, possibly paving the way for new treatments. The DNA fragment on chromosome 19 was found to be larger in affected individuals than in controls, and its size increased through generations in parallel with increasing severity of the disease, researchers at the Department of Energy's Lawrence Livermore National Laboratory and American, British and Dutch colleagues stated in Nature.

Feb. 7

Cleveland researchers alerted physicians that their patients are more likely to suffer obstructive sleep apnea if they have relatives with the disorder. A study of 154 relatives of 29 people with sleep apnea showed that the prevalence of symptoms associated with the disorder increased in proportion to the number of affected relatives, the Case Western Reserve team reported in the American Review of Respiratory Disease.

Feb. 10

A patient's speech may reveal heart-disease risk, a Cleveland researcher told the meeting for the American Association for the Advancement of Science. He performed computer analysis of the speech of 283 people and found that those who had two or more one-second pauses per minute were six times more likely to have heart attacks in the subsequent 10 years than those who did not. The micropauses may also signal stress or drug use, the researcher said.

Feb. 13

An Austrian researcher announced that direct exposure to light from a halogen lamp can irritate the eyes in 15 minutes. But reading by a 50-watt halogen lamp is safe for almost 11 hours, he commented in The New England Journal of Medicine. Afterwards, one is at risk of keratitis, he said.

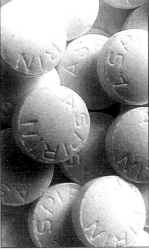

British data question the wisdom of taking aspirin with meals.

Feb. 15

Migraine sufferers can take a second dose of sumatriptan (Imitrex, Glaxo) to prevent headache recurrence, declared researchers from the Gothenburg Migraine Clinic in Sweden. Despite initial relief, 26 of 48 migraine patients who self-administered an injection of sumatriptan had another headache an average of 13 hours later, they reported in The Lancet. When the 26 patients administered a second shot within 24 hours of the migraine, only one sufferer had a recurrence.

Feb. 20

Corticosteroid therapy salvaged almost 90% of patients with severe alcoholic hepatitis, while fewer than half survived two months while receiving conventional therapy, revealed physicians from the Beaujon Hospital in Clichy, France. They gave 40 mg per day of prednisolone to 32 patients with biopsy-proved alcoholic hepatitis and either hepatic encephalopathy or a clinical measure of serious acute liver injury.

By the 66th day, four patients on steroids had died. By comparison, 16 of 29 patients receiving a placebo and standard hospital care died, the French clinicians reported in The New England Journal of Medicine. No serious side effects were noted.

Feb. 22

Researchers from Italy and Holland reported that patients with deep-vein leg thrombosis may be able to self-administer injections of a new version of heparin at home. In a study of 85 symptomatic patients, the frequency of recurrent venous thromboembolism did not differ significantly between the group given standard heparin therapy in a continuous intravenous infusion and those given low-molecular-weight heparin, the investigators reported in The Lancet. The ability to forgo regular laboratory monitoring and a longer plasma half-life suggest it is suitable for self-administration, said the researchers.

Feb. 23

Women were advised to look at their maternal relatives if they want to know whether they will develop varicose veins or spider veins on their legs. In a study of 500 women, 84% of those affected had at least one relative with the condition; four out of five of these were maternal relatives, according to a study team from Cornell University Medical College. Pregnancy, obesity, overexposure to the sun, oral contraceptive use and standing at a job for six or more hours also increased risk of varicose veins, the New York City researchers told a meeting of the North American Society of Phlebology.

Feb. 29

British researchers reported that patients on an aspirin regimen were able to avoid stomach ulcers by taking ranitidine (Zantac, Glaxo) along with their nonsteroidal anti-inflammatories. Twenty volunteers who took 600 mg of aspirin four times a day simultaneously took either a placebo or varying dosages of ranitidine. Those taking aspirin along with ranitidine developed fewer gastric ulcers, but only when the drugs were taken two hours before meals. At the maximum ranitidine dose, 600 mg, gastric erosion was cut by two thirds, according to data presented in the British Medical Journal.

Because the patients developed significantly fewer gastric erosions when they took aspirin on an empty stomach, the researchers from the University Hospital in Nottingham questioned whether the conventional advice to take the drug with food might be wrong.

March 1

Lyme disease is again on the rise, announced epidemiologists from the Centers for Disease Control. The disease, which had been increasing annually since 1986 until dropping in 1990, increased 17% to 9,308 cases in 1991, the CDC told Medical Tribune. The up-down-up pattern could mean that Lyme is stabilizing and near its peak in the U.S., said the medical epidemiologists.

March 11

A study of death certificates filed in New Mexico during the 1980s found that American Indians were eight times more likely to die from being struck by a passing motorist and 30 times more likely to die of hypothermia than other residents of that state, reported the New Mexico Department of Health. Most of these deaths occurred in men who were intoxicated and traveling along roads leading back to reservations, they explained in The Journal of the American Medical Association.

March 12

Hepatitis can be transmitted between hospitalized diabetic patients who share the same spring-loaded fingerstick device to test their blood-sugar levels, warned Centers for Disease Control investigators. They conducted an intensive investigation after 26 patients, 23 of them diabetics, contracted hepatitis B virus on one hospital ward. While nurses told the researchers they always changed the lancet, 30% of them did not always change the small plastic platform on which patients rest their finger when using the hand-held device, the CDC team reported in The New England Journal of Medicine.

March 13

The Food and Drug Administration licensed a more sensitive hepatitis C test that screens antibodies to three viral antigens. The nation's 2,400 blood banks had planned to replace the older, single antigen test with the newly licensed test (Ortho HCV 2.0 ELISA) by April 1, enabling them to eliminate 20% more potentially infected donors each year, according to the president of the American Association of Blood Banks. But even the new test will miss an estimated 10% of infected blood units from individuals who do not develop large amounts of antibodies, according to the National Institutes of Health.

March 14

Toxological findings in 5,106 poisonings, suicides and other violent deaths in Finland revealed that Halcion (triazolam, Upjohn) is no more likely to lead to suicide than other benzodiazepines, said University of Helsinki researchers. Halcion, while accounting for 29% of benzodiazepine sales, was present in 18% of suicides and 15% of other violent deaths. In contrast, oxazepam, usually considered a "safe" benzodiazepine, accounted for 20% of sales, but was the sole drug detected in 47% of suicides and 43% of other violent deaths, they wrote in a letter to The Lancet.

• • •

The bacille Calmette-Guerin vaccine reduced the expected incidence of leprosy by at least 50% in 83,500 Malawians, reported researchers from the London School of Hygiene and Tropical Medicine. The vaccine did not confer immunity against tuberculosis in the population studied, although it does protect against tuberculosis in other parts of the world, they noted in The Lancet.

March 15

The double dose of thyroid trouble suffered by President and Mrs. Bush was a coincidence, not the result of some environmental factor or bacteria, said a thyroid expert. Conjugal Graves's disease "may represent the chance occurrence of this relatively common disorder in married couples," the University of Massachusetts specialist wrote in the Annals of Internal Medicine.

March 16

Drugs derived from the Chinese herbal compound artemisinin (contained in the sweet wormwood plant) may be the only effective weapon against a deadly new strain of malaria resistant to available agents, said a director at the World Health Organization. WHO warned that the resistant malaria strain, which emerged

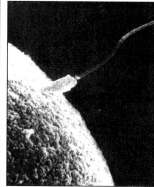

Sperm need PH-30 protein to identify and fuse with egg.

in areas along the border between Thailand and Cambodia and then spread west and north, had created an "extremely dangerous" situation.

March 19

Cystic fibrosis patients experienced significant improvement in lung function while taking a new genetically engineered drug, government researchers reported. The aerosolized drug, recombinant human deoxyribonuclease I (Genentech), or rhDNase, improved forced vital capacity by 10% to 20% among 16 cystic fibrosis patients, a team from the National Heart, Lung, and Blood Institute reported in The New England Journal of Medicine.

• • •

Scientists determined the structure of a protein needed for sperm to penetrate an egg, pointing the way to a male contraceptive that would knock out the protein to prevent fertilization, San Francisco researchers reported in Nature. The protein, PH-30, is found on the heads of sperm and may help them recognize and fuse with an egg, they said. In an accompanying editorial, a Scottish fertility expert said the lack of the protein also may explain male infertility.

March 21

German physicians added gardening to the many known causes of unilateral mydriasis. They traced a case of blurred vision to the angel's trumpet plant the patient was cutting; the plant, a member of the nightshade family, contains scopolamine, which can cause temporary dilation of the pupils, the investigators reported in The Lancet.

March 25

Indian physicians reported that 74% of 190 salmonella strains isolated from patients in the Bombay area are resistant to chloramphenicol, ampicillin, cotrimoxazole, tetracycline and streptomycin. The organisms are still sensitive to nalidixic acid and the fluoroquinolones, but widespread use increases the possibility of resistance to those drugs as well, they wrote in The Journal of the American Medical Association.

March 30

Levels of air pollution that are allowed by government standards are too high and have resulted in increased mortality from chronic lung disease, pneumonia and heart disease, claimed researchers from the Environmental Protection Agency. Death rates began to climb when particles reached levels as low as one third of the current standard of 150 mcg of particulate pollution per cubic meter of air, the research team noted in the American Review of Respiratory Disease.

APRIL

April 1
Patients can be told that contrary to popular belief, beta-blockers do not appear to cause depression, said Philadelphia geriatric specialists. Failure to consider confounding variables may have resulted in overestimating the link between the widely prescribed drugs and depression, reported the researchers from Presbyterian Medical Center. Their case-control study of 4,302 Medicaid recipients found that depressed patients were about 45% more likely to have taken beta-blockers in the year prior to diagnosis. But after controlling for such variables as benzodiazepine use, frequent outpatient visits and frequent use of other medications, there was no difference in use of beta-blockers between depressed patients and controls, according to The Journal of the American Medical Association report.

April 6
An Australian review of studies of the medicinal use of marijuana concluded that although the drug may relieve nausea, ease pain and enhance relaxation in seriously ill patients, its use should be tempered because of side effects. Marijuana has been used to treat epilepsy, Parkinson's disease, glaucoma and nausea caused by chemotherapy. Among the adverse effects cited in the Medical Journal of Australia: impaired mental function and an increased risk of leukemia in offspring of mothers who smoked just prior to or during pregnancy. Almost half of U.S. oncologists surveyed recently support the use of marijuana for chemotherapy-associated nausea, said the editor of the Australian journal.

April 7
A compound extracted from the leaves of the bitterbrush, Picramnia pentandria, a relative of the geranium, may yield a potent pain reliever, announced a researcher from the company Nova-Screen Inc. The extract of bitterbrush leaves contains compounds capable of blocking receptors for serotonin, dopamine and opium, the researcher told a meeting of the Federation of American Societies of Experimental Biology in Anaheim, Calif.

April 8
A new genetically engineered drug to treat cystic fibrosis was found to be safe in a Phase I study, researchers at the University of Washington in Seattle reported. No patient suffered allergic reactions or developed antibodies to the drug, rhDNase, after inhaling it three times a day for two weeks. Lung function and dyspnea also improved, according to the study in The Journal of the American Medical Association.

April 9
A Chicago investigator told Medical Tribune that the antidepressant fluoxetine (Prozac, Dista) may relieve the pain of chronic headaches. Over 65% of 52 patients with recurrent, severe headaches reported pain reduction after taking fluoxetine for two weeks to a few months, said the neurologist.

April 10
A new laser technique for the inner ear eliminated benign paroxysmal positional vertigo in all 14 patients on whom it was tried, its developer told the American Otological Society meeting. The laser procedure involves partitioning the labyrinth, resulting in the growth of a fibrous band that seals off the affected posterior semicircular canal, thus stabilizing the cupula, said the Fort Worth neurotologist. One patient experienced permanent partial hearing loss. Previous surgery for the condition, which involved severing the posterior ampullary nerve, carried up to a 40% chance of hearing loss.

April 12
Well over a year after receiving transplanted human islet cells, some type I diabetics remain insulin-free or on drastically reduced insulin dosages, announced researchers at the opening of the Joslin Diabetes Clinic at Baptist Hospital in Miami. However, of the more than 60 islet allografts that have been performed within the past two years, most have lasted only a few weeks or a few

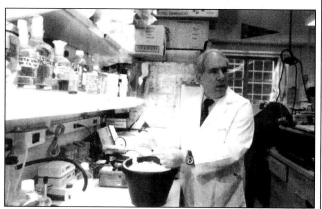

A new, genetically engineered drug to treat cystic fibrosis was found safe in Phase I study. Drug also improved patients' lung function.

months, cautioned researchers at the Joslin Diabetes Center in Boston and at the Diabetes Research Institute of the University of Miami.

April 15
Fish-oil supplements calmed the symptoms of ulcerative colitis and reduced the need for corticosteroids, announced researchers at Jewish Hospital of St. Louis. When 18 patients were given fish oil for four months, they had fewer symptoms and showed improvement on histological examinations compared with the four months when they received a placebo. Presenting the work in the Annals of Internal Medicine, the researchers theorized that fish oil works by blocking the production of leukotriene-B4, an enzyme promoting inflammation. During the fish-oil phase of the trial, leukotriene-B4 levels fell 61%.

April 23
A leading pulmonary expert called for a system of step-care that progresses from a warm bedside manner all the way to quarantine to ensure that tuberculosis patients comply with drug regimens. The specialist from the University of Medicine and Dentistry of New Jersey outlined to Medical Tribune the steps that must be taken to ensure that patients take their medication: First start with good communication; proceed to small payments for taking medicine; then to outreach workers; then, court-ordered outpatient therapy and finally, quarantine.

• • •

A mutation in the gene that regulates insulin secretion was pinpointed as the cause of some cases of type II diabetes. While the mutation on chromosome 7 affects no more than 5% of the estimated 11 million Americans who have this type of diabetes, it was the first time a specific genetic defect was linked to any form of the disease. The finding was reported in Nature by an investigator from the University of Chicago.

MAY

May 5

Daily light therapy was found to be helpful in reducing the incidence of binge-purge episodes in some bulimic individuals. At a meeting in Washington, D.C., of the American Psychiatric Association, University of British Columbia researchers said a half-hour each day in front of 10,000-lux white fluorescent light reduced the episodes by 43%, while exposure to a red light for the same period reduced the episodes by 12%. The therapy may be most helpful to bulimics who experience seasonal variations in their symptoms.

May 6

Doctors attending a meeting of the American Academy of Neurology in San Diego were told that positron emission tomography can spot brain abnormalities several years before the diagnosis of Alzheimer's disease. Researchers from Duke University evaluated 54 Alzheimer's patients three years after a PET scan and found that 28 with worsening symptoms had telltale signs in the temporal and parietal lobes in the original scan.

• • •

A neurologist from the University of California at San Francisco told the American Academy of Neurology meeting that patients who suffer head injuries may develop memory loss or epilepsy if cells in the hippocampus are damaged. The theory was based on experiments on rats with surgically induced concussions. If substantiated, it could lead to the development of drugs that would protect the hippocampus cells in head-injured patients, the researcher said.

• • •

Researchers who surveyed 5,426 doctors reported that physicians have a pattern of prescribing tranquilizers or pain relievers to themselves that could increase their chances of drug abuse or addiction. One of every nine doctors had prescribed his or her own tranquilizers in the past year,

and one in six had self-prescribed pain medicine in the past year without supervision from another doctor, investigators from the University of South Florida in Tampa reported in The Journal of the American Medical Association.

May 7

Many epileptics who take anticonvulsants say they experience a high incidence of side effects, revealed a Roper Organization poll of 500 epileptics. Nearly two out of three people said they experience some side effects from the drugs, while over half of the respondents reported 10 or more adverse effects. Two thirds of those polled complained of memory loss, while

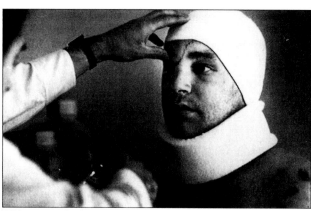

If hippocampal cells are damaged, memory loss or epilepsy may occur.

others reported depression, lethargy, weight gain and cognitive difficulty.

May 8

Physicians who prescribe estrogen to prevent osteoporosis should know that the patient has to stay on it for at least 10 years, an expert told the Advances in Managing Osteoporosis conference in New York. The specialist from Tufts' USDA Human Research Nutrition Center cited new studies showing that patients taken off estrogen after two years lost bone mass at the same rate as those on placebo. An exercise program must also be uninter-

rupted to halt bone deterioration, she said.

May 17

An alarming number of doctors working in large inner-city hospitals may be infected with tuberculosis, a survey by a Chicago physician indicated. She reported at the American Lung Association meeting in Miami that her team surveyed 128 staff physicians at Cook County Hospital and found that 12 of 26 doctors who had previously tested negative to TB on a skin test converted to a positive test. This percentage, 46%, was far higher than the conversion rates of 1% to 14% reported in the medical literature. The study also revealed that internal medicine special-

ists were at especially high risk for TB infection.

May 18

Men with sleep apnea who received continuous positive airway pressure were able to stay more alert on simulated road tests than apnea patients who did not get the treatment, University of Virginia researchers told the American Lung Association meeting.

May 21

Doctors in Los Angeles described to Medical Tribune what their lives were like during the hours that followed the verdict in the Rodney King beating trial.

Some lost everything, including their offices and records, while others worked straight through the riots or stayed in their hospitals because it was too dangerous to leave.

• • •

Hepatitis B vaccinations should be instituted to protect healthcare workers in emergency rooms, recommended the authors of a study in The New England Journal of Medicine.

In a study of 2,523 people who visited the Johns Hopkins Hospital, 5% were found to be seropositive for hepatitis B virus, 18% for hepatitis C virus, and 6% for HIV. Routine screening for HIV alone would identify only a small fraction of the patients with hepatitis B and hepatitis C infections, the researchers pointed out.

May 28

A new test can diagnose tuberculosis in 24 hours or less, compared with the three to 12 weeks needed for conventional tests, pathologists reported at the American Society for Microbiology meeting in New Orleans. In 300 sputum specimens, the new polymerase chain reaction test had a sensitivity of 91% and a specificity of 100%, said an Emory University team. Researchers at the University of Arkansas found that 93% of patients with active TB were PCR positive.

May 29

Diabetes may be prevented if insulin-producing tissue is implanted in the body at birth, suggested an experimental study from the University of Pennsylvania.

Researchers implanted a small volume of insulin-producing cells into the thymus of 18 newborn rats that were bred to be diabetes prone. None developed diabetes during a 210-day observation period, while seven of 14 controls developed the disease between 55 and 121 days of age, according to the report in Science.

Clinical Medicine

June 1

A MRFIT trial found that middle-aged men who drink more than three alcoholic beverages a day may have a significantly reduced incidence of coronary heart disease. A team from the University of Pittsburgh and the NHLBI followed a cohort of 11,688 middle-aged men at high risk for heart disease for seven years and recorded their drinking habits. Men who drank more than 21 alcoholic drinks per week had a death rate of 2.58 per 1,000 person-years, compared with 5.29 for nondrinkers.

June 11

Medicare carriers nationwide were examining randomly selected claims and sending out educational letters to physicians who miscoded claims under the new evaluation and management codes, the Texas Blue Cross/Blue Shield Medicare medical director told Medical Tribune.

Physicians were reportedly learning how to use the new codes, which went into effect on Jan. 1. But many were coding higher than they should be, he said.

As part of the six-month review program, no claims were being downcoded. Instead, physicians were being mailed educational letters to explain Medicare assessment and the reasons for it, he said.

•••

Radiologists at Brigham and Women's Hospital in Boston found that impaired blood flow through affected areas in cocaine users' brains improved when use of the drug was stopped. Previously, researchers had thought the drug permanently reduced the brain's blood flow by constricting blood vessels.

In a small study of 10 drug addicts who were evaluated with high-resolution SPECT and MRI, impaired blood flow increased by 11% after one week without the drug and by 23% after 17 to 29 days, the radiologists told a meeting of the Society of Nuclear Medicine in Los Angeles.

June 13

Diabetics often miss warning signs of hypoglycemia whether they take porcine insulin or human insulin, concluded researchers from New South Wales, Australia. After 50 patients complained that they could not feel the warning signs of hypoglycemia while on human insulin, they were enrolled in a double-blind crossover comparison. At the end of the study, only two patients could tell which insulin they were taking, the team reported in The Lancet. Diabetics failed to detect hypoglycemia 64% of the time when taking human insulin and 69% of the time when taking porcine insulin.

June 14

After receiving reports of 128 operative injuries and six deaths, the New York State Health Department issued an alert regarding the safety of laparoscopic cholecystectomy. The injuries, reported between August 1990 and March 1992, included a perforated aorta and serious injuries to the vena cava, liver, colon and common bile duct. Health department officials urged greater oversight by surgeons employing the popular laparoscopic techniques, now used in 75% of cholecystectomies.

Laparoscopists responded that individual hospitals or regions are able to provide adequate quality control, and the New York alert constitutes no reason to retrench from the use of keyhole surgery on a national basis.

June 20

Patients with chronic obstructive pulmonary disease may not be able to breathe as well after eating a diet high in carbohydrates, researchers at Churchill Hospital in Oxford, England, reported in the British Medical Journal.

Comparing the effects of a carbohydrate-rich drink, a fat-rich drink and artificially sweetened water on 10 COPD patients after a six-minute walk, they found that patients felt more breathless, had greater increases in minute ventilation, oxygen consumption and arterial blood gases, and could not walk as far after consuming the carbohydrate-rich drink.

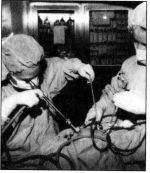

Six New Yorkers died, 128 hurt during keyhole cholecystectomy.

June 22

Harvard researchers announced that vigorous exercise may help prevent diabetes. Of the 22,000 male physicians in the Physicians' Health Study, the risk of non-insulin-dependent diabetes over a five-year period was 42% lower in those who exercised five or more times per week, compared with those who exercised less than once a week. The exercise has to be sufficiently vigorous to produce perspiration, the Boston team told the meeting of the American Diabetes Association in San Antonio, Texas.

•••

University of Wales researchers cautioned that white-water canoeing or rafting may result in gastrointestinal and upper respiratory ills when people inadvertently gulp spume from freshwater streams contaminated with bacteria and viruses.

In a study of 561 people who canoed in white waters, those who had paddled down a stream contaminated with runoff from a sewage treatment plant were twice as likely to develop stomach problems as those who used a purer stream, according to the report in The Lancet.

A scientist at the Centers for Disease Control commented that U.S. rafters are less at risk because most treatment plants in the United States do a good job of treating water.

•••

Blowing up a balloon 40 times a day reduced the breathlessness associated with chronic bronchitis, claimed researchers from Trafford General Hospital in Manchester, England.

Eleven patients who inflated an ordinary balloon 40 times a day for eight weeks had significantly less breathlessness compared with a control group, they reported in the British Medical Journal.

June 26

Two new studies presented at the Endocrine Society meeting in San Antonio revealed that testosterone replacement can improve hormone levels, muscle strength, libido and cognition in elderly men.

Free testosterone increased from 16 pg/ml to 24 pg/ml and total testosterone increased from 530 ng/dl to 683 ng/dl in 60 men aged 60 to 75 who wore scrotal testosterone patches for 16 hours daily, reported a team from the Oregon Health Sciences University in Portland.

Hematocrit, high-density lipoprotein cholesterol, osteocalcin and grip strength improved after three months in nine men aged 69 to 89 who received testosterone injections every two weeks, said physicians from St. Louis University. In addition, testosterone levels increased from 37 ng/dl to 323 ng/dl in these men, while remaining at 33 ng/dl in a control group of seven men, they said.

Clinical Medicine

July 1

A mutation of the gluco-kinase gene is a marker for non-insulin-dependent diabetes mellitus in African-Americans, researchers at Washington University in St. Louis reported in the journal Diabetes. They used polymerase chain reaction to study genetic factors in 112 African-Americans with NIDDM and 173 nondiabetics. The defective glucokinase gene was transmitted in an autosomal dominant manner, and those with the mutation were about three times as likely to have NIDDM, according to the report.

July 10

Bronchoscopy was found to speed diagnosis of pulmonary tuberculosis in patients at risk for HIV infection, a New York team concluded in a retro-spective study. Twenty-one HIV-positive male patients underwent bronchoalveolar lavage and transbronchial biopsy. All patients proved to have Mycobacterium tuberculosis on culture.

Bronchoscopic specimens led to immediate diagnosis of tuberculosis in 48%; TBB was the sole determinant of positivity in 24%.

The results indicate that bronchoscopic specimens, particularly TBB, allow for immediate diagnosis of HIV-related tuberculosis in almost half of infected patients, the researchers reported in the journal Chest.

July 13

Boston University investi-gators reassured the siblings and children of Alzheimer's disease patients that although they are at increased risk to develop the disease, it will likely occur late in life. In an evaluation of the relatives of 198 Dutch Alzheimer's patients, 10% developed the disease by age 65 and 13% by age 75. Overall, the risk to develop Alzheimer's was estimated at 39% by the age of 90, the team told the Third International Conference on

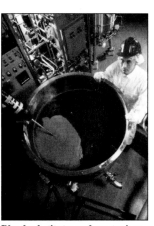

Blood substitute needs no typing or cross-matching, developer says.

Alzheimer's Disease in Pa-dua, Italy.

July 14

Investigators found that tacrine hydrochloride (Cog-nex, Warner-Lambert) produced at least a short-term gain in cognitive function in Alzheimer's patients. At the Third International Confer-ence on Alzheimer's Disease in Padua, Italy, the Warner-Lambert researchers said that more than 50% of 468 patients who received tacrine showed a four-point im-provement on the Alzheim-er's cognitive function scale at 12 weeks. Also, 23% of those treated with tacrine scored an eight-point gain on the cognition scale—the equivalent of avoiding about one year of cognitive decline. Elevations of transaminase resulted in the withdrawal of 25% of the tacrine patients from the study. Side effects such as nausea, vomiting and diarrhea forced another 10% to withdraw from treatment with the cholinergic compound.

July 15

A new blood substitute made from chemically mod-ified hemoglobin entered clinical trials. The substitute can be refrigerated for about a month, stored frozen for up to

a year and used immediately upon thawing, according to its developer, Baxter Healthcare Corporation in Deerfield, Ill. Cellular antigens are removed, eliminating the need for typing and cross-matching, according to the company.

July 17

The Food and Drug Admini-stration approved recombinant interferon alfa-2b (Intron A, Schering) to treat chronic hepa-titis B. The Department of Health and Human Services reported that interferon therapy for four months with 5 million IU per day or 10 million IU three times a week led to a loss of hepatitis B serum markers in about 40% of a study group. Side effects were reported by 21% to 44% of patients and included flulike symptoms.

July 20

A tiny metal implant shaped like a beehive enabled 11 of 16 patients suffering from chronic back pain to give up analge-sics, Israeli scientists reported. Indications for the implant include all those for posterior lumbar interbody fusion, metastatic disease of the spine, segmental instability, degen-erative spondylolisthesis and isolated disc resorption, re-searchers from Tel-Aviv-Sourrasky Medical Center told Medical Tribune. The highly porous implant is held in place by the normal pressure of the

vertebral column and becomes enmeshed with bone cells, fusing with and immobilizing the damaged vertebrae without pins, screws or other fasteners.

July 23

Medical Tribune reported that investigators have begun testing what conceivably could be the first drug to slow the course of amyotrophic lat-eral sclerosis. The new agent, Human Ciliary Neurotrophic Factor (Regeneron Pharma-ceuticals), is a genetically engineered version of a pro-tein found in small quantities in human nerve and muscle cells, the company said.

In preliminary testing of 12 patients injected with the drug over a four-month period, none experienced toxicity, said a researcher at the Cleve-land Clinic, one of four institutions where Phase I trials are under way.

July 24

The voracious Asian tiger mosquito, which entered the United States in 1985, has been found to be carrying eastern equine encephalitis virus, researchers at the Centers for Disease Control reported in Science.

Fourteen strains of EEE turned up in a sample of 9,350 mosquitoes taken from a giant tire dump located west of Disney World. No cases of EEE infection in people have been reported this year, a CDC official said.

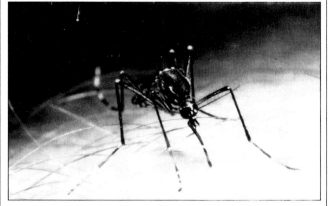

In a tire dump near Walt Disney World in Orlando, eastern equine encephalitis virus was detected in voracious Asian Tiger mosquitoes.

Aug. 1

The only islet-cell recipient to maintain normoglycemia for over two years following surgery was forced to resume insulin injections after her islet cells began to fail. The diabetic woman had received islet-cell implants during surgery to replace a failed kidney in 1990.

Many research groups are pursuing alternative treatments for the disease, including encapsulating islets in hollow acrylic fibers, disguising the cells wih HLA class I antigens and bioengineering the cells. Despite optimism that one of these approaches may work, experts told Medical Tribune that researchers still have a long way to go before a cure is found.

Aug. 5

A Houston company introduced a blood test it says can identify virally caused chronic fatigue immune dysfunction syndrome. The test, developed by Oncore Analytics, measures two enzymes that become elevated when the body fights a viral infection, the company told Medical Tribune. One CFIDS expert said the test is not specific for CFIDS, and could show a positive result for other chronic viral illnesses. But another expert said that while the test is not specific, it is sensitive and therefore useful as part of a CFIDS diagnosis.

Aug. 6

Johns Hopkins researchers reported that the incidence of hepatitis C infection from blood transfusions has decreased significantly since the introduction of improved screening tests.

In 1985, about one in 200 units of blood was infected with hepatitis C virus, they stated in The New England Journal of Medicine. In contrast, after an ELISA that detected HCV antibodies was licensed by the FDA in May 1990, fewer than one in 3,000 units contained the virus.

The researchers warned, however, that the test cannot eliminate the risk of HCV, because HCV antibodies may not develop in humans for three to 12 months, and ELISA would not detect the presence of the virus in such cases.

Aug. 12

University of Utah researchers warned that fluoridation of the water supply to 1 ppm, common in many areas in the U.S., increases the risk of hip

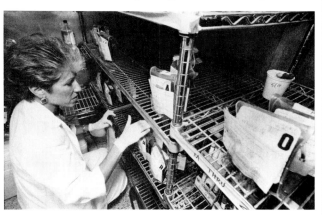

One in 3,000 units of blood must be dumped due to hepatitis C.

fractures in men and women after years of exposure.

The team compared areas in Utah with and without fluoridated drinking water and found the risk of fracture increased about 25% among women and almost 50% among men who had been exposed to the fluoridated supply for about 20 years.

In an editorial accompanying the study in The Journal of the American Medical Association, a physician at the Henry Ford Hospital in Detroit pointed out that some studies showed the opposite results, and no one has established a direct cause-and-effect relationship between fluoride levels and fractures. The FDA considers fluoride levels up to 8 ppm to be acceptable.

Aug. 13

English and French investigators speculated that a missing gene may be responsible for some cases of drug-resistant tuberculosis. Their report, which appeared in Nature, revealed that clinical isolates from patients infected with isoniazid-resistant TB were all missing the same gene, known as the catalase-peroxidase gene. The gene reportedly codes for an enzyme that enables anti-TB drugs to fight the infection. The investigators from London's Hammersmith Hospital and the Institut Pasteur in Paris noted that the genetic link could open the door to a molecular genetics approach to treatment.

Aug. 18

Adding evidence to the theory that a genetic predisposition may trigger the onset of Alzheimer's disease, a study in the American Journal of Psychiatry revealed that patients with a family history of Alzheimer's had a faster course of dementia. Evaluating 462 Alzheimer's patients, a team of psychiatrists from the University of Chicago, University of Miami and University of Wisconsin-Milwaukee found that 76.7% of patients with a familial history of dementia showed a rapid decline in neurological symptoms, compared with 56% among those who did not have a positive family history.

The patients who degenerated rapidly also were more likely to have a family history of psychiatric disorders (18.6% vs 7.2%), as reported by caregivers.

Aug. 20

Strings of antibiotic beads packed around bone show promise in the treatment of compound fractures with soft-tissue injury, orthopedic surgeons reported at a Musculoskeleton Infection Society meeting in Snow Mass, Colorado. The pea-shaped beads directly deliver 20 to 40 times the levels of antibiotics achieved intravenously, and in early trials halved the infection rate in open fractures. The beads surmount the problem of inadequate amounts of drugs reaching the wound because of damaged blood vessels, researchers from the University of Louisville in Kentucky reported. Phase II trials should begin shortly, the investigators predicted.

Aug. 29

University of Hong Kong researchers who studied 155 patients with endoscopically confirmed Helicobacter pylori and duodenal ulcers found that one week of bismuth, tetracycline, metronidazole and omeprazole (Prilosec, Merck Sharp & Dohme) is safe, eradicates H. pylori and reduces the number of recurrences. Seventy-eight subjects received the combination treatment and 77, only omeprazole. H. pylori was eradicated in 70 on the combo therapy, compared with four on omeprazole alone. Ulcers were found in four on the combo treatment and 16 on omeprazole, according to the report in the British Medical Journal.

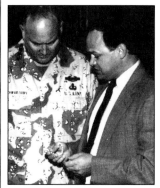

Desert Storm hero examines fracture-healing antibiotic beads.

Sept. 1

Fifty-seven cases of hepatitis A in Montana and Georgia were linked to a single contaminated batch of frozen strawberries packaged in a California processing plant. The infection probably was caused by a migrant field worker infected with the hepatitis A virus who picked the strawberries, Centers for Disease Control epidemiologists reported in the Journal of Infectious Diseases. They noted that contamination of foods with the hepatitis A virus is extremely rare in the United States.

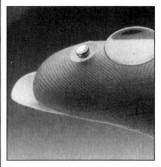

Hearing aid that looks like contact lens may be sound wave of the future.

Sept. 6

San Antonio researchers found that body fat distribution is the best predictor of insulin resistance in obese women, while total body fat is the best indicator of how glucose is metabolized in nonobese women. Past studies have suggested that a central pattern of fat distribution is linked to insulin resistance. But the University of Texas Health Science Center study of 18 obese and 18 nonobese, premenopausal diabetic women found that to be true only for obese women. In nonobese women, there may have been insufficient visceral fat accumulated to exert a major impact on whole-body glucose metabolism, the researchers suggested in the journal Diabetes.

Sept. 9

Diabetics were told that two aspirins a day could significantly reduce their five-year myocardial infarction risk. The recommendation stemmed from a 3,711-patient trial designed to determine if two 325 mg aspirins a day could reduce the rate of diabetic retinopathy. No such benefit was found. However, the researchers noted a 17% reduction in fatal and non-fatal MIs over subjects on placebo. The study, published in The Journal of the American Medical Association, followed the 1988 Physicians' Health Study that found aspirin could reduce a man's first-time MI risk by 44%.

Sept. 14

A futuristic hearing aid touted as a contact lens for the ear was unveiled at the American Academy of Otolaryngology-Head and Neck Surgery meeting in Washington, D.C. The tympanic contact transducer (Earlens), created at the California Ear Institute in Palo Alto, is placed on the surface of the tympanic membrane. An electromagnetic coil and sound processing electronics are placed in the ear canal.

The device was deemed to be stable, comfortable and safe to wear against the eardrum in small preliminary trials, according to the physician who developed Earlens. Hearing quality has yet to be tested.

Sept. 16

St. Louis University researchers told Medical Tribune that a combination of cell injections and electric stimulation may be the best way of healing chronic bone fractures that are resistant to conventional therapy. Under general anesthesia, osteocytes are aspirated from the marrow and centrifuged, then injected into the fracture site. A battery-operated device is worn over the fracture site for up to six months to stimulate bone and speed healing, according to the Missouri team.

Twelve patients with fractures of 1 cm or less have undergone the procedure. While healing time was similar to that with conventional therapy, patients reported less pain and inconvenience, said the researchers.

Sept. 21

Vermont researchers reported that quinine sulfate reduces the frequency, but not the severity, of nocturnal leg cramps. Researchers at the Veterans Affairs Medical Center in White River Junction followed 27 male veterans aged 38 to 73 who experienced at least six leg cramps per month. Subjects received quinine sulfate, vitamin E or placebo for four-week periods separated by four-week washout periods. Thirteen patients had a 50% reduction in the number of leg cramps while taking quinine sulfate compared with placebo, according to the report in the Archives of Internal Medicine. Vitamin E did not reduce cramp frequency. Side effects of the quinine were minor, the study found.

Sept. 24

The role of Helicobacter pylori in duodenal ulcers was shored up by recent studies, but physicians interviewed by Medical Tribune were still divided on whether to treat patients with combination therapy that includes antibiotics. A physician at the Veterans Administration Medical Center in Houston said he had no doubt that the future of ulcer therapy was combination treatment with bismuth, antibiotics and an H_2 receptor antagonist. Other physicians were more cautious, calling for a National Institutes of Health consensus conference or additional studies to confirm H. pylori's role.

Sept. 27

Rep. Joseph Kennedy (D-Mass.) held a public forum and congressional hearing to listen to testimony on a mystery ailment that some Persian Gulf war veterans claimed to be suffering. A spokesperson for the congressman said the office was inundated with calls from veterans from every state but Alaska, who said they too were suffering fatigue, intestinal problems, headaches, joint pain, painful gums or tooth problems, rash or loss of memory.

The hearings were prompted by an Army report released last month on 79 veterans who claimed to be suffering the same ills. The Army report concluded that 80% of the symptoms were related to stress. Occupational health experts told Medical Tribune that reports that the ill vets had been exposed to petroleum-contaminated shower water or noxious fumes from the thousands of burning oil wells would have to be further investigated to determine a cause-and-effect relationship.

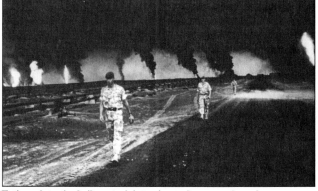

Fatigue, intestinal ailments, joint pains and memory loss plague veterans who returned from the Persian Gulf war.

Clinical Medicine

Oct. 1

British researchers found that adolescent females with insulin-dependent diabetes mellitus are heavier than their nondiabetic counterparts and diet more intensively to control their shape and weight. But they probably are not at increased risk of developing eating disorders, the investigators reported in the journal Diabetes Care.

Researchers from three hospitals in the United Kingdom studied 76 adolescents with IDDM and 76 matched controls. The incidence of eating disorders did not differ from group to group. Five females reduced or omitted their insulin use to control their weight, but only one had other features of an eating disorder, the researchers found.

Oct. 3

A new study in The Lancet added more evidence to support the use of lithotripsy to eliminate gallstones in patients who cannot tolerate surgery. The procedure may work best when the stones are small, reported researchers from Sheffield University in the United Kingdom. Of 163 patients studied, 65 had surgical cholecystectomy and 98 had lithotripsy for large or small stones. After a year, all patients had similar relief of symptoms and improvement in health. Lithotripsy was more expensive, but cost could be lowered if the procedure were given without bile salts on an outpatient basis, the researchers said.

Oct. 5

While car air bags are beginning to prove their worth, researchers said the design of the bags in some cars should be improved and certain safety precautions should be taken. Speaking at the annual meeting of the Association for the Advancement of Automotive Medicine in Portland, Ore., researchers said studies have shown that air bags used with seat belts reduced the death rate in accidents by 23%. To avoid injury from the bags, don't sit too close to the wheel, and wear a seat belt, advised a physician from the University of Louisville School of Medicine. He also suggested placing the hands on the rim of the steering wheel rather than over the hub where the bag is located.

Oct. 8

An Australian team from the Eliza Hall Institute of Medical Research in Victoria hypothesized that certain genes for the production of antibodies may trigger diabetes when stimulated by the release of interleukin-2. Their animal study in Nature concluded that the genes somehow evade

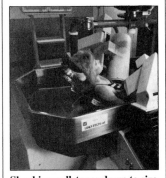

Shocking gallstones down to size spares surgery but costs more.

instruction by the immune system and therefore can't distinguish between their own antigens and those of foreign invaders. While the researchers said the study may help investigators understand the etiology of Type I diabetes, other investigators said that suppressing IL-2 is not the answer to curing diabetes and suggested that the work needs to be replicated in humans.

Oct. 12

A Phase II trial of a recombinant version of the natural protein interleukin-1 found that IL-1 receptor antagonist increased the survival time of patients with septic shock. Synergen Inc. reported the results of the agent, called Antril, at the Interscience Conference on Anti-Microbial Agents and Chemotherapy in Anaheim, Calif. The placebo-controlled study showed that IL-1ra reduced all-cause 28-day mortality in patients with sepsis syndrome. Survival was 56% in patients given placebo, 68% in those given low-dose IL-1ra (17 mg/hr), 75% in those given a mid-dose of 67 mg/hr and 84% in those given a high dose of 133 mg/hr. Phase III trials are under way.

Oct. 15

California researchers said that a nationwide screening program to identify people at risk of giving birth to a child with cystic fibrosis appears to be feasible. A preliminary program, involving about 5,000 pregnant women in California, laid to rest the concern that anxiety would cause people to avoid the tests. The study participants reported no increase in anxiety or stress, even if they were found to be at moderately increased risk of having a child with cystic fibrosis. CF screening can detect 85% of people carrying the gene, the Kaiser Permanente researchers said at the North American Cystic Fibrosis Conference in Washington.

Oct. 20

The California surgeon who tried to save a young woman's life on October 11 by using a pig liver as a "bridge" until a human donor organ could be found said the severe shortage of human organs is making the use of animals a necessity. Leonard Makowka, M.D., of Cedars-Sinai Hospital in Los Angeles, said the 26-year-old woman died of hepatitis-related complications because a human organ could not be located fast enough.

The bridge technique marked the first time a human was implanted with a porcine liver. Dr. Makowka said the case illustrates the severity of the organ-donor crisis.

Oct. 23

Physicians were warned that what may appear to be a case of gastroenteritis may, in fact, be the plague. The Centers for Disease Control said that 11 cases have been reported in the United States so far this year, including the first death from plague in the country since 1987. Four cases have been reported in Arizona, three in New Mexico, and one each in California, Idaho, Nevada and Utah. There were 11 cases in all of 1991; there was only one in 1990.

Most of the recent victims were infected with bubonic plague by a flea bite, and recovered. But one Colorado man was infected with pneumonic plague when he came face-to-face with a sick cat he was trying to rescue. After being prescribed medications for what appeared to be gastroenteritis, he went into shock and was hospitalized. He died 24 hours later.

The best treatment for both types of plague is streptomycin, according to an accompanying editorial in Morbidity and Mortality Weekly Report.

Oct. 29

A new study of the investigational Alzheimer's drug tacrine (Cognex, Warner-Lambert) found that it improved mental functioning, but so slightly that the patients' doctors failed to notice the change. Nonetheless, the head of the National Institute on Aging said that the study proves for the first time that Alzheimer's disease can be altered with drug therapy, and noted that other studies are under way to test whether tacrine might be more effective at higher doses.

As described in The New England Journal of Medicine, 215 patients were given either 40 or 80 mg of tacrine for six weeks, or placebo. Patients taking tacrine had a small, statistically significant improvement on the Mini-Mental State Examination and a smaller decline in activities of daily living than those on placebo.

Clinical Medicine

Nov. 3

Physicians at the American Fertility Society meeting in New Orleans were told that a 10-minute, no-incision, no-sutures vasectomy technique deserves its rising popularity in the United States. In the new procedure, first developed in China and used on more than 11 million men there, the surgeon makes a puncture hole and uses special instruments to clasp the vas deferens and pull it outside the scrotum. Once the tube is exposed, the pro-

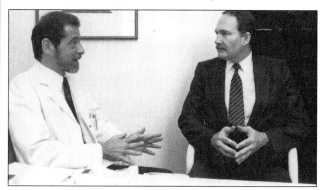

Patient counseled on new 10-minute, no-incision vasectomy technique.

cedure is the same as with a conventional vasectomy. A New York Hospital-Cornell Medical Center surgeon, who in 1986 was in the first group of Americans to learn the no-scalpel technique, reported that in 400 procedures, he has documented rates of bleeding, infection and hematoma one third of those encountered with the traditional approach to vasectomy, which requires a wide incision in the scrotum.

•••

Physicians were cautioned that carbon-monoxide poisoning may be misdiagnosed as a flulike syndrome. The leading cause of death by poisoning in the United States, carbon monoxide is characterized by symptoms—headaches, dizziness and nausea—that may also be confused with viral illnesses, food poisoning, depression and heart problems, a Baylor University researcher said. Physicians should be aware of the potential for mis-diagnosis, as one third of cases of carbon-monoxide poisoning

go undiagnosed, the physician told Medical Tribune. More severe symptoms of the poisoning include visual problems, confusion, seizures and coma, followed by heart failure and death, he noted.

Nov. 5

Drink for drink, the sons of alcoholics may feel less intoxicated than other men, placing them at greater risk for becoming alcoholics them-selves, a Los Angeles research-er reported. The University of Southern Caifornia investigator documented the pattern of reduced sensitivity to low and moderate amounts of alcohol in a meta-analysis of 10 research studies. The finding was striking enough that, in a report published in the American Journal of Psychiatry, the investigator advocated that physicians apprise the biological sons of male alcoholics of the phenomenon.

Nov. 6

The Centers for Disease Control and Prevention re-ported a fivefold rise in the number of diabetics with kidney problems severe enough to require dialysis or transplant. In 1980, 2,220 diabetics were reported to have end-stage renal disease; by 1989, the number had risen to 13,332, according to a study in Mortality and Mor-bidity Weekly Report. The government researchers re-ported that more diabetics are

living long enough to suffer from kidney disease, which can take years to develop. In addition, part of the rise was attributed to an increased availability of treatment and the expansion of Medicare criteria defining transplant or dialysis candidates.

A coauthor of the report advised that diabetics can preserve their kidney function by maintaining both their blood-pressure and blood-sugar levels within normal ranges, treating urinary-tract infections quickly and eating no more than the daily recom-mended allowance for pro-tein—about 56 g for a 150-pound adult.

Nov. 12

Adult children of people with Huntington's disease are likely to be relieved to find out the results of a genetic test that tells them whether they will develop the illness—even if the news is bad, a Canadian study reported. Researchers at the University of British Co-lumbia in Vancouver found that a year after 37 adults learned they had at least a 75% to 100% chance of developing Huntington's disease, they had less depression and a better sense of well-being than 40 others who declined the gene-tic test after counseling or received inconclusive results, leaving them with a 50:50 probability of developing HD.

Researchers carrying out the testing program had anticipa-ted that people might have difficulty coping with an in-creased risk, but were sur-

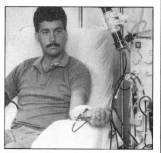

CDC predicts rise in diabetics who need dialysis or transplant.

prised to find that about 10% of the group of 58 who re-ceived good news—that chances were 10% or less that they carried the HD gene—had significant difficulty coping. A major hurdle for them seemed to be the realization that they are facing an unplanned future, the investigators suggested in The New England Journal of Medicine.

•••

Researchers at the Univer-sity of Maryland and the University of Indonesia re-ported that a single-dose, live oral cholera vaccine has been shown to produce a potent immune response, with mini-mal side effects, in more than 3,000 children and adults in worldwide trials.

If immunogenicity is con-firmed in Phase III trials, people in cholera-endemic areas, as well as travelers to high-risk areas, will benefit from the gen-etically engineered vaccine, one of its developers told Medical Tribune. The new vaccine, called CVD 103-HgR, affords at least several years of protection, based on studies of reinfection of wild-type cholera, the Univer-sity of Maryland investigator stated. Trials have indicated it triggers an immune response in around 90% of inoculees.

Nov. 17

The Nebraska Organ Re-trieval System was sued for breach of confidentiality by the family of an organ donor. The system had responded to a court order to provide infor-mation about a young man whose organs became avail-able for transplant after he died of a self-inflicted gunshot wound in 1985. The initial lawsuit was initiated by the family of a North Carolina man who died awaiting an organ transplant; the family charged that financial consi-derations kept their relative from being offered the liver from the Nebraska donor. The organ group stated that it will seek a protective order if sub-poenaed for donor information in the future.

Clinical Medicine

Dec. 1

New ultrasound techniques, including color Doppler, allow doctors to assess the kidneys more effectively, a Rhode Island Hospital researcher announced at the annual meeting of the Radiological Society of North America in Chicago.

Of 32 patients presenting with symptoms of acute renal obstruction, all 10 cases of complete obstruction were correctly diagnosed with ultrasound and kidney, ureter and bladder radiography. However, there was one false positive, as indicated in comparisons with intravenous urography. Eleven of 14 cases of incomplete obstruction were correctly diagnosed, as were seven cases diagnosed as having no obstruction, for an overall accuracy rate of 88%, the Providence research team reported. The techniques allow doctors to avoid the cost and risk of administering intravenous contrast material.

• • •

California researchers affirmed the efficacy of percutaneous methods of gallstone removal at the annual meeting of the Radiological Society of North America.

The investigators used percutaneous biliary drainage followed by fragmentation, dissolution and removal of stones in 23 patients with intrahepatic calculi, 20 with extrahepatic calculi and two with intra- and extrahepatic calculi.

Access to the stones was gained in 98% of patients, fragmentation and dissolution were achieved in 86% and stone retrieval was successful in 93%, a Stanford investigator reported. The new procedures are an important alternative to surgical or endoscopic techniques and increase the chances of successful therapy, the investigator concluded.

Dec. 2

Canadian researchers announced that using elevated prostate-specific antigen levels alone may not provide the best criteria for deciding when prostatic biopsy is warranted. The Toronto research team analyzed the impact of setting different PSA cutoff levels for biopsy in 151 men with both negative digital rectal examination and transrectal ultra-

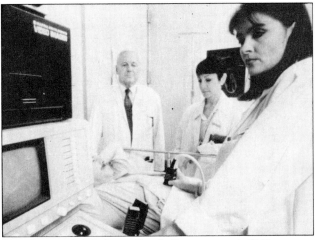

New ultrasound techniques allow better assessment of kidneys.

sound. A cutoff of 4 ng/ml would have resulted in 75 biopsies performed and all 10 cancers detected. A higher cutoff, 10 ng/ml, would have sent only 39 men for biopsy, and four cancers would have been missed, the researchers told the Chicago meeting of the Radiological Society of North America.

The investigators concluded that a formula correlating PSA levels with prostate volume provides the more fruitful approach to biopsy decisions. Applying the formula to these patients would have resulted in 56 biopsies to detect all 10 cancers, the investigators reported.

• • •

Korean researchers claimed that transrectal ultrasound can replace chain cystourethrography in the diagnosis of urinary stress incontinence. The Seoul investigators performed transrectal ultrasound on 10 control subjects and on 58 patients with urinary stress incontinence, evaluating the bladder base at rest and on maximal straining while the patient was in the left decubitus position with the hips flexed. The Yonsei University team told the Radiological Society of North America meeting that they tested several diagnostic criteria: a posterior urethrovesical angle greater than 149.6 degrees was 79% sensitive and 80% specific; a drop of bladder neck greater than 1.02 cm was 97% sensitive, but only 70% specific; and an opening of the bladder neck greater than 0.14 cm proved 83% sensitive and 90% specific.

Dec. 9

The American Society of Internal Medicine asked for a variety of legislative actions to boost public investment in primary care. In testimony before the Physician Payment Review Commission, the ASIM reiterated its support for the resource-based relative value scale (RBRVS) for Medicare payments, but asked that Congress block the higher surgical fee schedule update for 1992.

Unless it mandates a single volume performance standard, the government is contradicting the RBRVS' premise of equal pay for equal work, regardless of medical specialty, the ASIM stated. In lieu of a single standard, the ASIM requested that a separate and higher update floor be established for primary care.

To encourage young physicians to enter primary care, the ASIM asked for a variety of incentives, including low-interest loans, loan forgiveness, tax benefits and measures to alleviate the administrative burdens imposed on primary-care physicians.

Dec. 10

Physicians were told that breast-cancer patients' depression may be due not to their diagnosis or surgery, but to treatment with tamoxifen (Nolvadex, ICI Pharma). Doctors at Baylor University Medical Center in Dallas followed patients receiving adjuvant therapy for node-negative breast cancer.

Of 155 patients who had been receiving tamoxifen for three to six months, 15% reported symptoms of depression, compared with 3% of 102 who received no treatment or underwent chemotherapy without tamoxifen, the researchers reported at the

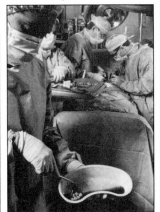

Percutaneous methods provide alternative to gallstone surgery.

15th Annual San Antonio Breast Cancer Symposium.

They concluded that depression is a more common side effect of tamoxifen therapy than was previously recognized, and advised physicians to thoroughly evaluate this possibility in patients receiving tamoxifen either as adjuvant therapy or in chemoprevention trials.

If one sumatriptan shot fails, try a second

FEB. 15—One third to one half of migraine sufferers who use an investigational injectable drug experience relief only to have the headache recur within 24 hours. But a second dose of the drug, sumatriptan, within 24 hours may prevent recurring headaches, Swedish migraine experts reported in The Lancet.

The researchers from the Gothenburg Migraine Clinic in Gothenburg, Sweden, found that 26 of 48 migraine sufferers who gave themselves one sumatriptan shot when they had a migraine had another headache an average of 13 hours later. Sometimes the second headache was worse than the first, the researchers reported.

When the 26 patients who had suffered recurrent headaches gave themselves two shots within 24 hours of a migraine, one sufferer had an additional headache, the researchers said.

A spokesperson for Glaxo Pharmaceuticals said about 35% of people in a company-sponsored study had another headache within 24 hours of the first shot.

An estimated eight million Americans suffer migraines, a majority of them young to middle-aged women.

A study published last year in The Journal of the American Medical Association found that injected sumatriptan reduced moderate or severe headache pain to mild or no pain in 70% of patients, and completely relieved the pain in half the study patients within an hour.

Seymour Solomon, M.D., director of the Headache Unit at Montefiore Medical Center in New York, said he and other researchers are treating migraine patients with oral sumatriptan in clinical trials.

Dr. Solomon is attempting to treat the recurring headache by using an initial injection of the drug followed by an oral dose when the second headache first begins. The oral dose being tested is 100 mg, compared with the 6-mg injectable dose.

Dr. Solomon explained that sumatriptan is eliminated from the blood quickly. Since migraines can last as long as 72 hours, long after the medication has been eliminated, some sufferers may require a second dose.

Interest in sumatriptan is high because it works quickly to relieve the pain, nausea and vomiting associated with migraines.

Rick Sluder, corporate communications manager for Glaxo, said some studies have reported that patients got relief from symptoms within 10 minutes of injection.

Sluder said that one Glaxo-sponsored study of 1,100 patients who received the drug found that 70% were pain-free after administration, but 35% of those patients reported recurrence of pain within 24 hours.

Sumatriptan is approved for use in Italy, the Netherlands, New Zealand, Portugal, Sweden and the United Kingdom. Glaxo applied to the U.S. Food and Drug Administration for approval of the injectable drug in June 1990 and for approval of tablets that December.

In October 1991, an FDA advisory panel recommended approval of the injectable form of the drug, but the FDA has yet to act. If approved in the United States, the drug would be marketed under the name Imitrex.

Steroid slows alcoholic hepatitis, raises survival

CLICHY, FRANCE, FEB. 20—Corticosteroid therapy is an effective treatment for patients with severe alcoholic hepatitis, according to French researchers.

Almost 90% of 32 patients who received a month-long prednisolone regimen were alive two months later, compared with about 46% of patients who received a placebo.

Bernard Rueff, M.D., of the alcoholic treatment center at the Beaujon Hospital here, reported the results of his study in The New England Journal of Medicine.

Conventional management of alcoholics with hepatitis includes forbidding alcohol, correcting dietary deficiencies and often hospitalization, he said.

But mortality, even in the hospital, is as high as 65%, according to Dr. Rueff.

The French study confirms the results of others that have found the steroid can help alcoholics with the liver disease, according to Charles Lieber, M.D., chief of the alcohol research and treatment center at the Bronx Veterans Affairs Medical Center in New York. "The study is helpful in that it identifies which patients should receive the treatment," he said.

"By using a liver biopsy and blood tests they have identified the very ill subgroup that could benefit," added Dr. Lieber.

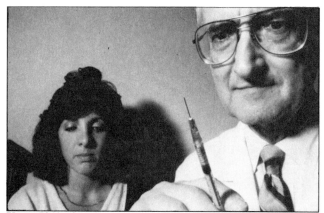

Up to 50% of patients may need second dose within 24 hours.

The French researchers studied 65 patients who had a discriminant function value above 32, spontaneous hepatic encephalopathy or both, reported Dr. Rueff.

"The discriminant function, which identified 57 of our 61 patients as having severe disease, appears to be a better index of severity than the presence of hepatic encephalopathy," wrote Dr. Rueff.

Researchers are not sure why corticosteroids have a beneficial effect on alcoholic hepatitis, according to the French investigator. "Corticosteroids stimulate the appetite, increase the production of albumin, and inhibit the production of collagen Types I and II," he wrote. In addition, they "decrease cytokine production, which may also play a part in the pathogenesis of alcoholic hepatitis," he added.

The prednisolone therapy had no serious side effects, according to the French team. "Infection and gastrointestinal bleeding were more common in placebo recipients than in corticosteroid recipients," Dr. Rueff said.

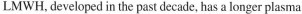

Self-administered heparin may control deep-vein thrombosis, eliminate need for hospitalization

By Luba Vikhanski

FEB. 22—Patients with deep-vein leg thrombosis may be able to self-administer injections of a new version of heparin at home, eliminating the need for hospitalization.

Italian researchers have found that a low-molecular-weight heparin (LMWH), administered subcutaneously every 12 hours, was as effective as standard heparin administered in a continuous intravenous infusion. Unlike the standard drug, LMWH was given without regular laboratory monitoring.

As part of the study, 85 symptomatic patients with proximal deep-venous thrombosis received standard heparin and 85 received LMWH for 10 days.

Oral coumarin was started on day 7 and continued for at least three months. The frequency of recurrent venous thromboembolism did not differ significantly between the two groups, according to Paolo Prandoni, M.D., of University Hospital of Padua, Italy, lead author of the study. Clinically important bleeding was infrequent in both groups, he reported in The Lancet.

"Anticoagulation is the treatment of choice for leg-vein thrombosis to prevent death from pulmonary embolism and to reduce morbidity from the acute event," he wrote. Heparin usually is administered by continuous intravenous drip, and the dose is adjusted on the basis of laboratory measurements.

LMWH, developed in the past decade, has a longer plasma

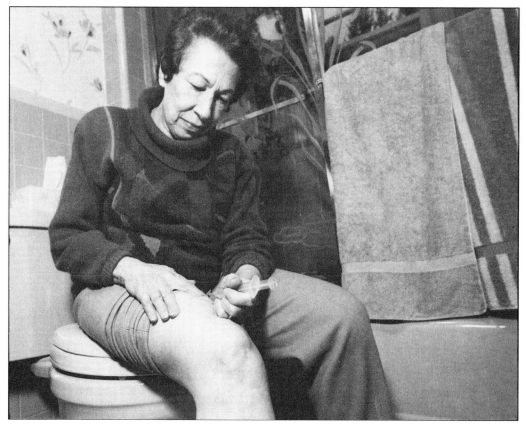

Self-injections of new heparin may control deep-vein leg thrombosis.

half-life, less variability in the anticoagulant response to fixed doses and a more favorable ratio of antithrombotic benefit to hemorrhagic risk, Dr. Prandoni said.

The study has confirmed these properties, suggesting that patients may be able to inject themselves with LMWH at home, avoiding hospitalization altogether.

"If [our] findings are confirmed, the treatment of venous thrombosis will be greatly simplified and much cheaper," he said.

LMWH has not been approved for use in the United States.

Even if the drug is approved, it may take several more years before patients will be treated at home rather than in the hospital, said Candice Kottke-Marchant, M.D., director of the coagulation laboratory at the Cleveland Clinic Foundation.

"Many studies will have to be conducted for the treatment of patients to change so drastically," she said.

The exact incidence of venous thrombosis is difficult to estimate because its signs and symptoms may be mistaken for other disorders, but the thrombosis is probably more common than generally believed, according to Dr. Kottke-Marchant.

Double thyroid trouble for Bushes 'coincidental'

MARCH 15—The double dose of thyroid trouble in the White House probably was a coincidence, not the result of some environmental factor or bacteria affecting both President and Mrs. Bush, according to a recent paper by a thyroid expert.

When the Bushes both were diagnosed with Graves' disease, physicians searched for an environmental factor, such as drinking water, but found no evidence of a cause for the disease, said Lewis Braverman, M.D., of the University of Massachusetts.

Dr. Braverman and colleagues published a report in the Annals of Internal Medicine describing a family he has treated since the 1960s in which the parents and two children have Graves' disease.

"We estimated that there could be anywhere from 20 to 1,500 couples with Graves' disease in the United States, but that's strictly an estimate and maybe a wild guess," Dr. Braverman said in an interview.

Conjugal Graves' disease "may represent the chance occurrence of this relatively common disorder in married couples," he wrote in his paper.

"I doubt that we will ever establish either an environmental or bacterial trigger for Graves'," he said. "I think it might be triggered by stress, but it would be very difficult to establish that link."

Some reports have implicated stressful events, which may facilitate expression of the disease in genetically susceptible people, possibly by disrupting the immune system, Dr. Braverman said.

"I don't think that there is any reason to screen a spouse for the condition when one member of the couple is diagnosed, but I do believe that children should be screened when a parent has Graves'," he said.

He encouraged physicians to report conjugal cases of the disorder so that insights can be gained into the relation between genetic and environmental factors in the etiology of Graves'. In his report on the family with Graves', Dr. Braverman said he diagnosed the disease in the wife in 1967, the husband in 1968, a daughter in 1971 and a son in 1972. In addition, two other daughters were diagnosed with thyroid problems, one with a nontoxic goiter in 1970 and another with Hashimoto's thyroiditis in 1976. Dr. Braverman said the children's thyroid problems are genetic.

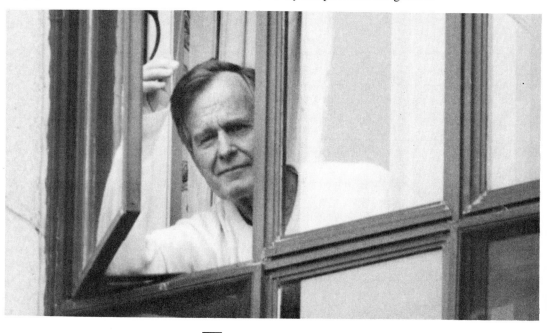

The Bushes' thyroid problems were not caused by environmental toxins or bacteria, according to an Annals report.

He had not considered publishing his case reports on the couple and their children until after he was contacted by a journalist who was writing an article about the First Family's condition.

"I was called by Larry Altman of The New York Times and asked about Graves' disease, and that's when I thought about this couple," he explained. Dr. Altman, who is a physician as well as a journalist, is a coauthor of the article.

Enzyme eases breathing in cystic fibrosis crises

By Marjorie Shaffer

MARCH 19—Cystic fibrosis patients experienced significant improvements in lung function while taking a new genetically engineered drug, a study has found.

The aerosolized drug, recombinant human deoxyribonuclease I, or rhDNase, improved forced vital capacity (FVC) by 10% to 20% among 16 cystic fibrosis patients, according to Ronald Crystal, M.D., of the National Heart, Lung and Blood Institute in Bethesda, Md.

This improvement is comparable to that seen after hospitalization and systemic antibiotic therapy for exacerbation of respiratory infection in CF patients, he wrote in The New England Journal of Medicine.

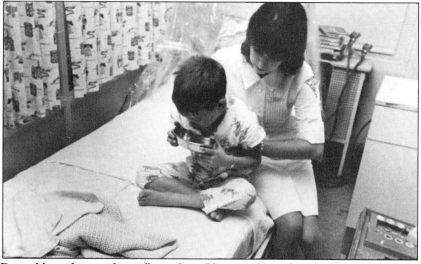

Recombinant human deoxyribonuclease I improved lung function by 10% to 20%.

"The drug offers a promising new strategy to help patients deal with their disease," said Dr. Crystal in an interview. "Theoretically the drug might decrease infection or even increase longevity."

Studies are under way in children and adults at more than 40 centers in the United States, according to Genentech, the drug's manufacturer.

Results are expected by the end of 1992. The company hopes to submit an application for marketing approval by 1993, a spokesperson said.

In Dr. Crystal's study, patients with airflow limitation due to purulent airway secretions received the drug or a placebo for six days, followed by a two- to three-week break from treatment. Study participants then switched therapies.

In addition to the objective improvements in airflow, 11 of the 16 patients commented that rhDNase inhalations noticeably improved their breathing ability.

No significant adverse effects were attributable to the drug, Dr. Crystal reported.

High concentrations of DNA in the airway secretions of CF patients contributes to the "tenacious and viscous" nature of the mucus, making it difficult to expectorate, Dr. Crystal said. The DNA is believed to come from the breakdown of inflammatory cells.

The drug is a genetically engineered version of the human enzyme DNase. In vitro, rhDNase cleaves DNA in sputum from patients with cystic fibrosis and reduces sputum viscosity.

In the study, patients' total volume of sputum was not significantly different with rhDNase and placebo, which

suggests that "simply increasing the volume of sputum cleared does not in itself improve lung function," Dr. Crystal wrote. The drug may enhance removal of small amounts of purulent mucus from critical sites in the lung, he hypothesized.

Study identifies no link between depression and beta-blockers

APRIL 1—Contrary to previous reports, beta-blockers do not appear to cause depression in patients, a new study has shown.

Failure to consider confounding variables may have resulted in overestimating the link between beta-blockers and depression in other studies, according to a report in The Journal of the American Medical Association.

In a case-control study of Medicaid recipients in New Jersey, the medical records of 4,302 persons diagnosed with depression were compared with controls matched for age, sex, race and nursing-home residency status.

The depressed patients were about 45% more likely to have taken beta-blockers in the year prior to diagnosis, consistent with results of a previous epidemiologic study by the same investigator, Daniel Everitt, M.D., a geriatric medicine specialist at the Presbyterian Medical Center in Philadelphia.

In all, 14% of the depressed patients and 10% of the controls had received beta-blockers during the year.

However, after controlling for confounding variables (including benzodiazepine use, frequent outpatient visits and frequent use of medications other than beta-blockers), there was no difference in use of beta-blockers between depressed patients and control patients.

"This study makes me less worried about depression when I select an antihypertensive," said Dr. Everitt. "However, I still have to consider it. There are good reports of patients who became depressed on beta-blockers and improved when the drugs were removed," he said.

The study design did not identify patients who received beta-blockers for a short period of time, and depression may have been one reason the medication was withdrawn, explained Dr. Everitt.

In case reports, onset of depression occurs two weeks to a year following onset of beta-blocker treatment.

The JAMA study weakens the link between beta-blockers and depression but does not completely rule it out, according to Stuart C. Yudofsky, M.D., chief of psychiatry at Baylor College of Medicine in Houston, Tex.

There still is circumstantial evidence supporting the link in 1% to 2% of people taking beta-blockers, said Dr. Yudofsky, who wrote an accompanying editorial.

In a depressed patient who is being treated for hypertension, captopril (Capoten and Capozide, Squibb) may provide an alternative to propranolol, suggested Dr. Yudofsky. He also suggested that when a beta-blocker is indicated, more hydrophilic compounds, such as atenolol (Tenoretic and Tenormin, ICI Pharma) and nadolol (Corgard and Corzide, Bristol Laboratories), may be less likely to cause depression and other central-nervous-system side effects. Compared with propranolol, these beta-blockers achieve lower concentrations in spinal fluid and brain tissue.

Step-care system for tuberculosis is proposed

By Bill Ingram

APRIL 23—Reacting to Congressional testimony that heroic efforts are needed now lest multidrug-resistant (MDR) tuberculosis reach epidemic proportions, a leading pulmonary authority called for a system of step-care that progresses from warmth and a bedside manner all the way to quarantine to ensure that patients comply with drug regimens.

"The technology exists to establish step-care now—the steps to make sure that every patient takes his or her medicine—and you either do it now or it will be much more costly later,"said H. Lee Reichman, M.D., of the University of Medicine and Dentistry of New Jersey.

"It starts as it would with the best private care—pouring a cup of coffee for them and asking how life is going. Maybe providing breakfast.

"If that doesn't work, suppose you pay $20, even $40 for the outpatient to take medicine? That's much cheaper than [multiple] hospitalization and infection of other patients and the spread of resistant strains.

"The next step is [outreach workers vouchsafing that the patient takes medicine at home, then] court-ordered outpatient treatment, and finally, restriction of freedom."

Agreeing with the proposal, TB clinicians in Miami and Chicago noted that they are already trying to follow a modified step-care model.

Joan Otten, director of the TB service at Miami's Jackson Memorial Hospital, reported that the use of such a model has reduced MDR cases, from 45 in 1990 to seven last year. There have been no cases since October.

In New York City, a spokesperson for the health department said steps such as encouragement and enticement "are in place." However, doctors in city TB clinics charged, anonymously, that step-care is not in place and that the

recommended six-month duration of TB treatment is seldom observed.

At Chicago's Cook County Hospital's TB service, which is trying to establish TB step-care, the rate of TB resistant at least to isoniazid and rifampin "is perhaps 1%," said Rebecca Wurtz, M.D. The MDR rate in New York City is 7%, said Thomas Frieden, M.D., of the Centers for Disease Control in Atlanta.

The overall drug resistance rate is 34%.

New York City has yet to take court action in this era to mandate TB treatment. In Miami, in the past year, "six or seven" noncompliant outpatients have been court-committed to the A.G. Holley Hospital in Lantana, said Otten.

Funded with federal money as a demonstration project, she said, the Jackson Memorial TB service has enlisted outreach workers and a public health adviser "to identify all MDR patients, follow up on all contacts and make sure they are compliant."

This ranges from phone reminders to home checks on no-shows to supervised drug administration at patients' homes. "We have done it without monetary incentives," she said.

New York City has had little federal funding for outreach programs. Last year, the city requested $15 million in federal funds and received $600,000.

"You do require funds to put step-care in place," said Dr. Reichman, president-elect of the American Lung Association.

William L. Roper, M.D., director of CDC, stated that the government would hire more outreach workers for compliance monitoring in 1992.

Dr. Reichman proposed the progressive compliance system in response to a warning issued by Allan Bloch, M.D., of the CDC at a hearing of the House Human Resources and Intergovernmental Relations Subcommittee early this month.

"Without immediate and massive efforts to address the

threat of [MDR] tuberculosis, this country faces the possibility of an epidemic of TB that is resistant to all available treatments.

"What is needed," said Dr. Bloch, "is a concerted effort to track down every case of TB, isolate all patients until they are no longer infectious and ensure compliance by directly observing drug administration."

Outbreaks of MDR TB were reported last year in three New York hospitals. Eight healthcare workers were found to have active TB. MDR strains were also isolated in the deaths of 13 prison inmates and one prison guard.

Nationwide, cases rose 9.4% last year to 25,701. The rate in children rose 39% between 1987 and 1990, when cases totaled 950.

The CDC has announced that limited quantities of streptomycin and para-aminosalicylic acid will be procured from Canada to help treat resistant cases. Production of both drugs had been halted in recent months.

Sustained estrogen suggested for osteoporosis

By Naomi Pfeiffer

MAY 8—Doctors who prescribe estrogen to prevent osteoporosis should know that the patient has to stay on it for at least 10 years, according to an osteoporosis expert from Tufts University in Boston.

Bess Dawson-Hughes, M.D., chief of the calcium and bone metabolism laboratory at Tufts' USDA Human Research Nutrition Center, cited new studies showing that patients taken off estrogen after two years lost bone mass at the same rate as those on placebo.

"Estrogen works only as long as it's taken," Dr. Dawson-Hughes said.

"When the placebo patients were put on estrogen, their bone loss stopped," she told a large Medical Grand Rounds audience at Memorial Sloan-Kettering Cancer Center, as part of a talk on "Advances in Managing Osteoporosis."

Similarly, an exercise regime must be uninterrupted to halt bone deterioration, she said.

An ongoing Tufts study of healthy postmenopausal women who exercised upright for an hour three times a week for a year revealed that their lumbar spine density increased by 5%, compared with a 2% decrease in sedentary controls.

"But when the women returned a year later for bone density measurements, those who stopped exercising had lost all the bone they had previously gained," Dr. Dawson-Hughes said.

Contrary to common belief, supplemental calcium is not always beneficial, because the rapid estrogen withdrawal overrides any impact of calcium, she said. "It just doesn't work during the first five years of menopause when an average woman loses half the total bone she will lose in her lifetime."

Later, women without osteoporosis should take 800-1,000 mg/day of calcium—i.e., their normal calcium intake plus supplements—while those with osteoporosis should take 1,400-1,500 mg/day, she said.

Supplementary vitamin D helps prevent bone loss in winter when women in northern latitudes are particularly vulnerable, Dr. Dawson-Hughes said, referring to a recent Swedish study of 250 people, half of whom took 400 units of vitamin D plus calcium supplements, while the rest took calcium alone.

"Both groups had an increase of 1.4% bone density in summer, but in the winter, those on calcium alone lost their gain," she said.

She prescribes 400-500 units of vitamin D all year to postmenopausal women, unless future vitamin D studies suggest otherwise.

And she discourages use of steroids, which cause severe bone loss by at least five different mechanisms, including increased urinary calcium excretion.

"When you know your patient is going on steroids—as part of chemotherapy, for example—have all your bone protection treatments in place. Don't wait until the fractures start," she said.

Since sodium further accelerates bone loss, physicians should always minimize sodium intake in patients going on steroids, Dr. Dawson-Hughes said.

Unfortunately, no treatment available today will stimulate bone regrowth, she said.

"We had high hopes for slow-release sodium fluoride, but it grew bone that was not fracture-resistant—so our hopes were dashed."

The dashed hopes actually were due to a misinterpreted study from the Mayo Clinic, said Joseph Zerwekh, Ph.D., of the University of Texas Southestern Medical Center, a co-investigator in the 1991 fluoride study showing new bone in 13 patients with osteoporosis.

"The Mayo study used a different type and dosage of fluoride, different kinds of patients and a different calcium supplementation," Dr. Zerwekh said.

He urged physicians to watch for the results of his team's larger controlled study, to be presented next year at the International Osteoporosis Society meeting in Hong Kong.

"Tamoxifen [Nolvadex, ICI Pharma] may be the answer in some cases of osteoporosis," said Dr. Dawson-Hughes. "The bone reads this drug as if it were estrogen."

But Lawrence Riggs, M.D., of the Mayo Clinic, is not enthusiatic about tamoxifen.

"Better drugs should be developed, perhaps from the same family," Dr. Riggs said. "While tamoxifen seems to offer weak protection against osteoporosis, there are too many side effects."

Calcitonin is one FDA-approved option for bone-sparing, but it must be injected three to seven times a week, Dr. Dawson-Hughes said. "It's inconvenient and expensive."

In some countries, calcitonin is delivered via nasal spray,

said Robert Heaney, M.D., of Creighton University's osteoporosis center in Omaha, Nebraska. "Two U.S. pharmaceutical companies will soon submit INDs for a nasal spray here," Dr. Heaney said.

A new vitamin D derivative, calcitriol, as well as other vitamin D compounds, are used widely for osteoporosis in Japan, "where they don't use female hormones at all," Dr. Heaney said. Calcitriol is approved in New Zealand and Australia. "Calcitriol is one of nature's most potent hormones and we don't know enough about it."

Dr. Dawson-Hughes said she was "skittish" about using the compound.

Hospital staffs' risk of tuberculosis may be high

MAY 17—An alarming number of physicians working in large inner-city hospitals are infected with tuberculosis, a new study suggests.

Hospitals serving large urban areas hit by the steep rise in tuberculosis cases need to implement more stringent TB control programs, said Linda Cocchiarella, M.D., a Chicago physician who led the new study.

The findings were released at the 1992 International Conference of the American Lung Association in Miami.

Dr. Cocchiarella and colleagues surveyed 128 staff physicians at Cook County Hospital in Chicago, a large urban hospital that treats mainly poor patients.

Twelve of 26 physicians who had previously tested negative to tuberculosis on a skin test converted to a positive test. None of the doctors who tested positive developed active tuberculosis, but many were no longer with the hospital and could not be examined, according to Dr. Cocchiarella.

The percentage of physicians who had converted to a positive test, 46%, was far higher than conversion rates of 1% to 14% reported in the medical literature, she said.

The study showed that physicians specializing in internal medicine were at especially high risk for TB infection, she said.

All healthcare workers are supposed to get periodic TB skin tests, but many neglect to take the test, Dr. Cocchiarella said.

The number of TB cases in the United States jumped nearly 16% from 1985 to 1990, fueled by poverty, homelessness and the AIDS epidemic. Last year, 26,283 people were reported to the Centers for Disease Control with full-blown TB, a jump of 9% from 1989. An estimated 10 million Americans are infected.

In the wake of the new epidemic, inner-city hospitals supported by public funds were unable to cope with the large number of TB cases and lack money for control programs. "Certainly the public hospitals are likely to be the most heavily impacted and are least prepared because of resource restraints," according to Dixie Snider, M.D., director of the TB division at the CDC.

There are no national statistics on the number of healthcare workers who were infected with TB on the job.

The American Hospital Association recommends that all hospitals identify TB-infected patients quickly and have appropriate isolation rooms available.

Federal health officials also recommend that doctors caring for TB patients wear airtight masks to filter out the bacteria causing TB, but there is some controversy over the masks' effectiveness, said Dr. Snider.

The TB specialist said that ultraviolet lamps, which kill the bacteria, also may help reduce the transmission of TB in hospitals.

L.A. riots placed MDs in the path of violence

MAY 21—As rioters in Los Angeles tore through the city after the Rodney King beating trial verdict, Gerald Fradkoff, M.D., watched on television as his second-floor office burned to the ground.

"The next morning, all that was left was ashes," Dr. Fradkoff said.

Gone too was six months' worth of Medi-Cal billing information needed for reimbursement. Because Dr. Fradkoff treated mostly poor patients, Medi-Cal, California's version of Medicaid, was his primary source of income.

"I've lost everything. My clinic, all my records, my capital. But I'm alive."

The only reminder of the riots at California Medical Center is the National Guard members who still come there for minor injuries they sustained on patrol. During the siege, staff there and at other area hospitals worked around the clock treating the thousands of injured.

Alan Heilpern, M.D., medical director of the hospital's emergency department, worked for two days straight. The hospital ran short of antibiotics and other supplies, and the pharmacy director had to drive to a sister hospital for more because suppliers refused to deliver.

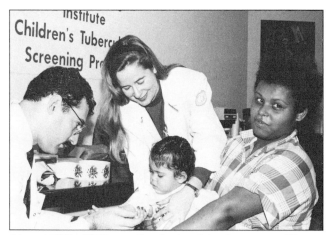

Almost 50% of TB-negative doctors later became positive.

Clinical Medicine

"It was a zoo," Dr. Heilpern said. "We squeezed extra beds into rooms. The hallways had people on gurneys on either side. We had some people in the driveway, waiting to get in."

Some hospitals called in all their staff, providing beds and food between shifts because in some cases it was too dangerous to leave the hospital, he said.

Bob Calverley, a spokesperson for the Los Angeles County Medical Society, said he had heard of only two or three physicians' offices being damaged during the rioting.

Hospitals, physicians and other health personnel now are resuming their normal routine. But for at least one institution, a specter still remains.

"This could scare away doctors," said Arthur Schapiro, M.D., vice president for medical affairs at Daniel Freeman Memorial Hospital.

"We're in the process of recruiting a neurosurgeon. This could make some very good candidate less willing to come here," he said.

Alcohol may protect heart, but heavy drinking poses overall health hazard, says MRFIT team

By Saralie Faivelson

JUNE 1—Middle-aged men who drink more than three alcoholic beverages a day may have a significantly reduced incidence of coronary heart disease, according to the Multiple Risk Factor Intervention Trial Research Group.

Increased alcohol consumption is associated with rising high-density lipoprotein cholesterol levels, reported Lewis H. Kuller, M.D., of the University of Pittsburgh School of Public Health in the Annals of Internal Medicine.

Dr. Kuller and colleagues at the National Heart, Lung and Blood Institute followed a cohort of 11,688 middle-aged men at high risk of heart disease for seven years and recorded their alcohol habits.

Men who drank more than 21 alcoholic drinks per week had a rate of death of 2.58 per 1,000 person-years, compared with 5.29 for nondrinkers.

Although it appears that moderate drinking can protect the heart without any ill effects, heavy drinking may increase the risk of car accidents or homicides, said Dr. Kuller.

"Our study excluded anybody with a drinking problem, or someone out of work or in jail because of drinking," he said. "It would be difficult to measure the adverse effects of alcohol based on this study."

In addition, as a recent British study has shown, men who drink heavily face an increased risk of sudden death.

The British Heart Foundation followed 7,000 middle-aged men and found that those who drank heavily and steadily, and those who drank between 13 and 27 cans of beer at one time were more likely to suffer sudden cardiac death.

"Sudden cardiac death after drinking large amounts of alcohol can happen to anybody," said Eric Rimm of the Harvard School of Public Health.

"Some of these people were perfectly healthy. It can happen to you or to me," he added.

Heavy drinking in the British study was defined as three or more pints of beer a day, six mixed drinks or six glasses of wine. Three pints of beer is equal to four cans of beer.

Previous studies, including a Swedish-German study of over 44,000 men, have added further weight to the theory that moderate amounts of alcohol protect men against heart disease.

Dr. Kuller and colleagues pointed out, however, that although these protective effects have been noted, "a public health policy to encourage nondrinkers to consume alcohol or occasional drinkers to increase alcohol consumption cannot be recommended, because of the known manifold adverse consequences of excess alcohol use."

Exercising to a sweat may help avert diabetes

By Luba Vikhanski

JUNE 22—Vigorous exercise, which is known to reduce the risk of heart disease, may also help prevent diabetes, according to researchers at Harvard University.

Of the 22,000 male physicians in the Physicians' Health Study, the risk of non-insulin-dependent diabetes mellitus (NIDDM) over a five-year period was 42% lower in those who exercised five or more times a week, compared with those who exercised less than once a week. The exercise had to be sufficiently vigorous to produce sweat, according to the Boston investigators.

But even breaking a sweat once a week, regularly, reduced the risk 23%; 38% for two to four times a week.

"Our results suggest that [late-onset] diabetes can now be added to the list of conditions that can be prevented or ameliorated by physical activity," said JoAnn Manson, M.D., assistant professor of medicine at Harvard Medical School.

The findings, presented at the American Diabetes Association annual meeting in San Antonio, Tex., were consistent with those of two other large prospective studies on exercise and diabetes that were published in 1991, Dr. Manson said.

The researchers say exercise may be the only practical way of preventing NIDDM since obesity, a dominant risk factor for the disease, is notoriously difficult to control.

Results in the physician group were unrelated to weight fluctuations.

In fact, overweight men who exercised at least once a week

had a diabetes risk 40% lower than those who exercised less than once a week.

"Thus men at greatest risk of diabetes were the ones who derived the greatest benefit," said David Nathan, M.D., of Harvard University, who is a coauthor of the study.

NIDDM is estimated to affect between 11 and 15 million Americans.

According to Dr. Manson, exercise may reduce the risk of diabetes through loss of fat tissue and by increasing the cells' sensitivity to insulin.

John Holloszy, M.D., from the Washington University School of Medicine in St. Louis, Mo., noted that in the early stages, NIDDM associated with abdominal obesity and insulin resistance may be reversed by exercise or a low-calorie diet.

But once a person becomes completely insulin-deficient, those measures are no longer effective, according to Dr. Holloszy.

He addressed a special session on exercise and obesity at the ADA meeting.

Tacrine shows promise in Alzheimer's patients

PADUA, ITALY, JULY 14—The results of a new multicenter trial suggest that tacrine may restore at least short-term cognitive function in patients with Alzheimer's disease.

The double-blind, placebo-controlled study of 468 patients with mild to moderate dementia found that after 12 weeks, more than 50% of patients receiving 80 mg of tacrine (Cognex, Warner-Lambert) showed a four-point improvement in the AD assessment (cognitive) scale.

"The primary explanation for better results in the present trial is its uncomplicated, straightforward placebo-controlled parallel design," Martin Farlow, M.D., associate professor of

neurology at Indiana University Medical School in Indianapolis, and co-investigator of the trial, said at the Third International Conference on Alzheimer's Disease and Related Disorders here.

Moreover, according to Stephen I. Gracon, D.V.M., clinical director of the pharmaceutical research division of Parke-Davis, 23% of the tacrine-treated patients scored an eight-point or one-year improvement on the ADA scale.

He said the findings may help satisfy some reservations that led to the drug's rejection by an FDA advisory panel last year.

"The problem with cholinergic compounds such as

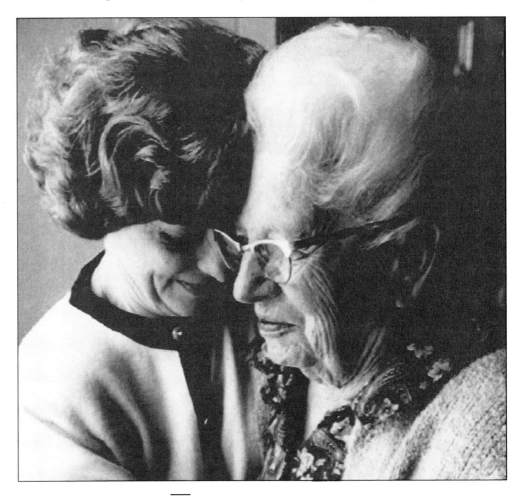

After 12 weeks, more than half of the patients given tacrine showed improvements in cognition; 25% withdrew due to elevated transaminases.

tacrine," said Zaven Khachaturian, Ph.D., associate director for Neuroscience and Neuropsychology on Aging, the National Institute for Aging, "is that if Alzheimer's disease patients are losing brain cells in large numbers and at an accelerating rate, such drugs will be effective only for a short period in the early stages of the disease. Delaying insti-

tutionalization for six months to a year and keeping people functional is better than nothing, and people may be willing to take the risk of side effects."

Approximately 25% of tacrine patients withdrew from the trial because of elevation in transaminase levels, and another 10% because of nausea, vomiting and diarrhea.

Chronic fatigue tests measure response to virus

Springer News Service

AUG. 5—A Houston company has introduced a blood test that it says can identify virally caused chronic fatigue immune dysfunction syndrome (CFIDS).

While some chronic fatigue experts say the test may not be specific enough, others contend it may be a useful confirmatory diagnostic tool.

Family physicians should familiarize themselves with CFIDS symptoms, since chronic fatigue patients often turn to their own physicians first, according to a physician who has treated more than 2,000 CFIDS patients.

"It's not a very long stretch between relative ignorance of the illness to being able to interpret the tests that are available," said Paul R. Cheney, M.D., Ph.D., director of the Cheney Clinic in Charlotte, N.C.

The new test, called 2' 5' Oligoadenylate Synthetase and RNase L, or 2' 5' A, measures two enzymes that become elevated when the body fights a viral infection, according to C.V. Herst, Ph.D., president of Oncore Analytics, Houston.

But according to Dr. Cheney, the Oncore test is not specific for CFIDS. "Any chronic viral infection such as a severe case of shingles, acute infectious mononucleosis or hepatitis will activate this intracellular biochemical pathway," he said.

Dr. Cheney advised that primary-care physicians "begin with the Centers for Disease Control case definition of CFIDS; then use the Oncore test to confirm the diagnosis. Very few people with CFIDS have a normal 2' 5'A RNA test."

Elaine DeFreitas, Ph.D., of the Wistar Institute in Philadelphia, has developed her own CFIDS assay that detects a retrovirus that she and colleagues have linked to the syndrome.

Dr. DeFreitas said the Oncore test "is one of the better assays. It's not specific, but it's sensitive. If I had CFIDS I would want that test."

Dr. Cheney said that he uses Dr. DeFreitas's test along with the 2' 5'A RNA assay.

No tests have been approved for confirming CFIDS, according to a spokesperson for the National Institute of Allergy and Infectious Diseases.

Dr. Cheney said that family physicians should have the CDC case definition for CFIDS handy when evaluating a patient with fatigue. "Xerox it, and check off the symptoms as you question the patient," he said. "Rule out other diseases that cause fatigue, such as diabetes, thyroid disease and hypertension."

One of the main problems in diagnosing chronic fatigue is that many of its symptoms also occur as a result of depression, according to John Stewart, M.D., of the Division of Viral Diseases at the Centers for Disease Control. Conversely, active, productive people who have not been able to function for three months because of CFIDS symptoms often become depressed.

"About 45% of the people referred to our four surveillance sites have had some pre-existing psychological or emotional problems," he said. "But even if some people are depressed to begin with, they can acquire chronic fatigue syndrome."

Physicians should take a careful history, perhaps even screening the patient for depression, Dr. Stewart said.

Once physicians are satisfied that the patient has CFIDS, they can begin treatment with nonsteroidal anti-inflammatories or acetaminophen, Dr. Cheney said. The difficulty occurs when the patient has bad pain; some of his patients require referral to a pain clinic, the majority of whom respond.

Dr. Cheney also uses a combination of antiviral immune modulators, such as gamma-globulin, and life-style changes to treat his patients. "Most of them will improve," he said.

The Charlotte clinician also uses Kutapressin (Schwarz Pharma), a "protein soup" made of porcine liver extract approved for the treatment of acne and other skin disorders. "It doesn't help the sickest patients, but it works in those who have already made a partial recovery," he said. "It can get people back to work and school."

The clinician also recommends mild exercise, "but if they exercise too much they'll relapse," he said. "There is no magic wand, but patients should be reassured that they'll slowly improve and recover."

Study advises diabetics to take daily aspirin

By Dan Hurley

SEPT. 9—Two aspirin tablets a day reduce diabetics' risk of dying or having a myocardial infarction during a five-year period, a study in The Journal of the American Medical Association has found.

The authors of the study concluded that diabetics at increased risk of having a heart attack or stroke should begin taking aspirin daily under the guidance of their physician.

Diabetic men have about two times the average risk of developing cardiovascular disease compared with non-diabetics, and diabetic women have three to five times the average risk of developing cardiovascular disease, said Charles H. Hennekens, M.D., professor of medicine and preventive medicine at Harvard Medical School in Boston.

In 1988, Dr. Hennekens published the first major study showing that aspirin could reduce the rate of heart disease. That study, the Physicians' Health Study, found that aspirin could reduce a man's risk of having a first myocardial infarction by 44%.

Led by Frederick L. Ferris III, M.D., of the National Eye Institute in Bethesda, Md., the new study, known as the Early Treatment Diabetic Retinopathy Study (ETDRS), was originally intended to test the effects of aspirin on diabetic retinopathy.

The ETDRS enrolled 3,711 diabetic men and women between the ages of 18 and 70 in a multicenter, randomized clinical trial. Thirty percent of the study subjects were defined as being Type I diabetics, and 31% as Type II. The type of the remaining 39% could not be definitely determined by the ETDRS group.

Half the patients were asked to take two 325-mg tablets of aspirin per day, while the other half were given a placebo.

The researchers found that aspirin had no effect, positive or negative, on a diabetic's risk for developing retinopathy.

They did find that the patients taking aspirin were 9% less likely to have died of any cause during an average five years of follow-up, compared with those on placebo, although that risk reduction was judged to be not statistically significant.

The patients taking aspirin also were 17% less likely to have a fatal or nonfatal myocardial infarction, compared with those on placebo.

Those figures were in the same direction as seen in previous studies of predominantly nondiabetics, although the ETDRS results were less dramatic than those of most previous studies.

Even so, Dr. Hennekens pointed out that the confidence intervals in both of those findings were wide enough to include stronger effects of aspirin.

"When you have small numbers, the confidence intervals become very wide," said Dr. Hennekens. "So they're compatible with the benefits we've seen in other studies."

And since diabetics as a group already have an increased risk of developing heart disease, even a seemingly small decrease in that risk can have a potentially wide effect on the diabetic population at large, Dr. Hennekens added.

Although the new study found no side effects from aspirin, Dr. Hennekens noted that his own study had found a slightly increased risk of gastrointestinal bleeding in some patients who took aspirin daily.

The study concluded, "Aspirin has been recommended previously for persons at risk for cardiovascular disease. The ETDRS results support application of this recommendation to those persons with diabetes at increased risk of cardio-vascular disease."

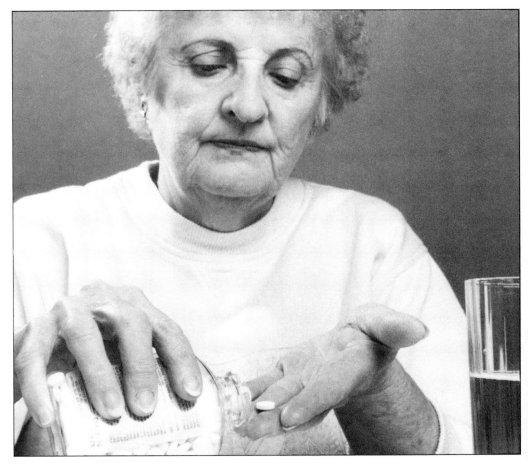

Diabetics taking aspirin were 17% less likely to have a fatal or nonfatal MI compared with those taking placebo.

Combination treatment may heal ulcers best

By Charlene Laino

SEPT. 24—Following new reports that add support to the role of Helicobacter pylori in the pathogenesis of duodenal ulcers, gastrointestinal experts contacted by Medical Tribune were divided about whether they would change the way they treat the disease.

David Graham, M.D., who performed one of the largest studies to date implicating H. pylori in duodenal ulcers, said that there is no doubt in his mind that in the near future all patients with duodenal ulcers will be treated with a combination therapy that includes antibiotics to eradicate H. pylori infection.

"Although not all physicians are currently aware of the role of H. pylori, they will be," said Dr. Graham, who is chief of digestive diseases at the Veterans Administration Medical Center in Houston.

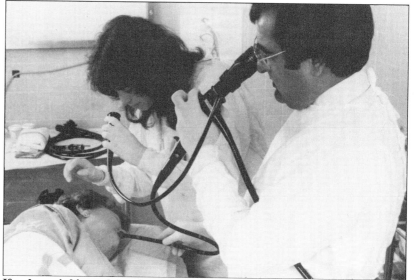

If endoscopic biopsy determines presence of H. pylori, antibiotics may be indicated.

More and more studies are providing evidence that H. pylori infection is responsible for ulcers and that getting rid of the bacterium with antibiotics can both cure ulcers and prevent their recurrence, he said.

His own study of 109 patients found that duodenal ulcers recurred in 12% of those taking ranitidine plus antibiotic therapy, while ulcers returned in 95% of those taking only ranitidine.

Other physicians were more cautious, however.

James Cooper, M.D., professor of medicine at Georgetown University in Washington, D.C., said that "the preponderance of the evidence suggests that H. pylori is the cause of the garden variety of ulcers suffered by most patients. But it's too early to make a blanket statement."

He said that there is a need for larger, double-blind, long-term studies to confirm the relationship between the bacterium and ulcers.

Dr. Cooper also suggested that a National Institutes of Health consensus conference be convened to give physicians more direction in treatment.

William Steinberg, M.D., professor of medicine at George Washington Hospital in Washington, D.C., said he is still skeptical of H. pylori's role.

The bacterium may be a causative agent in 15% of cases, but no more, he said.

"I would not treat my average patient for H. pylori," he said. For most of his patients, he said he prescribes drugs like ranitidine (Zantac, Glaxo) or bismuth.

Dr. Steinberg said he does not routinely recommend dietary changes for people with ulcers.

Only if a patient has complications—bleeding, or recurring or obstructive disease—does he perform an endoscopic biopsy to determine if H. pylori is present, said Dr. Steinberg. He noted that detecting H. pylori can be difficult, requiring repeated biopsies.

If the bacterium is detected, Dr. Steinberg said he proceeds to a course of combination therapy that includes antibiotics, bismuth and an H_2-receptor antagonist.

"Antibiotics are not without side effects," Dr. Steinberg pointed out in explaining why he does not automatically consider their use. And of course, there is always the risk of adding to the already burgeoning problem of antibiotic-resistant disease.

In the most recent report to appear in the literature, Arthur K. C. Li, M.D., of the Chinese University of Hong Kong and colleagues found that duodenal ulcers healed in all but four of 78 patients given a combination of antibiotics, omeprazole (Prilosec, Merck Sharp & Dohme) and bismuth four times a day for one week, followed by treatment with omeprazole alone for three more weeks.

Dr. Li used a combination of tetracycline 500 mg, metronidazole 400 mg, bismuth 120 mg and omeprazole four times a day for one week followed by three weeks of omeprazole alone.

A control group received omeprazole alone for four weeks.

Of 78 patients given the combination regimen, endoscopy revealed that only four still had ulcers after four weeks of therapy, compared with 16 of 77 patients given omeprazole alone.

Urease tests, microscopy and cultured antral biopsy were used to test for the presence of H. pylori. According to the Chinese researchers, infection was eradicated in 95% of patients on the combination therapy, compared with 4% on omeprazole alone.

Mild dizziness associated with omeprazole was the only side effect seen. It was reported by six patients in each treatment group and did not cause any patient to stop treatment.

Until now, most doctors thought that at least two weeks of antibiotic therapy was necessary, the Hong Kong team explained in a recent issue of the British Medical Journal. Shortening the length of treatment will mean better patient compliance, the researchers said.

But Dr. Graham called the difference in the length of treatment irrelevant. Unlike Dr. Steinberg, he said he considers antibiotic therapy to be without any significant side effects as well as inexpensive. "It makes little difference whether a patient is given the drugs for seven days, 10 days or two weeks," he said.

Dr. Graham commented that the 95% eradication rate seen in the Chinese patients was higher than would probably be seen in U.S. patients because "many Americans have taken a lot of antibiotics in their lives and may have developed resistance to treatment with the drugs."

It may be that the extra week of therapy is needed to completely eradicate the bacteria in American patients, he said.

At least 10% of the U.S. adult population suffers from duodenal ulcers, according to Mark A. Peppercorn, M.D., of Harvard Medical School.

Some Gulf veterans suffer mystery illnesses

By L.A. McKeown

SEPT. 27—An estimated 300 former Desert Storm personnel who are suffering from fatigue, arthritis, hair loss, rashes and other symptoms that they believe stem from their experiences in the Persian Gulf are being told by military experts that they are suffering from the stress of readjustment to civilian life.

But some of the soldiers and a prominent member of Congress are calling for a more thorough investigation in light of additional cases that have appeared since the war.

In June, a team from the Walter Reed Army Hospital issued a 60-page report on 79 veterans, most of them among a single group of reservists, in which the Army researchers concluded that 80% of the symptoms probably were related to stress.

The team, led by Major Robert DeFraites, an epidemiologist from Walter Reed Army Hospital, had been called in by an Army physician from the 123rd Army Reserve Command in Indianapolis who had seen 125 Gulf veterans with symptoms or concerns stemming from their experiences during the war.

The 123rd command, which sent 1,200 individuals to the Gulf, contains the largest cluster of such cases that the military has documented so far.

The physical complaints range from fatigue in 60% to intestinal problems in 56%, headaches in 47%, joint pain in 41%, painful gums or tooth problems in 35%, rash in 35% and loss of some memory in 35%, according to the official report.

About half of those reporting fatigue said the onset had occurred anywhere from 30 days before redeployment to 60 days after they returned home.

Major DeFraites said the most puzzling aspect of the Indiana cases is that while the complainants all are from the 123rd command, they belonged to various units and were deployed in different locations for a variety of duties.

All in the 123rd were, however, exposed for varying periods to the noxious plumes of black smoke from burning oil wells set ablaze when Saddam Hussein's troops fled Kuwait.

The military disputes exposure to airborne petroleum particulates as being linked to the myriad of health complaints.

"We don't think that the current illnesses are related to exposure to either the oil well fires or to any kind of petrochemicals," said Virginia Stepanoukis, a spokesperson for the Army Surgeon General's Office.

At a public forum last month organized by Rep. Joseph Kennedy (D-Mass.), an air pollution expert from the Center for Environmental Health Sciences at Massachusett's Institute of Technology said there is as yet no evidence to link the exposure to oil-fire smoke to the health problems.

"What I pointed out was that the conclusion that a particular set of symptoms are related is not justified from the information I saw," said William Thilly, director of the center. "There was not the kind of data set that one would associate with a cause and effect."

But Thilly added that there is no evidence indicating that there is not a relationship. Nor have experts had much experience with exposure on such a scale as existed in Kuwait.

Once in the Gulf, the 123rd was split up into various commands, further complicating the toxicologic sleuthing.

The 425th QM unit, for instance, was a personal service

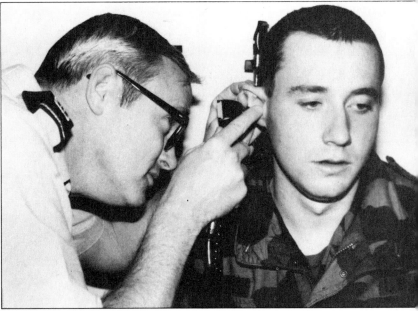

The military disputes claims that exposure to fuel spurred ills among veterans.

command that included truck drivers and fuel supply companies. Some veterans who now are ill say that the water they used for showering came out of tanks used to carry diesel fuel.

The Army's report said long-term exposure to fuel was not responsible for the health problems; however, an Army spokesperson said the panel may not have been told about the showering experiences.

The spokesperson, Steve Stromvall, said the first time he heard of the fuel in the shower water was from an Indiana reservist interviewed on the prime-time television program 20/20.

The investigators concluded that limited exposure to fuel oil, such as when filling and emptying tanker trucks, could cause mucous membrane and upper-respiratory-tract irritation, drying and irritation of skin, lightheadedness, dizziness and headache.

An occupational health expert from George Washington University, who has not seen any of the cases, said the exposure amount and duration would have to be documented before a conclusion could be drawn.

"People who are handling diesel fuel can get quite a bit on their skin and some of it can be absorbed," said Laura Welch, M.D., director of the occupational and environmental medicine department at the Washington, D.C., university.

Dr. Welch said oral, dermal or inhaled exposure to petrochemicals can cause symptoms similar to the veterans'. She pointed out that usually symptoms arise immediately after exposure.

"A long-term syndrome has been described, but it generally occurs from very high exposures over a short time or low exposures over a long time," she said. "I would be less concerned about their showering in it because it would be a short exposure and petrochemicals don't mix well with water."

Other possible explanations include side effects of the anthrax vaccine that many soldiers received before being deployed to the Gulf.

To that, Walter Reed epidemiologist DeFraites asked, "But then how do you explain symptoms in people who didn't get the vaccine?"

Leishmaniasis, endemic in the Persian Gulf area and carried by sandflies, has been tossed around as another explanation. DeFraites said all 79 Indiana reservists tested negative for this disease.

Thus the Army's reliance on the stress of readjustment to civilian life as an explanation.

Arthur F. Blank, M.D., director of the Readjustment Counseling Service of the Department of Veterans Affairs, said that up to 10% of Persian Gulf veterans need counseling for psychological stress, and most are getting it.

"The stress conclusion is very difficult for people to swallow," DeFraites admitted.

Kennedy is having an especially difficult time swallowing it. In addition to the public forum, he has held congressional hearings at which a group of soldiers from New England reported experiencing symptoms similar to those of the Indiana group.

"Once the word got out on what we were doing, we were literally inundated with calls," said Bea Grause, Kennedy's legislative aide for veterans affairs. "They [Gulf veterans] were calling from just about every state but Alaska."

Kennedy is drafting a bill to have the Gulf syndrome recognized as a medical ailment so that veterans can get prompt treatment at VA centers.

DeFraites said the problem comes down to a lack of commonality among the soldiers and their symptoms.

"We couldn't find the common thread that would tell us which way to go," he said.

Thilly of the MIT center said, "What we need to do is bring these medical records together, and then maybe some related experiences and related symptoms will pop out."

Dr. Welch, the occupational health expert from George Washington, said the Association of Occupational Health Clinics is considering drafting a letter to their 35 clinics asking if they have seen sick veterans of the Gulf. "Telling these people what didn't cause their problems is not telling them what they should do," Dr. Welch said. "Often they find their way to occupational exposure clinics, and we may be of some help to them."

Transplant of pig liver sparks ethics debate

By L.A. McKeown

OCT. 20—The California surgeon who tried recently to save a young woman's life by using a pig liver as a "bridge" to a human liver transplant says that the severe shortage of human organs is making the use of animals a necessity.

But some medical ethicists say the technique used by the California doctor puts critically ill people with little chance of survival ahead of other patients who need organ transplants and are more likely to survive.

The 26-year-old California woman, Susan Fowler, was brought to Cedars-Sinai Hospital in Los Angeles in a near coma, according to Leonard Makowka, M.D.

Fowler, who had a lifelong history of liver disease, was immediately put on a waiting list for a liver. But after 24 hours with no luck in finding a donor and with Fowler deteriorating, Dr. Makowka said a decision was made to use a pig liver to keep her alive until a human organ could be found.

"We approached the family and we let them know that we were ready to abort the pig procedure immediately if there was [a human liver] available," Dr. Makowka said. "Our approach was strictly to use the pig organ as a bridge. We were hoping all along that we would have the human liver."

Just prior to the surgery, Fowler's blood was passed through the kidneys of the pig and then returned to her. This procedure, xenoperfusion, acts as a filter to weed out antibodies that might cause the body to reject the organ.

But 32 hours later, when the pig organ was in place and a human donor had finally been found, the patient died of brain swelling brought on by the liver disease.

"Obviously we would have liked to treat her earlier and we would have gone ahead with a transplant as soon as she was brought in," Dr. Makowka said. "This whole effort just underscores the organ shortage in this country."

As of two weeks ago, there were 2,183 people in the United States waiting for a liver transplant. In the 19-to-45 age group, which included Fowler, there were 744 people waiting, according to the United Network for Organ Sharing based in Richmond, Va. On average, one person a day dies waiting for a liver.

One of those people who had reached the top of the list unknowingly forfeited the organ to Fowler, because by initiating the bridge procedure, the California doctors pushed the woman past other potential organ recipients, into what one medical ethicist calls the "hypersick" category.

Arthur Caplan, Ph.D., director of the Center for Bioethics at the University of Minnesota, said he believes that Fowler was too sick to get any benefit from the human liver. Dr. Caplan said the organs should be given to people who have the best chance of living longer with the transplant.

The human organ that would have been given to Fowler was eventually transplanted to another patient.

Martin Benjamin, Ph.D., a medical ethicist with the Center for Ethics and Humanities in the Life Sciences at Michigan State University, said Fowler's doctors were following the Hippocratic oath they took when they became doctors, which mandates them to do everything possible to save their patients.

While Dr. Benjamin said he sees nothing ethically wrong with using pigs to save human lives, he does have a problem with using scarce healthcare dollars to perform multiple operations on people whose lives have a small likelihood of being saved.

Fowler's doctors said they considered using the xeno-perfusion procedure alone, as Johns Hopkins surgeons did this summer when they saved a 25-year-old woman awaiting a liver transplant.

They said they hope that by splicing human genes into pigs, one day they will be able to have human-compatible pigs ready to donate organs.

Oral cholera vaccine proves superior to injectable

Medical Tribune News Service

NOV. 12—A single-dose, live oral cholera vaccine has been shown to produce a potent immune response with minimal side effects in trials of more than 3,000 adults and children worldwide, according to researchers at the University of Maryland School of Medicine in Baltimore and the University of Indonesia in Jakarta.

If immunogenicity is confirmed in Phase III trials, people in cholera-endemic areas, as well as travelers to high-risk areas such as some countries in Latin America, will benefit from the genetically engineered vaccine, called CVD 103-HgR, said one of its developers, Myron M. Levine, M.D.

The current cholera vaccine, around for about 100 years, consists of killed bacteria that are inoculated intramuscularly. "It's used very little because it is associated with only about four months of protection in less than half of the people who get it," said Dr. Levine, director of the Center for Vaccine Development at the University of Maryland.

CVD 103-HgR affords at least several years of protection, based on studies of reinfection of wild-type cholera, he said, and trials have indicated it triggers an immune reponse in around 90% of people.

A specialist in tropical medicine agreed that a better cholera vaccine is urgently needed and said the study results are encouraging so far.

"The next step is to look at whether the actual number of expected cases in endemic areas declines after people are given the vaccine," said John Ho, M.D., assistant professor of medicine at New York Hospital-Cornell Medical Center. So far, immunogenicity has been determined by levels of serum vibriocidal antibodies.

A Phase III trial to resolve that issue is planned for early 1993 in about 65,000 people in Indonesia.

Two recently published studies demonstrated the vaccine's safety and efficacy, said Dr. Levine.

In a double-blind, crossover trial, published recently in the journal Infection and Immunity, 94 U.S. college students did not suffer any more adverse reactions—chiefly diarrhea—when given the oral vaccine (5×10^8-CFU dose) than when given placebo. Ninety-seven percent developed a significant immune response as measured by serum vibriocidal antibody, Dr. Levine said.

In another study, 412 Indonesian children aged five to nine received single doses of various amounts of the vaccine or placebo. All doses were well tolerated, according to the report in The Lancet. While the 5×10^8-CFU dose did not produce a significant immune response in most children, the lone 5×10^9-CFU dose of vaccine elicited high rates of seroconversion in 87% of them.

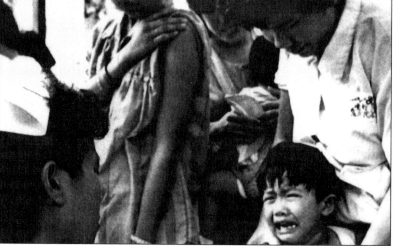

Painful intramuscular cholera inoculations may soon be a thing of the past.

COMMENTARY

Building bone with drugs and diet

By Theodore Fields, M.D.

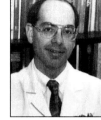

FOR OSTEOPOROSIS, 1992 brought clinicians such an encouraging expansion in our treatment armamentarium that we should be able to make a major impact on our patients' fracture rates. But many unanswered questions and controversies remain about this major health problem.

Estrogen. Estrogen replacement therapy is the most effective modality available today for the preservation of bone mass in postmenopausal women. In my opinion, any perimenopausal woman who has not made a commitment to estrogen therapy should have her bone density measured. This information may convince her to go ahead with estrogen or to consider other modes of protective therapy. High-risk patients, such as those with early menopause or those on corticosteroids, present the clearest case for determination of bone density and initiation of prophylactic measures.

And it is not too late to initiate ERT in patients who are several years past menopause. According to a helpful Mayo Clinic study released this year, women with osteoporosis who received an estrogen patch 10 or more years after menopause achieved a small increase in bone density and a 50% decrease in vertebral fracture rate during a one-year study period. Prior to these data, many physicians felt that estrogen was useful mainly in the two to three years following menopause, since those few years were when the greatest amount of bone turnover occurred.

Whether to administer estrogen orally or via transdermal patch is still an open question. The excellent results obtained by the Mayo Clinic team were supportive of the patches. Theoretically, the patches may reduce such problems as gallstones and thrombophlebitis by avoiding the enterohepatic circulation. Oral estrogen, however, is less expensive and raises HDL cholesterol, which is not true of the patch. The cholesterol effect may be a significant explanation for the apparent cardioprotective effect of oral estrogen. Putting the factors together, I tend to recommend oral estrogen for most patients, since the cardioprotective factor is an important counterbalance to a possible estrogen-related increase in breast-cancer risk (although there is some controversy about this as well).

Calcitonin. Calcitonin has consistently been found effective in preserving bone density and in reducing fracture rate. There is some resistance to calcitonin among patients because of the need for subcutaneous injection. However, now that we have a study demonstrating that this hormone, administered as a nasal spray, can also slow lumbar-spine bone loss, I expect that nasal calcitonin will become available in the next few years and will be well accepted by patients.

Diphosphonates. Etidronate has been shown in several studies to decrease fracture rate and to stabilize bone density. Unfortunately, because of a risk of osteomalacia with daily treatment, it can only be taken for 14 days out of each three-month period. I anticipate that within the next few years we will have new diphosphonates that can be taken continually, as well as more information on the long-term value of etidronate. At present, I consider prescribing etidronate in patients for whom estrogen or calcitonin are not appropriate or acceptable. This is not an insignificant group, and advancing our knowledge in this treatment category is very important.

Fluoride. Unlike other medications that reduce bone resorption, fluoride actually stimulates osteoblasts and can increase bone formation. Studies of fluoride have, in fact, demonstrated more dramatic increases in bone density than with any of the other agents above. Unfortunately, the fracture rate in patients receiving fluoride was actually increased, suggesting that denser but more fragile bone had been formed. These findings have markedly reduced the use of fluoride in the management of osteoporosis, but smaller doses may have a role in the future.

Diet. There is general agreement that all women, in the absence of hypercalcemia or kidney stones, should receive at least the minimal requirement of oral calcium: 1,000 mg daily for premenopausal and 1,500 mg daily for postmenopausal women. Vitamin D supplementation has shown promise in recent research, and women should receive at least 400 IU of vitamin D daily. In addition, some experts advocate a doubling of vitamin D intake and weekly supplementation with 50,000 units of 25-OH vitamin D_3, but most authorities consider these suggestions to be experimental.

Despite all that remains controversial in the field of osteoporosis, I believe that our treatment arsenal and fund of data have expanded to a point where there is little reason for any high-risk patient to go untreated.

Dr. Fields is associate professor of clinical medicine at New York Hospital-Cornell Medical Center and associate attending at the Hospital for Special Surgery in New York City.

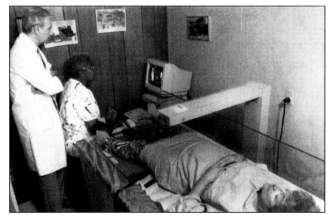

Densitometry evaluates bone loss in patients on corticosteroids.

1992 HIGHLIGHTS

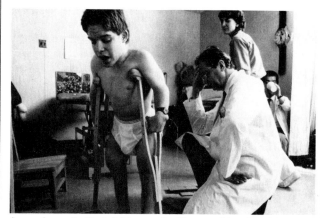

As much as a foot in height was gained by stretching dwarfs' bones.

Jan. 30

Antibiotics offered the best protection against surgical-wound infections when administered two hours or less before elective surgery, reported University of Utah researchers. The epidemiologists monitored 2,847 patients undergoing clean or "clean-contaminated" surgical procedures. Compared with preoperative prophylaxis, giving antibiotics within three hours after an incision carried 2.4 times the risk of infection. Waiting more than three hours conferred 5.8 times the risk, the team calculated.

Giving antibiotics more than two hours before surgery boosted infection risk almost sevenfold, according to the data presented in The New England Journal of Medicine.

Feb. 12

Researchers at the American Red Cross announced that blood banks may one day be able to store red blood cells at a regular refrigerator tempera-ture for 14 to 20 weeks, doubling or tripling the current storage limit.

Red Cross investigators have devised a method to keep red blood cells alive for up to 14 weeks by suspending them in a preserving solution stripped of negatively charged chloride ions, while Israeli researchers have extended the longevity of red blood cells to 20 weeks by adding mannitol to the preservation medium. Extended storage could be particularly useful for autologous transfusions requiring such large quantities of blood that it cannot be accumulated during the usual storage period, the head of the Israeli team told Medical Tribune.

Feb. 22

Five teenagers suffering from achondroplastic dwarfism gained as much as a foot in height after bones in their legs were fractured and then stretched, revealed University of California, Los Angeles, researchers. Using an experi-mental technique pioneered in the Soviet Union, surgeons insert instruments through a small incision in the leg and fracture the bone. A rod pinned to the bone at points above and below the break is gradually extended; as the bone segments are pulled apart, new bone grows to fill the gap, the investigators told the American Academy of Pediatrics meeting in San Francisco.

The UCLA team gained about six inches from most of the teenagers' shinbones over an 11- to 17-month period, and another five from their thigh bones over an 11-month period. One 18-year-old youth "grew" nearly a foot, as did a young girl. All five teens experienced adverse effects, including infections and temporary paralysis.

• • •

Surgeons at the Brooke Army Medical Center suggested that babies with broken bones could be treated more comfortably if removable canvas harnesses with adjustable chest and leg straps were used instead of traditional casts. Thigh-bone fractures in all of eight infants fitted with the new harnesses healed in about five weeks, the same length of time as for babies in a leg cast, but with much less discomfort, the San Antonio physicians reported at the annual meeting of the American Academy of Orthopaedic Surgeons in Washington, D.C.

• • •

Cigarette smoking may delay the healing of broken bones, Emory University researchers told the American Academy of Orthopaedic Surgeons. In a study of 29 osteomyelitis patients who had their tibias lengthened using a circular external fixator device, the smokers took five months longer to heal than nonsmokers, the Atlanta researchers said.

March 19

A surgical procedure, fundoplication, bested a variety of drugs in the treatment of daily, severe gastroesophageal reflux disease. But some gastroenterologists greeted the Veterans Administration report in The New England Journal of Medicine with caution, saying that the surgery is difficult and should only be performed on young people who face a lifetime of drugs or those who do not respond to medications.

March 28

A pain specialist described dramatic success using adrenal medulla grafts to treat severe chronic pain in terminal cancer patients. Five patients with bone metastases had portions of adrenal medulla harvested from cadavers injected into the spinal subarachnoid space, explained the director of the pain center at the University of Illinois Hospital in Chicago. Four achieved pain relief and were able to abandon narcotics; improvement correlated with increasing levels of norepinephrine and met-enkephalin stimulated after the injections. A fifth had complete pain relief at three weeks, but the pain returned after reoperation for a spinal lesion, the Chicago specialist told a meet-

Surgery

ing of the American Society of Regional Anesthesia.

April 7

Transplanting donor genes into organ-transplant recipients before the operation may free them from a lifetime of potentially dangerous immuno-suppressive drugs, a Harvard surgeon told a meeting of the Federation of American Societies of Experimental Biology. Studies of mice have shown that transplanting genes of the major histocompatibility complex from donor to recipient prior to organ transplantation guards against rejection of the organ, he said.

In the new technique, potential organ-transplant patients would have some of their bone marrow removed and then would undergo radiation to destroy the remaining marrow. MHC genes from the prospective organ donor's immune system would be inserted into the removed bone marrow before it is reinjected in the patient.

April 15

Surgeons from the University of California, San Francisco, told a meeting of the American Association of Neurological Surgeons in San Francisco that a balloon-tipped catheter can successfully open cerebral arteries clamped shut by vasospasm. The team has used the procedure for six years in patients who have failed to respond to standard treatment. Cerebral transluminal angioplasty involves threading a catheter tipped with an elastic silicone balloon from the groin through a carotid artery and into the brain. The balloon is gently expanded to stretch the arterial walls, and the maneuver is repeated along the length of the pinched blood vessel. Using the procedure, 20 of 31 patients showed marked improvement, with no restenosis evident at one year.

April 27

A thoracic surgeon described the first three reported cases of video-aided, thoraco-

scopic lobectomy at a meeting of the American Association for Thoracic Surgery in Los Angeles. The surgery was performed through three intercostal incisions in the chest. Lobar branches of the pulmonary artery and vein were stapled off and the excised lobe removed through a wide incision. The surgeon from St. Peter's Hospital and Medical Center in New Brunswick, N.J., said the procedure reduces pain, shortens hospital stay and allows normal function to return more quickly. However, a New York expert told Medical Tribune that he has reservations about the stapling instrument used in the procedure and does not advocate it for wedge resections.

May 7

Diagnostic MRI could replace diagnostic arthroscopy to confirm or rule out meniscal tears, predicted Yale University radiologists. Thirty-four patients with knee injuries underwent MRI immediately prior to diagnostic arthroscopy; in 32 patients, diagnoses based on MRI findings were confirmed at surgery. In 59 patients who did not undergo arthroscopy, treatment based on MRI information was successful in 89% and each patient saved an estimated $3,900 in medical costs, the investigators reported in Radiology.

May 11

Laparoscopic surgery is now being used to treat urinary incontinence in women, a British researcher reported at the American Urological Association meeting in Washington, D.C. Like traditional colposuspension surgery, laparoscopic surgery raises the bladder, but is performed through three tiny holes instead of a long incision.

Laparoscopic surgery can reduce in-hospital recovery time to two days, compared

with the seven days that follow conventional surgery, said the urologist from England's Sheffield University, who has performed six of the surgeries.

June 4

Teflon and silicone jaw implants, used to treat people with temporomandibular joint disorder, may themselves cause excruciating pain and bone deterioration, experts testified at a congressional hearing aimed at pressuring the Food and Drug Administration to require safety studies of the devices.

Like silicone-gel breast implants, which were sharply restricted by the FDA earlier this year, jaw implants were marketed before passage in 1976 of a federal law bringing medical devices under scrutiny. The most popular implant, made of Teflon, was recalled in 1988 under FDA pressure. But jaw implants made of silicone, acrylics and metal remain on the market.

June 10

Physicians at the annual meeting of Colon and Rectal Surgeons in San Francisco were advised that scalpel surgery is still the best bet for hemorrhoids.

Although laser surgery has been touted by some as superior to scalpel surgery for excisional hemorrhoidectomy, Grand Rapids, Mich., researchers said they found no added benefit from the technique and that scalpel-surgery patients actually healed slightly faster.

In a study of 64 patients who underwent internal-external hemorrhoidectomy, laser surgery did not reduce blood loss, length of surgery, postoperative pain or hospital stay, said investigators from Ferguson Hospital.

June 14

After receiving reports of 128 operative injuries and six deaths, the New York State Health Department issued an

alert regarding the safety of laparoscopic cholecystectomy. The injuries, reported between August 1990 and March 1992, included a perforated aorta and serious injuries to the vena cava, liver, colon and common bile duct. Health department officials urged greater oversight by surgeons employing the popular laparoscopic techniques now used in 80% of cholecystectomies.

Laparoscopists responded that individual hospitals or regions are able to provide adequate quality control, and the New York alert constitutes no reason to retrench from the use of keyhole surgery on a national basis.

June 27

Heart-lung transplants may greatly improve the breathing ability and quality of life of cystic fibrosis patients who survive, but the surgery is not without complications, researchers from Harefield Hospital in Middlesex, England, reported in The Lancet.

Forced vital capacity increased from 35% to 70% in 79 patients, and cystic fibrosis did not affect the transplanted lung. But 92%

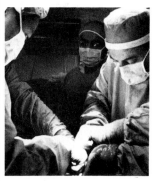

Surgeons transplant the first baboon liver into a human.

of patients had rejection episodes, and only 49% were living three years after surgery, the researchers said.

June 28

A team of surgeons at the University of Pittsburgh transplanted a baboon liver into a 35-year-old man dying of hepatitis. The operation was the first of its kind in an adult. If successful, surgeons commented, the operation could signal the start of an era in which xenografts would ease the shortage of human donor organs.

July 1

The first successful use of a 15-minute laser procedure to correct severe myopia was reported in the Archives of Ophthalmology.

Laser photorefractive keratectomy was performed at three centers on 16 severely myopic patients under local anesthesia with an excimer laser from the Visk Company in Sunnyvale, Calif. At six-month follow-up, 14 could see as well as they had preoperatively with glasses or contact lenses.

Other investigators have reported unpredictable results with the technique in patients with severe myopia, leading the Food and Drug Administration to limit clinical trials to mild or moderate cases.

July 6

British researchers announced plans to transplant transgenic pig organs into humans within five years, and said preparations had begun at Papworth Hospital in Cambridge, England, to insert parts of human genes into fertilized sow eggs. Once those pigs are born, they will be mated with normal pigs, eventually creating litters of pigs with human-ready organs, the researchers predicted.

July 11

Stem cells found in human umbilical-cord blood were more plentiful and of better quality than those found in normal bone marrow, British researchers reported in The Lancet. The Paterson Institute, Manchester, researchers said that their data from long-term laboratory tests convinced them that transfusions with umbilical-cord blood were an ideal alternative to bone-marrow transplants. They pointed out that cord

blood is in great supply, the procedure is painless and recipients do not have to be HLA-matched with donors. At least one company in the United States has been formed to create a human umbilical-blood cell "bank." The first successful cord-blood transplant was performed in 1988 at the Hôpital Saint-Louis in Paris, on a five-year-old boy with Fanconi's anemia.

July 27

A month after a 16-year-old from Texas underwent the world's first hand transplant, his physicians and therapists reported that the boy's condition was continuing to improve and that he was gradually becoming capable of moving his fingers and wrist. The boy, who was born with a grossly malformed right hand that was amputated at eight months of age, had been able to get along using a prosthetic hook worn on the right arm. Then a car accident resulted in irreversible paralysis of the left arm. In a 14-hour procedure, surgeons at Herman Hospital in Houston transplanted his usable left hand onto his right arm. They added that the boy would probably need further surgery to improve function in the hand.

Aug. 20

A new videoimaging technique may improve the safety of neurosurgery by allowing direct observation and high-resolution mapping of critical areas of the brain, suggested researchers at the University of Washington School of Medicine in Seattle.

The technique, optical imaging, has been used to map the cerebral cortex of 20 patients with intractable epilepsy, the investigators reported in Nature.

Fiberoptic light is shone through the skull while the patient is alert but quiescent. A

camera attached to the surgical microscope photographs the cortex to acquire control images, and comparative photos are taken while the patient performs tasks involving speech, movement and memory.

Sept. 16

A National Institutes of Health expert panel concluded that laparoscopic cholecystec-

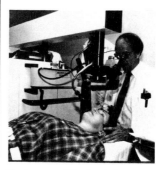

Doctor uses 15-minute laser procedure to correct myopia.

tomy is safe and effective, but recommended that training guidelines be developed. New York State issued its own guidelines earlier this year after a state panel reported that at least seven deaths had been linked to complications from the procedure. The most common complication was severed bile ducts. The New York guidelines recommend that doctors assist in the surgery at least 10 times and perform it under the supervision of another surgeon at least 15 times before doing it independently. The chairperson of the NIH panel said the 10- to 15-procedure training period would be a good national goal to shoot for. About 80% of the 500,000 gallbladder surgeries done each year are performed laparoscopically.

Sept. 21

In a development that broadened the applications of laparoscopy, surgeons reported performing keyhole surgery to widen the transverse carpal ligament in patients with carpal

tunnel syndrome. In a study presented at the meeting of the American Society of Plastic and Reconstructive Surgeons in Washington, D.C., the surgery was performed on 430 patients under local anesthesia; recovery time was cut from six weeks to three weeks. Surgeons from the Plastic, Reconstructive and Hand Surgery Center of Kansas City, Kansas, reported minor complications in three patients: one with an infection and two with bleeding from small arteries during surgery.

Oct. 13

Transplant pioneer Thomas Starzl, M.D., reported at the American College of Surgeons meeting in New Orleans that the potent immunosuppressive FK-506 has broadened the transplant surgeon's scope to include even the most complex "multivisceral" operations.

He and colleagues at the University of Pittsburgh described intestinal transplants in adults and children performed at the university since 1990. Twenty-four of the 29 transplant recipients have survived for more than two years. Several patients received multivisceral transplants, in which a cluster of intra-abdominal organs—liver, stomach, pancreas, spleen, and colon—is transplanted together, hanging from a central arterial stem.

Oct. 20

A New York surgeon reported that the best candidates for carpal tunnel syndrome surgery are those whose symptoms started after 50 years of age, who have been in pain for more than 10 months, who have a finger locked in the "trigger" position or who experience constant tingling or burning in the fingers. When none of these factors are present, about two thirds of people with carpal tunnel syndrome will improve without surgery, the St. Luke's-Roosevelt Hospital physician told a symposium in New York.

Surgery termed an option for severe reflux disease

MARCH 19—Surgery is more effective than drugs to treat daily, severe gastroesophageal reflux disease, a study published in The New England Journal of Medicine has found.

But one gastroenterologist, writing in a NEJM editorial, cautioned that the surgery is difficult and should only be performed on young people who face a lifetime of drugs or those who do not respond to medications.

Researchers found that patients who underwent fundoplication, in which a portion of the gastric fundus is wrapped entirely around the distal esophagus, experienced greater reductions in symptom scores (the "activity index"), esophagitis and acid reflux than patients receiving standard medical therapy.

In the Department of Veterans Affairs Gastroesophageal Reflux Disease Study Group trial, Stuart Jon Spechler, M.D., of Beth Israel Hospital, Boston, and colleagues compared medical therapy—life-style modifications and up to four medications—with surgery in 243 male and four female patients with peptic esophageal ulcer, stricture, erosive esophagitis or Barrett's esophagus. Drugs used in the medical-therapy group included antacid tablets, ranitidine (Zantac, Glaxo), sucralfate (Carafate, Marion Laboratories) and metoclopramide. The study began before approval of omeprazole (Prilosec, Merck Sharp & Dohme).

Patients were randomly assigned to receive either continuous medical therapy, treatment for symptoms only, or surgery. Among the findings were these:
• The activity index declined from 109 at baseline to 78 after two years among those in the surgery group, from 107 to 90 in the symptomatic-treatment group and from 108 to 88 in the continuous-medical-treatment group.
• The grade of esophagitis (as determined by endoscopy) declined from 2.9 to 1.5 in the surgery group, from 2.9 to 2.2 in the symptomatic-treatment group and from 2.9 to 1.9 in the continuous-treatment group.
• Acid reflux, given as the percent of a 24-hour day that esophageal pH was less than four, declined from 23 to 5 in the surgery group, from 23 to 14 in the symptomatic-treatment group and from 20 to 11 in the continuous-treatment group.

There was a high frequency of side effects in all groups, with 84% of patients in the surgery group and 88% of patients in the symptomatic- and continuous-treatment groups experiencing reactions that included abdominal fullness, diarrhea and impotence.

Some symptoms may have been due to disorders associated with reflux disease, such as delayed gastric emptying, Dr. Spechler said. Long-term treatment with four drugs also may have contributed to side effects. And the frequency of some symptoms "may have reflected their prevalence in a carefully studied, older population," Dr. Spechler wrote.

Commenting on the merits of surgery versus drugs, Joel Richter, M.D. of the University of Alabama, Birmingham and author of the NEJM editorial, said: "All the medications that we give just neutralize the effect of the acid, they don't fix the valve."

But if the esophagus is wrapped too tightly, the patient will have difficulty swallowing; too loosely, and the acid will continue to back up into the stomach, Dr. Richter noted.

Antireflux surgery should be limited to younger patients with severe disease or those with intractable conditions, he said.

Cross-sectional surveys suggest that 7% to 10% of Americans have heartburn daily, according to Dr. Richter. About a third of patients with heartburn who seek medical care have endoscopic evidence of esophagitis, and about 10% to 20% have severe complications.

Omeprazole is very effective, but is approved for use only for 12 weeks, Dr. Richter said. It also is expensive, costing between $100 and $200 a month.

Keyhole surgery linked to deaths; aggressive marketing blamed

NEW YORK, JUNE 14—Following reports of an alarming number of deaths and injuries associated with laparoscopic cholecystectomy, some physicians say aggressive marketing and eagerness on the part of the patient and physician for a simpler, faster surgical techique may have contributed to the problem.

Between August 1990 and March 1992, the New York State Health Department received reports of 128 incidents at 73 hospitals. Six patients died. Injuries included a perforated aorta and serious injuries to the vena cava, liver, colon and common bile duct.

State Health Department spokesperson Peter Slocum says that the total number of laparoscopic cholecystectomy procedures is not known, but the state's medical surveillance system identified "an unusually high number of incidents."

"We're reluctant to declare a crisis until we know what percentage of these surgeries are going wrong," he said.

Laparoscopic techniques are now used in 75% of cholecystectomies, according to the Society of American Gastrointestinal Endoscopic Surgeons (SAGES).

"The shift from open to laparoscopic cholecystectomy has not been the result of carefully planned and executed prospective trials designed to protect our patients; instead, in a free-market economy, patients wanted a treatment having less

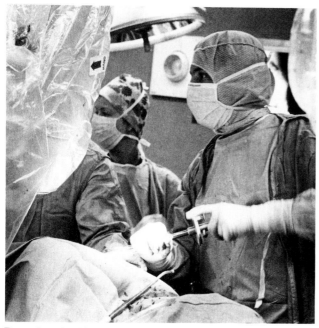

Procedure itself has not been the subject of attack.

pain, little or no hospitalization, a rapid return to life as usual and virtually no scar. Manufacturers of laparoscopic surgical equipment marketed the procedure to both physicians and patients," commented David Nahrwold, M.D., professor of surgery at Northwestern University Medical School in Chicago, in the Archives of Surgery.

But Frederick Greene, M.D., president of SAGES, believes that the reported complications in New York State represent "no reason to retrench [from the procedure] on a national basis."

"Each individual region and hospital must do their own quality assurance. If they find something, they can institute their own remedial action," said Dr. Greene, who is professor of surgery at the University of South Carolina at Columbia.

A recent prospective SAGES study of 1,771 laparoscopic cholecystectomies at 22 centers documented four bile duct injuries. A switch to an open procedure was required in 4.6% of patients.

By comparison, a review of open cholecystectomy at Cedars-Sinai Medical Center in Los Angeles revealed two ductal injuries in 1,200 procedures. Wound complications, which followed open procedures, would be expected less frequently after laparoscopic surgery, wrote George Berci, M.D., and his colleagues in the same issue of Archives of Surgery.

Injuries to the aorta, vena cava, iliac arteries, bladder, stomach, liver, colon and small intestines have all been documented.

Such injuries tend to occur either when trochars or other instruments are introduced into the abdominal cavity, or during manipulation of tissues around the gallbladder, Harvey Bernard, M.D., a surgical consultant in the Food and Drug Administration's Division of Health Care Surveillance and Standards said.

Calls to several state health departments in the midwestern and western United States revealed no programs to track

adverse effects relative to laparoscopic cholecystectomy. According to a spokesperson for the Food and Drug Administration, the only reports they receive are those relating to problems that occur because of a malfunctioning device.

New York State may be in a unique position to provide early warning of a more widespread problem with a procedure. Since 1985, the state has required hospitals to report and investigate any deaths or injuries (such as anesthesia deaths, falls or surgical mishaps) unrelated to the natural course of illness or treatment.

New York's probe began last year after a patient died during a laparoscopic cholecystectomy when the surgeon unintentionally perforated the aorta while inserting a trochar.

"To my knowledge, nobody has ever injured the aorta doing an open cholecystectomy," said Dr. Bernard.

A review of records showed that the problem of unintentional injuries and deaths is widespread. "There are some complications that are considerably increased over what we've seen previously with open cholecystectomy," said Dr. Bernard.

Injuries that occur during laparoscopic cholecystectomy usually necessitate repair via an open procedure, he said. "An injury to the common bile duct is difficult to repair, and is one likely to be followed by bad results even in the best of hands."

The New York State Health Department plans to issue an advisory to hospitals warning them about the types of injuries being observed, and encouraging greater oversight by surgeons.

Baboon transplant may help open xenograft era

By Marjorie Shaffer

NEW YORK, JUNE 28—The transplantation of a baboon liver into a 35-year-old man who had been dying of hepatitis brings closer the day when the acute shortage of human donor organs will be alleviated by xenografts, according to transplant surgeons.

At presstime, the unnamed recipient of the baboon liver was listed in serious condition at the University of Pittsburgh Medical Center, where a team of surgeons led by Thomas Starzl, M.D., performed the marathon operation on June 28.

"The patient is off the ventilator and is breathing on his own. The doctors are pleased with his progress, and there are no signs as yet of infection or rejection," said a University of Pittsburgh Medical Center spokesperson.

Transplant specialists said that a number of groups around the world are eagerly awaiting the long-term outcome of the surgery and are ready to move forward with their own experimental procedures.

"This is on the precipice of developing in a number of different organs," said Robert Michler, M.D., director of pediatric cardiac surgery and cardiac transplant research at Columbia-Presbyterian Medical Center in New York. The next most likely step is "the transplantation of a nonhuman primate heart into a desperately ill cardiac patient," Dr. Michler said.

In the last three decades, surgeons have tried 27 times to transplant organs from chimpanzees, monkeys and baboons into a human, but the longest a patient with a xenograft has survived is nine months.

The Pittsburgh operation marks the first time an attempt has been made to transplant a baboon liver into a human.

Due to advances in immunosuppressive therapy, especially the experimental drug FK-506 that the Pittsburgh team is using, transplant experts are hoping the biggest stumbling block to xenografts—rejection by the immune system—will be overcome.

"It is best to have a human organ, but unfortunately there are not enough to go around, and the problem will only get worse," said Ronald Ferguson, M.D., director of transplantation surgery at Ohio State University in Columbus.

"I give Dr. Starzl a great deal of credit for pushing forward with [the transplant] at this time," said Dr. Ferguson.

Nearly 40,000 Americans were waiting for an organ transplant last year, and only 16,012 received a transplant of a heart, kidney, liver, pancreas or heart and lung, according to the United Network of Organ Sharing, a private, nonprofit organization that operates a national system for organ transplants.

Of those waiting for an organ, 2,518 died last year, according to UNOS.

Unless more human donor organs become available (even under the best circumstances, experts say the need will far outpace the demand), the only way to save patients is by transplanting an animal organ or developing artificial organs.

Despite optimism about the Pittsburgh operation, experts are skeptical about the future use of baboons as a source of donor organs. Dr. Ferguson said that it is not simply a matter of collecting baboons from the wild, because the animals could harbor viruses that would endanger humans.

There are only a few hundred baboons currently available from research foundations for possible xenograft surgery, he said.

Many experts are looking to pigs to provide a plentiful supply of donor organs, because pig organs are the right size and the animals can be "genetically engineered" with human genes more easily than nonhuman primate species, said Dr. Ferguson.

By introducing human genes into the xenografts, the risks of organ rejection could be drastically reduced. Thus, the need for long-term immunosuppressives and their attendant side effects may be eliminated.

A group in England is reportedly breeding genetically engineered pigs carrying parts of human genes to provide organs for human transplant operations. And Dr. Ferguson said that a number of centers in the United States are contemplating the same approach.

However, he warned that there are many obstacles ahead, and scientists are still unsure "how to pick out the proper human genes."

While some progress has been made in the development of artificial organs, "the most useful treatment for end-stage organ failure is still organ transplantation," said Yukihiko Nosé, M.D., professor of surgery at Baylor College of Medicine.

Artificial devices are currently used extensively as "bridges" to maintain patients while they wait for transplant, said Dr. Nosé, a leading researcher in artificial liver devices.

Ultimately, artificial organs will provide the best chance at long-term survival for patients, Dr. Nosé said. "All of the immunosuppressive drugs have side effects because they affect the entire body and there is always some risk of rejection."

National Institutes of Health panel gives clean bill of health to laparoscopic cholecystectomy

By Fran Kritz

BETHESDA, MD., SEPT. 16—An expert panel convened by the National Institutes of Health concluded that laparoscopic cholecystectomy is safe and effective.

The panel, made up of surgeons, gastroenterologists, internists and other healthcare professionals, conducted an exhaustive review of the procedure in the wake of reports linking it with injury and death.

The panel recommended the development of guidelines for training and authorizing doctors to use the technique. But it did not spell out what it thought was adequate training or experience. Nor did the panel advise what patients should ask when contemplating undergoing the procedure.

It did call for additional long-term data and for various specialty boards, including the American College of Surgeons, to join together to develop guidelines quickly.

New York State recently issued its own guidelines after a state panel reported that at least six deaths had been linked to complications from the procedure. The most common complication was severed bile ducts.

The New York guidelines recommend that doctors assist in the surgery at least 10 times and perform it under the supervision of another surgeon at least 15 times before doing it independently. New York officials say the guidelines are meant for all endoscopic procedures.

Chairperson of the NIH panel, John Gollan, M.D., director of the gastroenterology division at Brigham and Women's Hospital in Boston, Mass., said the 10- to 15-procedure training period is a good national goal to shoot for.

Most of the laparoscopic cholecystectomy injuries have been in people whose procedures were performed by surgeons who had performed fewer than 10 procedures. That was the case in New York and in a study at Duke University Medical Center, Durham, N.C., which found similar results. That study of 10 patients referred to Duke with bile duct injuries suffered during laparoscopic cholecystectomy found that in every case, the surgeon responsible had performed fewer than 12 procedures. Since its introduction in the United States in 1988, the number of laparoscopic cholecystectomies has risen dramatically. About 80% of the 500,000 gallbladder surgeries done each year now are performed laparoscopically. About 15,000 U.S. surgeons now perform the operation.

The procedure cuts in-hospital recovery time from a week to about three days and at-home recovery time from three to four weeks to a few days.

Because the significant reductions in pain and recovery time were widely reported in the general media, some experts believe patient pressure spurred the rapid growth of the procedure.

But most experts on the panel backed the procedure. "Why should we traumatize the skin and muscles when all we want is the gallbladder?" asked Dr. Gollan.

Despite its approval of the procedure, the panel reached the conclusion that laparoscopic cholecystectomy not be done as a preventive measure for persons with gallstones but who have no symptoms, "so as not to risk unnecessary complications that any surgery may cause," said Joanne

A. P. Wilson, M.D., an associate professor of medicine at Duke University Medical Center.

The panel also said the new procedure is not appropriate for people with peritonitis, pancreatitis, end-stage cirrhosis of the liver or gallbladder cancer, nor for women in their third trimester of pregnancy, since the procedure could injure the fetus.

In two days of presentations, physicians and surgeons noted that mortality rates from laparoscopic and open cholecystectomy are well under 1%.

Complication rates range from 4% to 8% in the open procedure, perhaps because candidates for this procedure have more severely diseased gallbladders and other complications, and 2% to 5% in the laparoscopic technique.

At the consensus meeting, Keith Kelly, M.D., chairman of the department of surgery at the Mayo Clinic, said the procedure should be done only by board-certified general surgeons, who can switch to an open procedure should excessive bleeding occur during a laparoscopic cholecystectomy. Excessive bleeding occurs in about 5% of laparoscopic procedures, he said.

Potent immunosuppressive agent broadens transplant vista to include multivisceral operations

By Caroline Helwick

NEW ORLEANS, OCT. 13—The potent immunosuppressive FK-506 has broadened the transplant surgeon's scope to include even the most complex "multivisceral" operations, a University of Pittsburgh transplant team reported at the annual meeting of the American College of Surgeons here.

The team recently transplanted a baboon liver into a 35-year-old patient given FK-506 to prevent organ rejection. The man lived for 71 days. But Thomas Starzl, M.D., professor of surgery and director of the Transplant Institute at the University of Pittsburgh, said intestinal transplants are just as impressive.

"It's a spectacular achievement," he said. "A year or two ago these were not being done. Suddenly, they've become routine here."

Andreas Tzakis, M.D., associate professor of surgery, reported excellent results in adults and children who have received intestinal transplants since May 1990. About half the patients received cadaver donor intestine along with a donor liver.

Most other cases involved "solitary grafts" of intestine only, but several patients received "multivisceral" transplants, in which a cluster of intra-abdominal organs—liver, stomach, pancreas, spleen and colon—is transplanted together, hanging from a central arterial stem.

Half of the 29 organ recipients were children with congenital or neonatal defects. Adult recipients had vascular disease, Crohn's disease, trauma injuries or benign tumors.

Twenty-four patients have survived since May 1990: 10

of 14 pediatric patients and 14 of 15 adults. Three of the five deaths were due to sepsis, one to lymphoproliferative disease caused by immunosuppression and one patient died from organ rejection, reported Satoru Todo, M.D., associate professor of surgery at the university.

Before transplant, all patients were fed intravenously, but after transplant most have been able to take food orally and maintain weight, although children are often reluctant to eat, Dr. Todo said.

"This is a great treatment for patients who would otherwise die from short bowel syndrome or intractable intestinal failure secondary to Crohn's disease," he said.

Side effects of FK-506 included renal and neurotoxicity, he said.

Charles O. Elson, M.D., professor of medicine, division of gastroenterology, University of Alabama at Birmingham, said the transplants are a viable treatment approach for the small number of patients with inflammatory bowel disease who have failed to respond to conventional therapy. Without transplantation, he said, such patients become completely dependent on parenteral feeding.

He stressed, however, that most Crohn's patients don't need such an aggressive approach. "It's a focal, segmented disease; treatment has gravitated to limited resections that conserve as much bowel as possible, or stricturoplasty, where the intestinal narrowing is cut open and the bowel re-anastomized.

"Since these approaches have been adopted, we don't see many patients developing short bowel syndrome," said Dr. Elson.

Notes

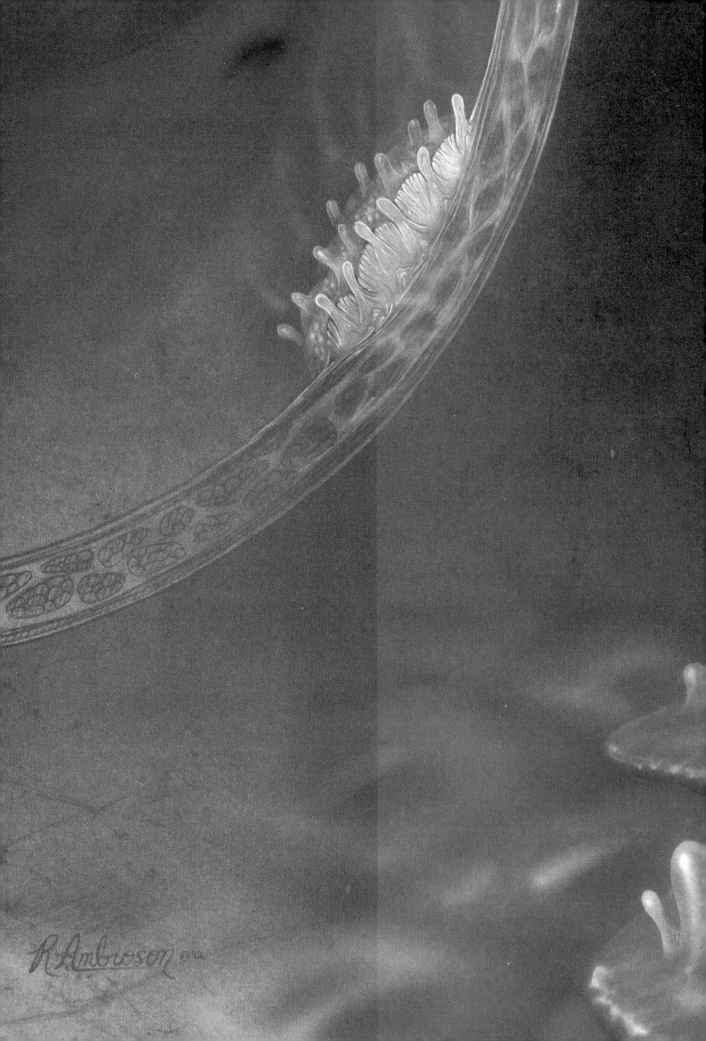

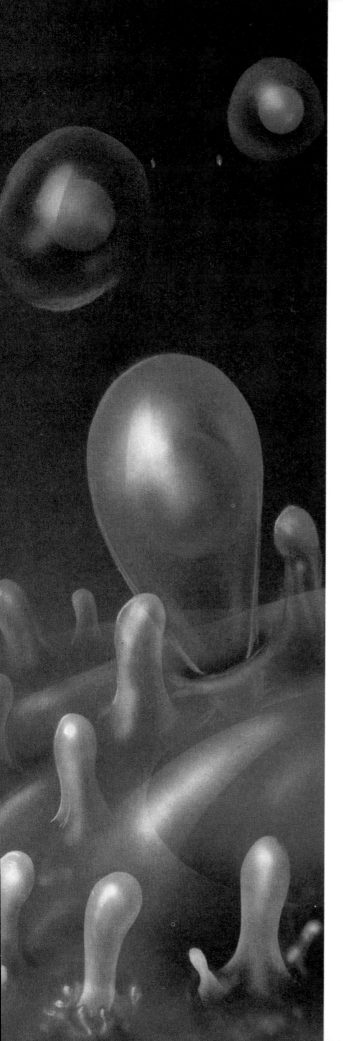

Oncology

Overview 222
Despite diagnostic and preventive strides, war on cancer is far from won

Month-at-a-glance 224

Reported at the Time 236
Drug news: more patients to get taxol; meta-analysis finds tamoxifen improves survival, but do benefits outweigh risks?...cancer strides challenged as spurious...vasectomy tie to cancer rebutted...PSA plus ultrasound favored for prostate exam...late-cycle mastectomies reduce recurrences...genetic test for colon cancer...monoclonal "bullet" curbs T-cell leukemia...mammography debated...new breast-screening reminders...umbilical-cord blood could supplant grafts for leukemia

Commentary 247
Molecular biology is wave of future
By David S. Ettinger, M.D.

Despite diagnostic and preventive strides, war on cancer is far from won

Mammography continued to be an underused method of detecting breast cancer, and the test became even more controversial after reports from the Canadian Breast Screening Study were published.

As successful treatments for many cancers continued to elude researchers and clinicians in 1992, prevention and early detection of these diseases became an even more important goal. Some scientists voiced the hope that by stopping early cancers or preventing them altogether, major neoplasia can be reined in. Others, however, noted that there is still a long way to go.

A healthy diet, regular cancer-screening tests and drugs used to treat late-stage cancer were proposed and reproposed as ways to inhibit cancer formation in its early stages.

Cancer screening moved forward with new studies of tests for colorectal and other cancers. Johns Hopkins University researchers in Baltimore announced that they have devised a genetic test that detects the mutant gene *ras* in stool samples. *Ras* is found in about 40% of people with colorectal cancer.

The prostate-specific antigen test, combined with a digital rectal exam, proved successful in detecting most cases of prostate cancer early, in studies at Washington University in St. Louis (see Urology, p. 175). Some urologists questioned any mass PSA screening of men over 50, however, saying that the test cannot distinguish between cancers that are likely to spread and those that will remain indolent.

Also this year, statistics from the Centers for Disease Control revealed that more than 42% of cervical-cancer deaths occurred in women over age 65, highlighting the need for routine Pap-test screening of elderly women.

Mammography continued to be an underused method of detecting breast cancer—some women say they cannot afford the test (up to $125), or that they fear the pain they believe it causes—and the test became more controversial after partial

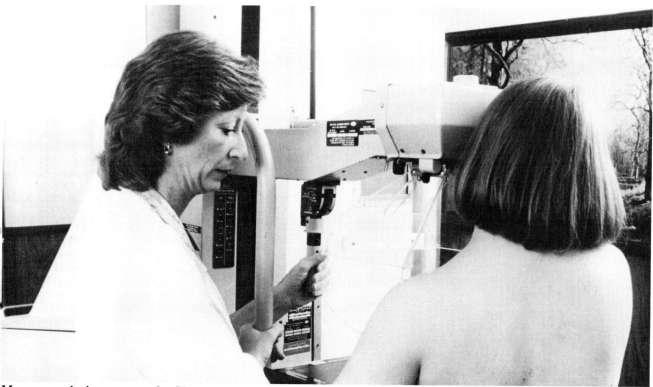

Mammography in women under 50 remains controversial, with pro and con studies clashing.

results of the Canadian Breast Screening Study were published in the lay media.

Initial reports said the Canadian study, led by the University of Toronto, found that women aged 40 to 49 were significantly more likely to die of breast cancer if they had mammograms than if they had only physical examinations. Those first reports are no longer valid, but when the study was published in November it showed no decrease in mortality rates with mammography in these younger women. The study authors used the findings to recommend against screening mammograms for women under the age of 50. But several U.S. radiologists said that the study's design and equipment flaws cast doubt on its results, and the American Cancer Society continues to recommend screening mammograms every one to two years for women, starting at age 40 and continuing up to age 49.

The benefit of mammograms for older women was not disputed in the study, even though mortality rates were not reduced in early follow-up, and in 1992, several agencies discussed methods of encouraging women to undergo the testing in accordance with ACS frequency guidelines.

The H. Lee Moffitt Cancer Center in Tampa, Fla., found that a small plastic card showing the date of the next appointment and stored in the wallet nearly doubled the percentage of women who returned for a second mammogram.

And at the ACS's National Conference on Cancer Prevention and Early Detection, computer programs were discussed that reminded both patients and physicians when mammograms and other cancer-screening tests were needed. One program generated a pamphlet and reminder postcard to mail to patients who missed their testing appointments, dramatical-

ly improving compliance with cancer screening, according to one physician.

With advances in detection, prevention and treatment came a paradoxical finding: The number of new cancer diagnoses cases is rising, due in part to early detection. Since 1950 the cervical cancer incidence has increased by 44%, according to one expert.

The prevention of cancer, particularly in high-risk women, also became the focus of a new trial of tamoxifen. Announced in April, the study is slated to enroll 16,000 healthy women at 270 medical centers across the country who are either over the age of 60 or are otherwise at high risk of the disease.

At the beginning of the year, a worldwide meta-analysis showed improved survival for thousands of women with early breast cancer who were treated with tamoxifen. Ten-year survival was 59% for women taking tamoxifen, compared with 53% for those in a control group.

Doctors now believe that tamoxifen may help prevent cancer. But at a congressional hearing later in the year, some experts testified that not enough is known about the drug's side effects to justify giving it to healthy women.

Apart from cancer prevention, physicians continue to study new therapies for treating early and later-stage disease. Taxol, the drug made from the bark of the Pacific yew tree, was studied on its own and in combination with other therapies for treating cancer. In November, an advisory committee recommended its approval for women whose ovarian cancer did not respond to standard chemotherapy. And because of the drug's scarcity, laboratories raced to develop a synthetic version so that more women might have access to the treatment.

Oncology

Jan. 1

Women told the Texas Breast Screening Project that concern about cost and lack of physician referral were the top reasons they had failed to receive mammography. In a survey of 36,000 women published in Cancer, 95% of women had had at least one clinical breast exam, but fewer than one third had had mammography prior to participating in the American Cancer Society's low-cost mammography program.

Jan. 4

Tamoxifen (Nolvadex, ICI Pharma) improved survival for thousands of women with early breast cancer, according to a worldwide meta-analysis of 75,000 women randomized to various systemic treatments. Ten-year survival was 59% for women receiving tamoxifen and 53% for controls. For women aged 50-69, standard chemotherapy plus tamoxifen beat standard chemotherapy alone in lowering the risk of recurrence and mortality, the Early Breast Cancer Trialists' Collaborative Group reported in The Lancet.

Jan. 11

British researchers reported that adjuvant ovarian ablation may be effective in the treatment of premenopausal women with breast cancer. A review of trials in which about 3,000 women were randomized to ovarian ablation revealed a reduction in the annual death rate of about 25%, similar to that associated with adjuvant polychemotherapy, the Early Breast Cancer Trialists' Collaborative Group stated in The Lancet. The reduction in annual mortality persisted even after 10-year follow-up.

Jan. 13

The American Cancer Society revealed that the number of new cancer cases in the United States is rising, partly because of earlier detection of the disease. An estimated 1,130,000 new cancer cases will be diagnosed in 1992, compared with 1,100,000 in 1991, according to the ACS.

Jan. 16

A Food and Drug Administration advisory panel recommended approval of a genetically engineered imaging agent for the detection of recurrent ovarian and colorectal cancers. The genetically altered antibodies (Oncoscint, Cytogen Corp.) are linked to radioactive particles and injected into the bloodstream, where they travel to the tumor site and can be detected with X-ray. In studies submitted to the FDA, Oncoscint identified colorectal cancers in 95% of cases and ovarian cancer in 70% of cases, aiding oncologists in staging tumors and perhaps avoiding "second look" surgery in some patients.

•••

New York City specialists determined that fewer than 60% of patients with acute myelogenous leukemia who are candidates for allogeneic bone-marrow transplantation actually receive the procedure. A review of 350 cases revealed that the procedure was frequently abandoned because of primary refractory disease, short complete remission, patient refusal and lack of a suitable donor, the Memorial Sloan-Kettering Cancer Center team stated in The New England Journal of Medicine.

Jan. 17

Among men, the death rate for malignant melanoma increased faster than for any other cancer from 1973 through 1988, according to statistics released by the Centers for Disease Control. During the 15-year period, the rate increased 50% among men, compared with 21% for women. Reasons for the difference: Men are less likely than women to use sunscreen or to examine themselves for lesions and are more likely to develop lesions on their backs, where self-detection is difficult, said the CDC.

•••

CDC statistics also revealed that more than 42% of cervical-cancer deaths occurred in women over the age of 65, highlighting the need for routine Pap tests in elderly women.

Physicians must correct the misconception that older women no longer need routine Pap tests because they are no longer sexually active or are beyond their childbearing years, commented a specialist at the Mayo Clinic in Rochester, Minn.

Jan. 25

An analysis of the cause of death in 95,217 British workers at nuclear facilities revealed an increased risk of death from cancer, particularly leukemia (excluding chronic lymphatic leukemia) and multiple myeloma. Death rates were positively associated with the quantity of radiation exposure, leading the researchers to conclude, in the British Medical Journal, that long-term low-level radiation increases the risk of all cancers. Although previous smaller studies have suggested a connection between low-level radiation and prostate cancer, this National Radiological Protection Board analysis found no evidence for such a link.

Jan. 27

Experts convened by the National Institutes of Health concurred that confusion exists within the medical community as to what constitutes the early stages of melanoma. With multiple terms for defining moles, lesions and cancerous cells leading to ambiguity, early melanoma may be overlooked, contributing to the 6,500 deaths due to the cancer each year.

The use of epiluminescence microscopy can improve diagnosis by up to 40%, said a specialist at New York University. He added that although his institution has the highest rate of melanoma detection in the United States, it is still only 62%.

Jan. 29

Radiation plus taxol may be more effective than taxol (Bristol-Myers Squibb) alone in destroying cancerous cells, researchers announced at a meeting of the Israel Cancer Research Fund. The first clinical trial combining taxol, which is derived from yew-tree bark, and radiation for women with advanced inoperable breast cancer is now planned at Columbia-Presbyterian Medical Center in New York.

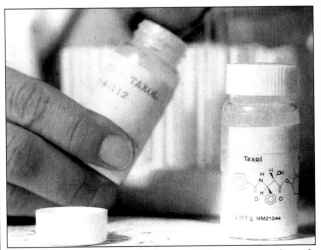

Trial of taxol plus radiation for inoperable breast cancer planned.

Oncology

Feb. 1

Patients with relapsed Hodgkin's disease recovered faster from chemotherapy and bone-marrow transplantation when they also received granulocyte macrophage colony-stimulating factor, said New York City researchers. Twelve Memorial Sloan-Kettering Cancer Center patients who

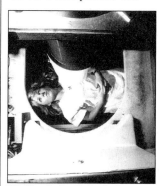

Likelihood of radiation for breast cancer found to depend on locale.

received GM-CSF spent less time in the hospital, required fewer transfusions of platelets and had shorter periods of neutropenia than 12 patients receiving a placebo adjunct to high-dose chemotherapy and bone-marrow transplantation. According to a report in the Annals of Internal Medicine, in-hospital charges for the patients on GM-CSF were dramatically lower, averaging $39,800, compared with $62,500 for the placebo group.

Feb. 4

Sixty experts in public health and oncology charged that the government and the American Cancer Society misled the public with repeated claims that we are winning the war on cancer. The group, including several former senior government officials, reminded a Washington audience that in 1960, cancer affected an estimated one in four Americans and killed one in five. Today, one in three Americans is getting cancer, and one in four is dying of it. The ACS and the National Cancer Institute were criticized for emphasizing cancer's relationship to

personal habits, such as smoking and dietary fat, while ignoring the causal role of avoidable environmental carcinogens.

Feb. 12

Despite the availability of effective prophylaxis, Pneumocystis carinii pneumonia continues to afflict patients with neoplastic disease, stated New York researchers. A 12-year review of cancer patients at Memorial Sloan-Kettering Cancer Center identified 142 cases of P. carinii pneumonia; of these, 87 had used corticosteroids, a known predisposing factor, they reported in The Journal of the American Medical Association.

The investigators thus suggested prophylactic measures for patients with solid tumors who receive corticosteroids, as well as for bone-marrow transplant recipients and any patient on steroids for more than two months.

Feb. 14

An American Cancer Society study found that where a woman lives drastically influences how her breast cancer will be treated. About 40% of women with breast cancer in New England underwent breast-conserving treatment, compared with fewer than 14% in some central and southern states. In mid-Atlantic, mountain and Pacific states, women had between a 20% and 30% chance of having breast-conserving treatment, consisting of a lumpectomy followed by radiation therapy. The study compared information on more than 41,000 women with breast cancer from 597 hospitals nationwide.

Feb. 15

Low cholesterol values predict which patients with Hodgkin's disease are at highest risk for a poor out-

come, claimed researchers from Tübingen, Germany. In an analysis of cholesterol levels at the time of diagnosis in 179 patients, those with total serum cholesterol below 140 mg/dl were 2.5 times more likely to be dead within five years than those with normal cholesterol levels. Patients with low cholesterol tended to respond poorly to therapy or relapsed sooner after remission, the investigators reported in Cancer. They suggested that provisions for intensified therapy, including bone-marrow transplantation, be made early in this high-risk group.

Feb. 17

British researchers told Medical Tribune that transfusions of umbilical-cord blood cells can generate healthy bone marrow cells in leukemia patients as effectively as bone-marrow transplants. Cord blood is readily available; thus the wait for transfusion can be as little as one week, compared with six months for a bone-marrow transplant, they said. Umbilical-cord blood cells also carry less risk of graft vs. host disease, in which transplanted cells attack the immune system of the recipient.

Feb. 19

A team at M.D. Anderson Cancer Center in Houston reported that oral retinoic acid plus subcutaneous alpha-interferon have proved valuable in the treatment of squamous cell carcinoma of the skin. Thirteen of 14 patients with advanced local disease responded to the treatment, as did four of six patients with regional disease and two of eight patients with distant metastases. Fatigue was the major limiting side effect, the team revealed in the Journal of the National Cancer Institute.

In a related development, the Houston researchers an-

nounced that the retinoic acid/alpha-interferon combination induced at least 50% tumor regression in 13 of 26 women with untreated, local advanced squamous cell carcinoma of the cervix. In both studies, treatment lasted a minimum of two months.

Feb. 20

In a study of 331 patients with inoperable non-small-cell lung cancer, cisplatin (Platinol, Bristol-Myers Oncology) plus radiation better controlled local disease and improved one- to two-year survival rates over radiation alone, researchers from the Netherlands Cancer Institute reported in The New England Journal of Medicine.

Feb. 24

Improvements in therapy of HIV infection that prolong survival are leading to in-

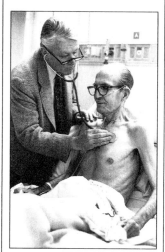

Treatment with corticosteroids can precede P. carinii pneumonia.

creases in HIV-associated lymphoma, reported researchers from the National Cancer Institute. In a study of 1,701 hemophiliac patients, 63% of whom were HIV seropositive, the incidence of non-Hodgkin's lymphoma after HIV seroconversion averaged 0.15 case per 100 person-years and rose exponentially after infection, they stated in The Journal of the American Medical Association.

Oncology

March 1

A new study of 4,665 patients with Hodgkin's disease supports the theory that radiation therapy to the mediastinum increases the risk of coronary artery disease, announced McGill University epidemiologists. The age-adjusted relative risk of death with any CAD was 1.82 after mediastinal irradiation and 1.28 after chemotherapy. Improvements in treatments for Hodgkin's disease, including the use of

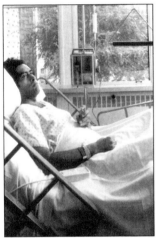

Mediastinal radiation boosts CAD risk in Hodgkin's patients.

less toxic forms of chemotherapy and lower doses of radiation, should reduce the probability of CAD, the researchers noted in Cancer.

March 6

Since reports of severe adverse reactions to silicone breast implants surfaced, women's preferences have shifted toward autologous tissue implants for breast reconstruction after mastectomy. A plastic surgeon from Emory University told a symposium on breast cancer on Long Island that more and more women are opting for $20,000 reconstruction using their own tissue from the abdomen, buttocks or back.

March 12

The human papillomavirus may be responsible for more than one quarter of penile cancers, declared Duke University researchers. The team detected HPV-16 in tumor specimens from eight of 29 patients with squamous cell carcinoma of the penis; HPV-18 was detected in one other patient. HPV was also detected in the metastatic lesions of three of six patients with more advanced disease, they reported in the International Journal of Cancer.

March 14

Cancer patients who receive psychological counseling after diagnosis feel less anxious and depressed about their disease, said researchers at the Royal Marsden Hospital in Surrey, England. The British team studied 156 people with cancer who all had been told they would live at least one year. Those who participated in brief, problem-focused, behavioral therapy reported feeling significantly less anxious, helpless, depressed and preoccupied with their disease after just two months; these feelings persisted at four months, it was reported in the British Medical Journal.

March 16

Two British cancer organizations announced they will proceed with a placebo-controlled trial of tamoxifen (Nolvadex, ICI Pharma) involving 16,000 women to assess its effectiveness in preventing breast cancer. The decision by the Imperial Cancer Research Fund and the Cancer Research Campaign was made despite withdrawal of support by the British government, which cited studies linking tamoxifen to liver cancer in rats.

March 18

The rate of brain cancer among the elderly doubled during the last 20 years, a University of Montreal study revealed. Only one fifth of the rise can be attributed to improved imaging techniques, the researchers stated in the Journal of the National Cancer Institute.

March 21

British researchers determined that contrary to earlier reports, men who have undergone a vasectomy do not face an increased risk of testicular or prostate cancer. The study of 13,246 men aged 25 to 49 years who underwent a vasectomy and 22,196 controls found no significant difference in cancer rates between the two groups, the Oxford University team reported in the British Medical Journal.

March 24

Cytologic analysis of cells in fluid aspirated from a healthy woman's nipple may help in predicting her risk of developing breast cancer, claimed University of California, San Francisco, researchers.

In a prospective study involving 2,701 nonpregnant, nonlactating women, those with abnormal cytologic findings in nipple aspirates were up to five times more likely to develop breast cancer than those with normal findings or women who produced no fluid, the team reported in the American Journal of Epidemiology. In addition, women aged 25 to 54 who produced breast fluid were almost seven times more likely to develop breast cancer than woman who did not produce fluid.

March 26

Postmenopausal women given tamoxifen (Nolvadex, ICI Pharma) to prevent breast-cancer recurrence gained a secondary benefit—better preserved bone mineral density in their lumbar spines, said University of Wisconsin researchers. Although tamoxifen blocks estrogen uptake in breast-cancer patients, it acts as an antiresorptive agent like estrogen to preserve trabecular bone, the investigators reported in The New England Journal of Medicine.

March 28

A pain specialist described dramatic success using adrenal medulla grafts to treat severe chronic pain in terminal cancer patients. Five patients with bone metastases had portions of donor adrenal medulla injected into the spinal subarachnoid space, explained the director of the pain center at the University of Illinois Hospital in Chicago. Four achieved pain relief and were able to abandon narcotics; improvement correlated with increasing levels of norepinephrine and met-enkephalin stimulated after the injections. A fifth had complete relief of pain at three weeks, which returned after reoperation for a spinal lesion, the Chicago specialist told a meeting of the American Society of Regional Anesthesia.

March 29

National Cancer Institute officials said that three times as many cancer patients will receive the experimental drug taxol (Bristol-Myers Squibb) this year, as compared with last year.

In 1992, more than 6,000 women with advanced breast or ovarian cancer are expected to receive taxol in clinical trials, an NCI director told the American Cancer Society Science Writers Seminar in St. Petersburg, Fla. Only 2,000 women received the drug last year.

In addition, 2,000 women will be able to get taxol on an individual basis through an NCI treatment referral center .

March 30

Knowing the prostate size enhances the predictive value of the prostate-specific antigen test in distinguishing between prostate cancer and benign enlargement of the gland, radiologists from St. Joseph Mercy Hospital in Ann Arbor, Mich., told an American Cancer Society seminar.

Oncology

APRIL

April 1

Waiting until the latter part of the menstrual cycle before performing mastectomy on premenopausal women could reduce the breast-cancer recurrence rate, claimed an epidemiologist at the Centers for Disease Control. In a 10-year retrospective analysis of 283 patients with primary breast cancer with positive nodes, women who underwent mastectomies during the follicular phase suffered recurrences at twice the rate of those operated on during the luteal phase, the specialist told a science writers' seminar sponsored by the American Cancer Society. Highest risk: days 7 to 14 of the cycle. Lowest risk: days 20 to 30.

• • •

Britain's Leukemia Research Fund began monitoring all new cases of cancer in children age 15 or younger living in the United Kingdom. In what they called the largest study ever to elucidate the causes of childhood cancer, the researchers said they plan to assess at least 4,000 new cases by 1997.

April 3

Johns Hopkins researchers announced that they had devised a genetic test with the potential to spot colon cancer early. The test analyzes stool samples for the presence of a mutant gene, "ras," found in about 40% of people with the cancer. The test detected the mutation in eight out of nine patients with benign or malignant colorectal neoplasms known to contain the mutation, according to the results presented in Science. No control stools were positive. It is estimated that the test, at a price under $100, could be ready for widespread use in about five years.

April 9

A leading cancer researcher announced that a new biochemical "bullet" shows promise in treating T-cell leukemia and other cancers.

Formed by fusing radioisotopes to monoclonal antibodies, the biochemical bullet achieved long-term remission in 11 of 14 patients with T-cell leukemia, a National Cancer Institute researcher told a Bristol-Myers Squibb symposium in New York.

April 13

In a new approach to gene therapy, Michigan researchers announced that they will inject liposome-wrapped

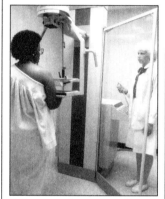

Better screening may partly explain rise in breast-cancer cases.

DNA directly into the tumor of a patient with metastatic malignant melanoma. The patient will receive injections of the gene coding for the transplantation antigen HLA-B7, with the goal of causing the patient's immune system to reject the entire tumor along with the foreign cells, the University of Michigan physicians explained.

April 15

Researchers at the National Cancer Institute warned that cigarette smoking substantially raises the risk of nasopharyngeal cancer among whites in the United States, with the risk increasing in proportion to the number of cigarettes smoked. In a case-controlled study, the risk of developing the relatively rare cancer was 50% higher among male smokers and 200% higher among female smokers, the

investigators disclosed in the Journal of the National Cancer Institute. The risk declined following cessation of smoking.

• • •

Despite concern about a possible link between cancer and electricity, a University of California physicist said there was no evidence that electricity causes leukemia or any other type of cancer. He wrote in the Proceedings of the National Academy of Sciences that an average person's exposure to low-frequency electromagnetic fields has increased 20-fold in the last 50 years, but the incidence of leukemia has not increased.

April 23

Two surveys in The New England Journal of Medicine found that lumpectomy use varied widely by state and by region of the country. The highest rates of lumpectomy were in New Jersey, New York and Pennsylvania, while Alabama, Kentucky, Mississippi and Tennessee had the lowest rates of the procedure. Larger hospitals were more likely than smaller hospitals to do the procedure, and younger women were more likely than older women to receive it.

April 25

With the most direct evidence to date, a Chinese study linked aflatoxin exposure to the development of hepatocellular carcinoma. In a prospective study of 18,244 middle-aged men in Shanghai, the presence of urinary metabolites of aflatoxin was associated with a 3.8-fold increased risk of liver cancer, the joint U.S. and Chinese research team reported in The Lancet.

• • •

Despite the widespread belief that severe stress is linked to cancer recurrence, researchers from several

hospitals in the United Kingdom reported that they found no such evidence. Of 204 female cancer patients, those who had lost a husband, child or grandchild were no more likely to have cancer recur than those who reported relatively stressless lives, the researchers wrote in The Lancet.

April 27

The rise in the incidence of breast cancer puzzled scientists at the National Cancer Institute. Breast-cancer cases, which had risen at a rate of 1% to 2% a year over the last 30 to 40 years, now are rising at the rate of 3% to 4%, reported the chief of NCI's Environmental Studies Section. While high-fat diets, delayed childbirth and better detection through mammography may partially account for the increase, other unexplained factors must be involved, she told the American College of Radiology's National Conference on Breast Cancer in Boston.

• • •

Irish researchers announced that they have identified a gene that may cause breast cancer. The gene, located on chromosome 11, is present in about 1 in 45 women, according to scientists from University College in Galway, Ireland. Of the more than 140 breast cancer patients they studied, 25% carried the gene. In contrast, none of 40 women without breast cancer had the gene, they told a press briefing in New York.

April 29

The National Cancer Institute announced the launch of a long-awaited trial of tamoxifen (Nolvadex, ICI Pharma) for the prevention of breast cancer. The trial plans to enroll 16,000 women at 270 medical centers across the country.

Researchers said they will also be looking at the potential for prevention of heart disease and osteoporosis.

Oncology

May 1

The risk of cervical intra-epithelial neoplasia increases with the number of cigarettes smoked daily, Italian researchers warned. The multi-center study of 366 patients and 323 controls also documented early age at the time of first intercourse and multiple sex partners as risk factors for CIN, the investigators reported in Cancer.

May 6

Women were told not to be concerned over an unpublished Canadian study that found that 52% more women under 50 who got mammograms died from breast cancer than women who had only a physical breast exam. American experts told Medical Tribune that the study of 90,000 women was flawed in that the screening procedures were outdated and patients were not properly randomized. However, the lead author of the study said she stood by the conclusion that mammography does not benefit younger women.

May 7

A report by the Physicians for Social Responsibility concluded that the Department of Energy's research on the health of nuclear weapons workers is seriously flawed. The report found that DOE used unreliable measurements of radiation and followed too few workers for too short a time for cancer to have developed. DOE studies found no higher than expected cancer rates among more than 600,000 workers involved in manufacturing nuclear weapons. DOE said it had not seen the report.

•••

A University of Michigan researcher announced that he had detected significantly higher concentrations of pesticides and polychlorinated biphenyls in the breast tissue of women with malignant breast tumors. When compared with samples from women with benign fibrocystic disease, he found 50% to 60% higher concentrations of PCBs in the women with cancer. The women were age-matched nonsmokers of comparable height and weight. The researcher told Medical Tribune that he would like to see a study comparing levels of suspected environmental carcinogens in women from countries with significantly different rates of breast cancer.

May 10

The prostate-specific antigen test combined with a digital rectal exam can detect most cases of prostate cancer early, a specialist told the American Urological Association meeting in Washington, D.C. In two studies of more than 17,000 men, only 27% of prostate-cancer patients screened with PSA and digital rectal exams had advanced cancers, compared with 67% of those tested with only the rectal exam, reported the Washington University School of Medicine urologist. But many other urologists questioned the value of mass screening in men over 50 with the PSA test because it is unable to distinguish between cancers that are likely to spread and those that will remain indolent.

May 11

Prostate cancer may affect more men than previously thought, reported researchers from Wayne State University in Detroit. Of 144 men aged 10 to 49 who had died of causes other than prostate cancer, 41% of those aged 40 to 49 had precancerous lesions of the prostate, as did 22% of those aged 30 to 39, they told the American Urological Association meeting in Washington, D.C.

May 12

Daily drinking can increase the risk of developing adenomas, reported University of North Carolina researchers. Unlike previous research, the new 236-patient study did not find a link between cigarette smoking and the risk of developing the condition, the team told a Digestive Disease Week meeting in San Francisco. The men in the study with the greatest risk drank at least four alcoholic drinks a day for at least seven years, the researchers said.

May 14

A four-year study of more than 37,000 postmenopausal women revealed that having a family history of breast cancer not only increases a woman's risk of developing the disease, but actually may multiply the effect of other risk factors. For example, women in the University of Minnesota study with a high waist-to-hip ratio (greater than 0.91) showed a slightly increased breast-cancer risk, but this body shape more than tripled breast-cancer risk in the subset of women who reported a first- or second-degree relative with the disease. Family history also multiplied the impact of other risk factors, including low parity, being older than 30 at the time of first pregnancy and being above average in weight and height, the team reported in The New England Journal of Medicine.

May 18

A lipid-based foam containing a chemotherapeutic drug delivered directly to the meninges vastly increased the drug's half-life and cleared some patients' cerebrospinal fluid of malignant cells, University of California at San Diego researchers announced.

The preliminary study of 12 patients found a 40-fold increase in the half-life of cytarabine (Cytosar-U, Upjohn) at doses ranging from 12.5 to 125 mg. The drug was encapsulated in the DepoFoam (DepoTech. Corp., San Diego) and injected through a surgically implanted reservoir into the lateral ventricle of the brain. Malignant cells were cleared from the cerebrospinal fluid of seven out of nine patients evaluated, reported the investigators at a meeting of the American Society of Clinical Oncology.

May 19

A small plastic card stored in the wallet nearly doubled the percentage of women who returned for a second mammogram, reported researchers at

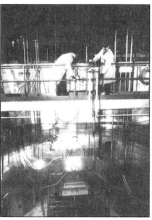

A physicians' group charged that a study on the health of nuclear workers is seriously flawed.

the H. Lee Moffitt Cancer Center in Tampa, Fla.

The credit-card-sized reminder had the date of the next mammogram engraved on it, the researchers told the American Society of Clinical Oncology meeting in San Francisco.

May 20

Megestrol acetate (Megace, Bristol-Myers Oncology) can be effective at one-tenth the commonly prescribed dose, thereby minimizing side effects such as weight gain or bloating in susceptible breast-cancer patients, a researcher from New York's Memorial Sloan-Kettering Cancer Center told the American Society of Clinical Oncology annual meeting in San Diego.

June 1

In postmenopausal women, overall obesity is associated with increased risk of breast cancer, but fat distribution—increased abdominal or central fat—is not, Dutch researchers concluded. Investigators at the University of Utrecht and Wageningen Agricultural University studied 16,355 postmenopausal women, aged 49 to 68 years, who were participants in a breast-cancer screening program. Women in the highest quartile on weight-height ratios had a 65% higher breast-cancer risk than women in the lowest quartile, the team reported in the journal Cancer, but no particular fat-distribution pattern gave an increased risk

June 5

University of Iowa researchers found that the risk of nosocomial pneumonia in patients having bone-marrow transplants was best predicted by a history of nosocomial infections, allogeneic unrelated bone-marrow transplant and the use of the anticancer agent methotrexate.

The mortality rate for 55 transplant patients with nosocomial pneumonia was 75.4%, compared with 12.7% in 55 transplant patients without pneumonia, they said.

Since preexisting nosocomial infections involve disruption of mucosal or cutaneous integrity, measures designed to preserve mucosal integrity could be a significant preventative, the investigators concluded in the journal Cancer.

June 11

Radiolabeled monoclonal antibodies aided in the detection and treatment of recurring or spreading breast cancers, two separate groups of researchers told the annual meeting of the Society of Nuclear Medicine in Los Angeles. In a study of 15 women with advanced breast cancer, the technique detected 86% of previously detected

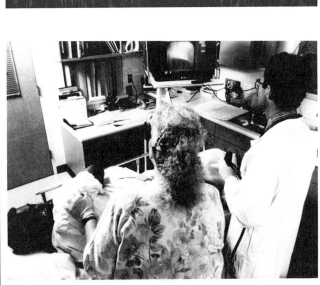

African-Americans twice as likely as whites to die of prostate cancer.

lesions, as well as five lesions that were unknown to researchers. A similar technique using a stronger radioactive substance was used by a University of California at Davis researcher to treat 11 patients who did not respond to conventional surgery and drug treatment. In four patients, tumors shrank 70% for up to five months, while in two other patients, the tumors shrank 40% for up to two months.

June 12

Using a high-tech version of the Trojan horse, National Institutes of Health scientists used gene transfer techniques to experimentally infiltrate brain cancer cells with herpesvirus and then destroy the tumors with the antiviral drug ganciclovir (Cytovene, Syntex Labs). Brain tumors regressed completely in 11 of 14 rats on which the technique was used; three had residual cancer, the team reported in Science. The NIH investigators have applied to the Food and Drug Administration for permission to test the method on humans.

• • •

Women over 40 who have two or more alcoholic drinks a day are 50% more likely to get breast cancer than women who drink less, Harvard

researchers told a meeting of the Society for Epidemiologic Research in Minneapolis. The multicenter study of nearly 14,000 women contradicted earlier findings of no link between alcohol and the cancer. Women in four states were interviewed by telephone about their diet, alcohol consumption, estrogen use and other factors.

• • •

The Centers for Disease Control reported that the rate of prostate cancer in American men has increased steadily, especially among white men, although African-Americans are twice as likely to die from the disease. From 1980 to 1988, the rate of the disease increased 30% among white men and 8% among African-Americans. During those years, death rates increased 2.5% in whites and 5.9% in African-Americans.

The rising rate of diagnosis may be due in part to greater availability of screening tests, said a CDC epidemiologist. He said the higher death rate in blacks may be due to postponement of therapy or less access to medical care.

June 15

Greek investigators warned that long-term administration of tamoxifen (Nolvadex, ICI

Pharma) can induce ocular toxicity. In a prospective study of 63 patients at the University of Ioannina, ocular toxicity occurred in four cancer patients 10 to 35 months after initiation of tamoxifen. At 20 mg/day, these patients had received a total of 6 to 21 g of the nonsteroidal antiestrogen, the team reported in Cancer.

Ocular findings included decreased visual acuity, bilateral macular edema and yellow-white dots in the paramacular and foveal areas of all patients; one developed subepithelial corneal opacities that did not reverse when tamoxifen was withdrawn.

• • •

Fluorescence in-situ hybridization may be an effective way to determine the number of ERBB2 and p53 genes in breast-cancer patients, researchers at the University of California, San Francisco, reported in the Proceedings of the National Academy of Sciences.

The method may also pinpoint which patients most need chemotherapy: Excess copies of ERBB2 are associated with a poor prognosis, and inactivation of p53 is linked with more aggressive tumors, the researchers said.

FISH relies on fluorescent genetic probes that bind to the genes in question, allowing investigators to count copies of genes within individual cancer cells.

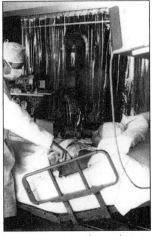

Bone-marrow transplant patients at high risk of nosocomial pneumonia.

July 1

Italian and Swiss researchers correlated approximately 8% of stomach cancers and 3% of colorectal cancers with a family history of these conditions.

In a case-control study of 628 cases of colon cancer, 456 cases of rectal cancer and 1,766 controls, the investigators found that a family history of gastric cancer more than doubled stomach cancer risk. A family history of intestinal cancer more than doubled colon cancer risk and almost doubled rectal cancer risk.

The findings suggest, but do not confirm, a genetic predisposition for the development of such cancers, the researchers concluded in the journal Cancer.

July 3

Italian researchers reported that myelotoxic agents in the environment may play a role in the genesis of acute myeloid leukemia. They studied patients with newly diagnosed AML—25 who had had prolonged contact with pesticides or organic solvents, and 34 who had not. Leukocyte count and blast cell percentage were lower for exposed patients. The clinicobiologic characteristics in the exposed patients were similar to those in patients who develop AML after chemotherapy for another tumor, suggesting that similar transformation pathways may underlie cytotoxic-drug-induced AML and AML caused by environmental exposure to some pesticides or solvents.

Conventional chemotherapy brought complete remission in one of 19 exposed patients, compared with 14 of 29 unexposed patients, researchers at the University of Ferrara reported in Cancer.

July 4

Iodine-131 treatments for hyperthyroidism or thyroid cancer did not increase the risk of leukemia among nearly 47,000 Swedish patients who were thus exposed to the ionizing radiation, Swedish and

JULY

American researchers reported. The findings suggest that those exposed to iodine-131-contaminated radioactive fallout from the 1986 Chernobyl nuclear accident in the Ukraine may not be at increased risk for cancer, the researchers wrote in The Lancet.

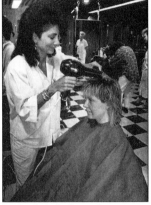

Dyeing hair dark may increase risk of non-Hodgkin's lymphoma.

July 9

Hydrocolonic sonography, a new method for detecting colon tumors, effectively spotted carcinomas and appeared less time-consuming and painful than colonoscopy, a researcher from the University of Frankfurt, Germany, reported in The New England Journal of Medicine. A prospective study of 300 patients compared the value of the water enema plus ultrasound method with conventional techniques using colonoscopy or the sonogram alone. The new hydrocolonic procedure detected 97% of carcinomas detected by colonoscopy, as well as 91% of polyps measuring at least 7 mm in diameter. However, it failed to detect 75% of polyps measuring less than 7 mm in diameter. Only 31% of carcinomas were identified with conventional sonography.

July 11

Stem cells found in human umbilical-cord blood were more plentiful and of better quality than those found in

normal bone marrow, British researchers reported in The Lancet. The Paterson Institute, Manchester, researchers said that data from long-term laboratory tests convinced them that transfusions with umbilical-cord blood were an ideal alternative to bone-marrow transplants. They pointed out that cord blood is in great supply, the procedure is painless and recipients do not have to be HLA-matched with donors.

July 13

Ten patients with cancer of the pancreas showed clinical improvement following the insertion of a new self-expanding metal stent designed to relieve malignant biliary obstruction, a Jerusalem researcher reported at the First Joint Spanish-Israeli Meeting on Liver and Biliary Diseases. The stent, composed of a nickel-titanium alloy, prevents tumor growth and can be removed endoscopically, according to its developer at Hadassah University Hospital. After the stent is inserted under guided X-rays, it can be expanded to 8 mm by tugging a thin wire on the catheter.

July 15

New York City researchers reported that while mammography often detects more local breast-cancer recurrences than physical examination, the two procedures can be complementary. In a group of women who had received conservative treatment for breast cancer, 42% of local tumor recurrences were only detectable by mammography, but another 25% would have been missed if mammography had not been supplemented by physical examination, the investigators reported in the journal Cancer.

All 42 women had undergone surgical excision, 16 had undergone axillary node dissections and five had received chemotherapy for

positive axillary nodes, according to the Memorial Sloan-Kettering team. Only 22% of women with node-negative cancer had same-site recurrences, whereas 57% of node-positive women had same-site recurrences.

July 20

Fine-needle aspiration cytology allows detection of breast cancer at a very early stage, thus offering a better prognosis for the patient, reported researchers from the Breast Clinic of Rochester in New York. The procedure also costs about one tenth that of biopsy, they pointed out in the journal Radiology. FNAC helped detect three unsuspected cancers in 222 patients with benign-appearing mammographic opacities, and eight unsuspected cancers in 2,248 symptomatic patients with clinically palpable masses and mammograms considered to be within normal limits. Although only one of every 225 nonsuspicious masses proved to be malignant, without FNAC there would have been no way to know which masses were newly surfacing carcinomas rather than benign conditions, the study reported.

July 25

Hair-coloring products were shown to be associated with over a third of non-Hodgkin's lymphomas in women who use them. Over a three-year period, National Cancer Institute researchers interviewed 583 men and women diagnosed with various types of cancer, including 385 with non-Hodgkin's lymphoma. Women who used hair-coloring products, specifically darker colors using permanent dyes, had a 50% higher risk of developing non-Hodgkin's lymphoma than women who did not color their hair, the investigators reported in the American Journal of Public Health. However, neither the NCI nor the Food and Drug Administration recommended cessation of hair-coloring use following publication of the report.

Oncology

Aug. 1

British researchers described a newly discovered mechanism of action for tamoxifen (Nolvadex, ICI Pharma). Already known to be an estrogen-receptor blocker in breast-cancer cells, tamoxifen also appears to spur healthy cells to produce a cancer cell-growth inhibitor called transforming growth factor beta 1, which targets adjacent malignant cells.

As reported in Cancer Research, tissue samples from 10 women with breast cancer were examined before and after three months of tamoxifen treatment. No growth factor was present in the samples before treatment, but it appeared in significant amounts after treatment, said investigators from the Royal Marsden Hospital in London and the U.S. National Cancer Institute. The factor is also present in normal, healthy tissue.

Aug. 3

Contrary to past reports that suggested a link between fluoridated water and bone cancer, the Food and Drug Administration found no link between water fluoridation and increased cumulative risk for bone cancer in North American or European cancer patients. FDA epidemiologists performed a statistical analysis of the cumulative risk of bone cancer in about 150 million patients, aged one to 74, enrolled in 40 cancer registries in the United States, Canada and Europe from 1958 to 1987. They found that deaths due to osteosarcoma did not increase as intake of fluoridated water increased in developed nations. Some bone metastases in the past may have been improperly coded as primary osteosarcoma, they theorized in the journal Cancer.

Aug. 5

A Milwaukee researcher found that bone-marrow transplants have not affected the relapse rate for most cases of leukemia. The marrow-transplant expert from the Medical College of Wisconsin reviewed the records of 7,788 bone-marrow transplant recipients who had acute lymphoblastic, acute myelogenous, or chronic myelogenous leukemia. While treatment-related mortality decreased from 32% in 1980 to 25% in 1988, the relapse rate remained constant at 18% for patients with early-stage disease and about 64% for those with advanced disease. Only transplant patients with intermediate stages of leukemia had a better chance of surviving in 1988, with a relapse rate of 38%, down from 46% in 1980, according to the report in The Journal of the American Medical Association.

Aug. 8

British pediatric epidemiologists cautioned that vitamin K injections to prevent hypoprothrombinemia of the newborn appear to double the risk of developing childhood leukemia by age 10. The team from the Royal Hospital for Sick Children in Bristol examined the medical records of 195 children with cancer who had been born in two major local hospitals between 1965 and 1987. About twice as many cancer patients had received vitamin K injections as those who had remained healthy, the researchers reported in the British Medical Journal. Oral vitamin K was not found to increase cancer

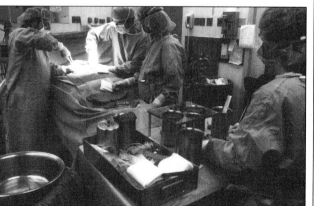

In study, marrow transplants did not reduce relapse rates appreciably.

risk; however, physicians were advised to wait for further evidence of a cancer link before substituting oral vitamin K for the injections.

Aug. 10

The Senate Subcommittee on Consumer and Environmental Affairs was told that radar guns that catch speeding motorists may cause or promote testicular, cervical, eye and brain cancers among police officers.

Scientists told the committee there is not enough evidence to conclude that the radar guns do in fact cause cancer, but said more scrutiny is needed. Officers testified that they often hold the guns in their laps, or rest them over their shoulders, exposing themselves to unshielded radiation emitted by the guns.

Aug. 12

Policies that limit but do not ban smoking in the workplace do not protect non-smoking workers from the health dangers of secondhand smoke, revealed a study in The Journal of the American Medical Association. Researchers from the University of California at San Diego and the Center for Behavioral Research in Cancer in Melbourne, Australia, analyzed data from 7,162 adult non-smokers who were asked about policies at their workplaces. Nonsmokers who worked in areas without smoking restrictions, or with limited restrictions, were more than eight times as likely to be exposed to environmental tobacco smoke than those who work at smoke-free work sites, the study found. At places that banned smoking in work areas but allowed it elsewhere, nonsmokers were about three times as likely to be exposed to passive smoke.

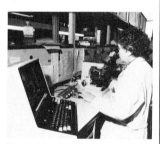

Tamoxifen found to spur cancer cell-growth inhibitors.

Aug. 20

Italian oncologists reported that adding tamoxifen (Nolvadex, ICI Pharma) to dacarbazine (DTIC-Dome, Miles Pharmaceuticals) may prolong the lives of women with disseminated malignant melanoma. However, the two-drug regimen did not increase the number of people who survived the cancer, nor did it significantly increase the lifespan of men with the disease, according to the report in The New England Journal of Medicine. The Italian Oncology Group for Clinical Research evaluated 117 patients aged 18 to 79, half of whom were randomized to receive dacarbazine alone and half to receive it in combination with tamoxifen. Among the women in the combination therapy group who lived, survival time more than doubled, from 30 weeks to 69 weeks.

In an editorial accompanying the study, University of Pennsylvania Cancer Center specialists argued that it was premature to say the combination therapy was effective.

S E P T E M B E R

Sept. 1

Computer programs to remind physicians and patients that it's time for various cancer-screening tests were discussed at the American Cancer Society's National Conference on Cancer Prevention and Early Detection in Chicago. One program for both IBM and Macintosh computers, called Check-up!, generates a report at the time of a patient visit, listing the dates of previous cancer tests

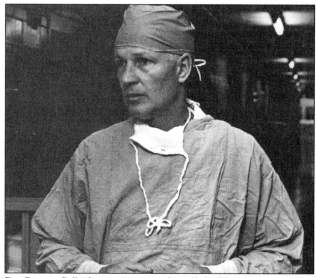

Dr. George Crile, lumpectomy catalyst, died of lung cancer at 84.

and what tests are called for based on ACS guidelines. If a patient skips an appointment, the program generates a pamphlet and postcard reminder that it's time for a test. The program dramatically improved compliance with screening, according to a physician from the University of California, San Francisco, who tested it.

Sept. 2

Female hormones appear to play a role in the development of some brain tumors, researchers at the German Cancer Research Center in Heidelberg found. The study of 127 women with meningiomas, gliomas and acoustic neuromas and 233 controls found that menopausal women had a reduced risk of developing meningiomas, especially when menopause

had been surgically induced by bilateral oophorectomy. Menopausal women were about twice as likely to develop gliomas or acoustic neuromas, except when menopause had been surgically induced. Pregnancy, and oophorectomy after menopause did not appear to influence risk of these cancers, according to data presented in the Journal of the National Cancer Institute.

Sept. 5

British researchers found that bone-marrow transplantation for children in the first remission of acute lymphoblastic leukemia is no better than chemotherapy and radiation at achieving five-year, event-free survival. Studying 183 children with ALL in first remission, they found that 69% of those who received BMT from an HLA-compatible sibling donor plus irradiation and cyclophosphamide experienced five-year, event-free survival. The rate was 52% for those who received cranial irradiation, late intensification and two years of continuous treatment, a difference that was not significant. However, significantly more treatment-related deaths

occurred in the BMT group, the researchers reported in The Lancet.

Sept. 10

The medical community mourned the death of George (Barney) Crile, Jr., M.D., the first surgeon in the United States to advocate lumpectomy. The noted surgeon and researcher performed his last radical mastectomy in 1954. Dr. Crile died of lung cancer at age 84. A graduate of Yale University and Harvard Medical School, he joined the Cleveland Clinic in 1937, where he chaired the department of general surgery from 1956 to 1968. In addition, he penned a dozen books and a humor column that appeared in Medical Tribune for two and a half years.

Sep. 11

A multicenter study began in Britain to evaluate the amount of electromagnetic radiation people are exposed to when using a cellular phone, Medical Tribune reported.

Exposure to the high-frequency radiation generated by mobile phones may amplify the effect of other carcinogens, said an expert with Britain's National Radiological Protection Board. Phones under development might work on frequencies twice as high as today's devices, he pointed out. And, because the antenna is held so close to the head, the waves of radiation can actually raise the temperature of the eyes and brain, the researcher said.

• • •

Breast-cancer surgery performed after the midpoint in the menstrual cycle may increase 10-year survival rates over surgery performed earlier in the cycle, a British team reported at the annual meeting of the Royal College of Physicians and Surgeons of Canada in Ottawa. A study of 86 premenopausal women treated for breast cancer found

that 79% who had the surgery at least 13 days after their last menstrual period were alive 10 years later, compared with 40% of women whose surgery was done between one and 12 days after their last period. Tumor size and the type of surgery did not affect survival, said the researchers from the London Regional Cancer Center.

Sept. 21

Harvard researchers launched the largest trial ever conducted on the prevention of cancer and heart disease in women. Over the next five years, investigators involved with the Women's Health Study are to examine the risks and benefits of aspirin and vitamins in preventing disease in 40,000 postmenopausal nurses. The 10-year, NIH-funded Women's Health Initiative of 140,000 women kicked off earlier this year.

Sept. 26

Jack Kevorkian, M.D., stood by as equipment he had invented was used in the suicide of a patient with lung cancer and metastases to the brain. With the approval of her general practitioner, oncologist and psychiatrist, the woman died after inhaling carbon monoxide through a masklike device. The patient, who had been told in April that she had only three months to live, reportedly found the pain of her illness intolerable.

Sept. 29

A University of California toxicologist reported that a compound found in barley leaves may be useful against skin cancer caused by sun exposure. The chemical, 2-0-G1, is an antioxidant that effectively inhibited cell damage in tests involving lipids in human skin, the toxicologist stated in the Journal of Agriculture and Food Chemistry.

He added that 2-0-G1 should have the same protective effects on lipids elsewhere in the body.

Oct. 9

University of California experts suggested that foods containing pesticides and other chemical residues that cause cancer in rodents should not be banned for human consumption. Writing in the journal Science, the Berkeley researchers said that giving large amounts of a chemical to animals in the lab may not be directly applicable to humans, whose diet contains very small amounts of the chemical. They argued that without some synthetic pesticides, fruits and vegetables would be more expensive and people would eat less of them. They suggested that more attention be paid to preventing smoking and exposure to high doses of chemicals in the workplace.

Oct. 15

Authorities warned that continuing ozone depletion is expected to cause a sharp rise in skin cancer. At a conference sponsored by the American Academy of Dermatology, an expert from the National Aeronautics and Space Administration predicted a 10% drop in atmospheric ozone in the United States and Western Europe by the year 2000. Such a drop could lead to a 10% to 20% increase in ultraviolet B rays during summer months. A Harvard University researcher added that for every 1% depletion of atmospheric ozone in this decade, melanoma incidence has gone up by 1.5%, basal-cell carcinoma by 3% and squamous-cell carcinoma by 5%.

Oct. 18

A Memphis family physician suggested that more generalists become willing to perform colonoscopies in the office or hospital to improve patient care, maintain the continuity of care and keep healthcare costs down. Speaking at the American Academy of Family Physicians annual scientific assembly in San Diego, the

OCTOBER

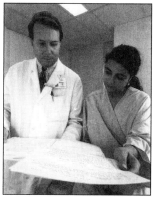

Some experts say tiny amounts of pesticides in food don't cause cancer.

University of Tennessee physician said that once more doctors become comfortable with performing the procedure in their higher-risk patients, premature death from colorectal cancer will be eradicated.

Oct. 20

Three medical groups released guidelines on which breast-cancer patients should be treated with lumpectomy instead of mastectomy.

The guidelines state that women whose breast cancer is detected by a mammogram and those with small lumps that have not spread to surrounding breast tissue should be offered breast-conserving therapy with lumpectomy, radiation, drug treatment or hormone treatment.

Even in some cases where the cancer has spread to surrounding tissue, the option might apply, according to the guidelines, cosponsored by the American Cancer Society, the American College of Surgeons and the American College of Radiology. A co-author said that at least one third of women with early breast cancer are candidates for lumpectomy.

• • •

An Ohio pain-management expert urged doctors to become more familiar with differential costs of drugs for relieving pain in cancer patients. At a meeting of the

American Society of Anesthesiologists, he said that one survey found that the monthly cost of pain relief ranged from $19 to $238 for oral opiate painkillers, based on equally potent dosages. The expert from the Arthur G. James Cancer Hospital and Research Institute in Columbus said many doctors don't know what these drugs cost. He added that some pharmacies charge far more than others for the same drugs, and that brand-name products often are three times more expensive than generic forms.

Oct. 22

A government-sponsored trial of the drug tamoxifen (Nolvadex, ICI Pharma) to prevent breast cancer in women at high risk of developing the disease may jeopardize the well-being of healthy women, critics of the study contended at a congressional hearing.

While the critics agreed that tamoxifen is a reasonable cancer treatment that produces relatively few side effects compared with other therapies, they maintained that too little is known about the drug's promise for preventing breast cancer and that the drug is too toxic to be used in healthy women. They also charged that many potential side effects have been down-

played by doctors enrolling women into the trial.

Six percent of centers have temporarily stopped enrolling patients because of such problems, and they are requiring more uniform consent procedures.

Oct. 31

A genetic test was found capable of detecting one cancer cell out of 10 million healthy cells in body fluids, British researchers reported in The Lancet. The test also distinguishes between the deadliest cancers that have spread beyond their original site and those that have not yet spread, the investigators found.

The Oxford University team took tumor tissue from 34 patients with cancer of the colon, breast or thyroid, and tissue or blood from 15 people without cancer. They then tested each sample for messenger RNA that are given instructions by the CD44 gene to synthesize various proteins located on many types of cells in the body. They found that when cancer is present, the CD44 gene produces variants of the usual messenger RNA. They found large quantities of the variants in patients with cancer but not in healthy patients.

In addition, the test distinguished between the 23 patients whose cancer had spread beyond the breast or colon from the eight whose cancer had not spread.

Uniform consent forms needed in tamoxifen trial, say critics.

NOVEMBER

Nov. 4

A new case-control study suggested that people who work in the field of auto mechanics, paint manufacturing and the rubber industry may be at increased risk of developing acute myeloid leukemia. People with AML were found to be nearly six times more likely than those without the disease to have worked at least five years in these occupations, reported researchers from the National Institute of Environmental Health Sciences in Research Triangle Park, N.C.

Further analysis of the 62 people with AML and 630 controls revealed that 10 people in the AML group had a ras oncogene mutation, according to the report in the Journal of the National Cancer Institute. Of AML patients with the mutated cancer gene, 60% had worked at least five years in a high-risk field, said the researchers. Of AML patients without the mutated gene, only 15% performed work considered high risk.

Nov. 5

Relatives of longtime smoker Rose Cipollone consented to the withdrawal of the lawsuit they had filed against the tobacco industry after her death from lung cancer. In June, the U.S. Supreme Court ruled that a 1965 federal law requiring cigarette warning labels did not shield the companies from personal injury lawsuits. However, the ruling said that smokers need to do more than prove that cigarette advertising and promotions tend to minimize the health hazards of smoking. Lawyers for the Cipollones and other cancer patients who had filed "toxic torts" against tobacco companies explained that they could no longer afford to pursue the protracted litigation.

Nov. 11

Medical facilities began to distribute a practical pain-

control brochure to cancer patients.

The pamphlet uses friendly drawings and clear, simple language to explain how pain control works, and it addresses the common fear of addiction, which often results in undertreatment. Offered by the National Council for the Right to Die, a patient advocate group in New York City, the pamphlet describes the wide range of therapies available for pain

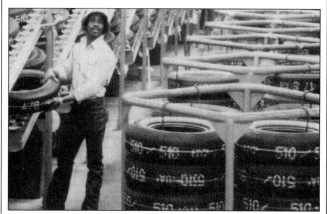

People in the rubber industry may be at increased risk of AML.

relief, including patient-controlled analgesia and at-home therapy.

The booklet also helps patients learn to describe their pain in concrete terms, so that caregivers can respond with appropriate therapy.

Nov. 13

Utah researchers announced that they may have located a gene that increases the risk for melanoma. Over a seven-year period, the investigators probed the genetic material of over 1,000 members of 10 families known to have a high rate of melanoma. In the journal Science, the Utah Medical Center group said they had pinpointed an area on chromosome 9 where they believe the gene or genes that render people vulnerable to melanoma are located.

Nov. 14

Environmental groups and medical advocacy organiza-

tions met to review the scientific literature on breast cancer and the environment. Scientific focus on causative factors in women's lifestyles—such as diet and reproductive decisions—blames the victim and ignores evidence concerning environmental contaminants, a University of Illinois College of Medicine investigator told the Greenpeace-sponsored meeting in Chicago. The discussion emphasized epidemiological and toxicological data that suggested a link between breast cancer and exposure to organochlorines, such as DDT, PCBs and dioxin.

Nov. 15

Scientists from New York's Memorial Sloan-Kettering Cancer Center announced that a differentiating agent induced complete remission in three of 41 patients with myelodysplastic syndrome or acute myelogenous leukemia. Another six patients achieved a partial remission when treated with hexamethylene bisacetamide, the investigators reported in the journal Blood.

Use of the agent represents a different approach to chemotherapy, as it works not by killing tumor cells, but by inducing the cancerous cells to differentiate and act more normally, the researchers explained.

The team also included investigators from Dana-Farber Cancer Institute in Boston and the Maine Medical Center in Portland.

Nov. 29

Japanese researchers announced that positron emission tomography imaging can delineate malignant lesions in the breast and the axillary nodes.

They administered PET plus F-18 fluorodeoxyglucose (FDG) to 21 patients with primary, metastatic or recurrent malignancies in the breast, chest wall and axillary region, and to six patients with benign lesions. Twenty of 21 malignancies showed up as an intense focal uptake of FDG, and the contrast ratios of the malignant group were significantly higher than those of the benign group, the investigators said at the annual meeting of the Radiological Society of North America in Chicago.

Nov. 30

Clinicians at teaching hospitals in Hamilton, Ontario, missed 6% of colorectal carcinomas in 257 patients, an investigator reported at the annual meeting of the Radiological Society of North America. He called the finding a "disturbingly high miss rate," and noted that standards of technique and interpretation have not improved in the last decade. The tumor was clearly visible in 93% of the missed cases, despite technical errors. Thirty-three cases were missed at barium enema and six at colonoscopy, the investigator reported.

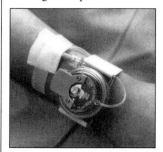

Patient-controlled analgesia described in new brochure.

DECEMBER

Dec. 2

Investigators from M.D. Anderson Cancer Center announced that a semisynthetic compound related to taxol (Bristol-Myers Squibb) showed promising antitumor activity in Phase I trials. After five consecutive days of one-hour infusions with taxotere (Rhone-Poulenc Rorer) in 39 advanced cancer patients, antitumor activity was observed in six out of 10 patients with ovarian cancer and in one with breast carcinoma, the Houston research team reported in the Journal of the National Cancer Institute. The dose-limiting side effect appeared to be granulocytopenia with oral mucositis, which developed in half of the patients on the highest taxotere dose, according to the investigators.

• • •

Chromosomal abnormalities were detected in the neoplastic cells of 23 of 28 patients with Hodgkin's disease, announced pathologists from the Cross Cancer Institute in Edmonton, Alberta. Rearrangements of the bcl-2 gene had previously been detected in up to 40% of cases of Hodgkin's disease. This study, published in the Journal of the National Cancer Institute, was the first to perform chromosomal analysis in Reed-Sternberg cells. These neoplastic cells of Hodgkin's disease generally constitute fewer than one percent of tumor cells.

Dec. 5

New York researchers announced that they had identified three antigens that are promising candidates for the construction of melanoma vaccines. Each is immunogenic in humans and preferentially expressed on melanoma, the New York University researchers told the American Academy of Dermatology meeting in San Francisco. In a study of 26 patients, the three antigens induced antibody responses in 62%, 27% and 19% of patients, respectively, the team reported.

Dec. 9

Seattle researchers reported that breast-cancer patients with poor prognostic features should receive radiation treatment within six months of their diagnosis. The University of Washington Medical Center researchers studied three groups of women: 65 women under age 50; 87 with positive axillary lymph nodes; and 53 with negative estrogen-receptor status. Patients in each group who received radiation within six months had better outcomes (improved local control, overall survival and disease-free survival) than those in whom radiation was delayed.

Although oncologists argue that chemotherapy should be maximized prior to initiating radiation, the doctors told the 15th Annual San Antonio Breast Cancer Symposium that the results of this investigation justify earlier radiation.

• • •

Breast-cancer surgeons were told that breast reconstruction performed immediately after a modified radical mastectomy is preferable to reconstruction done at a later date. Doctors from the Karolinska Hospital in Stockholm, Sweden, reported that patients who had immediate reconstruction had no greater rate of complications compared with those who had secondary breast reconstruction. The number of hospital stays and amount of time lost from work were less in the immediate surgery group, the doctors reported at the 15th Annual San Antonio Breast Cancer Symposium. The surgeons recommended that a general surgeon and a plastic surgeon operate simultaneously, to reduce operating time and complication rate.

Dec. 10

A comprehensive breast-screening center modeled after the Karolinska Hospital in Sweden has proved cost-effective and clinically advantageous in a U.S. hospital setting, its multidisciplinary team told the 15th Annual San Antonio Breast Cancer Symposium.

At the center, fine-needle aspiration and stereotaxic biopsy are available to immediately assess palpable and nonpalpable breast lesions, according to the Englewood Hospital Breast Center professionals. After diagnosis, preoperative treatment planning is initiated by a team that includes oncologists, plastic surgeons, pathologists and radiologists, the Englewood, N.J., physicians stated.

The team reported that 3,000 to 5,000 aspiration biopsies are performed at the center each year.

Dec. 16

The density of microvessels within malignant breast tumors was found to be a better prognostic indicator than axillary lymph node status, announced a pathologist from the University of California, San Francisco. In a prospective study of 165 patients, all patients with breast carcinomas having more than 100 microvessels/200x field experienced tumor recurrence within 33 months of diagnosis, compared with fewer than 5% of the patients with fewer than 34 microvessels/200x field. Among node-negative women, microvessel density was the only significant predictor of overall survival, the California researcher and an international research team reported in the Journal of the National Cancer Institute.

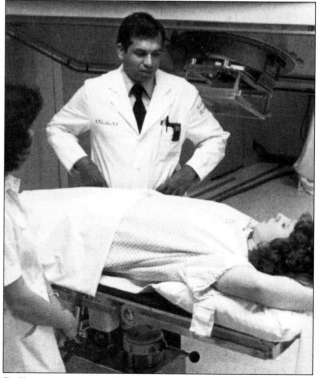

Radiation treatment within six months of diagnosis can benefit breast-cancer patients with poor prognostic features.

Meta-analysis finds that tamoxifen aids survival

JAN. 4—A meta-analysis of adjuvant therapy for early breast cancer in 74,652 women has confirmed that tamoxifen or chemotherapy may improve survival.

The Lancet analysis found that 59% of women who received tamoxifen (Nolvadex, ICI Pharma) were alive 10 years later, compared with 53% of controls. Ten years after polychemotherapy, 51% of patients were alive, versus 45% of controls.

Aman Buzdar, M.D., of the M.D. Anderson Cancer Center in Houston, pointed out some of the analysis' shortcomings.

The researchers found a 30%-40% reduction in mortality risk among middle-aged women who received combined chemo-endocrine regimens. "That was the softest data, because it was based on indirect comparisons," according to Dr. Buzdar.

As for chemotherapy, "in early breast cancer, I still have reservations about using it across the board," he added. Prognostic factors must be examined closely so that costs and benefits of chemotherapy can be weighed carefully, he said.

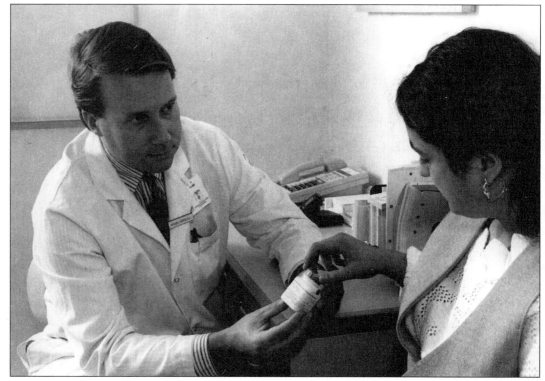

Fifty-nine percent of women given tamoxifen were alive 10 years later, vs. 53% of controls.

Cancer 'strides' challenged as spurious

By Bill Ingram

WASHINGTON, D.C., FEB. 4—A bitter debate has broken out, focusing on whether or not the seemingly relentless advance of cancer is being slowed. As it turns out, cancer officials themselves are divided on some of the issues.

An estimated 1.3 million new cases are expected this year, up from 1.1 million last year. Deaths are projected at 520,000, up from 514,000 last year.

At a press conference here, 60 physicians and scientists charged that even in the face of these discouraging data, the "cancer establishment confuses the public with repeated claims that we are winning the war...."

"Our ability to treat and cure most cancers has not materially improved," said the group of 60, led by Samuel Epstein, M.D., professor of occupational and environmental medicine at the University of Illinois.

Since 1950, the overall cancer incidence has increased by 44%, breast cancer and male colon cancer by 60% and prostate cancer by 100%, according to Dr. Epstein.

"For decades, the five-year survival rate for nonlocalized breast cancer has remained at 18%, and for lung cancer, 13%," he said.

The National Cancer Institute and the American Cancer Society were accused of "largely attributing [rising rates] to smoking and dietary fat, while discounting or ignoring the causal role of avoidable exposures to industrial carcinogens in air, food, water and the workplace."

Prevention studies and initiatives languish, Dr. Epstein charged: they are allotted only 5% of the $1.8-billion NCI budget. "Millions have died from what should be a preventable disease."

The ACS and NCI hit back hard at the charges.

"Dr. Epstein is irresponsible. He's hollering fire in a crowded theater where there's no fire," said John Laszlo, M.D., ACS senior vice president for research. "His claims about carcinogens in the air, for example: that's been looked at scientifically. There's no evidence to suggest a cancer cause there.

"Recent increases in rates are largely due to early detection—picking up cases this year that in the past would have been picked up three or four years later," Dr. Laszlo said. "And we're making treatment progress. With breast cancer, there are more cases, but the death rate remains the same. Adjuvant chemotherapy and tamoxifen constitute major advances that are just now starting to affect the statistics."

"Have we won the war? No," declared Richard Adamson, Ph.D., NCI chief of cancer etiology. "Have we made progress? Yes, particularly with childhood cancers, testicular cancer and Hodgkin's. The death rates for colon and rectal cancer have fallen 15 to 20% in the last two decades; ovarian has fallen 20%, bladder 30% and cancer of the cervix, 40%."

"The male death rate for lung cancer is now almost flat," said Clark Heath, M.D., ACS vice president for epidemiology.

On the issue of life-style factors, ACS president Walter Lawrence, M.D., reiterated the very etiologic assessment that Dr. Epstein had attacked. He insisted that "two thirds to three quarters of cancers are due to external things we might modify, such as tobacco and diet."

Drs. Heath and Laszlo would not go along with their superior, conceding a point to Dr. Epstein and the group of 60.

"I'm uncomfortable with those figures," said Dr. Heath. "I'm not uncomfortable with attributing 30% of cancer deaths to smoking, but those overall figures are pretty darned soft."

"I agree with Clark Heath," said Dr. Laszlo.

NCI's Dr. Adamson was also dubious. To reach the 75% figure, he said, "all environmental factors would probably have to be included—viruses, synthetic chemicals, radiation, fibers and so on, and I'm not sure you could modify all these factors."

The group of 60 also leveled the charge that the cancer establishment has "repeatedly grossly exaggerated their ability to treat and cure cancer. Claims [for drugs] are generally based on...[initial] tumor response rather than on prolongation of survival."

When asked, Dr. Epstein cited interferon and interleukin as examples.

Dr. Laszlo agreed that exaggeration is not uncommon. "People are not always objective," he said. "I object to exaggerations. I'm never happy when I see early reports like those on interleukin-2."

"There's a long list [of drugs] involving overexpectation," said Dr. Heath.

Though conceding these points, cancer officials were adamant about cancer-prevention efforts.

"In the coming year we will be spending not 5%, as Dr. Epstein maintains, but 33% of our $597-million budget on causation and prevention-related research—more than we spend on treatment," Dr. Adamson said. "We agree that occupational and environmental factors need serious consideration. We have 65 studies going in occupational groups."

"Whole environment factors" under NCI scrutiny, Dr. Adamson said, include chemicals and radiation, plus host factors—hormone levels, immunologic status and individual genetic endowment.

"Dr. Epstein says we should study substances in fat," the NCI official said. "We have. Halogenated pesticides, for example, have not been found elevated in breast cancer [patients], as compared with those with benign breast disease.

"Dr. Epstein doesn't even mention heterocyclic amines, which occur in cooking meat, poultry and fish at high temperatures and are among the most potent carcinogens known. We're studying them," Dr. Adamson said.

Counseling may ease anxiety of cancer

SURREY, ENGLAND, MARCH 14—Cancer patients who receive psychological counseling feel less anxious and depressed about their disease, according to British researchers at the Royal Marsden Hospital here.

An American psychiatrist supported the finding, saying support groups and patient networks can improve the quality of life for those stricken with cancer.

Psychiatrist Steven Greer, M.D., reported his findings in the British Medical Journal.

The British investigator studied 156 people diagnosed with cancer who all had been given at least one year to live.

After two months of psychotherapy, those who received counseling reported feeling significantly less anxious, helpless,

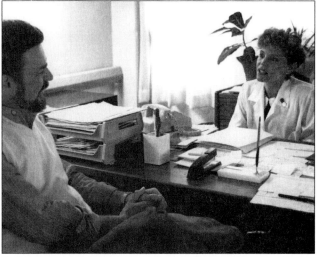

Support groups, patient networks and counseling may help mitigate depression in patients stricken with cancer.

depressed and preoccupied with their disease, according to Dr. Greer. They also showed more "fighting spirit," he added.

After four months of therapy, patients receiving counseling continued to report feeling less stress and anxiety than those who did not undergo counseling, he wrote.

"I'm delighted that we're getting good documentation that psychological counseling helps cancer patients," said Karen Ritchie, M.D., chief of the psychiatry section of the University of Texas M.D. Anderson Cancer Center in Houston. "We've suspected this for a while."

Patients at the Houston cancer facility can join support groups or patient-to-patient networks, according to Dr. Ritchie.

"People can do grieving work in therapy," she said.

"Grieving is frustrating if you can't do it. The patients can also learn coping skills."

Meeting other cancer patients in support groups also can lessen anxiety and bolster spirits, she said. "You realize you're not alone."

Too few studies have been done to conclude that psychological counseling improves the survival of cancer patients, according to Bernard Fox, Ph.D., professor of psychiatry at the Boston University School of Medicine.

But therapy may help ease anxiety and depression, according to Dr. Fox.

Vasectomy tie to cancer contradicted by study

OXFORD, ENGLAND, MARCH 21—Men who have undergone a vasectomy do not face an increased risk for testicular or prostate cancer, as some earlier research had shown, according to a study by British researchers.

Michael Goldacre, M.D., and colleagues at Oxford University compared 13,246 British men aged 25 to 49 years who underwent a vasectomy between 1970 and 1986 with 22,196 subjects who did not have the procedure. The investigators found there was no significant difference in rates of the cancers between the two groups of men.

The vasectomy findings were published in the British Medical Journal.

Although no biological reason for an increased risk of testicular cancer following a vasectomy has been identified, physicians became concerned when a Scottish study found a link between the two, according to Curtis Mettlin, Ph.D., chief of epidemiologic research at the Roswell Park Cancer Institute in Buffalo, N.Y.

"That study was weak, because men who had just had a vasectomy were under a doctor's care, and there's more of a chance of diseases being detected," he said. "This study is more rigorous, and it does not support the hypothesis that vasectomy increases the risk of two cancers."

Since prostate cancer occurs later in life than testicular cancer does, longer studies are needed to confirm that vasectomy does not increase the risk of that disease over the long run, according to both Dr. Goldacre and Dr. Mettlin.

Dr. Mettlin said that in a study he conducted involving more than 600 men, more subjects with prostate cancer reported having a vasectomy than did those who did not have the operation.

But most men who develop prostate cancer have not had a vasectomy, he added.

"The evidence is weak, but since so many men undergo vasectomy, that question must be investigated," Dr. Mettlin said.

An estimated 50 million men worldwide have undergone vasectomies.

A World Health Organization panel of experts from China, Denmark, India, Korea and the United States recently conducted a research review and found that the "weight of evidence is still that vasectomy is safe and effective," he said.

Men are most likely to get testicular cancer in their early 30s or their 70s, according to Dr. Mettlin. The only known risk factor is undescended testicles. In addition, "testicular cancer is more likely to be diagnosed in men of higher social class, and in white men," Dr. Mettlin said.

Prostate cancer is the most common cancer in men. About 106,000 American men are diagnosed and 30,000 die each year, according to the Prostate Cancer Education Council.

NCI: More patients to receive taxol

ST. PETERSBURG, FLA., MARCH 29—Three times as many cancer patients will receive the experimental drug taxol this year compared with last year, but many patients will still be unable to get it, according to National Cancer Institute officials.

The drug's manufacturer, Bristol-Myers Squibb, says alternative sources of taxol, which now comes exclusively from the bark of the Pacific yew tree, may become available within two years.

In 1992, more than 6,000 women with advanced breast or ovarian cancer are expected to receive taxol in clinical trials, compared with 2,000 last year, according to Michael Friedman, M.D., associate director of the Cancer Therapy Evaluation Program at the NCI, who spoke here at the annual Science Writers Seminar sponsored by the American Cancer Society.

In addition, 2,000 women will be able to get taxol on an individual basis through a treatment referral center set up by the NCI, he said. Patients can call the NCI hotline, 1-800-4CANCER, to find out about the availability of taxol.

Bristol-Myers Squibb, which has exclusive rights from the United States government to harvest yew trees on U.S. land, currently is searching for an alternative source of the drug as part of the agreement that it has with the NCI.

Testifying before a congressional hearing, company repreentatives said they have entered into over a dozen agreements with other companies, researchers and academic institutions and committed millions of dollars to the search for alternative sources of taxol.

Since environmentalists object to harvesting the centuries-old yews, four other methods are being tested: extracting taxol from twigs and needles of other tree species; chemically converting a natural material similar to taxol; using plant cell cultures produced in the lab from cells of yew trees such as roots and leaves; and total synthesis, namely, creating taxol in the laboratory.

At least one company, ESO Agenmetics of San Carlos, Calif., is leading an independent effort to manufacture taxol. Last week, the company announced that it would supply the NCI with taxol produced from its own cell tissue culture, and expects to supply hundreds of grams to the NCI and other companies by next year.

With partial funding from Bristol-Myers Squibb, researchers at the University of Kansas and Virginia Polytechnic Institute are also attempting to develop water-soluble versions of taxol and compounds similar to taxol that could be used in the future development of the drug.

PSA screen and ultrasound favored in prostate test

By Jean McCann

ST. PETERSBURG, FLA., MARCH 30—A new way of predicting whether a man has prostate cancer or merely a benign enlargement of the gland will avoid unnecessary biopsies, researchers say.

Currently, men are screened for prostate cancer by a digital rectal examination, measurement of the prostate-specific antigen (PSA) in the blood and transrectal ultrasound that is performed if PSA is high.

The new approach consists of comparing the size of the man's gland with PSA levels, according to Fred Lee, M.D., director of research in the department of radiology at St. Joseph Mercy Hospital in Ann Arbor, Mich., who presented his findings at the annual American Cancer Society Science Writers Seminar.

PSA levels above 4 ng/ml, as measured by the monoclonal assay, have until recently been considered abnormal, but Dr. Lee said elevated levels may be caused by a benign increase in the size of the prostate and not necessarily cancer.

"As males age, there is a growth of benign glandular tissue that causes an elevation of PSA," he said in an interview. "The danger of what's happening today is that many men with a high PSA are worried that they have prostate cancer unnecessarily."

Therefore, when the PSA is elevated, the next step is to correlate it with the size of the gland, which can be determined by ultrasound, he said.

For example, if a man's PSA is 10 ng/ml and his prostate is over 105 cc in size, such PSA levels may be normal, but if his

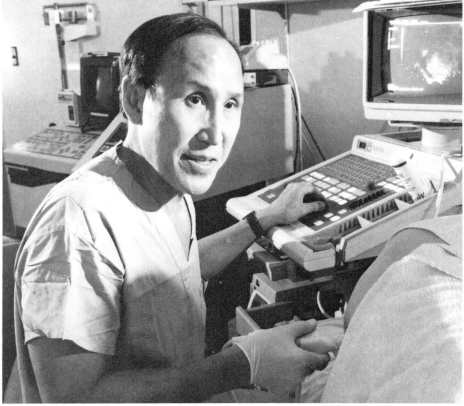

Dr. Fred Lee uses ultrasound to enhance the accuracy of prostate-cancer screening.

gland volume is only 25 cc, he almost certainly has prostate cancer, according to Dr. Lee.

"This helps determine whom really to biopsy," he said.

Dr. Lee has developed a formula according to which a man's PSA level measured by a monoclonal assay is considered normal if it is roughly equivalent to one tenth of the number that stands for the size of his gland measured in cubic centimeters.

Because of this new finding, he said, it is important for men not to have a biopsy of the prostate before its volume is determined by transrectal ultrasound, since the biopsy will reduce the size of the gland and throw off the calculations.

For the same reason, men should not take medicines that shrink the prostate before a PSA and ultrasound are done, Dr. Lee cautioned.

Correlating PSA levels with prostate size "should decrease the number of biopsies, at least at PSA levels below 10," reported Robert A. Kane, M.D., associate professor of radiology at Harvard Medical School in Boston.

He said the new approach will mostly affect men with PSA levels of 4 to 10 ng/ml, but all men whose PSA levels are above 10 ng/ml should still undergo a biopsy because their glands are so large they are difficult to feel and image adequately.

About 15% of men probably have PSA levels above 4 ng/ml but only 2% to 3% have PSA above 10 ng/ml, which signals a 50% or higher likelihood of cancer, according to Dr. Kane.

Prostate cancer is the second most common cancer in men after skin cancer, according to the American Cancer Society.

After age 50, the lifetime risk of developing a prostate malignancy that should be treated is about 10%, according to Dr. Lee.

Whether the cancer needs to be removed depends on its location, which might cause it to spread elsewhere in the body, and its size, he explained.

Late-cycle mastectomies may reduce recurrences in node-positive premenopausal women

St. Petersburg, Fla., April 1—Waiting until the latter part of the menstrual cycle before performing mastectomy on premenopausal women with positive nodes will reduce the recurrence rate, reported an epidemiologist at the Centers for Disease Control in Atlanta.

In a retrospective study of 283 women who had undergone mastectomies for primary breast cancer, the recurrence rate was twice as high at 10 years among those operated on during the follicular phase as among those operated on during the luteal phase, said Ruby Senie, Ph.D., at the annual Science Writers Seminar sponsored by the American Cancer Society.

"The rate of recurrence peaked among patients with positive lymph nodes who were treated between days 7 and 14 of the menstrual cycle, and was lowest between days 20 and 30," she said.

"Our study supports the hypothesis that the risk of recurrence may be affected by the hormonal milieu," Dr. Senie added, while noting that previous studies have sometimes supported and sometimes contradicted this view.

"It may be that unopposed estrogen early in the cycle enhances tumor cell dissemination, thus increasing the probability of metastatic disease," she said. "Or it may be that immune function is depressed prior to ovulation."

The group of women in Dr. Senie's study were a subgroup of 1,200 women who were treated between 1976 and 1978 at Memorial Sloan-Kettering Cancer Center in New York for primary breast cancer, and then followed for 10 years.

Women who were 25% or more over their ideal weight were at particularly high risk for recurrence, according to the CDC researcher.

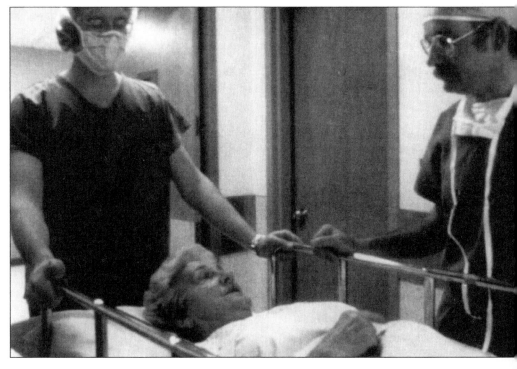

Follicular-phase surgery was associated with a twofold increase in breast-cancer recurrences at 10 years, compared with luteal-phase mastectomies.

In a group of women remaining in the study after exclusion of patients with metastatic disease at the time of diagnosis, or those with second primary breast tumors or tumors of unknown size, 42% of the obese women had developed a recurrence, and 34% had died by 10 years, according to Dr. Senie.

The recurrence rate was 32% in a group of women not markedly overweight, while the death rate was 24%.

"Overall, obesity increased the risk of recurrent breast cancer by 30%," she said.

"Among the 557 women free of cancer in the lymph nodes, the risk of recurrence associated with obesity is 60% greater than the risk in thinner women."

These findings indicate that obese node-negative women could be considered for the hormonal manipulation that tamoxifen (Nolvadex, ICI Pharma) provides, she said.

Genetic test may reveal colon cancer earlier

APRIL 3—After a decade of investigation into the molecular and genetic causes of cancer, scientists have hit pay dirt with a genetic test that has the potential to spot colon cancer early, Johns Hopkins researchers announced.

The test analyzes stool samples for the presence of a mutant gene that experts say is found in about 40% of people with the cancer.

"To our surprise, we were able to identify a significant percentage of mutant cells within the stool samples," reported David Sidransky, M.D., senior research fellow at the Johns Hopkins Oncology Center in Baltimore.

In results presented in the journal Science, the test detected the mutation in eight out of nine patients with colorectal neoplasms known to contain the mutation. No control stool samples were positive. Detection was successful in both benign and malignant neoplasms and was independent of tumor location.

The mutant gene, *ras*, is one of several genetic mutations associated with colon cancer.

Bert Vogelstein, M.D., also of Johns Hopkins, previously demonstrated that the *ras* gene is a cause and not simply a by-product of tumor growth.

"Our expectation is that as we look at other genes involved in colon-cancer progression, the number of patients we can identify should hit close to 100%," Dr. Sidransky said.

Curtis Harris, M.D., chief of the laboratory of human carcinogenesis at the National Cancer Institute, predicted that similar genetic tests may some day spot other cancers in their earliest stages.

Noninvasive gene-based detection is considered feasible for bladder tumors, which shed cells into the urine, and lung cancers, which shed cells into the sputum. Last year, the same researchers were able to identify the p53 gene mutation in urine samples from bladder-cancer patients.

However, the mutation only appears as the bladder tumors invade surrounding tissue, and is thus not expected to lead to development of a screening test.

Dr. Sidransky estimated that the colon-cancer test, at a cost of under $100, could be ready for widespread use within five years.

"It's a prime example of taking the latest in the molecular understanding of cancer from the laboratory to the bedside," Dr. Harris explained.

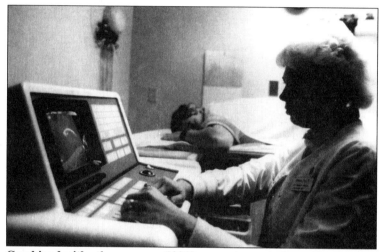

Combined with other genes, a 100% accurate screen is predicted.

Currently, the five-year survival rate for colon cancer is about 90% if diagnosed while it is still localized, compared with only 6% if diagnosed and treated after metastasis, according to the National Cancer Institute.

Monoclonal 'missile' disables IL-2 receptor, curbs T-cell leukemia

NEW YORK, APRIL 9—A noted cancer researcher told a Bristol-Myers Squibb symposium that he has developed a biochemical "bullet" that shows promise in treating T-cell leukemia and other cancers.

Thomas A. Waldmann, M.D., chief of the metabolism branch of the U.S. National Cancer Institute, Bethesda, Md., reported that he has found a way to fuse certain isotopes to monoclonal antibodies to disable the interleukin-2 receptor of leukemia cells and the T-cells of other diseases, while leaving normal cells alone.

In a clinical trial, the biochemical bullet was used to treat 14 patients with T-cell leukemia. All 14 responded favorably, including 11 who had long-term remission of the disease, Dr. Waldmann said.

Before the isotopes were linked to the antibodies, "they acted like guided missiles without a payload," said Dr. Waldmann. He said his new findings warrant further research into the potential uses of the technique in patients with related diseases.

In addition to leukemia and lymphomas, autoimmune diseases such as arthritis and lupus theoretically might be treatable using the technique, he said.

Mammography called neither a risk nor a help

By Laura Buterbaugh

MAY 6—Routine mammograms before the age of 50 will not increase the risk of developing breast cancer, despite published reports that a Canadian study found such a risk, an author of the study said.

The unpublished Canadian study found that 52% more women under 50 who got mammography died from breast cancer than women the same age who had only a physical breast exam, recent newspaper reports stated.

But new, revised study figures show that the death rates are no longer significantly higher among women aged 40 to 49 who got mammograms, said Cornelia Baines, M.D., of the University of Toronto. Researchers are constantly updating the number of deaths of women in the study, and will continue to do so into the next decade, she noted.

"We will not say that mammography kills," said Dr. Baines, who is deputy director of the Canadian National Breast Screening Study. "The conclusion that will be reached is that younger women do not benefit" from reduced mortality, she said.

Even when the study is published, it should be seen as preliminary, Dr. Baines said.

"The analysis has to continue as long as women with breast cancer are still around to be counted," she said.

Dr. Baines' findings contradict the recommendations of the American Cancer Society and the National Cancer Institute, which recommend mammograms every one to two years starting at age 40, and annually after age 50.

A spokesperson for the ACS said they will continue to recommend mammograms before age 50. "We've heard the study had some problems, and it hasn't been through peer review," said spokesperson Stacy Charney.

Guidelines in Canada do not recommend mammograms until age 50, according to Dr. Baines. Only British Columbia recommends them for younger women, she said.

One unfortunate effect of the rumors surrounding the Canadian study may be that women will be scared away from getting mammograms, according to Gerald Dodd, M.D., of the University of Texas M.D. Anderson Cancer Center in Houston.

"Every time you manage to get women aware of mammography and its benefits, someone comes along with something like this," Dr. Dodd said. "You have to start all over and repair the damage."

Dr. Baines said the danger of early mammograms is not from radiation, but from false-positive results, which can lead to unnecessary biopsies, resulting in scar tissue that can make later mammograms difficult to read.

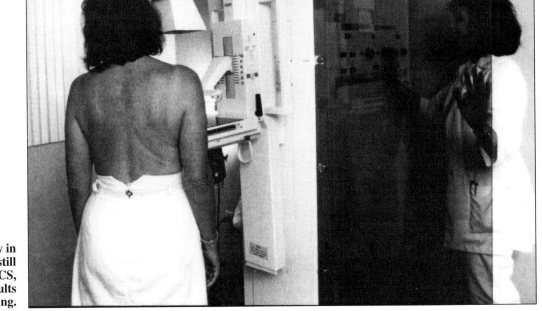

Mammography in women under 50 is still favored by ACS, Canadian results notwithstanding.

The study, one of the largest in the world to examine mammography, included nearly 90,000 women. Subjects received mammograms from 1980 to 1988.

Led by Anthony Miller, M.D., at the University of Toronto, the study is expected to be published within the next few months, Dr. Baines said.

Some American radiologists—several of whom were involved in the Canadian study in its early stages—have criticized it, saying that screening procedures were outdated and patients were not properly randomized.

"The combination of poor-quality mammography along with misassignment of women with late-stage breast cancer to the screening group has destroyed any value the study might have had," said Stephen Feig, M.D., director of breast imaging at Thomas Jefferson University in Philadelphia.

Dr. Feig was an adviser to the study for a year, but said he resigned in 1984 after his recommendations for improving the study were not heeded.

Sam Shapiro, M.D., a professor of health policy at Johns Hopkins University's School of Hygiene and Public Health, confirmed that the early-death figures in the Canadian study have been updated, removing any significant link between mammograms and the development of breast cancer.

"The radiologists attacking the study are still bearing in mind those earlier reports," said Dr. Shapiro, an adviser to the Canadian study.

"They haven't seen the results that are being pooled for the journal articles," he added.

John Bailar, M.D., a professor of epidemiology and biostatistics at McGill University in Montreal, also defended the study. "It's probably the best of the studies that's been done yet," he said.

Family history tops shape as breast-cancer risk

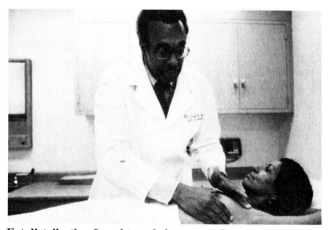

Fat distribution found to pale by comparison to genes.

MAY 14—Having a family history of breast cancer not only increases a woman's risk of developing the disease, but appears to multiply the effect of all other risk factors, including body shape, a new study has found.

So powerful is the effect of family history that without it, some other risk factors diminish to the point of insignificance, according to the study, published in The New England Journal of Medicine.

For instance, studies have found that women who have a top-heavy "apple" shape are at a greater risk for breast cancer than women with a bottom-heavy "pear" shape.

The new study found women with an apple shape without a family history of breast cancer have a 20% increased risk of developing the disease. But their risk is increased 320% if they have a family history of breast cancer, the study reported.

"This is the first study to find that the fat distribution appears to be important only for the women who have a family history of breast cancer," said Thomas Sellers, Ph.D., the study's lead author and an assistant professor of epidemiology at the University of Minnesota in Minneapolis.

The four-year study included more than 37,000 post-menopausal women aged 55 to 69. During the study period, 493 women developed breast cancer.

Researchers compared breast-cancer rates with survey information such as body measurements, family history of breast cancer and menstrual and reproductive history.

They found that a family history of breast cancer multiplies such risk factors as low parity, being older than 30 at the time of first pregnancy and being above average in weight and height.

Among women with no family history of the disease, those whose initial pregnancy was after age 30 were twice as likely to develop breast cancer as women who gave birth before 30. But the risk jumped by 575% for older mothers with a family history of breast cancer.

Wallet-card reminder boosts breast screening

By L.A. McKeown

SAN DIEGO, MAY 19—A wallet-sized plastic card that reminds women to get mammograms nearly doubled the percentage of women who returned for periodic screening, Florida researchers reported.

A pilot study of 220 women found that 72% of those given the cards at the time of their first mammograms showed up for subsequent mammograms, versus 40% given a written or verbal reminder from their doctors. Results of the program were reported at a meeting here of the American Society of Clinical Oncology.

The plastic credit-card-sized reminder has the date when

the woman should schedule her next mammogram engraved on it, said D.V. Schapira, M.D., of the H. Lee Moffitt Cancer Center in Tampa. The card displays the screening anniversary when placed in the wallet.

Mammogram screening has been shown to be effective in reducing mortality from breast cancer, she added.

The study included women between ages 40 and 70 who were undergoing their first screening mammography. At that time, they were assigned randomly to four groups.

One group of women received the plastic card, one received a card and a written reminder, one an appointment card and one a verbal recommendation.

A spokesperson for the American Cancer Society had not heard of the mammography card, but said it sounded promising.

"Certainly there are problems getting some women to come back for yearly mammograms," said ACS spokesperson Joanne Schellenbach. "Some women think because

their mammogram was negative they don't have to get another."

But one public health expert challenged the practice that the new reminder card promotes—widespread routine mammograms.

"There's no therapeutic benefit" to such testing in premenopausal women, said Samuel Epstein, M.D., professor of environmental and occupational medicine, University of Illinois at Chicago. In fact, the screening test "poses a serious added risk of cancer."

Premenopausal women "should destroy their [reminder] cards and forget about it," Dr. Epstein said.

The card could be useful, however, in promoting screening of postmenopausal women, provided radiation exposure is kept to a minimum, he added.

ACS recommends at least one mammogram by age 40, every one to two years for women aged 40 to 49 and annually for women aged 50 and older.

'Cord' blood could supplant marrow grafts

By Charlene Laino

MANCHESTER, ENGLAND, JULY 11—Umbilical-cord blood transfusions may replace bone-marrow transplants for people with leukemia, according to British researchers.

Cord blood transfusions hold several obvious advantages over bone-marrow transplants: the blood is in great supply with collection possible from any newborn, the procedure is painless and recipients do not have to be HLA-matched with

donors, the researchers from the Paterson Institute here wrote in The Lancet.

The blood also is rich in hemopoietic stem cells, making the transfusions an ideal alternative to bone-marrow transplants, they reported.

The use of umbilical-cord blood has proved so promising both in the lab and in 17 pioneering transplantations worldwide that at least one company in the United States has been formed to create a human umbilical blood cell "bank."

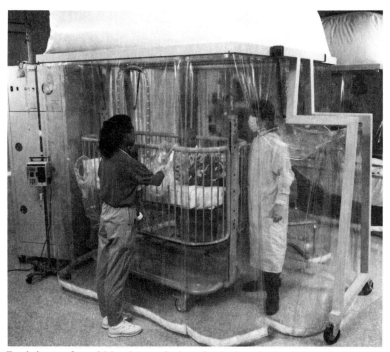

Similar to blood banks set up by the American Red Cross, it would have umbilical-cord blood readily available to patients who need transplantations for bone-marrow disorders.

The Paterson Institute researchers, in long-term laboratory tests, determined that the stem cells found in human umbilical-cord blood are actually more plentiful and of better quality than those found in normal blood marrow. American pioneers said that the results of the British study further justify the creation of an umbilical blood cell bank.

"They validate what a small number of actual transplantations have indicated," said Kenneth Moch, president of Biocyte Corp., the New York company that said it hopes to have a human umbilical-cord blood bank operating by early next year.

"Theoretically, an umbilical-cord blood bank would revolutionize the field," said George Santos, M.D., who oversaw the first U.S. transplantation.

He said that the umbilical-cord blood bank would especially benefit minorities, who have

Recipients of cord blood transfusions for leukemia don't have to be HLA-matched, unlike those treated with bone-marrow transplants.

the most difficulty in finding a donor with the same marrow type.

Biocyte plans to collect cord blood from all ethnic groups, Moch said. The first successful human umbilical-cord blood transplantation was performed in 1988 at the Hôpital Saint-Louis in Paris, on a five-year-old boy born with Fanconi's anemia.

In August 1990, the first U.S. umbilical-cord blood transplant was done on a child with chronic juvenile myelogenous leukemia at Johns Hopkins Medical Center in Baltimore. Almost two years later, the child is alive and well, said Dr. Santos, head of the Bone Marrow Transplantation Unit at Johns Hopkins.

The transplantation technique was successful in all but one of the remaining 15 patients worldwide, said Moch. He said the patient who died had complications unrelated to the use of umbilical-cord blood.

Some pro, much con on radar carcinogenicity

By Fran Kritz

WASHINGTON, D.C., AUG. 10—Radar guns that catch speeding motorists may cause or promote testicular, cervical, eye and brain cancers among police officers, according to officers testifying here before a Senate subcommittee.

Officers often hold the guns in their laps, or rest them over their shoulders, thus exposing themselves to the unshielded radiation emitted by the guns, they said.

Scientists testifying at the hearing, including Henry Kues, M.D., of the applied physics lab at Johns Hopkins University in Baltimore, told the committee that there is not enough evidence to conclude that the radar guns do in fact cause cancer.

The police officers' testimony "may well have some merit, but requires much more scrutiny," said William Ross Adey, M.D., consultant to the World Health Organization for health problems related to electromagnetic radiation and a physician at Pettis Memorial VA Medical Center in Loma Linda, Calif.

About 70% of the radar detectors used by police are mounted inside or outside the patrol car, usually at a safe distance from the officer. But 30% are the radar-gun type, and half of those cannot be turned off, but emit a constant stream of radiation.

Gary P. Poynter, research officer of the National Fraternal Order of Police, told the Senate Subcommittee on Consumer and Environmental Affairs that he had compiled a list of 89 officers who used radar guns over a period of years and later developed cancer.

Industry representatives and a spokesperson for the Institute of Electrical and Electronics Engineers, which developed voluntary standards, say the radiation emitted by the devices is well below the level deemed safe by current standards, and well below that emitted by other devices.

According to the IEEE, "Most of the police units...have an output range of 10 to 25 milliwatts. By comparison, cellular hand-held phones operate at hundreds of milliwatts."

According to Bryan Hardin, director of the National Institute for Occupational Safety and Health, "We do not have sufficient scientific information to evaluate the health risks posed by radar-gun use or low-level microwave radiation because limited research has been conducted."

Sen. Joseph I. Lieberman (D-Conn.), the subcommittee's chairman, said his committee would quickly ask for funds, estimated at about $1.5 million, to allow NIOSH to conduct research on the possible link between radar guns and cancer, which Hardin said could take at least two years.

Do tamoxifen benefits outweigh its risks?

OCT. 22—Most experts agree that the cancer drug tamoxifen is effective in treating breast cancer. What they do not agree on is whether the drug's use should be pushed into the prevention arena—whether its risks to healthy women outweigh its benefits.

A five-year, $68-million government-sponsored trial of tamoxifen (Nolvadex, ICI Pharma) to prevent breast cancer in women at high risk of developing the disease may jeopardize the well-being of healthy study participants, critics of the study contended at a congressional hearing.

While the critics agree that tamoxifen is a reasonable cancer treatment that produces relatively few side effects compared with other therapies, they maintain that too little is known about the drug's promise for preventing breast cancer and that the drug is too toxic to be used in healthy women.

Tamoxifen therapy has been associated with an increased risk of blood clots, uterine and liver cancers and ocular toxicity.

"There is little evidence to support the protective effects claimed," Adriane Fugh-Berman, M.D., of the National Women's Health Network, told the House of Representatives' Human Resources and Intergovernmental Relations Subcommittee.

"Women eligible for enrollment are not truly at high risk

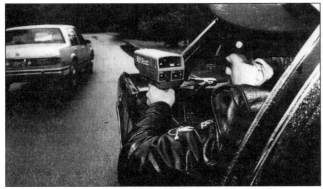
Police group submitted a list of 89 radar gun-wielding officers who later developed a variety of cancers.

for breast cancer. Tamoxifen is too toxic for use in healthy women," she said.

Under the auspices of the National Cancer Institute, the Breast Cancer Prevention Trial will be conducted at 270 centers in the United States and Canada and will include 16,000 women deemed to be at high risk of developing breast cancer.

The trial will accept two groups: women over 60 and those between 35 and 59 with two known risk factors for breast cancer, such as family history of the disease or having had at least two noncancerous breast tumors. Half the women in the study will receive 20 mg of tamoxifen a day and the other half a placebo.

Proponents of the study say the trial is essential to determine the effectiveness of tamoxifen in preventing breast cancer in high-risk women before it gains widespread use in the community.

"Anecdotal evidence suggests that some physicians are already prescribing tamoxifen to individual women as a preventive approach," said Peter Greenwald, M.D., director of NCI's Division of Cancer Prevention and Control.

Large studies of the drug indicate that it reduces the incidence of cancer in the second breast in postmenopausal women with cancer in one breast. But only one unpublished study shows a reduction in tumors in premenopausal women, said Dr. Fugh-Berman.

Helen Rodriguez-Trias, M.D., president-elect of the American Public Health Association, argues that "in order to ensure truly informed consent, it is essential that the risk and benefits be clearly spelled out and thoroughly understood by the person imparting the information, as well as the person who will enter the study. With the tamoxifen study, the central weakness lies in a consent form that does not sufficiently emphasize the probable risk." Each of the 270 centers collaborating in the study may make up its own consent form.

Rep. Donald Payne (D-N.J.), who chairs the subcommittee, said that a recent review of such forms found that two thirds did not mention the risk of blood clots.

Six percent of centers have temporarily stopped enrolling patients because of such problems, and are requiring more uniform consent procedures.

Study questioning early mammography rebutted

Nov. 15—Results of the much-awaited Canadian National Breast Screening Study have added more fuel to the controversy over whether younger women should have routine mammograms.

The study, published in the Canadian Medical Association Journal, found that annual mammograms for women aged 40 to 49 did not reduce mortality or improve survival rates—prompting its authors to recommend against the test for these women.

At least one U.S. physician agrees, contending that the risk of mammography in premenopausal women outweighs any benefits. But many U.S. radiologists said the Canadian study is too flawed to be used as a guide for when to offer mammograms.

The Canadian study, one of the largest in the world to examine mammograms and breast cancer, followed nearly 90,000 women aged 40 to 59 at 15 hospitals across Canada for an average of eight years. About 50,000 women participated in the aged-40-to-49 arm of the study.

The study found that while annual mammography combined with a physical breast examination detected more node-negative, small tumors than a control group that received only physical breast exams, early detection had no impact on the mortality rate from breast cancer. In fact, during the study period, 38 women died in the mammography group while 28 women died in the physical-exam-only group, although the difference was not statistically significant.

The aged-50-to-59 arm of the study found a similar lack of reduced mortality. But the study's deputy director, Cornelia Baines, M.D., of the University of Toronto, said she expects a mortality difference to emerge eventually in the older group.

The American Cancer Society, the National Cancer Institute and nine other institutions recommend mammograms every one to two years starting at age 40, and annually after age 50. They have called for U.S. women to continue to follow those guidelines until an international breast-cancer screening conference is held in February 1993. That conference will review all screening trials worldwide.

Daniel Kopans, M.D., director of breast imaging at Massachusetts General Hospital in Boston, said that if anything, the guidelines should be more aggressive; women aged 40 to 49 should be screened annually.

Dr. Kopans warned that in a two-year interval, cancer may develop in a younger woman's breast and progress to a later stage before the next mammogram. "I would suggest that doctors not do anything based on the Canadian study," he said. "The validity of the data is questionable."

Dr. Kopans and other reviewers of the mammograms have criticized the quality of the films, saying that much of the mammography equipment was outdated and therefore caused cancers to be missed. Dr. Baines countered that the equipment used at the beginning of the study—the period most criticized in terms of film quality—was similar to American equipment used then.

Dr. Kopans added that an unusually high seven-year survival rate for women who did not receive mammography—88% to 91%—may point up a problem with randomization in the study.

But Samuel Epstein, M.D., a professor of occupational and environmental medicine at the University of Illinois in Chicago, said that women who use the Canadian study's results to refrain from mammograms until age 50 "will be absolutely right in reaching that conclusion."

"Routine mammography for women under age 50 is a highly hazardous undertaking," Dr. Epstein said. He believes that breast tissue in premenopausal women is more sensitive to potential carcinogens, and therefore younger women are more at risk from mammography-caused cancer than they are from breast cancer that might naturally occur.

COMMENTARY

Molecular biology is the wave of future

By David S. Ettinger, M.D.

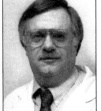

IN THE ONGOING EFFORT TO detect, treat and someday cure cancer, molecular biology has taken center stage.

Molecular biology may lead to some of the most significant advances in the future of oncology, particularly potential early detection and gene therapy.

In the area of screening, for example, scientists are looking at gene mutations as tools to identify people at risk for development of cancer even before it's clinically apparent. At Johns Hopkins, we analyzed the mutant gene *ras* in stool samples and found it to be present in 40% of patients with colorectal carcinoma. This may prove to be another way of detecting patients at risk for the disease.

With gene therapy, we hope to manipulate the immune response to increase the chance of cure and to decrease toxicity.

Techniques have been developed to use genes to encode cytokines, which increase the systemic immune response against tumor-specific antigen, thereby killing the cancer. Protocols soon will be approved to test this hypothesis.

The gene-transfer method is under investigation experimentally to treat brain tumors. The strategy is to infiltrate brain-cancer cells with herpesvirus, then destroy the tumors with the antiviral drug ganciclovir.

One of our major concerns is whether gene therapy will also affect normal cells and increase the patient's risk of cancer later on. But the possible benefits of such therapy are monumental.

New drugs also will play a strong role in oncology's future. To date, colon, breast and lung cancer treatments are not particularly effective, and we will continue to see protocols using taxol, topotecan and CPT-11, to determine against what disease sites they will be effective.

Taxol will be approved by the Food and Drug Administration, with the primary role of treating refractory ovarian carcinoma. But I feel it will eventually be expanded to treat breast cancer, non-small-cell lung cancer and head and neck cancer. Before long, the drug will be synthesized to ensure its availability on a larger scale.

Since we also have to be concerned about why drugs don't work, we will look at pharmacological approaches to overcoming drug resistance. Studies already are looking at how we can use old drugs more effectively.

Etoposide and anthracyclines, which are natural products, induce drug resistance. There is a multidrug-resistant phenotype found in certain tumors that is associated with expression of the p-glycoprotein. The p-glycoprotein acts as a membrane-efflux pump and ejects the drugs trying to reach the cancer cell.

Drugs that can reverse the membrane-efflux pump, such as angiotensin-converting-enzyme inhibitors, will be tested with anticancer agents such as etoposide, vinca alkaloids, anthracyclines and doxyrubicin.

Verapamil, along with the immunosuppressant, cyclosporine-A, is being examined for use with etoposide to see if the combination is more effective against the specific cancer than the anticancer agent itself.

Research efforts at overcoming drug resistance will continue. We know for a fact there are drugs that are active, but not after one or two cycles of therapy. If you can overcome that problem and continue to use the effective agent, you have a better chance of curing the patient.

Finally, another key area to watch in the 1990s and beyond will be combined modalities—not just using therapies in sequence, but utilizing various therapies concomitantly. For instance, in treating esophageal cancer, physicians will use chemotherapy and radiation followed by surgery, instead of just surgery with the possible addition of chemotherapy if there is a relapse.

Single modalities are better tolerated, but combinations increase the gain. The ultimate goal is not palliation, but cure.

Dr. Ettinger is professor of oncology at Johns Hopkins Medical School, Baltimore.

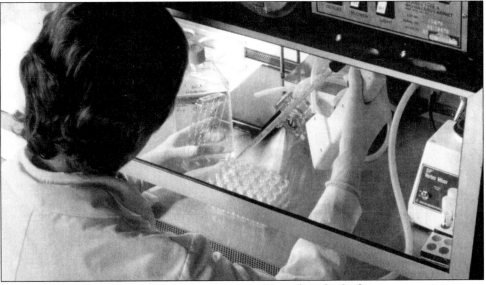

Research efforts at overcoming drug resistance will continue in the future.

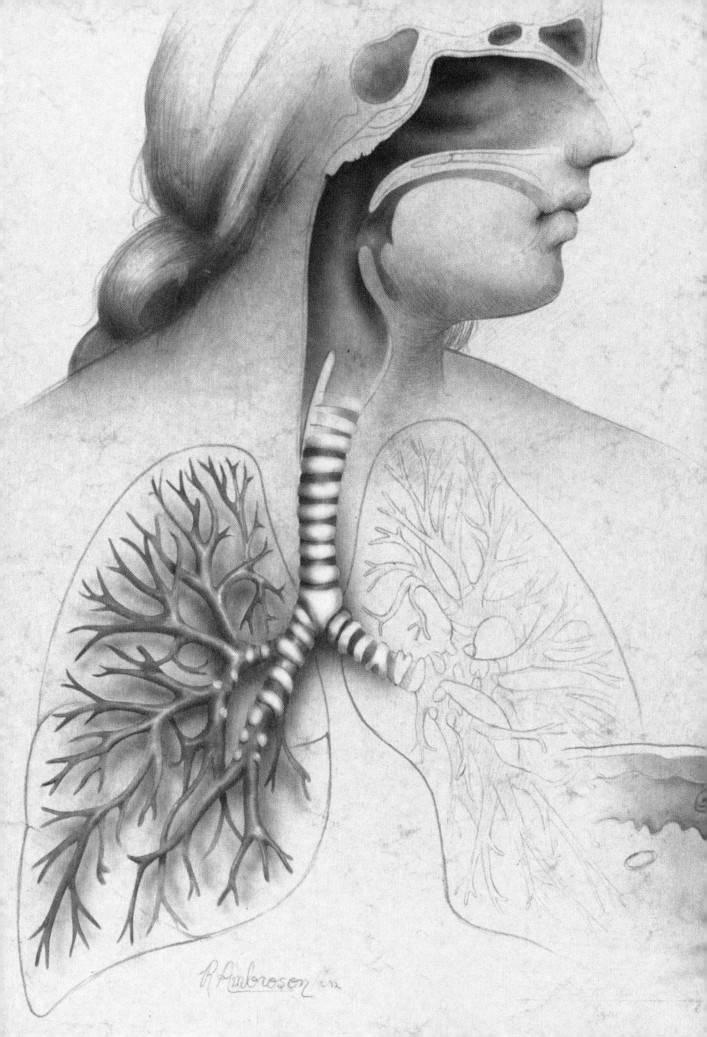

R. Ambroson

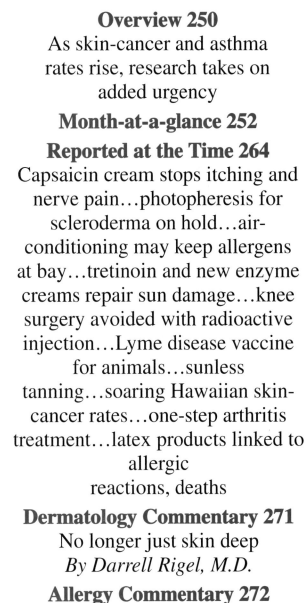

Overview 250
As skin-cancer and asthma rates rise, research takes on added urgency

Month-at-a-glance 252

Reported at the Time 264
Capsaicin cream stops itching and nerve pain…photopheresis for scleroderma on hold…air-conditioning may keep allergens at bay…tretinoin and new enzyme creams repair sun damage…knee surgery avoided with radioactive injection…Lyme disease vaccine for animals…sunless tanning…soaring Hawaiian skin-cancer rates…one-step arthritis treatment…latex products linked to allergic reactions, deaths

Dermatology Commentary 271
No longer just skin deep
By Darrell Rigel, M.D.

Allergy Commentary 272
Breathlessly awaiting drugs for better control
By Robert N. Hamburger, M.D.

OVERVIEW

As skin-cancer and asthma rates rise, research takes on added urgency

In rheumatology, Cambridge University researchers reported that they had taken the first step toward curbing arthritis with a single treatment.

In 1992, allergic and dermatologic diseases showed alarming rises in numbers and in severity, adding urgency to researchers' pursuit of advances in treatment and prevention.

In dermatology, ozone levels continued to fall, skin-cancer rates continued to rise and research continued to offer new insights into treatments and preventive strategies.

In one Swedish town, researchers reported that the incidence of basal-cell carcinoma doubled between 1970 and 1986. In Scotland, melanoma rates jumped 82% between 1979 and 1989. Those increases fit with predictions made by a physician from the University of California, San Francisco, School of Medicine, who warned in January that depletion of the protective ozone layer will cause rises in rates of all types of skin cancer.

However, there was good news in preventing and treating sun damage. A cream that contains a synthetic melanotropin to stimulate the production of melanin is currently in Phase I trials to learn if it protects the skin from sun damage.

Other topicals offered promise for the reversal of sun damage. The Food and Drug Administration Dermatologic Drugs Advisory Committee recommended that approval of tretinoin be expanded to include the treatment of sun-damaged skin, fine facial wrinkles and roughness. Sunscreen containing 5-methoxypsoralen, a chemical found in the peel of a bitter Mediterranean orange, reduced DNA damage in the skin by one half in a British study. And other British researchers reported that they are testing an experimental skin cream containing liposome-encapsulated endonuclease for its ability to enhance and speed DNA repair in skin cells exposed to ultraviolet radiation.

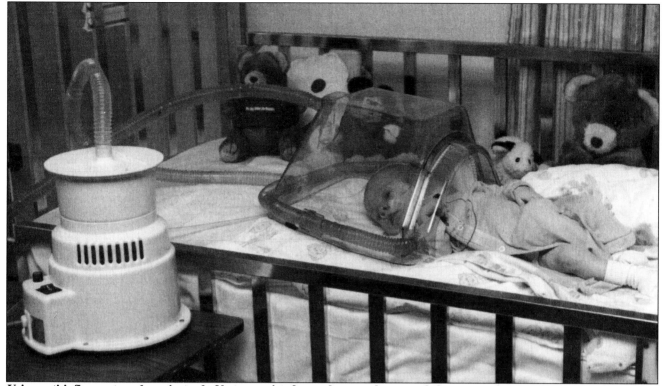

Using anti-inflammatory drugs instead of beta-agonists for moderate asthma may help prevent attacks that require a respirator.

In rheumatology, Cambridge University researchers reported that they had taken the first step toward curbing arthritis with a single treatment, using humanized monoclonal antibodies to target and destroy cells that cause the crippling disorder.

Seven of eight patients treated for 10 days with the drug, called anti-CD 52, showed a marked improvement, with a reduction in joint swelling and inflammation lasting from three to eight months. Four patients were then given a second course consisting of three times as much of the antibiotics over a five-day period. The hope is to keep increasing the dose until a single course controls the disease.

Children with resistant juvenile rheumatoid arthritis may find eased joint pain and improved mobility with low doses of methotrexate, a joint U.S./Russian trial confirmed.

In allergy and immunology, both asthma incidence and mortality are rising sharply. Government researchers reported that asthma deaths increased by 54% among women in the past decade, compared with 23% for men. Every year throughout the 1980s, African-Americans were twice as likely to be hospitalized for asthma as whites. And the number of people who saw a doctor for asthma increased from 6.5 million in 1985 to 7.1 million in 1990.

For children, the increase in asthma rates has been even more severe, researchers from the Mayo Clinic in Rochester, Minn., reported. The number of young children with asthma has increased as much as 200% in the past two decades, they reported, with children aged one through four showing the most startling increases.

But new insights into underlying disease mechanisms may help reverse those trends. Two studies confirmed the impor-

tance of using anti-inflammatory drugs such as inhaled steroids rather than beta-agonists as the treatment of choice for moderate asthma.

The first, by researchers from McGill University in Montreal, concluded that regular use of beta-agonists may mislead both patients and their doctors into thinking that the asthma is under control when it is not.

The second, published in the American Lung Association's Review of Respiratory Diseases, found that airway constriction caused by muscle tightening is unlikely to cause shortness of breath unless the airways are also inflamed. The study helped explain why inflammation plays so central a role in asthma, and why inhaled steroids are fundamental in its treatment. In line with that growing view, the National Asthma Education Program of the National Heart, Lung and Blood Institute told physicians that they should rely more heavily on inhaled anti-inflammatories such as corticosteroids and cromolyn, rather than on beta-agonists, to control asthma in sufferers with moderate disease.

Latex allergies also grabbed headlines. Baffled by news of severe, occasionally anaphylactic reactions to the synthetic rubber, health officials gathered at an FDA conference in Baltimore to discuss a phenomenon that was virtually unknown a decade ago. At least 16 deaths linked to latex exposure had been reported to the FDA by year's end. All were hospital patients who were having barium enemas with latex-tipped tubing.

In 1992, then, rising morbidity and mortality rates reminded dermatologists of the importance of continued advances in basic research and the transfer of hard-won research insights into improved strategies for treatment and prevention.

Dermatology/Allergy/Immunology/Rheumatology

Jan. 2
A prominent dermatologist warned that depletion of the protective atmospheric ozone layer would lead not only to a dramatic increase in the incidence of malignant melanoma, but also to a greater number of basal- and squamous-cell carcinomas. The University of California, San Francisco, School of Medicine physician made his prediction after scientists aboard a converted spy plane flying over New England and eastern Canada detected the highest levels of a potent ozone-depleting chemical, chlorine monoxide, ever recorded in the world (1.5 parts

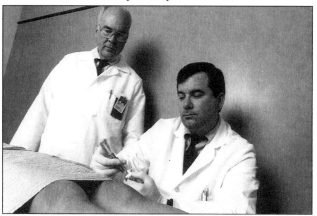

One approach: soaking up interleukin-1 in inflamed arthritic joints.

per billion). NASA calculations indicate that these levels, combined with smaller amounts of bromine monoxide, are high enough to destroy ozone at a rate of 1% to 2% per day.

Jan. 6
Elderly osteoarthritis patients cut their pain by more than half with home laser treatments. In an Israeli trial presented in the the Journal of the American Geriatrics Society, 50 patients held laser instruments to their arthritic knees twice a day. After 10 days, the low-intensity infrared or red light resulted in a 50% reduction in pain and a 40% improvement in joint mobility, while patients using sham devices did not improve. Benefits lasted four to six months after treatment,

according to researchers at Shmuel Harofe Hospital in Beer Yaakov.

Jan. 9
A topical cream derived from chili peppers relieved pruritus in eight of nine long-term hemodialysis patients, Ohio researchers announced. The cream, capsaicin, has also shown promise in relieving nerve pain associated with herpes, diabetes, rheumatoid arthritis and psoriasis, dermatologists from the University of Cincinnati reported in the Journal of the American Academy of Dermatology.

Jan. 13
Immunex, Inc., announced clinical trials of a new drug to relieve the pain and joint inflammation of rheumatoid arthritis. The new drug, called IL-1 receptor, is designed to act as a sponge to soak up interleukin-1 in inflamed joints.

Jan. 15
Extensive analysis of 183 patients in the first cluster of chronic fatigue syndrome cases in Incline Village, Nev., revealed that they may have been experiencing an immunologically mediated inflammatory process of the central nervous system. Beginning with a flulike illness, the syndrome resulted in

immune dysfunction and the consequent reactivation of latent viruses, particularly the active replication of human herpesvirus type 6, a national collaborative group reported in the Annals of Internal Medicine. Based on laboratory and neurological findings, they concluded that chronic fatigue syndrome is probably a heterogenous illness that can be triggered by multiple different factors, including stress, toxins and exogenous infectious agents.

Jan. 16
Tattooing should be regulated, asserted a Massachusetts General Hospital dermatologist. He warned that the practice carries a risk of infection, allergic reaction and transmission of hepatitis B, tuberculosis and HIV. Although tatooing is legal in almost half of the states, there is no tattoo-parlor inspection and little or no regulation regarding adequate training or the sterilization of instruments, he wrote in The New England Journal of Medicine.

Jan. 18
An annual flu vaccine should not be administered to stable asthmatics because of the potential side effects, warned specialists at the Royal Infirmary in Sunderland, United Kingdom. Bronchial reactivity can be increased and asthma exacerbated by

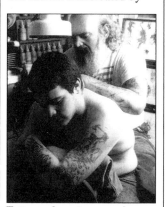

Tattoo-parlor patrons may bear the mark of HIV, hep B or TB.

the vaccination, they wrote in The Lancet.

Jan. 21
The Asthma and Allergy Foundation of America kicked off a campaign to educate teachers and coaches about how to recognize signs of

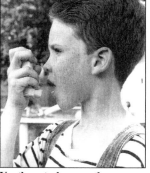

Youth controls own asthma care.

asthma in schoolchildren. Nationally, three million children and teenagers suffer from asthma, resulting in 30 million lost school days per year.

• • •

Therakos, a subsidiary of Johnson & Johnson, withdrew its request to the Food and Drug Administration for approval of its photopheresis therapy for severe scleroderma. The FDA had indicated that there were problems with the new drug application due to poor study design.

Jan. 23
Patients with steroid-resistant inflammatory bowel disease were invited to participate in a University of Pittsburgh clinical trial of a new immunosuppressive agent. FK-506, a substance isolated from soil fungus, had already shown promise in preventing rejection and other serious complications following liver transplantation. An estimated 75% of IBD patients not helped by steroids are responsive to immunosuppressive agents, but cyclosporine creates serious side effects. Previously, FK-506 appeared to ameliorate pyoderma gangrenosum, the purulent inflammatory skin condition associated with IBD.

Feb. 3

The World Health Organization announced that a new therapy scheduled for widespread testing could help eliminate Hansen's disease (leprosy), the disorder that disfigures an estimated five to six million people worldwide. The combination of the powerful oral antibiotics ofloxacin (Floxin, Ortho) and rifampin may be able to slash treatment time to four weeks, making it more acceptable than current drugs that require months or years to work, according to the WHO.

Feb. 6

Tretinoin lightened or eliminated liver spots on the arms and faces of older people, University of Michigan dermatologists announced. After 10 months, actinic lentigines had lightened on the faces of 83% of patients using 0.1% tretinoin cream (Retin-A, Ortho), compared with 29% of the patients on a placebo moisturizer. All had instructions to avoid sun exposure and to use sunscreens appropriately. In a study presented in The New England Journal of Medicine, the researchers found that liver spots that completely disappeared during tretinoin treatment did not return during a six-month post-treatment follow-up.

• • •

Swedish researchers bolstered a long-held suspicion that people suffering from polymyositis or dermatomyositis are at increased risk of cancer. In a population-based study of 788 patients, men with dermatomyositis had 2.4 times the cancer risk of men without the disease. Dermatomyositis conferred a 3.4-fold increased overall cancer risk in women, including a 17-fold higher risk of ovarian cancer. Patients with polymyositis also were at moderately higher risk of cancer, but researchers from the Karolinska and Huddinge Hospitals in Stockholm said they thought that careful

cancer screening in these patients might have been enough to account for the observed difference. Writing in The New England Journal of Medicine, they recommended that physicians more diligently screen for cancer in persons with dermatomyositis.

Feb. 8

Adults with chronic severe asthma obtained significant relief during a 12-week trial of oral cyclosporine (Sandimmune, Sandoz). The 33 patients had had asthma for an average of 27 years and had

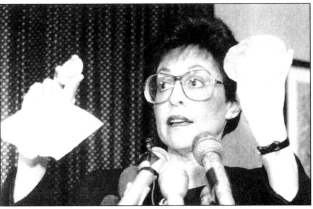

Breast and testicular implants on stage at FDA hearing.

been on oral corticosteroids for an average of nine years. While receiving 5 mg/kg/day cyclosporine in the double-blind crossover trial, patients had a 17.8% increase in forced expiratory volume and had 48% fewer disease exacerbations (severe enough to require an increased prednisone dose).

The results, presented in The Lancet by researchers from London's National Heart and Lung Institute, were said to provide evidence that activated T-lymphocytes are involved in the pathogenesis of chronic severe asthma.

Feb. 12

School-age children with a history of wheezing as toddlers may already have impaired lung function, cautioned researchers from the

University of North Carolina, Chapel Hill. Airway function was affected most in those who also presented with an allergy to dust mites, according to their study of 126 children detailed in the American Review of Respiratory Disease.

Feb. 19

Silicone-breast-implant manufacturers told the Food and Drug Administration that it was extremely unlikely that leaking silicone could cause autoimmune diseases. Rebutting previous expert testimony that up to 6% of the implants ruptured, manufacturers said the rupture rates are 0.13% to 0.5%.

Feb. 22

Patients who have allergies to certain fruits should be tested for latex allergies, advised two groups of researchers in the British Medical Journal. A French physician described the case of a man allergic to bananas and avocados who collapsed every time he underwent a surgical procedure that exposed him to latex. Belgian doctors wrote about nurses allergic to latex who developed symptoms after eating bananas, avocados and chestnuts.

• • •

Almost 100 cases of facial rash were traced to ingredients in the laundry detergent used at a British holiday resort, reported public health authorities in Taunton. Insufficient rinsing of sheets washed in detergent containing an optical brightener, caustic soda and potassium hydroxide was blamed for the irritant dermatitis, they reported in the British Medical Journal.

• • •

Thalidomide, the drug that caused phocomelia in children born in the 1960s, successfully relieved skin and joint symptoms of lupus in three women treated at Hôpital Saint-Charles in Montpelier, France. Moderate doses of thalidomide (25-200 mg/day) generated a good clinical response and allowed corticosteroid doses to be lowered substantially, physicians reported in The Lancet. However, because of thalidomide's extreme teratogenicity and its neurologic side effects (peripheral neuropathy in one woman and drowsiness in two in this study), American researchers deemed the approach somewhat drastic, particularly since it had not been tested against organ-threatening lupus.

Feb. 25

Preliminary data from Phase II clinical trials suggested that a topical non-steroidal antiandrogen may be effective in the treatment of both acne and male-pattern baldness. In trials of 295 patients with moderate to severe acne, those who applied a 0.5% Cyoctol solution daily for three to six months had 21.9% fewer acne lesions than those applying placebo, according to the manufacturer, Chantal Pharmaceutical Corp.

In a study of 40 patients with male-pattern baldness, hair counts increased 83% in those receiving 0.5% Cyoctol. There was a 20% net gain in those applying 0.1% Cyoctol and a loss of 8.9% in those on placebo. The only side effect reported was mild scalp dryness.

March 7

A North Carolina pathologist warned that potentially deadly fire ants could reach as far north as Canada in the West and New Jersey in the East. Over decades, fire ants have caused 32 deaths in the United States. The ant's venom, which is 5,000 times more deadly than the venom of bees, is considered the most powerful allergen ever identified, the investigator told the annual meeting of the American Academy of Allergy and Immunology in Orlando, Fla.

• • •

Patients who attribute their outbreaks of hives, itching or swelling to aspartame may be mistaken, declared Harvard researchers. The Boston team studied 17 women and four men who had documented allergic reactions they attributed to eating or drinking products containing the artificial sweetener. They received tablets of either aspartame or placebo on different days, and four of the 21 sustained allergic reactions that lasted from 30 minutes to 12 hours. Two of the reactions occurred after taking aspartame and two after taking placebo, the researchers told the American Academy of Allergy and Immunology meeting.

• • •

A woman allergic to penicillin suffered a hypersensitivity reaction after eating chicken that had been fed antibiotic-containing medicated chicken feed, physicians from East Surrey Hospital in England reported in The Lancet. The patient was treated with an antihistamine and hydrocortisone; her symptoms resolved three days later.

• • •

Australian researchers said they may have solved the puzzle of post-thunderstorm asthma epidemics. Although dry grass pollen particles are too large to penetrate the lower airways and trigger a grass attack in pollen-sensitive asthmatics, the particles burst when wet, releasing microscopic

MARCH

allergen-containing starch granules into the air, the University of Melbourne team reported in The Lancet. This means that people with allergies or asthma should stay inside, with their air conditioners on, the day afer a rainstorm, commented a New Jersey allergist.

March 8

Two Oxford University scientists are close to locating a gene that causes asthma, declared the British press. After analyzing blood samples from 1,000 people from 100 families with a history of asthma, the scientists were said to be closing in on one small area of chromosome and focusing on three possible genes. Without published results or corroborative data available, American allergists were cautious in greeting the news.

March 9

Allergy shots may prevent people from sneezing around cats and dogs, but they are not a cure, reported Swedish researchers. They studied 32 people who received the shots every six weeks for three years. Five years after cessation of therapy, four felt their allergies were worse. Bronchial histamine and allergen challenges revealed, however, that the condition of 23 subjects had actually worsened. Their allergies were probably not bothering them because they avoided animals, the Karolinska Institute pediatricians told the meeting of the American Academy of Allergy and Immunology.

March 10

Central air conditioning bested room air conditioners in keeping mold and bacteria from the homes of persons with allergies and asthma. When University of Michigan researchers assessed mold and bacteria levels in 12 homes,

single-room models provided no improvement over no air conditioners at all. To gain the most effectiveness from room air conditioners, doors and windows should be kept closed and potential allergen sources removed from the room, the team reported at an American Academy of Allergy and Immunology meeting.

In a related study from

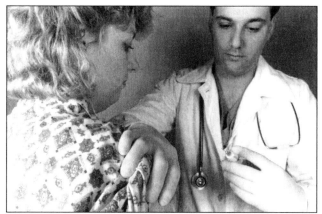

Allergy shots against cat and dog allergens appear ephemeral.

France, three pricey vacuum cleaners touted for their ability to remove cat dander and other troublesome allergens proved no more effective than regular, inexpensive vacuums.

• • •

The president of the American Academy of Allergy and Immunology told the society's annual meeting that asthmatics are more likely to have difficulty breathing when levels of ozone in the air are high. A study of 10 asthmatic and eight nonasthmatic subjects indicated a dose-response relationship between ability to breathe and ozone levels in asthmatics only. Ozone may also worsen hay fever and ragweed allergy, he added.

March 12

A hand-held "gene gun" firing microscopic DNA-coated gold pellets may provide a simplified method for genetic immunization,

announced University of Texas researchers. When the gun was used to shoot growth-hormone-coated pellets into mice, 88% of the mice mounted a long-lasting immune response to the hormone, according to a report in Nature. The technique avoids the time-intensive process of protein purification needed for traditional immunization, the researchers said. It also may have the potential to improve immunization against viral infections and to trigger the immune system of cancer patients into destroying their tumors.

March 13

A dermatologist poohpoohed the highly publicized theory that earlobe creases are a harbinger of heart disease. Speaking at a meeting of the American Society of Dermatologic Surgery, a Johns Hopkins University physician offered evidence for a more prosaic explanation of the creases: They occur in people who sleep on their sides. In a study of 212 adults, people who favor sleeping on one side were likely to have an ear crease on the same side, while those who slept equally on both sides had bilateral creases, she explained. About half of all people have creased earlobes, and people with heart disease may be more prone to the creases because they spend more time lying in bed.

Dermatology/Allergy/Immunology/Rheumatology

April 2

Swedish researchers determined that infants with a strong family history of eczema are less likely to develop the disorder if breast-fed for the first three months by a mother consuming no egg whites, cow's milk or fish products. By four years of age, 19 of 65 children whose mothers followed the antigen-avoidance diet had developed atopic dermatitis, compared with 28 of 50 children whose mothers consumed a regular diet. Rates of asthma, bronchial obstruction and rhinoconjunctivitis were similar in the two groups, researchers from the Central Hospitals in Boras and Skovde reported in Pediatrics. Children in both groups were started on cow's milk at six months of age, and eggs and fish were introduced after nine months.

April 6

A substance extracted from starfish suppresses T-cell division and maturation in vitro and may yield a unique immune-suppressing medication, researchers told the Federation of American Societies for Experimental Biology meeting in Anaheim, Calif. Dubbed sea-star factor, the substance might be used to prevent rejection of donor organs or to treat uveitis, asthma and allergies, a Johns Hopkins University professor stated.

April 9

Two popular acne medications received favorable recommendations from the Food and Drug Administration Dermatologic Drugs Advisory Committee. The panel unanimously recommended that approval for tretinoin (Retin-A, Ortho) be expanded to include the treatment of sun-damaged skin.

In addition, they advised that benzoyl peroxide, a non-prescription ingredient in acne preparations used by one quarter of American teenagers, remain on the market pending the outcome of studies assessing its cancer-causing potential. The panel could have recommended restricting benzoyl peroxide to prescription use only or banning it altogether until additional research is completed.

•••

The quest for thin thighs landed a woman in the hospital suffering from acute tenosynovitis, reported physicians at St. Vincent's Medical Center in Staten Island, N.Y. The patient had exercised 15 minutes a day for six weeks using a popular spring-like device promising thin thighs in 30 days. The device is positioned between the knees and squeezed, providing resistance for repeated hip adduction exercises. Tenosynovitis affected both the right hip joint and the adductor muscles, an overuse injury the doctors dubbed "thigh-thinner's thecitis" in their letter to The New England Journal of Medicine.

April 16

A joint U.S./Russian trial confirmed that low doses of methotrexate can ease joint pain and improve mobility in children with resistant juvenile rheumatoid arthritis. During the six-month study, 63% of children receiving weekly, low-dose (10 mg per square meter of body-surface area) methotrexate improved, as compared with 32% of those given half as much methotrexate and 38% of children receiving a placebo. During the multicenter study of 127 children from 23 pediatric rheumatology centers, all participants were allowed to receive prednisone and nonsteroidal anti-inflammatory drugs.

While short-term results are encouraging, further study is needed to determine whether methotrexate prevents joint erosion or is safe for long-term administration, arthritis experts commented in The New England Journal of Medicine.

April 18

Melanoma rates jumped 82% in Scotland over an 11-year period, revealed the Scottish Melanoma Group. Between 1979 and 1989, the annual incidence rate per 100,000 population increased from 3.4 to 7.1 in men and from 6.6 to 10.4 in women, they reported in The Lancet. The greatest rates of increase were seen in lesions of the superficial spreading histogenetic type on the female leg and the male trunk.

April 23

First dog Millie and her owners, George and Barbara Bush, inspired a study of autoimmune disorders in pets, a British researcher told a conference on systemic lupus erythematosus in London. Investigators compared

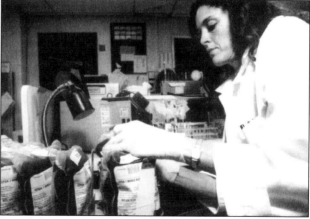

Transfusion-spread Chagas disease is turning up in the U.S.

the immune systems of 15 dogs of lupus sufferers, nine dogs of healthy people and 10 dogs themselves diagnosed with lupus. Blood from the dogs of lupus owners contained levels of autoantibodies similar to those of dogs diagnosed with lupus, revealed the investigators from Queen's Medical Center in Nottingham, leading them to conclude that something in the environment may trigger the disease.

•••

The World Health Organization announced that Chagas disease may be spreading to large cities in Central and South America, threatening up to 90 million people. According to WHO, the disease is now being spread through blood donations. Transfusion-acquired cases also have been identified in California, New York, Washington, D.C., and Winnipeg, Canada.

April 27

In preliminary studies in London, a unique skin cream showed promise in repairing DNA damage from ultra-violet radiation. The cream (T4N5 liposome, Applied Genetics) delivers liposome-encapsulated endonuclease to the basal-cell level, where the supplementary enzyme enhances and speeds the DNA repair process, according to researchers from St. Thomas's Hospital. The preliminary trials were conducted on persons with xeroderma pigmentosum, an inherited disorder of DNA repair that carries a 5,000-fold increased risk of skin cancer. The manufacturer stated that the cream would also be able to prevent skin damage after sun exposure in persons without the disorder.

MAY

May 1

Parents who have watched a child suffer with painful sunburn are far more likely to insist on sunscreen use, announced dermatologists from the University of Texas in Galveston who surveyed 82 parents with beach-going children. However, since just one blistering sunburn in childhood is believed to double the risk for malignant melanoma in adulthood, parents need to heed the sunscreen warning sooner, the team warned in the Archives of Dermatology.

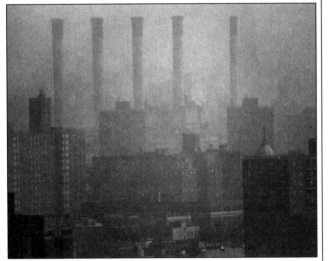

The EPA reported that even low levels of smog can worsen asthma.

May 4

Researchers at Brigham and Women's Hospital in Boston described a 10-minute radiation treatment as an alternative to surgical removal of inflamed synovial tissue. In the procedure, already used widely in Canada and Europe, the radioactive isotope known as [165]Dy-FHMA (Dysprosium, Ferric hydroxide Macroaggregate) is injected into the knee. Of some 400 patients treated in the United States, about 65% experienced relief in pain and inflammation and improvement in the knee's range of motion, the researchers told Medical Tribune. The mechanism by which the isotope works is not yet known, according to the investigators.

May 8

German researchers reported that hyperactive children whose symptoms may be triggered by allergic reactions to certain foods may not have to avoid those foods if they receive food-extract injections. The Universitatskinderklinik of Munich team gave three 0.2-ml doses of an extract of foods, food coloring and food additives to 20 children who had previously become more hyperactive after eating certain foods. Another 20 received a placebo. Parents reported that 16 of the 20 children who received the extract did not show an increase in hyperactive symptoms after eating foods that normally produced hyperactivity. Four children in the placebo group became similarly more tolerant of trigger foods, the team reported in The Lancet.

May 12

High doses of a genetically engineered cytotoxin reduced the number and severity of swollen joints in a small group of rheumatoid arthritis patients resistant to other therapies, announced Seragen Inc., the drug's manufacturer. An expert in rheumatology at Beth Israel Hospital in Boston told Medical Tribune that the cytoxin could potentially be a major therapeutic advance against arthritis.

In a preliminary clinical trial, 19 patients received five to seven days of daily intravenous infusions of the cytotoxin, a protein that contained diphtheria toxin and interleukin-2 fused together. Eleven of the 13 patients treated with higher doses improved, but none of the six patients given lower doses did, the company said. Five of the responses amounted to greater than a 50% reduction in both the number of tender joints and the number and severity of swollen joints, the company noted.

May 17

An Environmental Protection Agency survey conducted in Seattle found that low levels of particulate air pollution can cause serious health problems for asthmatics. While city air quality met government standards, the particulate level appeared to be responsible for 11% of asthma-related emergency-room visits during a 13-month period, the EPA reported at the American Lung Association meeting in Miami.

The number of visits to hospitals by asthmatics in the Seattle area was associated with the previous day's measurements of particulate air pollutants, especially particulates that were 10 mcg or smaller.

May 21

The Food and Drug Administration warned that serious injury can result when patients try to achieve younger-looking skin by applying chemical skin-peeling products. The agency announced that it is investigating four injury reports involving Peelaway, a phenol-containing product manufactured by Global Esthetics of Seattle. In one case, a woman suffered seizures, shock and second-degree burns after Peelaway was applied to her legs by a beautician. An FDA spokes-person suggested that patients consult a dermatologist if they are seeking treatment for wrinkles, age spots or acne scars.

May 27

Symptoms of asthma, including wheezing and shortness of breath, were found to be common among elite swimmers and postulated to be caused by irritants in pool water. At least one symptom of respiratory distress was reported in nearly 92% of a group of 251 elite swimmers, according to a Canadian survey presented at a meeting of the American College of Sports Medicine. Of the 35 swimmers with documented asthma, 74% said they had been diagnosed after they had started swimming competitively. The athletes swam 12 to 56 miles a week for 37 to 51 weeks a year for a mean of 9.5 years.

May 28

The antiviral drug interferon alfa-2a (Roferon-A, Roche) may successfully shrink hemangiomas in infants, which until now have been untreatable in up to two thirds of cases, announced researchers at the Dana-Farber Cancer Institute in Boston.

When injected daily for about eight months, the drug shrank life-threatening hemangiomas in 18 of 20 newborns by 50% or more, they reported in The New England Journal of Medicine.

May 31

Two Scottish researchers reported on a mouse study that may hold the key as to why some people prematurely go gray. Studying a mouse strain called light, the researchers found that genetic alteration in a gene that codes for tyrosinase-related protein-1 causes the hair to pigment only at the tip and may affect the way cells store melanin. A similar defect in the analogous human gene may be responsible for familial forms of premature graying, as well as vitiligo, the researchers hypothesized in the journal Nature Genetics.

JUNE

June 1

Skin testing is not helpful in predicting which children will have an adverse reaction to the measles, mumps and rubella vaccine, claimed Johns Hopkins pediatric allergists.

MMR vaccine contains albumin, posing the risk of reaction among egg-sensitized children. In a reevaluation of the safety of the MMR vaccine, 100% of 140 children known to have egg sensitivity were safely vaccinated. Additionally, two children who suffered an anaphylactic response to MMR, despite no history of egg sensitivity, showed no prick skin test reaction to egg, the investigators said.

Presenting their data in the journal Pediatrics, the investigators called on the American Academy of Pediatrics to consider revising its current policies on MMR.

June 4

Nine out of 10 children with atopic dermatitis were found to have skin colonization with Staphylococcus aureus, reported German and French immunologists. Of 41 children tested, 38 harbored S. aureus, compared with 13 of 41 controls, according to a

report in the Journal of Infectious Diseases. The investigators were particularly concerned about the prevalence of toxigenic strains of the bacteria, found in 37% of atopic dermatitis patients and 5% of controls. Previously, outbreaks of staphylococcal toxin disease have been

traced to S. aureus-carrying atopic dermatitis patients.

Antibiotic therapy aimed at eliminating S. aureus has been attempted in atopic dermatitis patients, but recolonization recurs immediately, according to the European researchers.

June 12

A George Washington University photobiologist warned that sunscreens with sun protection factors of 15 or more don't offer complete protection against the damaging effects of ultraviolet radiation. Twelve of 13 sunscreens tested did not effectively protect against UV radiation-induced immune suppression, he told a Senate subcommittee on Consumer and Environmental Affairs. However, an official of a leading sunscreen manufacturer told the subcommittee that his company's research showed that the higher SPF products did provide protection against immune suppression.

June 13

Synthetic versions of magainins, natural antibiotics

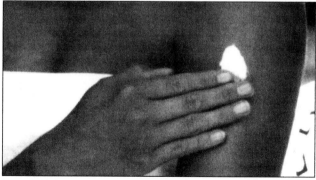

Even SPF 15 suncreens may not completely protect against UV rays.

found in the skin of African clawed toads, display potent antitumor properties, a University of Pennsylvania researcher told the 18th World Congress of Dermatology.

In a two-month study of mice with intraperitoneal ovarian carcinoma, magainin injections cleared the animals

of detectable cancer, the investigator said at the New York meeting. The magainins proved as effective as adriamycin, and killed a variety of laboratory-grown human cancers on contact.

Previously, magainins had proved cytotoxic to numerous organisms, including bacteria, fungi, the malarial parasite Plasmodium falciparum and acanthamoebas, which can infect the corneas of contact-lens wearers.

June 15

A two-year study by Yale and Harvard researchers suggested that a new vaccine may break the Lyme disease infection cycle at the animal vector stage—before humans are exposed. The vaccine protected mice from becoming infected when they were bitten by Lyme-infected ticks, the team reported in the Proceedings of the National Academy of Sciences. At the same time, the Borrelia burgdorferi bacteria were killed in the ticks who fed on vaccinated animals, while 72% of recovered ticks remained Lyme-infected after feeding on control mice. Similar vaccines have been used to fight malaria.

June 16

An Australian skin cancer expert dismissed predictions of a dramatic rise in skin cancer rates due to ozone depletion. He pointed out that predictions of the rise are based on estimates of the number of people in their 50s and 60s who had suffered repeated sunburns when they were children. Younger people, in contrast, are heeding education campaigns and covering up when in the sun, the coordinator of the Australian Cancer Society said at the World Congress of Dermatology meeting in New York.

June 17

The active ingredient in the acne drug isotretinoin

(Accutane, Roche) may help in the treatment of potentially cancerous oral lesions, announced researchers at the M. D. Anderson Cancer Center in Houston.

Leukoplakia was reversed in 67% of 33 people who received 13-cis-retinoic acid, they told the American Association for Cancer Research meeting in San Diego.

June 18

Since blood tests for Lyme disease may produce false-positive results, physicians must look for symptoms such as bull's-eye erythema, and may also need to do more extensive tests of the nervous system before diagnosing Lyme disease, said a Lyme disease expert from Tufts University School of Medicine in Boston.

Speaking at the 18th World Congress of Dermatology in New York, he said that a diagnosis based on physical symptoms alone may also be inaccurate, since the patient may actually have arthritis or chronic fatigue syndrome.

Maintaining that Lyme disease is an overdiagnosed illness, he said that physicians must weigh both clinical symptoms and blood and neurological tests before making a diagnosis.

June 24

People whose basal-cell or squamous-cell carcinomas had been successfully treated were reported to have up to a 50% chance of a subsequent cancer within five years. Data from a six-year multicenter study of 1,805 patients in The Journal of The American Medical Association indicated that the risk of a subsequent malignancy was greatest among men over age 60 at the time of first diagnosis, fair-skinned people and those with severe actinic sun damage. Current smokers were twice as likely to have a subsequent cancer as those who had never smoked, said the Dartmouth Medical School investigators.

JULY

July 4

British researchers announced that an ancient Chinese herbal remedy may relieve symptoms of allergic dermatitis. About half of 40 patients with intractable dermatitis who were given a tea containing an extract of 10 herbs said that they itched less and slept better, according to the report in The Lancet. Dermatitis was reduced, and there were no side effects aside from the unpleasant taste of the tea, the researchers from the Royal Free Hospital asserted. Despite the encouraging results, an American dermatologist told Medical Tribune that the treatment must be further tested for potential toxic effects and strict guidelines must be developed before it could be prescribed to the general public.

July 7

At the request of the Food and Drug Administration, Marion Merrell Dow, Inc. announced plans to send letters to 600,000 healthcare professionals warning them that some allergy patients who use the antihistamine terfenadine (Seldane) may be at risk of life-threatening cardiac arrhythmias. The new warnings, upgraded from precautions, come as a result of a new study conducted by Marion Merrell Dow and FDA consultants that confirmed the link. Patients thought to be at risk are those who use the antihistamine while also taking erythromycin or the antifungal drug ketoconazole (Nizoral, Janssen), patients with liver disease and those who take an overdose of terfenadine, including a single dose of 360 mg. The recommended dose for adults is 60 mg b.i.d.

July 10

Seattle researchers successfully protected three bone-marrow transplant patients against a deadly virus by transfusing donor immune cells trained to attack the virus. Although the study involved few patients, immunologists said it could open the way to new treatments for cancer and AIDS.

T-cells from the patients' bone-marrow donors were cultivated and exposed in vitro to cytomegalovirus-infected cells; they were then infused

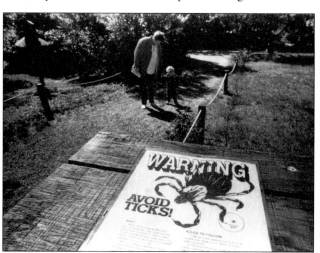

CDC: Lyme disease cases dropped but reached over 23 states.

once a week for four weeks into patients. The T-cells retained their ability to attack the virus for up to 12 weeks, and none of the patients developed CMV infections, researchers from the Fred Hutchinson Cancer Research Center reported in Science. Ordinarily, the virus infects about 50% of bone-marrow recipients.

July 13

The incidence of basal-cell carcinoma in one Swedish town doubled from 1970 to 1986, researchers revealed. In the review of histologically diagnosed BCC cases in Malmo, approximately two thirds of the tumors were found on the head and neck, the Allmanna Sjukhuset researchers reported in the journal Cancer. As populations age, greater allocation of medical resources to BCC treatment will be required, they warned. The investigators hypothesized that the rise could be due to increased screening, increased exposure to sunlight resulting from increased leisure time, exposure to chemicals or other unknown factors.

July 15

Seven patients who took an herbal preparation, germander, to promote weight loss developed hepatitis-like symptoms, underscoring the dangers of self-treatment with herbal remedies, reported a researcher at Saint-Eloi Hospital in Montpellier, France. It is not known how the herb, part of the mint family, damages the liver, but some scientists speculated that it may trigger an immune or allergic reaction. The patients' symptoms included jaundice, abdominal pain and dark urine, which gradually disappeared when the germander was discontinued, according to the report in the Annals of Internal Medicine.

July 18

The number of Lyme disease cases reported so far this year was down 15% compared with the same time last year, said the Centers for Disease Control. However, the figures—2,997 this year versus 3,582 last year—may be misleading: The real number of cases is undoubtedly much higher, and the tick-borne disease has spread into 23 states, warned CDC experts. Tighter standards for diagnos-

ing the disease and less media coverage, along with a public that is better educated in avoiding the disease-carrying ticks, were included as possible factors in the apparent leveling-off of prevalence, said the coordinator of the Lyme disease program at the CDC.

July 20

The Food and Drug Administration warned that allergy sufferers taking the antihistamine astemizole (Hismanal, Janssen Pharmaceutica) should not exceed the recommended dosage of one daily 10-mg tablet. The announcement followed reports of nine deaths and 44 serious cardiovascular events from the drug's use. Most cases were associated with substantial doses, including three deaths from intentional overdose. However, some cases of arrhythmia occurred at doses as low as 20 to 30 mg, the FDA said.

Because astemizole does not become effective until blood levels build up, some physicians start patients on higher doses. Following the FDA announcement, the president of the American Academy of Allergy and Immunology called on his colleagues to stop this practice.

July 26

A Chicago geriatric specialist reported an outbreak of pediculosis among tenants of a Chicago retirement home. Because topical lindane (Kwell, Reed & Carnick) treatment for pediculosis is thought to be associated with greater toxicity in very old and young patients, the Northwestern University Medical School investigator emphasized the importance of discerning and correcting likely modes of transmission. In this case, the outbreak was traced to the linens, which had been brought to a local laundromat. Clean and soiled linens were found next to each other, and bags used for clean and dirty linens were not differentiated, the investigator reported in the Journal of the American Geriatrics Society.

AUGUST

Aug. 1

Administration of pulse-released albuterol sulfate (Proventil Repetabs, Schering) to asthmatics at bedtime significantly improved their overnight pulmonary function and morning peak-flow readings, announced researchers at the National Jewish Center for Immunology and Respiratory Medicine in Denver. As reported in Chest, the scientists studied 10 patients in a randomized, double-blind, placebo-controlled, crossover study. Placebo patients experienced a significant overnight drop in forced expiratory volume, while those taking albuterol sulfate did not. Albuterol patients also reported less nighttime wheezing and awakening.

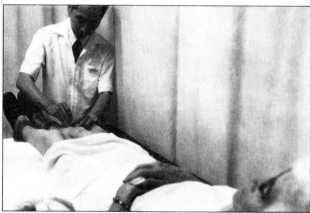
Severe knee arthritis found to respond well to acupuncture.

Aug. 5

British investigators announced progress using photodynamic therapy to remove cutaneous tumors. The method involves the use of a light-sensitive cream containing aminolevulinic acid. The cream, which is applied to the cancerous area and wiped off several hours later, triggers the production of large amounts of porphyrins in tumor cells, the University of Leeds researchers told Medical Tribune. Laser irradiation for five to 30 minutes activates the compound, inducing tumor necrosis.

In 30 patients with either basal-cell carcinomas or Bowen's disease, 90% of the Bowen's patients reportedly had a complete response, and 80% remained clear a year later. Ninety percent of the patients with basal-cell carcinomas had an initial complete response, and 63% were clear a year later, said the Leeds team.

Aug. 6

Children with severe food allergies are more vulnerable than ever to anaphylaxis from "hidden" ingredients used by increasing numbers of manufacturers, Johns Hopkins University researchers reported in The New England Journal of Medicine. In a study of 13 children with asthma and food allergies, six died and seven anaphylaxed after accidentally ingesting foods such as peanuts, eggs and milk proteins in commercial bread, cookies and candy. One expert called for greater use of emergency epinephrine and education about the signs of anaphylaxis to prevent death from accidental allergen ingestion.

Aug. 10

Acupuncture can ease pain and improve joint movement in cases of severe knee arthritis, researchers at the University of Copenhagen in Denmark reported in Acta Anaesthesiologie Scandinavica.

Researchers randomly assigned 29 patients with severe arthritis who were candidates for knee replacement surgery to receive either traditional Chinese acupuncture, in which needles are inserted for 20 minutes into specific points under the skin, or standard painkillers twice a week for nine weeks.

Acupuncture patients had significantly less pain and better function in tests of walking 50 feet and climbing 20 steps, with seven of them responding so well they declined surgery. Improvements continued during yearlong follow-up.

Aug. 15

Ten healthcare workers became tuberculin positive while caring for an 84-year-old woman with a weeping leg sore positive for Staphylococcus epidermidis and Candida, reported a University of Rochester physician. Although extrapulmonary TB is not usually considered contagious, this case and others point to an increased risk of transmission for hospital personnel, the Rochester, N.Y., physician warned in the Annals of Internal Medicine.

Aug. 19

Doctors at the Arizona Cancer Center in Tucson announced that they are testing whether a cream that stimulates the production of melanin can protect the skin from ultraviolet radiation damage. The cream, a synthetic analogue of alpha-melanotropin, is called Melano-Tan II.

If found safe and effective, the cream would be particularly useful in photosensitivity disease and albinism, the researchers stated in the Journal of the National Cancer Institute.

Aug. 25

University of Colorado researchers reported that varicella zoster vaccine might prevent shingles in older people who had had varicella infection years earlier.

Immunization with live attenuated VZV seems to renew the body's immunity to the virus after the body's cell-mediated immune response

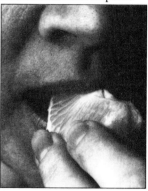
Chemical in discarded orange peel may protect against skin cancer.

wanes with age, the researchers stated in the Journal of Infectious Diseases.

The study of 202 volunteers aged 55 to 87 injected with the vaccine showed significantly increased levels of anti-VZV antibodies and VZV-specific proliferating T-cells during the first year. At 24 months, no patients had developed shingles; several cases would have been expected without treatment.

Aug. 31

A chemical found in the peel of a bitter Mediterranean orange may protect fair-skinned people from skin cancer, investigators at the Cancer Research Campaign in Manchester, England, reported. They studied a group of fair-skinned people who were given either a standard sunscreen or a sunscreen fortified with the chemical, 5-methoxypsoralen, and then were exposed to artificial sunlight to simulate sun exposure equivalent to two weeks in the Mediterranean. Skin samples taken at the end of two weeks indicated that those who used the fortified sunscreen had one third to one half the DNA damage as those who used standard lotion, the researchers told Medical Tribune.

Sept. 10

Massachusetts researchers said that they are hoping a full-thickness living skin substitute they have developed will one day replace self-donated grafts in burn victims, the Medical Tribune reported.

Graftskin, manufactured by Organogenesis of Cambridge, is produced by constructing a dermal layer of collagen with fibroblasts, which is then overlaid with epidermal cells from donated neonatal fore-skins. These cells are placed on top of the dermal layer to grow into a multilayered human skin equivalent. It has not provoked any infections or immune responses in five burn patients after 18 months, according to a researcher at the company.

The fully differentiated four-by-eight-inch Graftskin patches are immunologically neutral and can be grafted without tissue matching or immune suppression. Five centers are now recruiting 100 patients for further studies.

•••

An outbreak of Tricho-phyton tonsurans infection of the scalp and trunk affected eight of 22 members of a school wrestling team, diag-nosing physicians reported in The New England Journal of Medicine. The Johns Hopkins University School of Medicine team suggested that sharing protective headgear, as well as skin-to-skin contact during wrestling holds, may have contributed to the fungal in-fections. They recommended that coaches exclude wrestlers with infected skin and scalp lesions from practice and competition, a precaution already suggested for wrestlers with herpesvirus sores.

Sept. 16

Caucasian men and women living on the Hawaiian island of Kauai have the highest rate of basal-cell carcinoma in the United States, a Dayton, Ohio, researcher reported at an American Academy of Derma-tology meeting in New York. The incidence is 422 per 100,000 people, compared

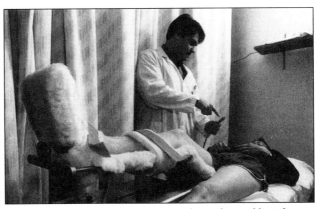

SEPTEMBER

Arthritis patients who used a continuous passive motion machine at home after surgery had less swelling, more flexibility and lower medical expenses.

with 317 per 100,000 in Tucson and 185 per 100,000 in San Francisco, the Wright State University scientist said. The cancer occurs more often in middle-aged and older people. White Kauaian men over age 75 have basal-cell carcinoma about twice as often as women of the same age. At younger ages, however, rates between men and women are more similar.

•••

Boston researchers an-nounced that arthritis sufferers who require total knee arthro-plasty can save nearly $7,000 in rehabilitation expenses by utilizing a home physical ther-apy machine. Ninety-three patients with end-stage rheu-matoid or osteoarthritis re-ceived either standard physical therapy or were discharged with a continuous passive mo-tion machine after surgery at Brigham and Women's Hos-pital. The home PT machine gently bends and extends the leg in slow increments while the patient lies in a supine position. Patients receiving the continuous motion (between 6.3 and 12.4 hours a day) had less swelling, achieved earlier motion and, at six weeks after surgery, had three degrees more active flexion than pa-tients who received traditional therapy, the team reported in The Journal of the American Medical Association.

For the six weeks of ther-

apy, the total cost for users of the machine was $53,160, compared with $59,924 for standard therapy, which in-volved having the knees for-cibly flexed under anesthesia.

Sept. 21

Autoimmune disease is the least likely consequence of silicone breast implants, an immunologist from Johns Hopkins Medical Center told the annual meeting of the American Society of Plastic and Reconstructive Surgeons. Expert panelists said that based on current data, they believe that immune disorders only occur in the small fraction of implant recipients who are genetically predisposed to the conditions. A Los Angeles authority said the implants should not be removed in the vast majority of women.

Sept. 23

University of Miami aller-gists announced that Hurricane Andrew had unleashed a torrent of allergy and asthma misery in southern Florida. The initial downing of trees boosted pollen counts. With the cleanup came airborne irritants to many asthma and allergy sufferers, including dust, dirt and ashes from fires set to burn rubble. Finally, water damage encouraged mold growth in the carpets and walls of affected homes, they reported, and residents were

unable to use air conditioners to counter high humidity.

Sept. 25

A new hair transplant technique called linear grafting produced more aesthetic re-sults for 32 patients with male pattern baldness than conven-tional grafting, its developer told Medical Tribune.

Small, linear grafts about 2 to 5 cm long by 2 mm wide are placed in a curved manner be-hind and parallel to the frontal hairline, ensuring a smooth, continuous appearance, said the dermatologic plastic surgeon from the University of Arkansas. Other advantages include preservation of exist-ing hair, good graft yield and minimal scarring, he claimed.

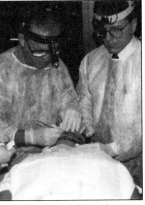

Small, linear hair transplants produced more aesthetic results.

Sept. 26

British researchers reported that they have used humanized monoclonal antibodies to treat rheumatoid arthritis. The Cambridge University investi-gators used genetic engineer-ing to convert rodent mono-clonal antibodies to a human form less likely to cause immune system rejection.

Seven of 8 patients with rheumatoid arthritis unrespon-sive to drug therapy improved clinically after a 10-day course of anti-CD52 (Campath-1H, Burroughs Wellcome), with a reduction in joint swelling and inflammation lasting from 12 weeks to eight months; there were no appreciable side effects or signs of rejection, stated the report in The Lancet.

Dermatology/Allergy/Immunology/Rheumatology

Oct. 1

Australian researchers found that laundering bedding in the hottest cycle of the washing machine will kill dust mites. But most commercial detergents do not kill mites, the University of Sydney team reported in the Journal of Allergy and Clinical Immunology.

The Australian team put live mites in capsules and exposed them to water at varying temperatures with different detergents. They found that water temperatures of 131 degrees Fahrenheit killed all mites, 122 degrees killed half, and below 113 degrees, there was virtually no effect at all. None of 11 commercial laundry products tested killed mites at the lowest temperatures; however, eucalyptus oil, an Australian product, killed mites at 122 degrees when used in concentrations 30 times that recommended by the manufacturer.

Oct. 2

Government researchers reported that asthma incidence and mortality in the United States have risen sharply in the past decade, especially among women and African-Americans. Asthma deaths increased by 54% among women, compared with 23% for men, a Centers for Disease Control epidemiologist wrote in Morbidity and Mortality Weekly Report. Deaths were consistently more prevalent in African-Americans than in whites, and every year throughout the 1980s African-

Americans were twice as likely to be hospitalized for asthma as whites. The researcher added that the number of people who saw a doctor for asthma increased from 6.5 million in 1985 to 7.1 million in 1990.

Oct. 8

Researchers from the Mayo Clinic in Rochester, Minn., reported that the number of young children with asthma has increased as much as 200% in the past two decades. Indoor air pollution, maternal smoking and respiratory-tract infections all are important factors in the increase, the researchers said at a New York press conference sponsored by the American Lung Association. Children ages 1 through 4 had the most startling increases in asthma diagnosis.

Oct. 12

A session of the American College of Rheumatology meeting in Atlanta was told that children with arthritis should be encouraged to exercise regularly and participate in gym classes at school. Researchers at Hahnemann Hospital in Philadelphia studied five children aged 5 to 13 years—four with rheumatoid arthritis and one with another unspecified form of joint disease. A one-hour exercise program three times a week for six weeks improved the children's aerobic capacity, increased their exercise tolerance

and decreased joint pain and stiffness. Four of the five children improved significantly in their ability to do sit-ups and long-distance running; none suffered injuries. The amount of pain reported by the children and the number of joints affected by arthritis was cut by almost half, they said.

Oct. 14

San Francisco researchers found that estrogen may ease the symptoms of rheumatoid arthritis. Of 154 postmenopausal women with RA, those who reported long-term estrogen use had significantly better function and fewer swollen and painful joints than women who had discontinued the hormone, according to study results presented at an Arthritis Foundation meeting in Atlanta. Researchers from the University of California at San Francisco said the study was prompted by the long-standing observation that the majority of women with RA have fewer symptoms when they are pregnant, followed by a worsening of symptoms within the first four weeks after giving birth.

Oct. 22

To spot patients with rheumatoid arthritis, physicians should watch for a gradual onset of pain, swelling and tenderness in small and large joints, fever, fatigue and morning stiffness, a North Carolina researcher told Medical Tribune. The swollen soft tissue may feel spongy, but the patient may not have redness or heat, so sometimes doctors miss the diagnosis, the Duke University expert said. He also recommended a complete blood count, as inflammation will lower the blood count and the hematocrit.

• • •

British and Dutch researchers reported that asthmatics who regularly used an inhaled

beta-agonist to open their airways built up a tolerance to the drug that made them more vulnerable to the effects of substances that can trigger an asthma attack. Their findings, reported in The New England Journal of Medicine, added to the concern that regular treatment with beta-agonists alone may make it more difficult to control patients' asthma, according to the study's lead author.

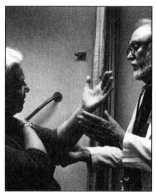

Pain, swelling and fatigue can signal rheumatoid arthritis.

Oct. 29

Baltimore researchers found that patients who are allergic to fish and other foods may be able to satisfy their fish craving by eating canned tuna. Eating canned tuna produced no hives or other symptoms of allergies in 45 children and adults who were allergic to various foods, the researchers reported in the Journal of Allergy and Clinical Immunology.

About half of the 45 people in the study were allergic to cooked fish, and others were allergic to various other foods. None of them developed allergy symptoms after consuming 3 to 6 ounces of chunk-light tuna, and they continued to eat the canned fish for at least six months after the first attempt without experiencing any adverse reactions. The fish proteins responsible for allergies appear to be destroyed during the canning process, said the Johns Hopkins researchers, who added that the findings may also apply to canned salmon.

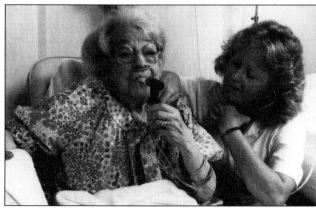

CDC reported that asthma deaths have increased 54% in women.

Dermatology/Allergy/Immunology/Rheumatology

Nov. 5

Health officials meeting in Baltimore expressed concern over an increasing number of reports of dangerous allergic reactions to latex products. The U.S. Food and Drug Administration sponsored the conference after receiving reports of 16 deaths linked to latex exposure during barium enemas. In 1991, doctors in Milwaukee reported a cluster of severe latex allergies in 10 children who had undergone surgery as newborns. At the meeting, a Milwaukee researcher said that in some people even indirect exposure to latex, such as being in a room with an open box of latex gloves, can provoke a powerful allergic response. Those at highest risk of latex allergies are operating room personnel and children who have surgical procedures, according to reports at the meeting. No serious risk of latex allergies is thought to exist from the use of condoms in the general population.

Nov. 15

Several studies presented at the 50th Anniversary Meeting of the American College of Allergy and Immunology concluded that asthma patients need closer monitoring and more information to reduce their risk of hospitalization and death. At the Chicago meeting, a San Francisco physician reported that 20% of asthmatics he had studied significantly underestimated the severity of their asthma. A Colorado doctor found that children with asthma who were pretreated and monitored throughout a daylong ski trip showed an improvement in their asthma at the end of the day. And a Sylvania, Ohio, doctor reported that adult asthma patients who attended a self-help management program showed significant long-term improvements in their knowledge of the disease and in their confidence about managing the illness.

Nov. 16

Denver allergists announced that they had successfully desensitized five patients to rifampin and five to ethambutol (Myambutol, Lederle). The treatment enabled the tuberculosis-positive patients to resume optimal antibiotic treatment, the investigators reported at the 50th Anniversary Meeting of the American College of Allergy and Immunology in Chicago.

During the desensitization protocol, patients were given increasingly larger oral doses of each drug at 45-minute intervals over a nine-hour

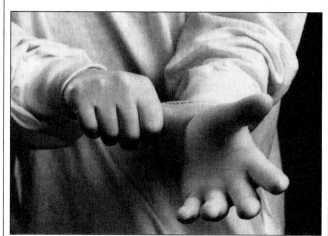

Latex gloves can pose severe problems for some healthcare workers.

period. Full-strength doses were then administered over the next three days.

Four patients developed a rash during desensitization; three responded to antihistamines and one required prednisone. No patient required cessation of antibiotic therapy.

Nov. 17

A Milwaukee allergist told the 50th Anniversary Meeting of the American College of Allergy and Immunology that some U.S. healthcare workers appear to be becoming increasingly sensitive to latex and are at risk of potentially life-threatening allergic reactions. Researchers from Columbia Hospital tested for latex-specific allergic anti-

bodies in healthcare workers with contact dermatitis, contact urticarial syndrome or systemic reactions such as hives or anaphylaxis. Most of the patients with a history of systemic reactions, but one with a localized reaction, tested positive for the antibodies, the allergist reported.

• • •

A Memphis allergist announced that many coaches of school athletic teams lack knowledge about exercise-induced asthma and unnecessarily restrict affected children from participating in sports.

In a survey of 49 public-school coaches, 35% did not allow children with asthma to participate in any sports, including bowling and golf. Six percent of the coaches said they thought children with asthma were less competent at sports, according to the researchers.

The survey also showed that many of the coaches were misinformed about how to prevent and treat exercise-induced asthma. For example, 51% of the coaches said they didn't know the proper time children should use a metered-dose inhaler to prevent exercise-induced asthma. In addition, only 8% knew that cold, dry air can trigger an attack; 57% actually thought that warm, dry air was a more likely trigger.

Nov. 18

New Orleans physicians reported that a processed fish product used in imitation crab and a variety of meatless foods may cause severe allergic reactions in fish-sensitive patients. Known as surimi, the fish product is derived from Alaskan pollock and poses a significant health risk, since most foods that contain surimi are not labeled as containing fish or fish products, the investigators reported at the American College of Allergy and Immunology's 50th Anniversary Meeting in Chicago.

They described the case of a 39-year-old woman with asthma, rhinitis and fish allergy who experienced several episodes of wheezing, oral pruritus and hives within minutes of ingesting imitation crab meat.

The investigators urged manufacturers to list surimi as an ingredient in foods that contain the fish product, such as meatless hotdogs, sausages and pizza toppings.

Nov. 30

A government study found that asthma has a significant impact on the health and well-being of children.

Compared with nonasthmatic children, American children with asthma miss an additional 10.1 million days of school each year, visit the doctor 12.9 million additional times and are hospitalized 200,000 additional times, the researchers reported in Pediatrics. The estimates were based on a survey of 17,110 households conducted by researchers at the Centers for Disease Control and Prevention in Atlanta and the University of California at San Francisco.

Almost 30% of kids with asthma were limited at least somewhat in their activities, compared with 5% of children without asthma, the researchers found. African-American children with asthma had significantly greater restrictions in activity; they had fewer doctors' visits but were hospitalized more frequently than white asthmatic children.

DECEMBER

Dec. 5

A Houston dermatologist reassured physicians that skin pigmentation need not be a factor when considering phototherapy treatment for hyperbilirubinemia of the newborn. Phototherapy is not contraindicated in infants with albinism or neonatal lupus, the dermatologist told the American Academy of Dermatology meeting in San Francisco. Additionally, increased skin pigmentation does not reduce the effectiveness of the treatment, the University of Texas Health Science Center physician stated.

Dec. 7

Austrian investigators suggested that people with allergies to nuts may have similar reactions to tree pollens because of structural similarities between the respective allergens. A study of 25 patients with tree pollen allergy and intolerance to hazelnuts found a cross-reactivity of pollen-specific IgE antibodies. The results, reported in the Journal of Clinical Allergy and Immunology, provide a basis for the theory that food and pollen allergy are frequently associated. The researchers pointed out that other studies have indicated a more pronounced sensitivity to nuts during and after tree pollen season.

Dec. 8

A Barcelona dermatologist reported that subdermal implants made of polytetrafluoroethylene (Gore-Tex Soft Tissue Patch) can be used to permanently correct facial skin irregularities. In 53 patients, small pieces of Gore-Tex patches or threads were used to correct deep nasolabial folds, smooth facial wrinkles or augment the rim and middle section of the upper lip, the physician told the American Academy of Dermatology meeting in San Francisco.

In 10% of the patients, a slight and transitory papulo-erythematous reaction occurred at some point along the trajectory of the threads.

Allergy tests before surgery were not required, and no patient had to have the implants removed for incompatibility, said the dermatologist from the Centro Clinico Disciplinario de Laser y Dermocosmetica.

• • •

A Mayo Clinic dermatologist reminded colleagues that sun-damaged skin can be rapidly and successfully treated with a facial chemical peel. By destroying the epidermis and upper dermal layers, a chemical peel with trichloroacetic acid can dependably improve fine cross-hatched wrinkles and often improves moderately deep wrinkles as well, the dermatologist told the American Academy of Dermatology meeting. Following treatment with the TCA peel, re-epithelialization occurred within seven days and remodeling of dermal collagen continued for up to six months, the physician said.

• • •

A dermatologist from Poland announced that a one- to six-week course of azathioprine (Imuran, Burroughs Wellcome) eased atopic dermatitis in 22 of 24 patients who had suffered with the condition since childhood. Azathioprine (200 mg/day) fully relieved pruritis, inflammation and lichenification in 15 patients and achieved partial improvement in eight others, the Wroclaw physician told the American Academy of Dermatology meeting in San Francisco. One patient's condition worsened on the immunosuppressive therapy and another withdrew from treatment because of abdominal pain, the physician reported. The patients' mean age was 30, with a mean disease duration of 20 years.

• • •

At the American Academy of Dermatology meeting, Swedish dermatologists familiarized their American counterparts with a cutaneous hallmark of longstanding chronic Lyme disease—acrodermatitis chronica atrophicans. The condition is characterized by a bluish-red discoloration and, in some cases, swelling of at least one extremity; Borrelia spirochetes have been cultivated from skin biopsies of the affected areas, said the researchers. The majority of patients also complain of peripheral sensory neuropathy, intermittent pains, muscle cramps and weakness in the muscles of the affected limbs. Over many years, the affected areas of the skin gradually become atrophic and develop a "crumpled cigarette paper" appearance, said dermatologists from the Karolinska Institute in Stockholm. Acrodermatitis chronica atrophicans has been diagnosed almost exclusively in Europe or in European immigrants to the United States.

Dec. 9

An Emory University physician reminded dermatologists to look for underlying bowel pathology when erythema nodosum or pyoderma gangrenosum are diagnosed. Erythema nodosum occurs in up to 9% of patients with ulcerative colitis and 15% of patients with Crohn's disease; it responds best to surgical or medical treatment of the underlying colitis, said the Atlanta specialist. The researcher told the American Academy of Dermatology meeting that pyoderma gangrenosum occurs in 12% of patients with ulcerative colitis but only 2% of those with Crohn's disease. The cutaneous ulcerations of the lower extremities or face, or at the parastomal site, that accompany pyoderma gangrenosum are often unresponsive to treatment.

Dec. 16

Canadian investigators reported that the natural history of occupational asthma appears to be different depending on the sensitizing agent. In a 661-worker study of occupational asthma, persons sensitive to Western red cedar or to isocyanates were twice as likely to have a rapid onset of symptoms (within a year after exposure) than were persons sensitive to high-molecular-weight agents (such as crabs, flour, and laboratory animal antigens), the investigators wrote in the Journal of Allergy and Clinical Immunology. The findings may be helpful in understanding symptom development in common IgE-mediated allergies, stated the University of Vancouver researchers.

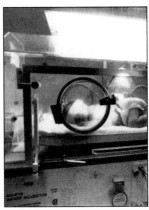

Phototherapy is said to be safe and effective in albinism.

Dec. 21

Liquid and powder laundry detergents containing enzymes were not found to be associated with skin irritation in most consumers. Ohio researchers working for the Proctor & Gamble company conducted fabric- and garment-exposure tests with mens' briefs and T-shirts, wrist bands, infant wear and cloth diapers. The study of 100 volunteers, reported in Cutaneous and Ocular Toxicology, found that even when the clothing was washed in an excess amount of the detergents and worn damp on the wrist, people were no more likely to complain of irritation than if the detergents had no enzymes. Enzymes have been added to various laundry detergents in the United States and Europe for at least the last 20 years.

Capsaicin cream stops itches and nerve pain

JAN. 9—Topical capsaicin may relieve the pruritus associated with long-term hemodialysis, according to Ohio researchers.

The cream, derived from chili peppers, has also been used to treat nerve pain associated with herpes, diabetes, rheumatoid arthritis and psoriasis, wrote Debra L. Breneman, M.D., of the University of Cincinnati Medical Center, in the Journal of the American Academy of Dermatology.

Eight of nine hemodialysis patients who applied 0.025% cream four times daily for six weeks reported relief or complete cessation of the itching sensation, according to Dr. Breneman.

Capsaicin has been shown to deplete and prevent the reaccumulation of substance P, a principal neurotransmitter involved in the transmission of the itch sensation, she said.

The patients applied the cream (Zostrix, GenDerm Corp.) to their chests, arms or legs. Aside from a slight, temporary burning sensation, none of the participants experienced any adverse side effects, Dr. Breneman reported.

"Pruritis is very common among hemodialysis patients, and in some it actually impairs their quality of life," said Joel Kopple, M.D., of the Harborview-UCLA Medical Center in Los Angeles. "They scratch themselves while they sleep, tear their skin and develop skin infections. They're very uncomfortable."

Doctors have tried to treat the condition with moisturizers, topical steroids, UVB light, antihistamines, cholestyramine and intravenous lidocaine, but either the treatments are ineffective, or the patients cannot tolerate the side effects, according to Dr. Breneman.

In a separate study, Geraldine M. McCarthy, M.D., a rheumatologist at the Medical College of Wisconsin in Milwaukee, found that the cream significantly reduced pain in the finger joints of people with osteoarthritis.

"The drug won't change the progression of the disease, but it will make patients feel better," she said. The drug may be particularly beneficial to people who experience gastrointestinal symptoms after taking nonsteroidal anti-inflammatory medications, she added.

In studies of 101 patients conducted at six medical centers, Zostrix relieved pain in arthritic patients, according to Patrice Flynn, associate director of clinic research at GenDerm Corp., Lincolnshire, Ill.

"In four-week double-blind studies, rheumatoid arthritis patients experienced an average 57% reduction in pain, while osteoarthritis patients reported a 33% reduction in pain," she said.

Photopheresis for scleroderma on hold

By Patty Williams

WASHINGTON, D.C., JAN. 21—Members of the Food and Drug Administration's Arthritis Advisory Committee found themselves with no application to consider when company sponsors abruptly withdrew a request for approval of its photopheresis therapy for the treatment of severe scleroderma.

Therakos, a subsidiary of Johnson & Johnson, had sought approval for the combination treatment, but in a letter asked the agency to withdraw its request and keep recent study data confidential. As a result, advisors found themselves discussing data from an earlier study reviewed last year, as well as other treatments being studied for the disease and how best to design trials to determine the effectiveness of therapy.

Many of the problems associated with the new drug application for photopheresis were attributed to poor study design, said Janet Woodcock, acting deputy director for Biologics Evaluation and Research at the FDA.

Because the trial was initiated after observing a dramatic and immediate improvement in two seriously ill scleroderma patients who had undergone photopheresis, study designers apparently believed a large treatment effect would be seen in the study as well and did not make adequate provisions to detect smaller effects, she said.

In its application, Therakos cited a study of 56 patients from eight medical centers. Thirty-one patients received photopheresis plus D-penicillamine and 25 received D-

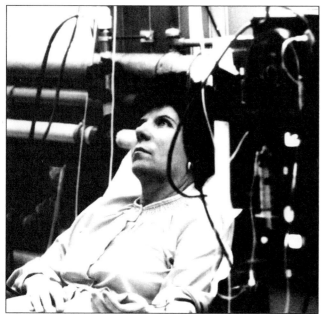

Hemodialysis patient may benefit from topical capsaicin.

penicillamine alone. Two thirds of the patients on the combination therapy improved and only 10% got worse. Of the 25 treated with D-penicillamine alone, one third improved and one third got worse.

Photopheresis is approved for cutaneous T-cell lymphoma and is being studied in patients with AIDS-related complex, rheumatoid arthritis and cardiac transplant rejection.

The technique involves giving 8-methoxypsoralen (8-MOP), and removing a pint of blood and cycling it through a machine that treats it with ultraviolet light. The blood is then returned to the patient and the light-activated 8-MOP latches on to diseased T-cells and keeps them from multiplying.

"We continue to believe that this therapy is safe and effective for the treatment of systemic sclerosis," a Johnson & Johnson spokesperson said. "However, we feel that it would be fruitless to pursue this application further."

Rep. John D. Dingell (D-Mich.), chairman of the Subcommittee on Oversight and Investigations, recently held a hearing on the FDA's handling of the application. In the official transcript, Dingell called the matter "confusing, at best."

Central air conditioning keeps allergens at bay

ORLANDO, MARCH 10—Room air conditioners appear to be less effective than central air in keeping harmful mold and bacteria from getting into homes and causing breathing problems in people with asthma or allergies.

University of Michigan researchers who studied 12 homes with either type of air conditioners found that higher levels of mold and bacteria were found in homes that had only room air conditioners.

The levels of the mold and bacteria found in these homes were comparable to the levels that would be expected in homes with no air conditioning, lead researcher Harriet A. Burge reported at the American Academy of Allergy and Immunology annual meeting.

She said that while the study does favor the use of central air, particularly in homes of people with allergies or asthma, room air conditioners are not all bad.

"If you remove all the allergen sources in a room and keep the doors and windows closed, I think that is an effective way of using a room air conditioner," Burge said.

The study was part of a larger study of the effects of indoor pollutants on school-age children done in conjunction with Harvard University.

In another presentation, French researchers reported that expensive so-called antiallergic vacuum cleaners that are purported to clean all troublesome particles, including cat dander, from carpeting are no more effective than standard, inexpensive vacuum cleaners.

In a study of three of these special vacuum cleaners, a carpet in a home with two cats was cleaned for 15 minutes and the air in the room was sampled for 30 minutes.

Frederic de Blay, M.D., of the Hospices Civils Hôpitaux at the Universitaires de Strasbourg, found similar levels of cat dander in the air after using the special cleaners and after using the inexpensive vacuum cleaner.

"We conclude that allergists and patients should be careful

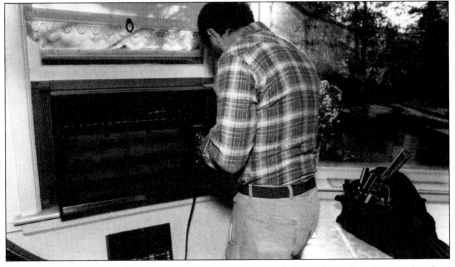

Room air conditioners found less effective than central air for lowering allergen levels.

about buying very expensive antiallergic vacuum cleaners," Dr. de Blay said. The models used in the study were all European brands.

Panel supports use of Retin-A to smooth skin damaged by sun

By Jane Anderson

BETHESDA, MD., APRIL 9—In unanimous votes, two popular acne medications received favorable recommendations from a Food and Drug Administration advisory panel.

The FDA Dermatologic Drugs Advisory Committee recommended that approval of tretinoin (Retin-A, Ortho) be expanded to the treatment of sun-damaged skin. In addition, they recommended that benzoyl peroxide, a nonprescription ingredient in acne preparations used by one quarter of American teenagers, remain on the market pending the outcome of studies assessing its cancer-causing potential.

The committee considered restricting benzoyl peroxide to prescription use only or banning it altogether until additional research is completed.

Over the past decade, several studies have shown that benzoyl peroxide promotes tumor growth in rodents. Citing those, the National Consumers League had petitioned the FDA for a warning label on products containing the ingredient.

But panel members decided that not enough evidence exists indicating that benzoyl peroxide causes or promotes cancer in humans to warrant either limiting its use or adding a warning label to the product.

Scientists at the meeting told FDA panel members that at least one large retrospective study of benzoyl peroxide users showed no evidence that it causes cancer.

"The bottom line is, it was a totally negative survey," said Mark Greene, M.D., an oncologist at the Mayo Clinic in Rochester, Minn.

In the decision on Retin-A, the advisory committee recommended that Ortho be allowed to market the drug as Renova to treat fine facial wrinkles, roughness and uneven skin coloration resulting from sun exposure.

Barbara Gilchrest, M.D., professor of dermatology at Boston University School of Medicine, told the panel that about 80% of patients in three clinical trials showed improvement in these parameters when using Renova once a day for six months. About half of the participants reported excellent improvement, while half reported fair to good improvement.

Nearly twice as many patients improved on Renova as

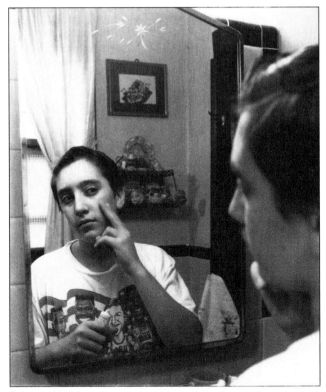

Teens still able to buy creams containing benzoyl peroxide.

improved on a traditional regimen of moisturizers and sun avoidance.

"Patients felt that small wrinkles improved, skin tone improved and skin color improved," said FDA expert Ella Li Toombs, M.D.

When the drug was applied daily for an additional six months, patients' skin condition continued to improve slightly.

After a year, application of Renova three times a week maintained the improvement.

Side effects, which peaked after two weeks and declined afterwards, included mild irritation and peeling in a majority of patients, Dr. Gilchrest said. Five percent of patients stopped using Renova because of the side effects.

The panel cautioned that Retin-A should not be seen as a cure for wrinkles.

However, the panel's consumer representative, Joanne Cossman, cautioned: "The way it will be perceived in the marketplace is as a miracle drug, no matter what."

Enzyme cream repairs skin damaged by sun

APRIL 27—British researchers are testing an experimental U.S.-made skin cream that can repair severely sun-damaged skin, according to the manufacturer.

The cream, known as T4N5 liposome, would also be able to prevent skin damage after sun exposure, said Daniel Yarosh, Ph.D., president of Applied Genetics Inc. in New York.

The cream penetrates to the bottom skin layers, delivering extra doses of the cell-repairing endonuclease that occurs naturally in the body, but is produced too slowly or in insufficient amounts to heal severely damaged skin, according to Dr. Yarosh. The cream also triggers the natural production of endonuclease.

It takes about 12 hours for endonuclease to repair half the damage done to DNA by a severe sunburn, Dr. Yarosh said.

The cream prods the enzyme into action in four to six hours, he said.

Speeding the repair process could reduce the risk of skin cancer from overexposure to the sun.

The London trials of the cream included people with xeroderma pigmentosum.

The rare condition, caused by insufficient supplies of endonuclease, increases the risk of skin cancer 5,000-fold and increases the risk of malignant melanoma 2,000-fold.

Within 10 minutes, the cream began penetrating the skin cells, Dr. Yarosh said.

Although the cream is being tested in people with a rare skin disorder, Dr. Yarosh said he hopes the FDA will approve its use for general public use. The cream is not available on the market.

The cream can also be used after sun exposure, before skin damage occurs, according to Dr. Yarosh. The cream should be applied when the skin is feeling hot, he said.

Fast radioactive injection obviates surgery, provides relief for inflamed synovial tissue

By Fran Kritz

MAY 4—Researchers at Brigham and Women's Hospital in Boston are investigating a 10-minute radiation treatment as a replacement for knee surgery to remove inflamed synovial tissue.

Thousands of surgeries are done each year, either with a traditional incision or laparoscopically, and can cost between $5,000 and $20,000, not including the rehabilitation therapy usually needed.

The new procedure, a 10-minute injection done on an outpatient basis, requires no rehabilitation and is expected to cost far less, according to Clement Sledge, M.D., chairman of Brigham and Women's department of orthopedic surgery.

Initially, however, only research centers near medical nuclear reactors can perform the treatment, because the half-life of the radioactive isotope used in the treatment is only two hours, said Dr. Sledge.

In the procedure, already used widely in Canada as well as in Europe, the radioactive isotope known as ^{165}Dy-FHMA (Dysprosium, Ferric hydroxide Macroaggregate) is combined with an inert carrier that is designed to home in on the synovial tissue.

During the procedure, the radioactive isotope is injected into the patient's knee following administration of a local anesthetic, according to Dr. Sledge.

He said the exact mechanism by which the isotope works is not yet known. About 400 patients in the United States have been treated with the isotope, which can be produced at only 10 nuclear reactors in the country, according to Dr. Sledge.

Researchers are trying to develop similar radioactive substances that last longer and thus could be shipped from reactors to medical centers across the country, he noted.

Some experts are considering building regional nuclear generators to produce the isotope.

Brigham and Women's gets its isotopes from the nearby Massachusetts Institute of Technology.

In the treatment, patients are hospitalized for about eight hours after the injection, with a brace on the knee for part of that time to prevent radiation leakage.

The amount of radiation is thought to be small and poses no harm to the patient. Hospital personnel don't have to take special precautions to avoid radiation either, said Dr. Sledge. They simply avoid long exposure.

About 65% of those treated have had relief in three categories: pain, inflammation and the knee's range of motion.

Success rates aren't higher, according to Dr. Sledge, because the patients have varying degrees of disability prior to treatment.

Paul Lotke, M.D., professor of orthopedics at the University of Pennsylvania School of Medicine, who has referred two patients to Brigham and Women's for the radiation treatment, thinks it has great potential.

He cautioned, however, that pockets of synovial tissue can often be both in front of and behind the knee, making it hard for the isotope to reach all the tissue.

The research team is now studying animal models and both pre- and posttreatment MRI films to see which patients can most effectively be treated with the procedure, Dr. Sledge said.

Unlike arthroscopic surgery, no posttreatment rehabilitation is needed after the radioactive injection, other than a slow return—up to three months—to normal activity, he added.

After surgery, the synovial tissue typically grows back in three to four years, necessitating another operation.

The synovial tissue is likely to grow back even after the radiation treatment, but it can take up to six years for that to occur, according to Dr. Sledge.

At that time, the course of action can be another outpatient injection instead of surgery.

Vaccinating mice may curb transmission of Lyme disease

By Laura Buterbaugh

JUNE 15—A two-year study by Yale and Harvard researchers suggests that a vaccine may break the Lyme disease infection cycle at the animal vector stage—before humans are exposed.

The study also found that the vaccine killed the Borrelia burgdorferi bacteria in ticks that spread the disease, potentially preventing the ticks from infecting other animals and humans.

The study using mice, led by Erol Fikrig, an associate research scientist in immunobiology at Yale University School of Medicine, was published in the Proceedings of the National Academy of Sciences.

"It sets up the possibility that you may be able to eliminate the organism in nature," said Robert Edelman, M.D., associate director for clinical research at the University of Maryland Medical School's Center for Vaccine Development in Baltimore.

The Lyme vaccine, using outer surface protein A (OspA) of B. burgdorferi, follows the pattern of other "altruistic" vaccines, in that it immunizes the animal or insect that spreads the disease rather than protecting the host.

Similar vaccines have been used to fight malaria, by injecting a host with an antibody, Dr. Edelman said. When a mosquito bites the host, the antibody immunizes the mosquito against malaria, making it unable to spread the disease.

"If you can immunize mice, which are the natural reservoirs of Lyme in the environment, you may be able to prevent transmission to man," Dr. Edelman said.

Studies already have shown that a vaccine will protect

mice that are injected with Lyme bacteria. But no previous studies tested the vaccine against Lyme bacteria transmitted naturally: from the bite of a Lyme-infected tick.

Fikrig and his colleagues injected outbred mice with B. burgdorferi. Three weeks later, larval Ixodes dammini ticks were infected with the organism by allowing them to feed on the blood of the mice until they were engorged. The ticks then were collected and grown to the nymphal stage.

Researchers then immunized 30 four-week-old mice with 10 mcg of recombinant OspA, and booster injections on days 14, 28 and 42. Twenty-six control mice were similarly immunized with glutathione transferase.

Fourteen days after the last booster, three or eight ticks were placed on each mouse and allowed to feed until engorgement. The ticks were examined for spirochetes four or 10 days later.

After 10 days, 72% of the recovered ticks remained Lyme infected after feeding on control mice, while none of those feeding on OspA-immunized mice remained infected—evidence that the blood sucked from the vaccinated animals killed the bacteria.

Fikrig said he now is using the vaccine with ticks from different geographical areas, to see if they respond similarly. He also is testing different antigens on the spirochete, such as OspB, for possible alternative vaccines.

He said it could be three to five years before the vaccine is tested in humans.

Dr. Edelman said the vaccine could be used to inoculate wild mice in areas where Lyme disease is prevalent, by putting it into food left for the animals.

Human application must be researched carefully, he said, because the vaccine could cause a severe arthritic autoimmune reaction in people who are genetically predisposed to such a reaction.

But David Volkman, M.D., a professor of medicine at State University of New York at Stony Brook, said oral immunization of wild animals has not been successful in the past, and that immunizing humans may prove more promising.

Sunless tanning method may provide UV shield

AUG. 19—A cream that stimulates the production of melanin may protect the skin from damage caused by ultraviolet rays, Tucson researchers reported in the Journal of the National Cancer Institute.

Since having a tan or being naturally darker-skinned protects against skin cancer, the hope is that the new cream will have the same effect, said one of the researchers, Robert T. Dorr, Ph.D., director of the Cancer Pharmacology Research Program at the Arizona Cancer Center.

The cream, a synthetic analogue of alpha-melanotropin, called Melano-Tan II, is currently in Phase I study.

Previous studies have shown that injections of Melano-Tan I over a two-week period provide a safe way to tan the skin. The effects were seen within two weeks and faded by the seventh week, according to Dr.

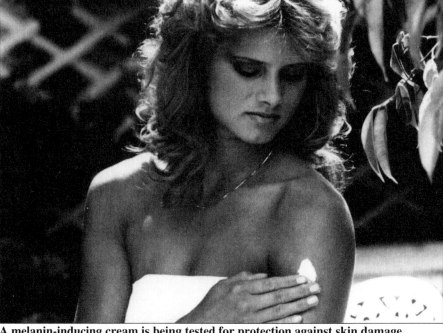
A melanin-inducing cream is being tested for protection against skin damage.

Dorr, who coauthored a paper on the subject last year with Norman Levine, M.D., also of the Arizona Cancer Center.

Side effects included vague gastrointestinal discomfort and a flushing sensation that lasted for about an hour after injection.

According to Dr. Dorr, Melano-Tan II contains half the amino acids of the original and is absorbed 10 times better.

"What normally happens is you get sun damage and, as a delayed response to that, you get a tan," said Dr. Dorr.

"We're trying to tell the cells to make pigment without damaging them first," he said.

Some commercial sunless tanning products contain the carotenoid canthoxanthin.

Although products containing the chemical give the appearance of a tan, they provide no protection against damaging ultraviolet rays.

Dr. Dorr said the ultimate goal of his research is to show that the products protect against skin cancer.

"The objective of the researchers is worth pursuing," said Mahjukar Pathak, M.D., a senior associate in dermatology at Harvard Medical School. He emphasized the need, however, for carefully designed studies to prove the drug's effectiveness.

Ultimately, Melano-Tan II might be useful for albinos, who lack pigment in their skin; for people who develop photosensitivity as a result of taking certain drugs; or for fair-skinned people.

Skin-cancer rate on island of Kauai on the rise

By John Dinolfo

NEW YORK, SEPT. 16—A new study on skin cancer suggests there may be trouble in paradise for the Hawaiian island of Kauai.

Caucasian men and women in Kauai have the highest rate of basal-cell carcinoma in the United States, according to Tsu-Yi Chuang, M.D., associate professor of dermatology at Wright State University in Dayton, Ohio.

For whites in Kauai, the incidence of basal-cell cancer is 422 per 100,000 individuals, compared with 317 per 100,000 in Tucson and 185 per 100,000 in San Francisco, Dr. Chuang said here at a meeting sponsored by the American Academy of Dermatology.

In Kauai, basal-cell carcinoma occurs more often in middle-aged and older people, increasing with age, according to Dr. Chuang.

White Kauaian men above age 75 have basal-cell carcinoma about twice as often as women of the same age. Among white Kauaians aged 35 to 44, however, men and women have roughly the same rates of this cancer.

Basal-cell carcinoma affects an estimated 450,000 people in the United States.

Fair-skinned men and women are at greatest risk of the carcinoma, especially those exposed to the sun for prolonged periods of time.

With residents exposed to intense, yearlong sun, Kauai is the ideal place to study the risk for basal-cell carcinoma.

"A Caucasian who spends his life in Kauai has about a 50% chance of developing basal-cell carcinoma by the age of 82," Dr. Chuang said.

For a white male or female living in Minnesota, the odds of developing this form of cancer are approximately 17%, he said.

Dr. Chuang said that Caucasian Hawaiians may have the highest rate in the nation because they may be exposed to stronger and more prolonged doses of potentially cancer-causing ultraviolet A and B sun rays than other Americans.

Experts do not know whether the findings reported by Dr. Chuang mean the predicted increase in skin cancer this decade will be even worse than expected in sunbaked parts of the United States.

Dr. Chuang speculated that any extra rise in basal-cell cancer should not be dramatic. But he cautioned that Hawaiian residents, as well as vacationers who spend a great deal of time in the state, should think preventively when it comes to sunburns.

"Tourists are very vulnerable," he added, "especially those with lighter complexions."

Physicians should suggest that their patients follow the American Academy of Dermatology's recommendations, which state that one should:
• Stay out of the sun between 10 a.m. and 3 p.m., when the sun's rays are most intense.
• Apply sunscreen liberally and frequently; reapply every two hours when working, playing or exercising outdoors.
• Use a sunscreen with a sun protection factor (SPF) of at least 15, even on cloudy days when 80% of the sun's rays penetrate the clouds.
•Keep babies under six months of age out of the sun. Apply sunscreen on children older than six months, and minimize their sun exposure.

Working toward controlling arthritis with one treatment

By Charlene Laino

CAMBRIDGE, ENGLAND, SEPT. 26—British researchers have taken the first step toward controlling rheumatoid arthritis with a single treatment.

John Isaacs, M.D., of Cambridge University here, reported that he has used humanized monoclonal antibodies to target and destroy cells that cause the disease. He described the technique in The Lancet.

People who suffer from the crippling disease now must take medication for the rest of their lives to control pain and swelling of the joints.

"The results are exciting and promising," said David Pifetsy, M.D., medical advisor for the Arthritis Foundation in Atlanta.

"They suggest that these antibodies may produce long-term results in rheumatoid arthritis sufferers," said Dr. Pifetsy, who is also a professor of medicine at Duke University in Durham, N.C.

About 1% of Americans suffer from rheumatoid arthritis, according to the Arthritis Foundation.

Previously, monoclonal antibodies that were used in an attempt to destroy these extra disease-causing cells were derived from rodents. The rodent antibodies appeared foreign to the human immune system, which rejected them, said Dr. Isaacs.

The British researchers overcame this problem by re-shaping the monoclonal antibodies through genetic engineering, thus converting Chinese hamster antibodies to a human form unlikely to cause rejection.

In the preliminary study, eight patients whose arthritic symptoms had not improved despite drug treatment received intravenous infusions of the modified monoclonal antibodies called anti-CD 52 (Campath-1H, Burroughs Wellcome) two hours a day for 10 days.

Seven of the eight patients showed a marked improvement, with a reduction in joint swelling and inflammation within one week and lasting from three to eight months.

There were no significant side effects or signs of rejection.

Four patients were then given a second course of treatment, which consisted of three times as much of the monoclonal antibodies over a 5-day period. Three showed improvement for up to 200 days, said Dr. Isaacs. However, one patient developed low blood pressure and nausea and had to stop treatment.

The results are encouraging for the ultimate goal of using a single course of treatment to control arthritis or other auto-immune diseases, he said.

The British pharmaceutical company Wellcome thought the results were so promising that it purchased the rights to the drug and is now planning larger studies in rheumatoid arthritis patients, according to Dr. Isaacs. It also will test the drug in another autoimmune disease, lymphoma.

Latex products linked to allergic reactions, deaths; U.S. health experts perplexed

Nov. 5—Health officials are baffled by the increasing number of reports of dangerous allergic reactions to natural rubber latex products, according to experts meeting in Baltimore today through Nov. 7.

Doctors at the conference, sponsored by the U.S. Food and Drug Administration, said the problem of latex allergy was virtually unknown a decade ago.

"This is an unusual, if not unique, problem," said Lauren Charous, M.D., an allergist at the Milwaukee Medical Clinic in Wisconsin.

"Ten years ago, if I'd asked somebody about latex allergies, they would have looked at me like I was crazy," Dr. Charous explained.

Health officials first became aware of the problem last year, when doctors reported a cluster of severe latex allergies in 10 children treated in a Wisconsin hospital.

All of the children had undergone surgery as newborns, and are believed to have become allergic to latex at that time.

The most common allergic reaction to latex is a rash and itchiness, although many victims develop breathing problems or go into shock, Dr. Charous said.

At least 16 deaths linked to latex exposure have been reported to the FDA. All were patients who were having barium enemas with latex-tipped tubing.

In some people, even indirect exposure to latex can provoke a powerful allergic response. "We're talking about people who walk into a room where there is an open box of latex gloves and have asthmatic symptoms, [and] people who touch something and go into shock," Dr. Charous said. "These are profound degrees of reaction."

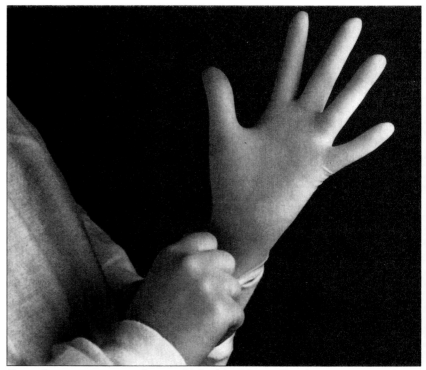

Operating-room personnel are at high risk of latex allergies, experts say.

Those at highest risk of latex allergies are children who have surgical procedures and operating-room personnel, experts say.

Industry representatives at the conference discussed the possibility that a change in the manufacture of latex is introducing allergy-provoking chemicals into the process.

Health officials cannot explain why severe latex allergies have emerged as a problem, according to the Milwaukee researcher.

"That's the big question," Dr. Charous said.

Experts say there is no serious risk of latex allergies from the use of condoms among the general population.

COMMENTARY

No longer just skin deep

By Darrell Rigel, M.D.

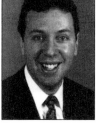

TEN YEARS AGO, A DERMA-tologist might have diagnosed a melanoma and then sent the patient out to a general surgeon for treatment. Today, dermatology has expanded dramatically and we are no longer just diagnosers.

With no condition is this clearer than melanoma. At current rates, one in 105 Americans can be expected to develop melanoma. With the rate of this insidious cancer increasing faster than any other malignancy in the United States or the world, dermatologists must keep abreast of important advances in computer-aided diagnosis. I am most enthusiastic about epiluminescence microscopy, in which a 40-power microscope is placed directly on an oil-covered skin lesion to identify patterns in the lesion that may indicate melanoma. With the development of computer techniques to do some of the analysis, it will be the first time in many practices that computers are used for dermatological diagnosis.

In treating melanoma, narrower and narrower surgical margins are being used. Ten years ago, it was not uncommon for 3- to 5-cm margins to be used for surgically removing melanomas. At the recent National Institutes of Health consensus conference, 1-cm margins were recommended for thin, early melanomas. Soon, narrow margins will become generally accepted for early melanomas.

Better prognostic models are also being developed. The best-known individual prognostic factor is tumor thickness. Now, two new factors have been noted to have a significant impact on survival prediction: tumor volume, which can be computer-estimated based on size and thickness, and tumor growth phases. Tumors first grow radially, and they're not really dangerous at that stage. When they begin to grow vertically, their metastatic potential increases markedly.

One of the biggest controversies in dermatology is the significance of dysplastic nevi, or atypical moles. Are they potential precursors of melanoma, or a vaguer marker for increased risk?

The problem is that dermatopathologists have yet to agree on uniform histological definitions as to what these nevi really are. I personally believe nevi are potential precursors of melanoma as well as markers of increased risk. No matter what pathologists say, people who have many dysplastic nevi are at increased risk.

In regard to pediatric lesions, there is still varied opinion as to whether small congenital nevi must be removed because of melanoma risk. My point of view is that the risk does not justify prophylactic removal. If a clinician believes these should be removed, it is best to wait until a child is 8 or 9 years old and can tolerate local anesthesia.

In less life-threatening areas of dermatologic practice, several satisfying advances in treatment options are emerging. Stronger topical steroids are becoming available, as well as milder topical retinoids. For acne, the continuing development of new retinoids will continue to optimize treatment. Initially, retinoid treatment was only suitable for cystic acne with multiple lesions. Now we're seeing gentler retinoids that can be used to treat milder, papular acne.

I predict a breakthrough in treatments for fungal infections of the nail, a common and disfiguring problem, in the near future. Currently, they are difficult to treat. Oral medications have a significant risk of side effects, while topical medications haven't worked very well. But as major research continues into topical medications for fungus of the nails, I believe improved products will be released — probably in the next year or two.

In conclusion, it's obvious that the scope of dermatology is expanding dramatically to include issues related to oncology, pathology, infectious disease and cosmetic concerns. So I think it's fair to declare that dermatology is no longer skin deep.

Dr. Rigel is clinical associate professor of dermatology at New York University Medical Center.

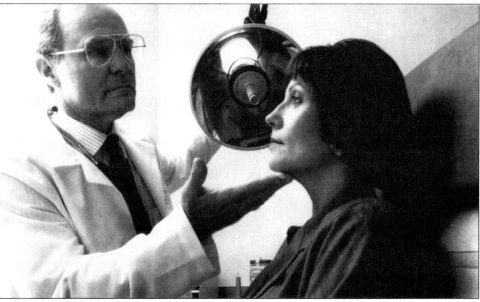

Diagnosing and treating melanoma will be improved with new techniques.

COMMENTARY

Breathlessly awaiting drugs for better control

By Robert N. Hamburger, M.D.

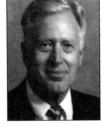

ALLERGISTS, AS WELL AS THE millions of asthma sufferers, are breathlessly awaiting the release of new drugs that hold the promise of better control of both early- and late-phase disease. Some of the therapies are expected to be released as early as 1993 and if they live up to even some of their expectations, the year could mark the turning point in decreasing asthma mortality.

The first development to look for is the expected U.S. Food and Drug Administration approval of two long-acting bronchodilators. Insiders predict that the Food and Drug Administration will give the nod to two 12-hour preparations, Salmeterol (Glaxo) and Formoterol (Ciba-Geigy).

Their twice-a-day dosing regimens hold the promise of reducing asthma-related deaths. Some of us in the field believe that asthma mortality, which has risen from about 2,800 deaths a year in the mid-1980s to about 4,500 in 1990, can be traced to an overreliance on beta-agonists. The drugs, which are very effective at relaxing constricted bronchi, do nothing to relieve the underlying respiratory inflammation, which has come to be known as the hallmark of the disease. Left unchecked, this underlying inflammation can flare up, causing an acute and severe bout of breathing difficulty that cannot be controlled with a beta-agonist.

It is often difficult for asthmatics to keep track of the number of times they have used a beta-agonist in a day, especially if they are having a difficult time breathing. I believe that with these 12-hour agents, asthmatics will know immediately whether they have gone over the recommended dose. They can then get themselves to their doctor, who can put the patient on inhaled anti-inflammatories to control the underlying disease.

We have come a long way toward better controlling asthma and I believe 1993 will also see more physicians using a combination of inhaled anti-inflammatories and beta-agonists as first-line therapy. Physicians must learn to rely on inhaled steroids or cromolyn for their patients with moderate disease. I classify moderate disease as necessitating daily use of a beta-agonist. But to make diagnosing and treating the disease more precise, the National Asthma Education Program of the National Heart, Lung and Blood Institute has released a series of charts that physicians can use like a cookbook for treating asthma. I believe the charts should be in the office of every physician who sees at least one asthma patient in his or her practice. They guide the practitioner through the treatment of all forms of asthma, indicating when it is appropriate to step up therapy to perhaps a short course of oral steroids.

These guidelines to care are based on the new realization that asthma is a two-phase disease, consisting of an acute phase and a late-phase response. The acute attack primarily is orchestrated by IgE and mast cells. The mast cells release broncho-constricting and proinflammatory mediators such as histamines, prostaglandin D2, leukotrienes, cytokines and perhaps platelet-activating factor, which lead to the late phase.

The chief effect of late-phase response appears to be the maintenance of inflammation rather than the promotion of bronchoconstriction. T-lymphocytes release cytokines and lymphokines, which in turn spur eosinophils to infiltrate and inflame the lungs by secreting protein factors that are damaging to respiratory epithelium.

Asthma therapies being developed for the future focus on using this knowledge to attack the disease earlier than is now possible. The agents consist of leukotriene receptor antagonists, lipoxygenase inhibitors and phosphodiesterase analogues. These agents hold the promise of intervention far earlier in the disease process than agents currently available. They are designed to hit the mediators that many asthma experts believe begin the cascade of events that leads to airway inflammation. But it may be many years before the agents are proven safe and effective.

I believe the future will also bring FDA approval of pentapeptide (Pentide, Dura Pharmaceuticals). The agent has proven significantly effective in clinical trials of over 1,000 atopic patients.

Dr. Hamburger is professor emeritus of pediatrics of the allergy and immunology division at the University of California at San Diego, and head of the allergy and immunology laboratory at UCSD.

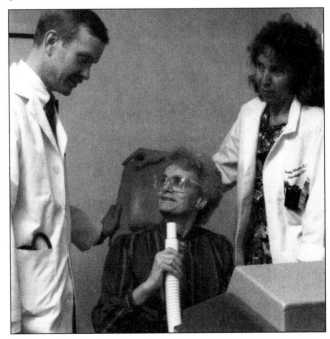

Asthma sufferers will benefit from combination therapies.

Notes

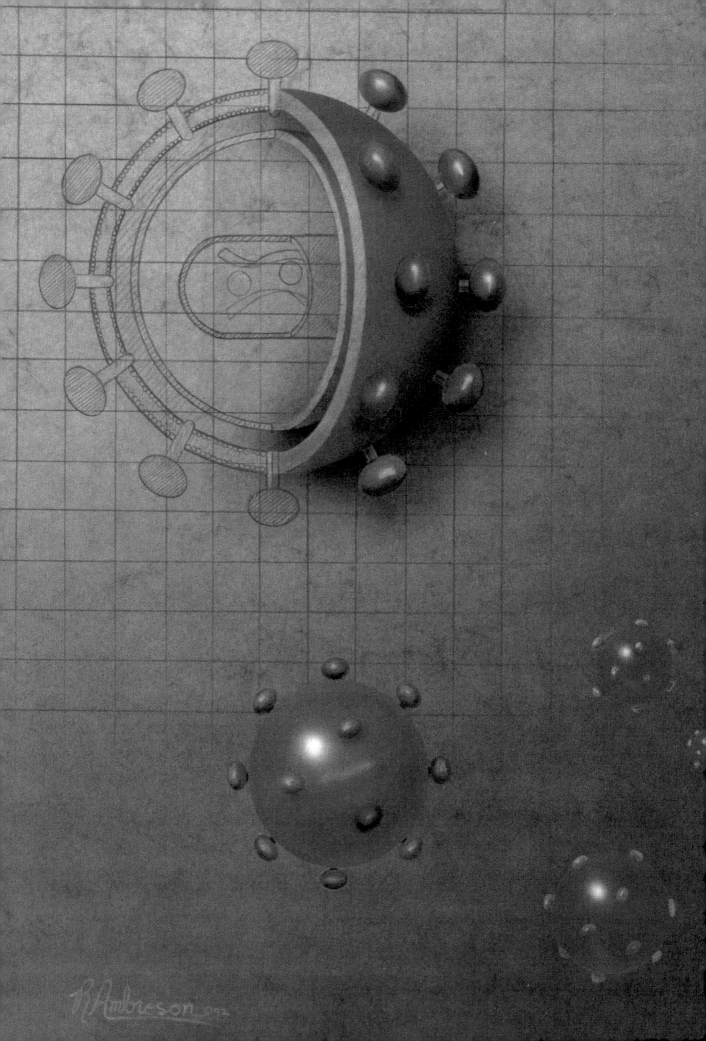

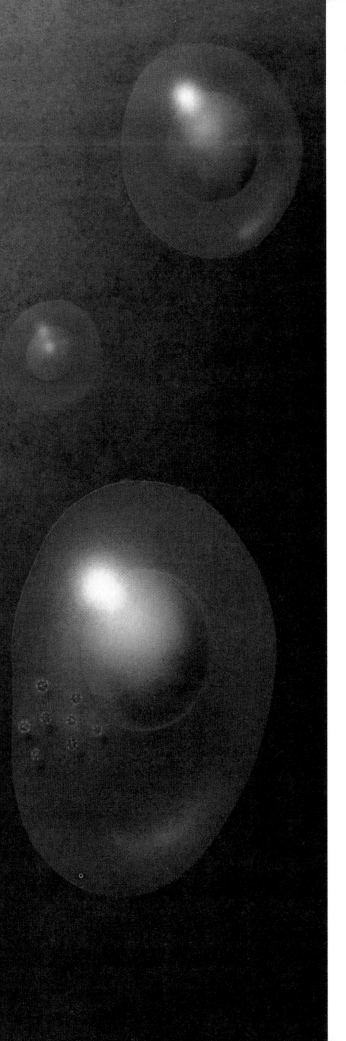

Overview 276
AIDS penetrates the heartland;
women fastest-growing population
of victims

Month-at-a-glance 278

Reported at the Time 290
Long-term HIV survival…AZT,
DDC, other drug news…new
vaccine approaches…HIV risk from
donor blood…WHO's estimates of
AIDS cases challenged as too
low…reports from 8th International
Conference on AIDS: AIDS-like
illness without HIV infection, new
urine test, women at higher
risk…CD4 test for in-office
screening…resistant TB spreading
among AIDS patients…the orphans
of AIDS

Commentary 303
New AIDS-like illness remains
elusive
By Jeffrey Laurence, M.D.

AIDS penetrates the heartland; women fastest-growing population of victims

President Bush was chided for his failure "to say clearly and forthrightly that we have a crisis on our hands, that it has killed more Americans than Vietnam and Korea combined."

The reality that AIDS is no longer confined to the larger cities or to the eastern or western coasts of the United States has hit home; AIDS has penetrated the heartland. In 1992, a Gallup poll reported that four out of five American physicians have treated at least one AIDS patient.

We also saw evidence that education on prevention is not keeping up with the spread of AIDS. A University of California, San Francisco, study found that teenagers are not using condoms regularly, nor are they being instructed to use them in their AIDS education classes. Teens with the greatest number of sexual partners were found to be the least likely to use condoms.

The rising incidence of tuberculosis was one topic that dominated AIDS news in 1992. By some estimates, up to 50% of all people infected with HIV may also be infected with TB. HIV-positive patients are also at high risk for drug-resistant TB, which carries a mortality rate as high as 80%. The Institute of Medicine concluded in a special report on emerging microbials that the United States needs to increase its efforts to monitor and combat AIDS, drug-resistant TB and drug-resistant malaria, or risk an epidemic equal to the flu outbreak of 1918-1919, when 20 million people died.

The major drug-approval news on the AIDS front this year was DDC (Hivid, Hoffmann-La Roche). The drug was approved in June for use in combination with AZT (Retrovir, Burroughs Wellcome) for advanced AIDS. In some studies, DDC plus AZT produced greater boosts in CD4 counts than AZT alone.

In other drug news, a large multicenter study concluded that DDI (Videx, Bristol-Myers Squibb) should become a standard second-line therapy for HIV-infected patients, whether or not they respond to AZT. And a Food and Drug Administration

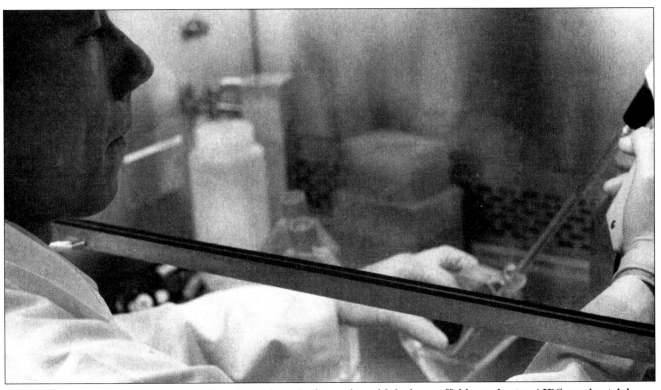

Three-dimensional computer-generated model and synthetic vaccine with lysine scaffold may hasten AIDS vaccine trials.

advisory committee recommended that atovaquone (Mepron, Burroughs Wellcome) should be approved for the treatment of mild to moderate Pneumocystis carinii pneumonia.

In research, a Seattle team announced a promising animal model for AIDS. Studies of Indonesian pigtail macaques found that they could be readily infected with HIV-1, and that within days cell cultures taken from them would demonstrate evidence of viral replication in CD4 cells and the presence of HIV-1 DNA in peripheral blood mononuclear cells. Previously, only endangered chimpanzees and gibbon apes had shown HIV-1 susceptibility.

Another first occurred this year when a three-dimensional, computer-generated picture of reverse transcriptase was achieved. Yale researchers said that having an image of the enzyme will help lead to the development of drugs to inhibit HIV replication.

And another stumbling block in the design of a vaccine may have been overcome by the development of a synthetic vaccine with a lysine scaffold to which any number of protein fragments could be attached to test which are most effective. The synthetic vaccine mobilizes both neutralizing antibodies and killer cells. Being able to attach different fragments to the scaffold would save researchers from having to test various fragments individually before incorporating them into a vaccine.

Earlier in the year, Medical Tribune was one of the few publications in the United States to report that French researcher Luc Montagnier, M.D., had questioned HIV as the sole cause of AIDS. Just three months later, that theory was announced at the Eighth International Conference on AIDS in Amsterdam. Jeffrey Laurence, M.D., (see Commentary, p. 303) and others (including Dr. Montagnier) reported patients with low CD4 counts and AIDS-like illnesses but no evidence of HIV infection.

David Rogers, M.D., the vice chairman of the National Commission on AIDS, commented in an op-ed piece in Medical Tribune that Dr. Montagnier had found HIV via urinalysis, which suggests that these were simply variations on a multifaceted disease. "Put the chain of cases alongside half a million bona fide AIDS cases and the reality is something that is probably trivial, although it deserves careful study," he wrote. In the same piece, he chided President Bush's failure "to say clearly and forthrightly that we've got an AIDS crisis on our hands, that it has killed more Americans than Vietnam and Korea combined," and to suggest measures to deal with the crisis.

Also confirmed this year was a report that Florida dentist David Acer had infected five patients with HIV. The most widely known of his patients was college-student-turned-AIDS-activist Kimberly Bergalis, who died in 1991 at age 23. The CDC could draw no conclusion as to how Dr. Acer had transmitted the virus. A few months after the CDC report, Georgia researchers revealed that dental hand-pieces and their attachments are possible sources of HIV contamination.

Finally, after a long delay, the CDC announced it would implement an expanded clinical definition of AIDS in January 1993 to include invasive carcinoma of the cervix, pulmonary tuberculosis and two or more episodes of bacterial pneumonia. The new definition could double the number of AIDS cases reported next year and significantly increase the number of women and drug abusers reported as having the disease. Women in the United States have become the fastest-growing segment of the AIDS population, said the CDC, which estimates that by the year 2000, more than half of all new AIDS cases will be women.

JANUARY

Jan. 1

Patients with AIDS and ARC maintained their T-lymphocytes at higher levels for longer periods of time while on combination anti-viral therapy. Compared with AZT (Retrovir, Burroughs Wellcome) alone, 10 weeks of therapy with AZT and dideoxycytidine (Hivid, Hoffmann-La Roche) boosted CD4 counts as much as 121 cells/mm^3 in 56 patients, researchers at the University of California at San Diego reported in the Annals of Internal Medicine.

Jan. 4

Is AZT adequate long-term antiviral therapy for children with AIDS? In a new study of 23 children who had been on AZT for 9 to 39 months, plummeting in-vitro sensitivity to AZT accurately predicted which children were headed for deterioration or death during the next six months. Children who develop decreased AZT sensitivity may be candidates for alternate antiretroviral therapy, Duke University researchers suggested in The Lancet.

Jan. 9

Ninety-three percent of persons with HIV failed to notify their sexual or needle-sharing partners, according to epidemiologists at the University of North Carolina. In a 310-person study described in The New England Journal of Medicine, partners were successfully notified 50% of the time when specially trained counselors were assigned to the task, but only 7% of the time when patients were asked to initiate the conversation. In North Carolina, people with HIV are legally required to inform partners of the infection.

Jan. 13

Researchers failed to detect HIV in perspiration, leading experts to declare that no evidence justified restricting Magic Johnson from playing basketball in the 1992 summer Olympic games. No trace of HIV was detected in perspiration collected from 50 AIDS patients during workouts, reported researchers from New York Medical College in the Journal of Infectious Disease.

Jan. 14

Former Surgeon General C. Everett Koop announced that museums across the country will host exhibits to teach children how HIV-1 invades the human body. The exhibits, which will include interactive videos, computers and games, are funded by a federal grant of $1.5 million and could reach 10 million visitors a year.

Jan. 15

Johns Hopkins University epidemiologists cautioned that federal guidelines for tuberculosis testing may be inadequate to detect the disease in persons infected with HIV. A study of 260 HIV-

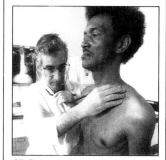

CDC warns that drug-resistant TB can kill in one to four months.

positive and HIV-negative intravenous drugs users revealed that the Centers for Disease Control's definition of skin test positivity (induration of 5 mm or greater in diameter) misses TB in a significant number of HIV-positive people. In The Journal of the American Medical Association, switching to a cutoff of 2 mm or greater was recommended.

Jan. 17

A recombinant vaccine successfully protected monkeys from infection with the HIV-like simian immunodeficiency virus. In an experiment reported in Science, monkeys were immunized with SIV surface glycoproteins carried by live vaccinia viruses and later boosted with other glycoproteins. Within two weeks of boosting, all animals showed a 30-fold or greater increase in antibody response against SIV surface antigens, and all animals later injected with SIV virus remained virus-free.

• • •

A Japanese and American team developed a two-step vaccine approach that may help scientists overcome a major obstacle to AIDS vaccine development—the ability of HIV to avoid complete destruction by constantly changing its protein makeup. The system, described in Science, involves priming the immune system with injections containing protein fragments from the surface of HIV. A booster would then introduce laboratory-altered HIV fragments in order to sharpen the immune system's recognition of HIV viruses of widely different protein makeups.

Jan. 20

A World Health Organization official warned that AIDS threatens the lives of tens of millions of people in Asia and the Pacific and could jeopardize economic development efforts in the area. Heterosexual sex and intravenous drug use appear to be the prime modes of HIV transmission in the region, where the number of persons infected with HIV jumped from 500,000 to one million last year, a meeting of economic aid coordinators in Manila learned.

Jan. 23

On the 10th anniversary of their diagnosis, a California AIDS expert attributed 65 HIV-positive patients' longevity and high quality of life to aggressive care. Despite lab results indicating alarmingly deteriorated immune systems, he told a WHO teleconference that the long-term survivors are active and feeling well on a program that includes medication and stress reduction. When CD4 counts drop below 500 cells/mm^3, patients are started on AZT and prophylaxis against Pneumocystis carinii pneumonia.

Jan. 24

The Centers for Disease Control announced that the death rate from drug-resistant tuberculosis can be as high as 80%, with progression from diagnosis to death taking one to four months. HIV-infected people and those living in hospitals and correctional facilities have shown the highest rate of TB resistant to rifampin and isoniazid, the two major drug treatments, said the CDC. The agency also disclosed plans to release several million dollars to help states cope with AIDS.

Jan. 25

A new study challenged existing guidelines for determining when HIV-infected people should begin antiviral treatment. Since 1990, a CD4 count below 500 cells/mm^3 has been considered reason enough to initiate AZT treatment in asymptomatic people. But during a 30-month multicenter follow-up of 555 HIV-infected hemophilia patients, only 4% to 5% of those with CD4 counts between 300 and 500 developed AIDS. In contrast, about 50% of those with CD4 counts below 200 developed AIDS, participants in the Transfusion Safety Study reported in the British Medical Journal.

The researchers concluded that antiviral treatment of asymptomatic people with CD4 counts of 300-500 cells/mm^3 is "questionable" if predicated on near-term progression to AIDS. However, AIDS experts commented that until better predictive guidelines are developed, most physicians will not change their prescribing habits.

FEBRUARY

Feb. 3

Kenyan health workers predicted that the AIDS epidemic will require changes in strategies to prevent and treat measles in endemic areas. In their report in the Journal of Infectious Diseases, infants born to HIV-seropositive mothers were four times more likely than other infants to contract measles before being vaccinated at nine months of age. In the study, measles was associated with serious complications and poor growth in all affected infants.

Feb. 6

A retrovirus that may accelerate the course of HIV infection was found to be prevalent among intravenous drug users, reported Centers for Disease Control researchers. The virus, human T-cell lymphotropic virus Type II, was detected in 17.6% and 14.4% of intravenous drug users at Los Angeles and New Orleans sexually transmitted disease clinics, they wrote in The New England Journal of Medicine.

Feb. 10

The CDC announced that it is testing a new AIDS prevention program with a new kind of role model—high-profile local people who have changed their risk-taking habits. Brochures, posters, audiotapes and videotapes prominently display pictures and quotes from the role models. The five-city test program is targeted at groups considered to be difficult to reach: men who have sex with men but do not identify themselves as bisexual or gay, drug users not in treatment programs, female partners of these two groups and prostitutes.

Feb. 12

The World Health Organization announced that an estimated 10 to 12 million people worldwide have become infected with HIV, and the numbers have increased by more than a million in only

eight months. About 90% of the new infections have been in adults and 90% of the adults were infected through heterosexual sex, reflecting a continuing trend toward heterosexual transmission of HIV not only in developing countries but in the industrialized world as well, according to the new WHO report.

• • •

A study of 1,309 people who were tested for HIV suggested that one post-counseling session may not be enough to promote condom use, warned a Johns Hopkins researcher. Almost 10% contracted sexually transmitted diseases within two years of post-test counseling, which suggests continued high-risk behavior, he reported in The Journal of the American Medical Association. Both those who tested positive and those who tested negative for HIV had about the same rate of STD infection.

Feb. 13

A Veterans Administration study raised questions about the timing and effectiveness of AZT (Retrovir, Burroughs Wellcome) therapy. In a four-year evaluation of 338 patients, early AZT treatment delayed the onset of AIDS but did not improve survival over patients who did not receive AZT until they developed symptoms of infection. According to the report in The New England Journal of Medicine, HIV-infected adults who began taking AZT presymptomatically also experienced more anemia, leukopenia, nausea, vomiting and diarrhea.

Feb. 17

Heterosexuals who are infected with herpes genitalis learned that they are at increased risk of being infected with HIV. In a study of 368 heterosexual men and 103 women, those who tested positive for herpes simplex

virus type 2 were twice as likely to have been infected with HIV as HSV-2-negative patients.

To help prevent HIV transmission, University of Maryland infectious disease specialists called for prompt diagnosis and therapy of all diseases causing genital ulcers, including genital herpes, syphilis and chancroid. Using condoms with a nonoxynol-9-containing spermicide and avoiding sex when a partner has visible herpes lesions can

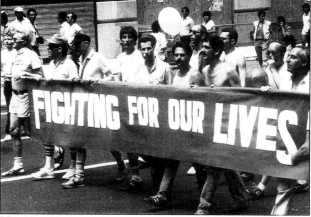

Marching to bolster public awareness. HIV now infects 10-12 million.

reduce the risk of transmission, they reported in the Journal of Infectious Diseases.

Feb. 20

Antibodies raised against a component of HIV-1 had both preventive and protective effects, claimed an international team. They developed a vaccine from a purified version of a monoclonal antibody specifically targeted against the V3 loop of the HIV-1 envelope glycoprotein 120. One chimpanzee given the vaccine and then injected with HIV-1 did not become infected; another injected with HIV-1 and then given the vaccine 10 minutes later also did not become infected during an eight-month period, they reported in Nature.

• • •

Hoffmann-La Roche Inc. announced plans to make DDC (Hivid) more widely

available to AIDS patients through their physicians.

Feb. 22

Blood tests that measure triglyceride and interferon levels better predicted the efficacy of AZT therapy than currently used tests which determine CD4 counts, suggested a study from Beth Israel Medical Center in New York. In a placebo-controlled trial of 19 patients with AIDS or AIDS-related complex, rapid and significant decreases in interferon and triglyceride levels were observed only in those given

AZT, the researchers reported in The Lancet. Concentrations of the substances at four months were inversely correlated with subsequent length of survival.

Feb. 27

Prevention experts gave failing grades to school AIDS education programs for neglecting to promote condom use among teenagers. Out of 1,899 junior high school students in San Francisco, only 37% of sexually active teens used condoms regularly. An equal percentage said they rarely or never used condoms, according to a survey published in Pediatrics.

The University of California researchers found that teens with a greater number of sex partners were less likely to use condoms than those with a steady partner.

March 2

A new British vaccine stimulated the immune systems of 12 of 16 healthy people to make antibodies to an HIV protein. The vaccine is not designed to protect people against HIV, but it may be able to lengthen the time that it takes for an HIV-infected person to develop AIDS, a researcher at St. Mary's Medical School in London told Medical Tribune.

March 4

Patients with AIDS live longer if they take AZT (Retrovir, Burroughs Wellcome), reported Italian researchers. In a study of 271 AIDS patients at the Instituto Superiore di Sanita in Rome, nearly 46% of people receiving AZT were still alive after two years, compared with 21% of those not receiving the drug. More than half of those studied were thought to have acquired the disease through intravenous drug use, which some studies have correlated with a shorter survival time, the researchers noted in The Journal of the American Medical Association.

• • •

Measles can be fatal in people with AIDS or cancer, reported infectious disease specialists. People who come into close contact with AIDS or cancer patients, especially family members, should be vaccinated against measles, said the University of Chicago physicians. In addition, all children infected with HIV and some with cancer can safely be vaccinated themselves, they wrote in The Journal of the American Medical Association.

March 5

A new study from Madrid found that people with HIV are in danger of developing tuberculous meningitis. Of 455 people infected with HIV, 37 also had tuberculous meningitis, determined a research team from the Hospital Gregorio General Mar-

anon. Of 33 who were treated, seven died, according to a report in The New England Journal of Medicine, emphasizing the need for early detection and treatment.

March 11

Government officials revealed that transplanted tissues from an HIV-seronegative donor transmitted HIV-1 infection to at least seven of 48 recipients. The donor was a 22-year-old male gunshot victim with no known risk factors for HIV infection and who had tested negative prior to the removal of his tissues

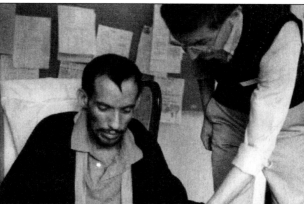
Experts warn that measles can kill AIDS and cancer patients.

and organs. HIV was, however, detected in lymphocytes from tissue that had been stored after the donor died. Of 41 identified recipients tested for HIV antibodies, four who received organs and three who received unprocessed fresh-frozen bone were subsequently found to be infected. Centers for Disease Control investigators announced that they are considering improvements for HIV testing, quarantine and treatment of donated tissues as well as better tracking of tissues after donation.

March 18

Newark researchers reported that healthy children have higher levels of CD4 cells than adults, suggesting that children infected with HIV may need to start treat-

ment sooner. A study of 208 healthy children revealed CD4 counts ranging from 1,800 cells/mm³ of blood for children 59 months old to 2,950 for those between the ages of 12 and 23 months, said the University of Medicine and Dentistry of New Jersey team. Median CD4 counts for healthy adults has been reported at 760 cells/mm³ of blood. Currently, the recommended CD4 threshold to begin AZT therapy in adults is 500 cells/mm³ of blood; however, the researchers suggested in The Journal of the American

Medical Association that AZT therapy in infants be instituted at CD4 counts of 1,500 cells/mm³ or less to avoid the development of P. carinii pneumonia.

March 21

London researchers reported that HIV-infected patients are more likely to develop Pneumocystis carinii pneumonia when it rains or is humid. They recorded the amount of rainfall, average temperature and number of people admitted to Middlesex Hospital from October 1989 to January 1992. Their study showed that the number of people with PCP was highest in June, July and December of 1990 and September of 1991—rainy or humid months.

Fungal spores are more likely to be spread and inhaled in warm soggy weather, the researchers explained in The Lancet.

March 25

Contrary to previous reports, intravenous drug users infected with HIV did not get sick faster than patients who were infected through sexual behavior, reported Johns Hopkins researchers. A study of 621 drug users revealed that they had about the same number of CD4 cells as homosexuals with the disease, they stated in The Journal of the American Medical Association.

March 26

A 17-center study determined that AZT is well tolerated by pregnant women who are infected with HIV.

Two of 43 women who received AZT in doses of 300 to 1,200 mg per day during some portion of pregnancy suffered toxicity episodes, one hematologic and one gastrointestinal. All the babies were born alive. No teratogenic abnormalities were noted in the 12 infants with first-trimester AZT exposure, the physician noted in The New England Journal of Medicine.

Still unknown is whether the drug can protect the fetus from transmission of the virus.

March 31

The Centers for Disease Control postponed indefinitely adopting an expanded definition of AIDS, which was to have been released on this date. It was the second time this year the federal agency delayed issuing the broadened definition, which would have doubled the number of people officially classified as having the disease, according to the AIDS Action Council. A major component of the expanded definition would have been the inclusion of HIV-infected people who have fewer than 200 CD4 cells/mm³ of blood.

APRIL

April 7

A European study revealed that pregnant women co-infected with hepatitis C virus (HCV) and HIV can transmit HCV to their offspring. Polymerase chain reaction detected HCV in six of eight HIV-positive mothers and four of eight infants, according to the study in the Journal of Infectious Diseases. The authors called for prospective studies of infants born to women seropositive for HCV and HIV and said additional studies should address the issue of increased HCV viremia by coinfection with HIV. The extent of vertical transmission of HCV is not known.

April 10

A Science magazine investigation found that at least five companies have abandoned, or been hampered in, their efforts to develop an AIDS vaccine due to fears of lawsuits.

April 13

The AIDS Clinical Trials Group was informed that DDI may be more effective than AZT for people with asymptomatic HIV infection or AIDS-related complex. In a University of California-San Francisco study, more than 900 subjects took AZT (Retrovir, Burroughs Wellcome) for at least four months and then were randomly assigned to remain on the drug or switch to 500 or 750 mg/day of DDI, dideoxyinosine (Videx, Bristol-Myers Squibb). DDI led to a greater delay in the development of the first AIDS-defining illness and also was associated with higher CD4 counts and 33% fewer new opportunistic infections than AZT, even at the lower dose. There was no difference in patient survival, the researchers told the group at a meeting in Washington.

April 15

Johns Hopkins University researchers reported that, among Haitian women, smokers have a higher risk of HIV infection than nonsmokers. In a survey of Haitian women, smoking was associated with more high-risk sexual behavior, and, even after adjusting for this factor, appeared alone to increase the risk of HIV, the researchers revealed in The Journal of the American Medical Association. Smoking may make the vagina more susceptible to viral infection, the researchers speculated.

April 16

An analysis of deaths among men in the Multicenter AIDS Cohort Study revealed that men lived longer if they started taking AZT and anti-pneumonia drugs before they developed full-blown AIDS. In a study of 2,568 HIV-positive men, the risk of dying within six months after entering the study was reduced by 57% in people who took AZT early, with or without drugs to prevent Pneumocystis carinii pneumonia. After two years, the risk of dying was reduced by 40% in patients taking both AZT and prophylaxis for PCP, researchers reported in The New England Journal of Medicine.

April 21

After eight hours of discussion and an 8 to 3 vote, the Food and Drug Administration's Antiviral Drugs Advisory Committee recommended that the agency grant conditional approval to the anti-HIV drug dideoxycytidine (Hivid, Hoffmann-La Roche), to be used only in combination with AZT for people with advanced HIV infection. Relying heavily on a study showing that patients who took AZT survived longer and were less likely to experience HIV-related infections, the committee decided to recommend against approving DDC for use alone in patients who cannot tolerate or who do not respond to AZT.

April 25

A European Collaborative Study clarified the risk factors for perinatal transmission of HIV. In an analysis of 721 children born to 701 mothers, the overall transmission rate was 14.4%, the 19-center team reported in The Lancet. Infected mothers with p24-antigenemia or a CD4 count of less than 700 were more likely to pass on the virus. Infants born before 34 weeks gestation, and those who were breast-fed, were more likely to have become infected.

April 26

Medical Tribune reported that HIV codiscoverer Luc Montagnier, M.D., had said that he believes AIDS can occasionally develop without HIV. He denied making the claim, but said he had come to believe that certain essential cofactors probably are needed in order for HIV to cause AIDS. One likely cofactor is mycoplasma infection, he claimed.

April 27

AIDS education programs have largely failed to reach women of reproductive age who use illegal drugs, Philadelphia physicians told colleagues at the American College of Obstetricians and Gynecologists annual meeting in Las Vegas. After comparing surveys of pregnant drug users in 1990-1991 with those conducted in 1988-1989, investigators at Thomas Jefferson University found that AIDS knowledge had not increased.

April 30

A team from the New York Psychiatric Institute found that addressing socioenvironmental influences on risky behaviors may prove to be the most effective AIDS preventive strategy among adolescents. A survey of 531 tenth-graders residing in a New York City borough revealed that 56.8% had had intercourse in the past year. Of these, 67.3% reported unprotected intercourse with low-risk partners, 1.3% reported unprotected intercourse with high-risk partners and 6.6% had had a sexually transmitted disease in the past year.

Further analysis showed that students whose friends

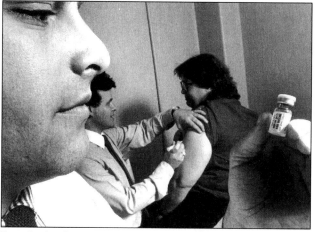

Investigation showed lawsuit fears hamper AIDS vaccine development.

had intercourse and never or inconsistently used condoms were more than five times more likely to be engaged in behaviors that placed them at high risk for acquiring AIDS, the New York team reported in the American Journal of Public Health. Students who believed that the majority of their peers had intercourse were almost four times as likely as the others to exhibit such high-risk behavior.

May 1

A stumbling block in the design of an AIDS vaccine—finding one which stimulates the broadest possible immune system response to HIV—appears to have been circumvented by creating a synthetic structure that mimics the surface coat protein of HIV, reported Rockefeller University researchers. After guinea pigs and mice were injected with the vaccine, they produced both neutralizing antibodies and killer cells, the team explained in the Proceedings of the National Academy of Sciences.

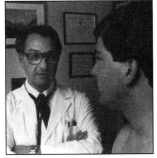

HIV-positive patients who have not yet developed AIDS are straining resources, says report.

May 10

Although the human immunodeficiency virus may not be detected in the ejaculate of vasectomized men who are HIV-positive, they may still be able to transmit the virus during unprotected sex, a University of Washington, Seattle, urologist reported at the American Urological Association meeting in Washington, D.C. In a study of 46 HIV-positive men, he detected HIV in the ejaculate from 18 of 44 men who did not have a vasectomy, but in no samples from four vasectomized men. The data are still early, so men must continue to use a condom to prevent HIV transmission, said the researcher.

May 13

A study conducted by the National Health and Hospital Institute found that patients infected with HIV who have not yet developed full-blown

AIDS are placing a significant toll on resources from public hospitals. This finding rebuts the tenet that people infected with HIV do not develop serious health problems until they develop AIDS, according to the report in The Journal of the American Medical Association.

The study determined that, whereas in 1988, one third of HIV-positive patients admitted to 300 public hospitals did not meet the CDC definition of AIDS, that proportion has since risen to one half, said the Institute's president.

May 14

The Centers for Disease Control confirmed that five people had been infected with HIV from a Florida dentist. But after reviewing the records of the deceased dentist, interviewing his former employees and conducting HIV testing on about 1,100 of his former patients, the CDC said it still has not been able to figure out how the dentist transmitted the virus to the patients.

May 18

Up to half of the people infected with HIV may also be infected with tuberculosis, San Juan researchers reported at the American Lung Association meeting in Miami. Between 22% and 49% of 1,399 people infected with HIV tested positive for TB infection, compared with an estimated TB infection rate of 5% in the general population, said the director of the Community Programs for Clinical Research, a 17-center consortium. The team also found that those patients infected with HIV had a 36% chance of developing active TB after exposure to another patient with TB.

May 23

Following the Centers for Disease Control's decision to

postpone expanding the definition of AIDS, French researchers said doing so in Europe could lead to underreporting of the disease. People with low CD4 counts who had not yet developed AIDS-related diseases might not seek healthcare or testing and therefore would not be counted as having AIDS, they explained. Expanding the definition could also skew the comparison of AIDS data among countries, the University of Bordeaux researchers wrote in The Lancet.

The 12-country European Community Project Management Group on AIDS Epidemiology decided last September not to adopt the proposed CDC change.

May 26

More than four out of five American physicians have treated at least one AIDS patient, according to a recent Gallup poll.

Doctors under age 35 and those practicing in the Northeast and in urban areas were the most likely to treat HIV-infected patients, the poll found.

The poll also revealed that 81% of doctors believe they have a right to know whether a patient is HIV-positive before offering treatment, while 87% believe that a physician who is HIV positive should not perform invasive procedures without getting a patient's informed consent.

May 27

The antiviral drug AZT (Retrovir, Burroughs Wellcome) reduces the amount of HIV in semen, but men should still consider themselves infectious and take precautions against transmission, said researchers at Harvard Medical School in Boston.

A study of 95 HIV-positive men, presented in The Journal of the American Medical Association, detected the virus in 13% of men not treated with the drug, compared to 3% of those treated.

•••

The CDC received 158 state health department reports of people who contracted AIDS from blood transfusions in the five years since blood screening began in 1985. However, only 15 cases could be confirmed, since most of the transfusion recipients had other risk factors for HIV infection, the CDC researchers stated in The New England Journal of Medicine.

May 29

A study of the seroprevalence of HIV infection in heart-attack victims outside the hospital indicated that performing cardiopulmonary resuscitation on these victims is safe, the Centers for Disease Control reported.

Only five of 604 Seattle-area heart-attack victims who received CPR were infected with HIV, the CDC noted.

But even in cases of infected people, the risk of transmission is low unless blood is present from an injury, the CDC concluded.

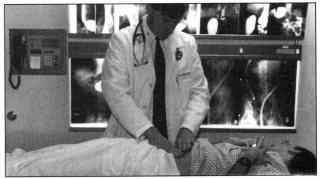

About 80% of doctors have treated at least one AIDS patient.

June 3

Projected figures by the World Health Organization on the number of worldwide AIDS cases by the year 2000 could be greatly below the true number, claimed Harvard researchers.

WHO has estimated that 40 million people will be infected by the year 2000, whereas a forthcoming book, written by researchers at the Harvard-based Global AIDS Policy Coalition, puts the figure at between 38 million and 110 million adults, plus 10 million children.

The Harvard team based its estimates on interviews with experts, whereas WHO based its figures on national reports, which some countries are believed to suppress for political reasons.

June 4

The Centers for Disease Control blamed some of the national tuberculosis outbreak on a failure to follow federal guidelines in treating hospitalized AIDS and TB patients.

The CDC recommends that people with active TB be isolated in negative-pressure rooms with individual air supply and exhaust systems. But in a study of 18 AIDS patients with drug-resistant TB, a CDC team found that while patients were isolated, they were in rooms without adequate safeguards. Air was escaping into the hallway instead of being ventilated and pumped out of the building, the researchers stated in The New England Journal of Medicine.

June 9

Amid the nationwide increase in tuberculosis and with little relief in sight, the Centers for Disease Control held a discussion of whether all healthcare workers should be vaccinated with bacille Calmette Guerin to protect against TB. One stumbling block is that the vaccine produces tuberculin positivity so that it would be impossible to determine previous

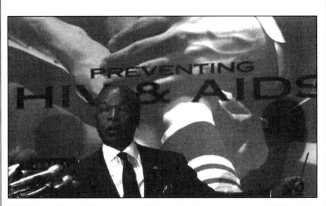

JUNE

HHS head Dr. Sullivan was criticized for his response to AIDS crisis.

exposure to the mycobacterium causing TB, infection-control experts said. The vaccine could also be harmful to HIV infectives and raises the controversial issue of HIV testing of healthcare workers, they noted. Also still in question was the vaccine's effectiveness; of eight BCG TB clinical trials, only half showed some protective effect, said an investigator from the National Institutes of Health.

June 13

In the first five years of HIV infection, the concentration of serum beta 2-microglobulin—which has been shown to reflect the degree of immune system activation—emerged as the strongest independent predictor of the development of AIDS. In 214 men from the San Francisco City Clinic Cohort Study, each with a well-defined date of seroconversion, beta 2-microglobulin provided important prognostic information, regardless of CD4 lymphocyte count or the use of AZT (Retrovir, Burroughs Wellcome), researchers disclosed in The Lancet. Another advantage: Beta 2-microglobulin can be measured by equipment available in standard laboratories and requires no special handling.

June 15

When high doses of AZT are given to HIV-positive

people with mild symptoms, its side effects may offset any quality-of-life benefit to taking the drug, asserted researchers from the AIDS Clinical Trials Group. The onset of AIDS-related symptoms was 27 days later in 360 mildly symptomatic HIV-infected people given 1200 mg/day of AZT for 18 months, compared with 351 patients given placebo. However, the AZT-treated patients suffered from severe adverse side effects for about 33 days, the 32-center team reported in the Annals of Internal Medicine.

The investigators predicted that at currently recommended doses (500 to 600 mg/day), AZT treatment would yield a more favorable balance of benefits to risks in this patient group.

June 18

The Centers for Disease Control sent a letter to state health officials announcing its decision not to create a list of procedures that HIV-infected healthcare workers would be prohibited from performing.

The American College of Physicians, the American Hospital Association, the American Dental Association and the American Medical Association all have approved or proposed policies that call for a case-by-case review of what procedures an infected healthcare worker may perform.

June 22

The Food and Drug Administration approved dideoxycytidine for use in combination with AZT in adults with advanced HIV infection. The approval of DDC, or zalcitabine (Hivid, Hoffmann-La Roche) was based on two studies involving fewer than 100 patients under the FDA's "conditional approval" program.

In the studies, the combination therapy produced a greater increase in the number of CD4 cells than AZT alone. The drug has not been shown to prolong survival, lower the incidence of opportunistic infections or halt the progression of HIV.

June 25

The National Commission on AIDS criticized the Bush administration for failing to lead the fight against the AIDS epidemic.

The commission said that Health and Human Services Secretary Louis Sullivan, M.D., was unresponsive to the AIDS recommendations it issued last September.

Dr. Sullivan issued a statement that called the commission's charge "a total misrepresentation of the facts," and maintained that AIDS is one of the highest government public health priorities.

June 26

For the first time, a three-dimensional, computer-generated picture of reverse transcriptase has been obtained, Yale University researchers reported in Science.

They said the discovery may speed development of drugs to inhibit HIV. Knowing the structure of the enzyme will narrow the focus for researchers so they can better target potential therapies, according to the report.

In the study, the researchers also found that the experimental anti-AIDS drug nevirapine paralyzed reverse transcriptase in a similar fashion to AZT, DDI and DDC, but with fewer side effects.

AIDS

July 2

The number of AIDS cases rose 5% last year, with women, minorities and residents of the South experiencing the highest proportionate increases, the Centers for Disease Control reported.

Of 45,506 cases of AIDS reported to the CDC in 1991, more than half were transmitted among homosexual or bisexual men, reflecting past trends. But the proportion of these cases dropped by about 0.5%, while the percentage of cases among female and male drug users rose almost 10%.

July 3

Seattle researchers announced the discovery of a promising animal model for AIDS. Pigtail macaques, common in Indonesia, proved readily infected with HIV-1, within days demonstrating viral replication in CD4 lymphocytes and the presence of HIV-1 DNA in their peripheral blood mononuclear cells, according to a report in Science.

Previously, chimpanzees had been successfully infected with HIV-1, but because they do not develop AIDS they were considered a less than ideal model for the human infection. Rhesus monkeys are susceptible to SIV but not HIV-1. Whether pigtail macaques remain infected more than a few months has yet to be determined, the University of Washington researchers said.

July 15

A monoclonal antibody that holds HIV replication in check may prevent HIV-positive patients from developing or dying from full-blown AIDS, Thomas Jefferson University researchers speculated in the Proceedings of the National Academy of Sciences. The Philadelphia scientists used the antibody to block the action of endotoxin—a potent trigger for HIV replication—in a cultured cell line of monocytes.

JULY

July 20

A World Health Organization official predicted that more than half of newly infected AIDS patients will be women by the year 2000. Researchers at the 8th International Conference on AIDS in Amsterdam said far more attention must be paid to the detection and treatment of AIDS in women in light of accumulating data that women have poorer survival rates once they are diagnosed and are less likely to receive appropriate medication. One group presented data showing women with very low levels of CD4 cells were significantly less likely to get AZT (Retrovir, Burroughs Wellcome) than men with similar levels.

July 21

An AIDS expert set off a chain reaction by announcing that he has seen patients with an AIDS-like syndrome who are not infected with HIV. Other researchers came forth one by one to tell a hastily assembled press conference at the 8th International Conference on AIDS in Amsterdam that they, too, have seen patients with low CD4 counts and signs of impaired immunity.

A researcher at Cornell University Medical College revealed that he had seen five such cases, a physician with the Centers for Disease Control said he knows of another six in the U.S., and a researcher from the University of California at Irvine reported two other cases in the Proceedings of the National Academy of Sciences.

While the National Institutes of Health urged doctors with information of similar cases to come forward, researchers debated whether the reports suggest the existence of a new, HIV-like virus or whether the patients simply have an undetected cancer. The American Association of Blood Banks, meanwhile, said that the nation's blood supply is still safe, and that screening of CD4 counts is not warranted.

• • •

An experimental HIV urine test may be less expensive, more convenient and just as accurate as current blood tests, California researchers announced at the Amsterdam meeting. The urine test, developed by Calypte Biomedical Corp. of Berkeley, Calif., proved as accurate as current blood screens in a study of 530 people who were tested with both methods, the University of California, San Francisco, researchers claimed. The company plans to submit to the Food and Drug Administration a request to market the urine test, they added. But researchers at the meeting were skeptical, warning that if urine tests are approved by the FDA, they could readily, and perhaps secretly, be used by employers or insurers to test for the virus.

July 22

Researchers at the 8th International Conference on AIDS predicted that it will be a long time before an effective therapeutic vaccine for AIDS is found.

One promising vaccine, composed of the envelope protein gp160, induced a sustained antibody response in 27 of 28 patients who completed a trial at the Walter Reed Army Institutes of Research in Rockville, Md. Another study found that the vaccine does not seem to interfere with AZT therapy. A double-blind randomized trial of the vaccine was set to begin in the fall.

• • •

A new drug proved as effective against Pneumocystis carinii pneumonia as trimethoprim/sulfamethoxazole (TMP-SMZ) and caused fewer side effects, a Memphis researcher reported to the Amsterdam meeting. At St.

Jude's Children's Hospital, the investigational drug atovaquone (Burroughs Wellcome) was compared with TMP-SMZ in the treatment of 320 PCP patients. Among 226 patients with mild disease, 63% responded in each treatment group. In 96 patients with moderately severe PCP, treatment was considered a success in 59% on atovaquone and 66% on TMP-SMZ. Only 6% of patients on atovaquone experienced leukopenia, rash, fever, liver disorders or vomiting, compared to 19% of those on the TMP-SMZ regimen, he said.

July 23

A 10-minute office test to count CD4 cells may eliminate the need to send out blood samples for flow cytometry, predicted immunologists at the Amsterdam meeting. The test, manufactured by the Coulter Corporation, uses latex beads coated with anti-CD4 monoclonal antibody, and requires only that a physician have a light microscope and hemacytometer. In a study of more than 500 healthy and infected people, the new test proved 90% as precise as laser-operated flow cytometry in counting CD4 cells, said an immunologist at Rush-Presbyterian-St. Luke's Medical Center in Chicago.

July 31

The Centers for Disease Control released information it had obtained on five more cases of infection with a new AIDS-like virus, bringing the total to 26. The CDC's report coincided with a report in tomorrow's issue of The Lancet on four men and one woman with AIDS-related disorders and CD4 counts ranging from 552 cells/mm^3 to 76 cells/mm^3 but no evidence of HIV. While no trace of HIV could be found, reverse transcriptase was identified in the two patients in whom PCR testing for reverse transcriptase was performed, according to the Cornell University Medical College researcher.

AUGUST

Aug. 1

University of Miami physicians exhorted colleagues to screen for tuberculosis in HIV-infected patients and to adhere to strict acid-fast bacilli isolation precautions when treating patients with HIV infection and TB. The Florida researchers discovered that 71% of 62 patients with multidrug-resistant TB had had previous contact with an HIV clinic, compared with HIV clinic contact in 27% of 55 patients with single-drug-resistant or susceptible bacilli. In the Annals of Internal Medicine, they called the emergence of multiple drug-resistant strains of M. tuberculosis among patients with HIV infection and their close contacts "alarming," with "serious public health implications."

• • •

The New York Department of Health revealed that 22% to 50% of healthcare workers who had previously tested negative became positive on tuberculin skin-testing after being assigned to wards housing patients with multidrug-resistant TB. In the Annals of Internal Medicine, Centers for Disease Control and Health Department investigators stressed the need for rigorous infection-control procedures, not just in hospitals, but also in prisons, hospices and shelters for the homeless.

Aug. 10

A proposal to charge user fees to prescription-drug manufacturers could cut the review time for AIDS drugs from 12 to six months, testified Food and Drug Administration Commissioner David Kessler, M.D., at a hearing of the Health and Environment subcommittee of the House's Committee on Energy and Commerce.

While the plan would cost drug companies several hundred thousand dollars a year, it could restore the millions companies lose when a drug approval is delayed, FDA and drug manufacturers agreed.

Aug. 13

Centers for Disease Control researchers concluded that routine voluntary HIV tests in hospital patients would uncover thousands of previously unknown carriers.

Testing of specimens from anonymous donors left over from other medical tests at 20 hospitals found that 4.7%, or 9,286 of 195,829 specimens, were HIV positive, according to the CDC report in The New England Journal of Medicine. Hospital patients aged 15-54 are most likely to be carrying the AIDS virus and should be offered the routine AIDS tests.

In an accompanying

editorial, it was speculated that 60% to75% of the 750,000 Americans infected with the AIDS virus may not know it.

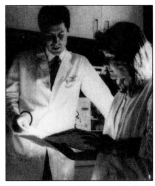

Healthcare workers at risk for drug-resistant tuberculosis.

Aug. 14

The physician who first called for screening the nation's blood supply for HIV in 1980 urged the use of tests to detect unexplained CD4 T-lymphocyte depletion.

Speaking at a packed meeting on CD4 depletion without evidence of HIV infection at the Centers for Disease Control in Atlanta, the Memorial Sloan-Kettering Cancer Center physician said the mysterious AIDS-like cases could have implications for the nation's blood supply.

But many other experts at the meeting questioned the wisdom of installing costly new equipment, training workers and alarming the public until more is known.

Aug. 24

Novopharm Inc. filed an Abbreviated New Drug Application for a generic version of AZT and is seeking fast-track approval from the Food and Drug Administration, the company president announced. Although Burroughs Wellcome holds the patent on AZT (Retrovir), Novopharm is challenging the patent's validity, asserting that the drug was discovered and tested by researchers from the National Institutes of Health.

This background was omitted in the Burroughs Wellcome patent filings, the Novopharm executive said. Burroughs Wellcome executives responded that its scientists had conceived of the idea to use AZT to treat HIV infection.

• • •

An Arkansas biomedical company reported that it is studying enzymes that can inhibit HIV replication. The enzymes, myeloperoxidase and eosinophil peroxidase, would help prevent the spread of AIDS and other sexually transmitted diseases by killing the virus after it enters the vagina or anus during sexual intercourse, according to the company, ExOxEmis. The enzymes, extracted from cows and pigs, act against certain viruses without harming normal tissue and bacteria, the company claimed. Laboratory testing is still in the early stages.

Aug. 27

A large multicenter study by investigators from both the private and public sectors concluded that DDI (Videx, Bristol-Myers Squibb) should become a standard second-line therapy for HIV-infected patients, whether or not they respond to AZT. DDI has been used to treat AIDS patients who did not respond well to AZT. But the new study of 913 people found that switching to DDI benefitted patients who had responded well to AZT for 16 weeks by keeping their immune systems stronger and delaying the development of AIDS-related infections. Life expectancy was not extended, however, according to the report in The New England Journal of Medicine.

Although doses of both 500 mg and 750 mg of DDI increased CD4 counts and decreased the number of infections, the 500-mg dose caused fewer side effects, which included peripheral neuropathy, elevated amylase levels and decreased leukocytes.

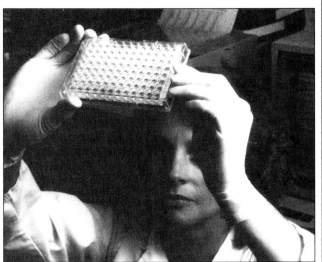

Some experts urged CD4-depletion screening by blood banks.

Sept. 2

The Centers for Disease Control conducted a special hearing to receive alternatives to its proposed new definition of AIDS. Members of AIDS advocacy groups proposed that three conditions be added to the CDC's definition: pulmonary tuberculosis; recurrent bacterial pneumonia; and cervical cancer or precancerous lesions of the cervix. By including these conditions, the groups contended that doctors will become alerted to the possibility of HIV infection in more women and intravenous drug users. However, the CDC maintained

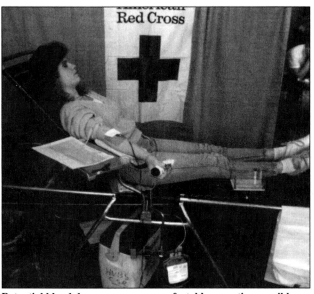

Potential blood donors are more comfortable reporting possible AIDS risk factors to a computer than to a human, study finds.

that too few studies have been done to reliably link the conditions to HIV infection.

Sept. 6

The first man to receive the liver of a baboon died of intracranial bleeding, and it was revealed that he was HIV positive. The revelation sparked debate over the ethics of using the terminally ill in medical experiments. Physicians at the University of Pittsburgh, where the transplant was performed on June 28, said they knew prior to the procedure that the man was infected but said he showed no signs of AIDS.

Sept. 9

Doctors at Beth Israel Hospital in Boston found that potential blood donors may be more comfortable revealing possible AIDS risk factors or symptoms to a computer than to a human. In a study of 294 blood donors, a computerized self-conducted interview identified 12 people who reported either symptoms suggestive of AIDS or behaviors that increased their risk of HIV infection. None of the 12 had been so identified by standard Red Cross written questionnaires or by face-to-face interviews, the doctors noted in The Journal of the American Medical Association.

Sept. 15

Oral polio-vaccine developer Albert Sabin, M.D., predicted that a preventive or therapeutic vaccine against AIDS will never be successful as long as researchers concentrate purely on eradicating cell-free virus from the body. The importance of virus-infected cells, which are found in high concentrations in the lymph of blood and semen, is being ignored by current vaccine researchers, he wrote in the Proceedings of the National Academy of Sciences. Dr. Sabin added that rectal transmission of HIV introduces large numbers of virus-infected cells that persistently infect the portal of entry, presenting one of the biggest challenges to immunization.

Sept. 18

A Brigham Young University ethnobotanist reported that a medicinal plant found in Samoa has yielded a promising anti-AIDS drug. The drug, prostratin, is used by native healers to cure yellow fever, he told a symposium on healing plants at the New York Botanical Garden.

Sept. 19

French researchers cautioned that the prevalence of HIV infection in pregnant women may be underestimated because testing excludes both pregnant women who will go on to have an abortion and those with ectopic pregnancies. Researchers at the European Centre for the Epidemiological Monitoring of AIDS in St. Maurice studied more than 11,000 women who were tested for HIV at the end of pregnancy, regardless of pregnancy outcome. They found that HIV rates in women who had an ectopic pregnancy were more than seven times higher than among women who gave birth. The rate among women who had an abortion was more than twice as high as in women who gave birth, according to the report in The Lancet. Women who had a miscarriage had rates similar to those who gave birth.

Previously, U.S. government investigators reported that they had begun using polymerase chain reaction testing to better determine the rate of woman-to-fetus transmission of HIV.

Sept. 23

An advisory committee of the Food and Drug Administration recommended that atovaquone (Mepron, Burroughs Wellcome) be approved for the treatment of mild to moderate Pneumocystis carinii pneumonia.

In a 39-center trial, 322 AIDS patients with mild to moderate PCP received either atovaquone or trimethoprim/sulfamethoxazole. Seventeen percent of patients on atovaquone failed to respond compared with 6% given TMP/SMX. However, 20% of the TMP/SMX patients experienced drug failure because of side effects, compared to 7% of atovaquone patients.

Sept. 24

Screening the nation's blood supply for a mysterious AIDS-like illness is not warranted at present, concluded a Food and Drug Administration Advisory Panel. The FDA convened a meeting of its Blood Products Advisory Committee following reports of an AIDS-like illness—in 47 people, at this point—with no trace of HIV. The panel voted 8 to 1 against screening, but agreed unanimously to study levels of CD4 cells in random donors and in people at high risk for blood-borne diseases, such as people with hemophilia.

Sept. 28

Herpes simplex virus can stimulate HIV replication and spur progression to AIDS in persons infected with clinically latent HIV, Harvard researchers reported. In laboratory cultures of CD4 lymphoid cells, cells superinfected with HSV exhibited augmented HIV-1 replication, the investigators wrote in the Journal of Infectious Diseases. The team was unable to determine precisely how HSV activates latent HIV, but they cautioned that either de novo infection or reactivation of HSV could have the effect.

Oct. 1

Johns Hopkins researchers estimated that the risk of contracting HIV from a blood transfusion is about one in 60,000 units of blood, higher than a prior estimate by the American Red Cross of one in 225,000. Reporting in the Annals of Internal Medicine, the researchers said that two of 12,000 surgery patients who received 120,000 units of blood contracted HIV through a transfusion, although the virus was not detected in the blood before transfusion.

A Red Cross scientist commented that once the differences between the two studies that generated those numbers are taken into account—the differences being that the Red Cross study was larger and involved many centers around the country—the risk rates actually are similar.

Oct. 3

Basketball legend Magic Johnson's disclosure that he was infected with HIV increased public awareness of AIDS, a Medical College of Wisconsin psychologist reported. In the study, 361 Chicago commuters were asked about their concern about AIDS before and after Johnson's disclosure. More than half said they were very interested in getting more AIDS information after the disclosure compared with a little over one third before the announcement, the psychologist reported in the American Journal of Public Health.

Oct. 10

Australian researchers reported in The Lancet that they may have found a less virulent strain of HIV that has not produced AIDS symptoms in five people, seven to 10 years after they received infected blood transfusions from a single donor. The recipients and the donor of the infected blood continue to have normal levels of CD4 cells and no

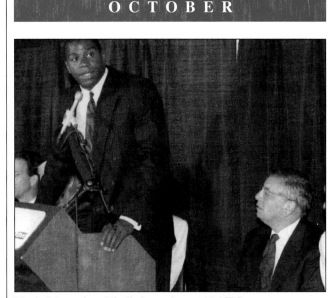

OCTOBER

Magic Johnson's public disclosure increased AIDS awareness.

p24 antigenemia. Theirs is the first report of what appears to be a nonvirulent strain of HIV that seems to remain nonvirulent after being transmitted, said the scientists, from the New South Wales Red Cross Blood Transfusion Service. Such information could be vital in developing a vaccine against the disease, they said.

Oct. 15

A panel of physicians concluded in a new report that the United States needs to increase its efforts to monitor and combat AIDS and other infectious diseases. Without improved public health initiatives for HIV and drug-resistant malaria and tuberculosis, an epidemic equal to the flu outbreak of 1918-1919, when 20 million people died worldwide, is likely to recur, they predicted. At a press conference convened by the Institute of Medicine in Washington, D.C., collaborators outlined 15 specific proposals for protecting the public, including offering incentives to drug companies to develop drugs and vaccines for diseases that might not yet be widespread.

Oct. 18

The Multicenter Candida

Esophagitis Study Group concluded that fluconazole (Diflucan, Roerig) is associated with significantly greater rates of endoscopic and clinical cure than ketoconazole (Nizoral, Janssen) in patients with AIDS and candida esophagitis. Reporting in the the Annals of Internal Medicine, they added that both drugs appear to be safe and well tolerated.

In the study, 169 AIDS patients were randomly assigned to receive fluconazole (100 mg/dl) or ketoconazole (200 mg/dl); doses were doubled if no symptomatic improvement occurred during a week. Endoscopic cure occurred in

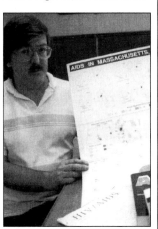

AIDS, other infections require better monitoring, said panel.

91% of patients treated with fluconazole and in 52% of those given ketoconazole. Esophageal symptoms resolved in 85% of fluconazole-treated patients and 65% of ketoconazole-treated patients. Side effects were minimal and comparable between the two groups, according to the report.

Oct. 22

Burroughs Wellcome told Medical Tribune that it had filed a complaint in U.S. District Court alleging patent infringement against Novopharm Inc., which had announced that it planned to manufacture and sell generic AZT if given the nod from the Food and Drug Administration. The president of Novopharm said that the patent for AZT (Retrovir) is invalid since the drug was discovered and tested by researchers from the National Institutes of Health. Burroughs Wellcome, however, said it was awarded the patent because of "creative insight''—that is, conceiving of the idea of using AZT for the treatment of HIV infection.

• • •

A French collaborative study found that viral culture at birth can correctly identify about half of newborns with HIV infection. Researchers at the Hôpital Necker-Infants Malades in Paris and other centers studied 181 infants born to HIV-infected mothers. Viral cultures at birth were positive in 19 of the 40 infants later found to be infected and in none of the uninfected infants, yielding a sensitivity of 48%. The sensitivity of p24 antigen testing at birth was only 18%.

The fact that the usually sensitive viral cultures failed to identify about half the infected neonates suggests that vertical transmission of HIV can occur late in pregnancy or during delivery, the researchers wrote in The New England Journal of Medicine.

AIDS

Nov. 2

Infection with herpes zoster was not found to be predictive of faster progression to AIDS in HIV-infected patients, scientists from the Centers for Disease Control and Prevention reported. Several previous studies have suggested that herpes zoster is a significant predictor of more rapid progression.

In statistical analyses, controlling for age, development of herpes zoster was not significantly associated with rate of progression to AIDS (relative risk:1.2; 95% C.I.)

The report in the Journal of Infectious Diseases found the overall incidence of herpes zoster in HIV-positive men to be 29.4 cases/1,000 person-years, which was significantly higher than the incidence in HIV-negative men and age-matched population controls.

The researchers noted that one of these studies suggesting that herpes zoster is a harbinger of AIDS progress lacked a control group of men without zoster.

Nov. 5

New York University researchers reported that HIV infection in children can result in a prolonged clinical latency and can masquerade as other pathologic conditions. They studied 181 HIV-infected children, 32 of whom were diagnosed when they were 4 years of age or older.

Of 32 asymptomatic children referred for testing because of HIV infection in their mothers, 24 had a history of recurrent infections, including otitis media, sinusitis, pneumonia and bacteremia. The absence of classic clinical symptoms in older children at risk for HIV infection should not deter HIV testing, the researchers concluded in Pediatrics.

Nov. 7

Celebrity disclosure of HIV or AIDS status was credited with reducing discrimination against HIV-

infected people and in motivating people to take an interest in their own health by a group of California researchers. In a letter in the British Medical Journal, representatives from the Orange County Health Care Agency said that Rock Hudson, Liberace and Earvin "Magic" Johnson helped heighten awareness among Americans about the importance of safe sex. Johnson was credited for an unprecedented rise in HIV testing in California for several months after his disclosure. The researchers suggested that physicians encourage celebrities to disclose their HIV or AIDS status.

Nov. 10

The National Institutes of Health announced that it has asked its scientists studying drug and alcohol abuse and mental illness to participate in the government's five-year plan on AIDS research. Inclusion of the additional NIH branches will boost the NIH budget for AIDS programs from $873 million to about $1 billion, according to Anthony Fauci, M.D., head of the AIDS advisory committee, who is also head of the National Institute of Allergy and Infectious Diseases.

In the new participating branches, the National Institute of Alcohol Abuse and Alcoholism plans long-term studies on alcohol's effect on the immune system. The National Institute of Drug Abuse will attempt to educate IV drug users on risks inherent in sharing needles and in drug use itself. The National Institute of Mental Health already has 25 studies under way to test ways to change risky behavior.

Nov.11

AIDS deaths in women between the ages of 15 and 44 surged dramatically during the 1980s, reported

epidemiologists at the Centers for Disease Control and Prevention in Atanta. In 1988, AIDS was the eighth leading cause of death in women in this age group, as compared with 1991, when it was the fifth leading cause of death, said the researchers.

In 1988, there were 1,365

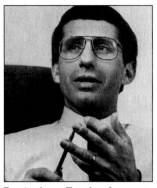

Dr. Anthony Fauci seeks more funds for AIDS programs.

deaths in women aged 15 through 44 attributed to HIV infection on death certificates: 202 deaths with HIV infection listed as an associated cause and 149 excess deaths due to conditions highly associated with HIV infection. Ascertaining the cause of death from death certificates is thought to identify between 55% and 80% of actual HIV-related deaths in women.

Nov. 12

Seattle researchers suggested that condom-giveaway programs at drug abuse treatment centers may decrease high-risk sexual behavior. At the time a giveaway program was started at the Seattle Veterans Affairs Medical Center, 27% of the male addicts in the study used condoms for vaginal intercourse. After condoms were placed in rest rooms, waiting rooms and group therapy rooms, 44% of the men said they used condoms. Most of the condoms were taken from the men's rest rooms.

More clients who had multiple sexual partners in the

previous year took condoms than those who were monogamous, said the researchers.

Nov. 16

The Centers for Disease Control and Prevention announced that it plans to implement an expanded case definition for AIDS in January 1993. Under the new definition, AIDS will be diagnosed if a patient has CD4 cell counts of less than 200 cells/mm[3]. The definition still uses the 23 clinical conditions already in use but will now include pulmonary tuberculosis, recurrent pneumonia and invasive cervical cancer. The expanded definition is expected to significantly increase the number of women and drug abusers reported as having the disease. The proposal for the changes was based on information presented by healthcare workers and AIDS advocates.

Nov. 18

The Israeli government announced that it will bar the immigration of HIV-positive people.

Nov. 21

University of Georgia researchers revealed that dental handpieces and their attachments for drilling and cleaning teeth are possible sources of HIV contamination and transmission. The investigators obtained samples from the inside channels of 12 new high-speed drills and 30 rotary attachments used to clean and polish teeth. After use on HIV-infected persons, HIV proviral DNA was detected in samples taken from inside the equipment and from their attached air/water hoses, the investigators reported in The Lancet. The investigators recommended that all states adopt regulations requiring that reused high-speed, air-driven handpieces and dental hygiene equipment be cleaned and heat-treated between each patient to prevent transmission of HIV, as well as hepatitis B virus. Five states already have such regulations, the investigator said.

AIDS

Dec. 1

On the occasion of World AIDS Day, the Centers for Disease Control and Prevention launched its new HIV education program, called Business Responds to AIDS. In the program, business executives were encouraged to undertake employee education and training aimed at primary prevention of HIV infection. Business leaders were also asked to develop written HIV policies for the workplace and to encourage employees to volunteer in community HIV-prevention activities.

To assist business and labor leaders, a manager's kit for the development of HIV policies and education programs became available from the CDC National AIDS Clearinghouse.

Dec. 5

If dermatologists vigorously evaluate even mild skin lesions in HIV-infected patients, they can speed the diagnosis of disseminated opportunistic infections and allow for more rapid institution of antibiotic therapy, asserted a New York dermatologist. Biopsies should be performed on even banal-appearing lesions (particularly if a patient is febrile) and bisected to allow for culture as well as histopathologic examination, the New York University Medical Center researcher told the American Academy of Dermatology meeting in San Francisco. Gram staining of a touch preparation from a skin specimen may reveal the etiology of an infection immediately, according to the dermatologist.

Dec. 7

Disability insurers should consider HIV-positive physicians "totally disabled" even if they have no symptoms, asserted the Missouri delegation to the American Medical Association House of Delegates interim meeting in Nashville. The delegation asked the AMA to require the "total disability" designation from all disability insurance carriers that provide coverage under the AMA name, endorsement or control. The action is necessary because of the loss of income when physicians inform patients of their seropositive status and are no longer able to perform invasive procedures, the physicians argued.

Texas representatives, while advocating that insurers voluntarily change their disability criteria (instead of being required to do so), noted that even if no invasive procedures are involved in HIV-positive physicians' clinical practices, they should not treat highly

American Academy of Dermatology meeting in San Francisco. Additionally, HIV proviral DNA has been detected in the smoke plume of the CO_2 laser, and HIV-specific antigens have been detected through cultures of collection tubing used in dermatologic procedures on HIV-positive individuals. The professor, from Cornell University Medical College, recommended that dermatologists wear eye protection and masks capable of removing particles as small as 0.2 mm, and that they adopt the use of special evacuation systems for laser and electrosurgery.

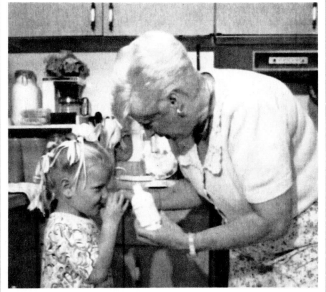

With more than 80,000 AIDS orphans predicted by the year 2000, grandparents may called on to become primary caretakers.

contagious patients because of their suppressed immune systems.

Dec. 8

A New York specialist cautioned dermatologists that rigorous precautions should be taken to prevent HIV transmission during dermabrasion and laser surgery. Particles produced during dermabrasion are of sufficient size to allow inspiration and pulmonary retention of HIV, the researcher told the

Dec. 11

The CDC's expanded definition of AIDS will force clinics that treat HIV-infected people to do gynecological exams on their female clients, predicted the author of "The Invisible Epidemic: The Story of Women and AIDS." Previously, even the few women—8.6% of total participants—being treated in AIDS clinical trial groups (ACTG) did not receive Pap smears or pelvic examina-

tions, she told Medical Tribune. Currently, there is no requirement that ACTG study teams include a gynecologist, and there is only one ACTG pilot study that includes a gynecological protocol, the researcher stated.

Dec. 15

Pediatricians at Ohio State University warned that sharing earrings may spread blood-borne infections, including HIV and hepatitis B. They wrote in a letter to Pediatrics that even teenagers who are aware of the risks associated with the sharing of needles and sexual activity may not be aware of the risk of sharing earrings, which could become contaminated with blood.

The physicians suggested that practitioners include questions and warnings about the practice of earring sharing in their interviews.

Dec. 23

Children of patients who have died of AIDS will become one of the fastest growing and hardest-to-care-for segments of the AIDS population, reported New York researchers. By the year 2000 there will be more than 80,000 orphans of AIDS patients, many of whom will themselves have AIDS, an epidemiologist from the Sophie Davis School of Biomedical Education/City University of New York Medical School revealed in The Journal of the American Medical Association. Collaborating researchers from the Orphan Project suggested that new social services are needed to help these traumatized and displaced children who will require mental health support and to aid family members who have become their guardians.

New York City currently has the largest number and the highest proportion of AIDS orphans in the country—a situation that is predicted to continue.

'Wellness program' helps long-term HIV survival

By Naomi Pfeiffer

SAN FRANCISCO, JAN. 23—Aggressive medical care and life-style changes are largely responsible for the long-term survival of 65 HIV-positive patients in vigorous health 10 years after diagnosis, according to the physician who treats them.

"Our long survivors have had no clinical findings that could be defined as AIDS," said Marcus Conant, M.D., of the University of California School of Medicine here.

Yet, he stressed, their immune systems have deteriorated alarmingly over the years. "We're amazed when we see their lab results. We shake our heads and say, 'This individual should be very sick. Five years ago he would have been dead [with such low CD4 cell counts].'"

Dr. Conant begins intervention when the patient's CD4 counts are well above 500 cells/mm³. "We work through a 'wellness program,' including stress reduction, rest, exercise, elimination of recreational drugs," he said.

At CD4 counts of 500, he starts AZT 600 mg/day plus trimethoprim sulfamethoxazole to prevent Pneumocystis carinii pneumonia.

"These interventions have altered the natural history of PCP and HIV disease," he said. "Average life expectancy in my patients with AIDS has tripled."

At CD4 counts below 100, Dr. Conant adds aerosolized pentamidine to the PCP prophylaxis, and starts fluconazole (Diflucan, Roerig) to prevent cryptococcal meningitis, as well as clarithromycin (Biaxin, Abbott Laboratories) to prevent Mycobacterium avium infection.

Attitude is also important, he said, adding that aggressive, positive patients live longer than those who take a passive attitude.

"I really push exercise," Dr. Conant said. "Studies show that exercise helps sustain HIV-infected people both physically and emotionally."

Ronald Grossman, M.D., a New York internist with a large AIDS practice, agrees that antiretroviral therapy, prophylaxis and a sensible life-style add up to long-term survival in some patients. But he recommends only basic aerobic and muscle-building exercises three times a week. "Overexertion can cause weight loss. Weight loss often turns out to be secondary to an infection," he said.

Brady Allen, M.D., an HIV specialist from Baylor University, Dallas, said that after years of AZT (Retrovir, Burroughs Wellcome) alone, long-term survivors often ask for combination therapy with AZT plus DDC (Hivid, Hoffmann-La Roche) or DDI (Videx, Bristol-Myers Squibb) when their CD4 counts fall below 100 or 200. "There's no clinical data yet showing these combinations are safe and effective, although there's synergy in vitro."

Donald Abrams, M.D., assistant director of AIDS activities at San Francisco General Hospital, believes strong CD8 suppressor cell activity may add to long-term survival.

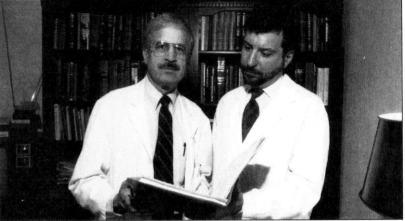

Dr. Grossman (left) recommends basic aerobic exercises three times a week.

Some 5% of 442 HIV-infected patients he follows show no clinical signs of the disease nine to 13 years after diagnosis. Their CD4 cell counts range from 4 to 1,200 and their CD8 level is uniformly high.

He recommends Dr. Conant's "wellness program," and PCP prophylaxis when CD4 counts go below 200.

He added that antiretroviral therapy "is a choice. We ask the patients to educate themselves about their treatment options. If they ask for AZT, they get it."

Study questions when to start AZT therapy

WASHINGTON, D.C., FEB. 13—A new Veterans Administration study suggests that AZT delays the onset of AIDS but does not improve the chances of patients living longer when drug treatment is started early in the course of HIV infection.

While the study raises new questions about the timing and effectiveness of AZT therapy, an FDA spokesperson said the agency would not change its recommended labeling for the drug.

The FDA currently recommends that patients infected with HIV routinely take AZT as soon as their CD4 cells drop to a blood count below 500. "At this point we are not considering changing the labeling," said FDA spokesperson Brad Stone.

The new study also showed that HIV-infected adults who

began taking AZT early, experienced more anemia, leukopenia, nausea, vomiting and diarrhea than those who waited until they developed symptoms. The study appears in The New England Journal of Medicine.

The four-year study evaluated 338 patients at VA medical centers across the country.

The study compared AZT therapy in patients who were symptomatic but had CD4 blood counts between 200 and 500 with those whose CD4 counts were below 200 or in whom AIDS had developed.

After two years, 28 people in the early-therapy group had developed full-blown AIDS, compared with 48 in the late-therapy group.

Deaths totaled 23 in the former group and 20 in the latter group. The researchers said the data raise anew the debate over the best time to start AZT therapy in HIV-infected patients with CD4 blood counts above 200.

They said that early therapy when CD4 counts are below 500 is an option that warrants much consideration.

But because of the uncertainty about the long-term effects of AZT, doctors may consider delaying the beginning of treatment in patients whose conditions are stable and whose CD4 blood counts are between 200 and 500, according to the researchers.

Early therapy compared with late therapy does not improve survival, said John Hamilton, M.D., of the Durham, N.C., Veterans Administration Medical Center, who led the study.

But the drug may still prolong life, he stressed.

AZT prolongs life compared with taking nothing at all, said Michael Simberkoff, M.D., of the Veterans Administration Medical Center in New York City, who also worked on the study.

He said he would follow the FDA's recommendation, but had some "doubts and hesitations."

FDA committee okays DDC with condition

BETHESDA, MD., APRIL 21—An advisory committee has recommended that the FDA grant conditional approval to the anti-HIV drug dideoxycytidine, to be used only in combination with AZT for people with advanced HIV infection.

The recommendation, passed by vote after eight hours of discussion and data analysis by committee members, was based on preliminary findings of ongoing studies. It is considered a test of a new federal policy to speed approval of vitally needed drugs.

The Antiviral Drugs Advisory Committee decided to recommend against approving DDC (Hivid, Hoffmann-La Roche) for use alone in patients who cannot tolerate or who do not respond to AZT (Retrovir, Burroughs Wellcome). The vote was eight to two with one abstention.

The committee specified that if continuing clinical trials fail to support DDC used in combination with AZT, it should be removed from the market.

In deciding to reject DDC monotherapy, the committee

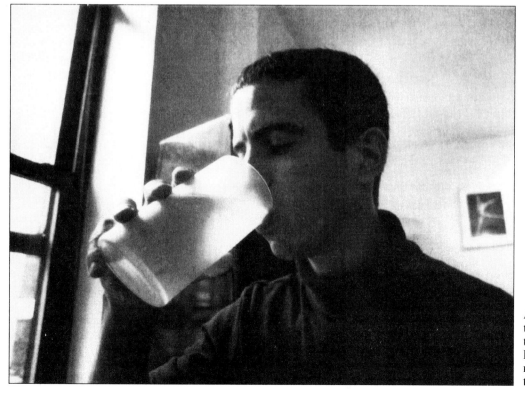

A patient unresponsive to AZT can be switched to combo therapy with DDC or DDI monotherapy, according to one FDA official.

relied heavily on a study showing that patients who took AZT survived longer and were less likely to experience HIV-related infections than those on DDC, according to David Feigal Jr., M.D., director of the division of antiviral drug products at the Food and Drug Administration.

The study also showed that up to 20% of people on DDC may develop peripheral neuropathy.

In deciding to approve combination treatment, committee members relied heavily on a study involving about 90 patients comparing AZT and DDC with AZT alone. Patients who took the combination experienced about twice the increase in CD4 cells as those who took AZT alone, Dr. Feigal said.

The problem with the study, however, was that none of the patients had taken nucleoside drugs before. This means that it is not known for sure whether patients will benefit from adding DDC to an existing daily regimen of AZT, he said.

How should physicians and patients act on the committee's recommendations?

"AZT remains the first-line drug," he said. "No one has shown that another drug is equivalent or superior as an initial therapy."

But a patient who has been on AZT for a period of time and feels that his or her immune system is continuing to deteriorate can switch to dideoxyinosine (Videx, Bristol-Myers Squibb), an option that has been shown to be effective, he said. "The other option would be to try combination therapy."

The committee decided to recommend making this option available despite the paucity of data "because of what the HIV community has been telling us," Dr. Feigal said. "They're the ones who have the infection and they're the ones who want to make the choice."

But Dr. Feigal did have some advice: "I hope that as physicians and patients make their choices, they consider the evidence and the potential uncertainty of starting combinations when we really don't know quite how they will turn out."

Vaccine may offer wider immune responses

MAY 1—A stumbling block in the design of an AIDS vaccine—finding one that stimulates the broadest possible immune system response to HIV—appears to have been circumvented with the development of an oligomeric lysine scaffolding for testing potentially effective protein fragments, according to a new report.

"This approach obviously has a lot of promise," said Jonathan Allen, M.D., an AIDS researcher at the Southwest Foundation for Biomedical Research in San Antonio.

The synthetic vaccine is made from peptide antigens from a glycoprotein on the AIDS virus's outer coat. The pieces are stitched together at one end of a chemical scaffold made up of lysine.

On the other end of the scaffold, the researchers attached a nontoxic oligomeric compound made from bacteria.

The compound enhances the immune response and anchors the entire structure to a liposome, which carries the structure into cells, eliciting an immune response against the virus.

The study was published in the Proceedings of the National Academy of Sciences.

In animal tests, guinea pigs and mice injected with the synthetic vaccine produced neutralizing antibodies against the virus pieces, said James P. Tam, Ph.D., assistant professor of biochemistry at Rockefeller University in New York, who led the study.

AIDS researchers said the important part of Dr. Tam's vaccine is that it mobilizes both antibodies and killer cells, the two arms of the immune system.

Many groups are attempting to make an AIDS vaccine out of harmless protein fragments taken from the virus.

But the fragments by themselves only elicit an antibody response and it is not clear which fragments fight the virus best.

To that end, Dr. Tam's vaccine may help in the search for the proper fragments.

According to Dr. Tam, the vaccine would provide a scaffold to which any number of protein fragments could be attached so doctors could see which one worked the best.

He said the next step is to test the vaccine in monkeys exposed to the AIDS virus.

HIV risk from donor blood: 1 in 225,000 transfusions, CDC says

MAY 27—The Centers for Disease Control has received 158 state health department reports of people who contracted AIDS from blood transfusions since blood testing began in 1985, but has been able to confirm only 15, according to a letter in The New England Journal of Medicine.

Most of the people had other risk factors for AIDS infection, according to the CDC survey of cases reported between April 1985 and March 1990.

Other patients may have received blood before March 1985, when widespread testing of the nation's blood supply began, but were not diagnosed with AIDS until later because of the long latency of the virus.

Seven of the 15 confirmed cases of transmission occurred in states with a "low" incidence of AIDS: Indiana, Alabama, Kentucky, Michigan and Oregon. Eight patients received the transfusions in states with a "high" incidence: California, Texas, Florida, Nevada and New Jersey. The CDC researchers concluded that risk of infection from blood

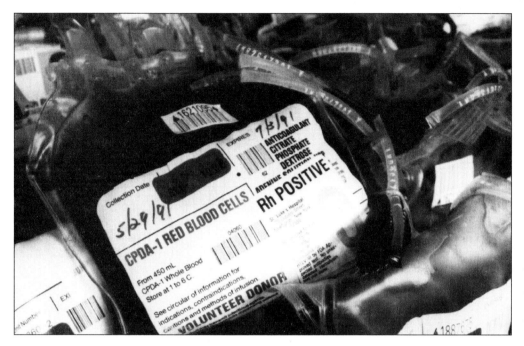

About 2% of all reported AIDS cases are linked to blood transfusions, according to the CDC.

transfusions is no greater in high-incidence areas than in ones with lower rates of the disease.

The rates of HIV transmission through screened blood is about one in 60,000 transfused units, concluded the government researchers.

The number of confirmed transfusion-based AIDS cases may have risen to 20, but the risk of infection from a transfusion still is low. "What that means is that the risk of getting AIDS from a blood transfusion is about one in 225,000 transfusions," said American Red Cross spokesperson Liz Hall.

The American Red Cross provides approximately half of the nation's blood supply, or six million units a year.

Hall noted that according to the CDC, about 2% of all reported AIDS cases, or 4,770 AIDS patients, are linked to blood transfusions. Almost all of those cases occurred before screening measures were implemented, she said.

There has always been some concern that infected blood might slip through the testing net because of the latency period during which the HIV virus is present but not detectable. Newer tests can now detect HIV in the blood less than 40 days after a person becomes infected, compared with about three months for previous tests, she said.

The test also has been upgraded to include screening for HIV-2, an AIDS strain common in Africa.

Last August, a Gallup poll commissioned by the American Association of Blood Banks found that 71% of people surveyed believed that the nation's blood supply was somewhat to very safe, but only 25% said they had "a lot of confidence" that it was very safe.

The CDC report concluded that since HIV infection from transfusions is very rare, "this very small risk should not discourage patients who need transfusions from receiving them."

WHO's estimates of AIDS challenged as too low

Medical World News Report

JUNE 3—A new report by AIDS researchers challenges the World Health Organization's projected figures for the number of worldwide AIDS cases that have been predicted for the year 2000.

The researchers urge government leaders and health experts to develop a new global strategy to prevent the spread of the disease and to provide treatment for those already infected.

"The gap between lagging national and international efforts against AIDS and the expanding pandemic is widening rapidly and dangerously, and a new global strategy for the 1990s is urgently needed," said Jonathan Mann, M.D., director of the International AIDS Center at the Harvard School of Public Health. He is also the coordinator of the Global AIDS Policy Coalition, a privately funded group based at Harvard that serves as an informational network for AIDS policy and program research and analysis.

Dr. Mann is one of the editors of the new report, titled "AIDS in the World 1992," which was funded by the GAPC and will be published by Harvard University Press.

WHO has estimated that 40 million men, women and children will be infected with the virus that causes AIDS by the year 2000, according to Susan Holck, M.D., chief of policy for the organization's Global Program on AIDS.

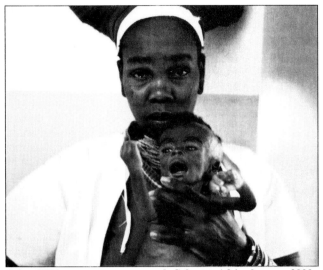

Asian HIV cases may surpass sub-Saharan Africa by year 2000.

The GAPC report projects that by the year 2000, between 38 million and 110 million adults and over 10 million children will become HIV infected.

The WHO numbers are based on country reports, though it is thought that some countries suppress reports on AIDS and other diseases. The GAPC numbers are based on interviews with experts around the world.

The 40-member team that developed the report includes physicians, AIDS activists and members of the non-governmental health and social agencies.

"In 1992, no one really knows what will happen eight years from now," said Dr. Holck, responding to the new report. "It's hard to predict, and a lot depends on how successful national programs will be. What really matters is that we don't get to either number."

"It matters that we get the numbers right so that we can plan both prevention and care," said Mindell Seidlin, M.D., director of the AIDS program at Bellevue Hospital in New York City, which cares for the largest number of AIDS cases in the United States. "You have to start thinking about the global economic impact, and what effect it will have on local economies when so many people can no longer work and will need assistance," she added.

What especially concerns the GAPC is that the spread of HIV has not been stopped in any community or country, and that the disease is spreading to new countries, often with great rapidity.

An explosion of HIV has recently occurred in southeast Asia, Thailand, Burma and India, where in just a few years over one million people have become infected, according to the report. By the year 2000, the largest proportion of HIV infections will develop in Asia (42%), surpassing sub-Saharan Africa (31%), Latin America (8%) and the Caribbean (6%).

Daniel Tarantola, M.D., an epidemiologist and the scientific editor of the report, said that the group hopes to have a yearly report that will address priorities and detail progress in both treatment and prevention.

To stem the pandemic, countries must focus on the groups at highest risk, according to Dr. Tarantola.

Many countries often ignore prevention and treatment strategies among intravenous drug users and prostitutes. These groups often make up the largest number of AIDS cases, he said.

One roadblock to prevention and treatment is that planning and coordination in many countries is often done through the ministries of administrative affairs, the groups with which WHO is most likely to work, instead of coordinating efforts with the departments of education, tourism, defense (for HIV infections in the military), social affairs and finance, added the report's editor.

It's also important to put some AIDS issues into the hands of community groups and nongovernmental agencies, according to Dr. Tarantola. Discrimination against women, the poor and minority populations in many countries often results in a lack of treatment.

"In such cases, we need to work with human rights groups to see to it that everyone who needs it is getting treatment," he said, "especially now that the number of women infected with HIV has grown to 40% of the total worldwide."

"Low tech" therapies that don't require constant monitoring would be a major breakthrough in the developing world, according to Bellevue's Dr. Seidlin. Because AZT can cause toxic side effects and its users must be monitored frequently, it is a poor choice for treatment in countries where regular blood tests can't be run.

Right now, "nothing qualifies" as a less time- and resource-consuming alternative, according to Daniel Hoth, M.D., director of the AIDS division of the National Institute of Allergy and Infectious Diseases in Bethesda, Md.

Getting the prevention message across, even in countries where sex education is prohibited, may prove to be easier than developing therapies and vaccines to treat and prevent the disease.

Scientists are stymied in their efforts to develop new drugs to treat the disease because every time they find a new medication to beat the virus, at least one mutant version, and often a whole colony resistant to therapy, will emerge, according to researchers. "Right now, the virus is smarter than we are," said Mark Goldman, an AIDS pharmaceutical researcher formerly with Merck & Co.

Anti-HIV agent granted conditional approval

June 22—Following an advisory panel's recommendation, the Food and Drug Administration has approved the anti-HIV drug dideoxycytidine for use in combination with AZT in adults with advanced HIV infection.

The approval of dideoxycytidine, or zalcitabine (Hivid, Hoffmann-La Roche), was based on two studies involving fewer than 100 patients, under the FDA's new "conditional approval" program. Under that program, the drug can be pulled from the market if further studies find it to be ineffective.

In studies, DDC with AZT, also called zidovudine (Retrovir, Burroughs Wellcome), increased the number of CD4 cells better than AZT alone. It is the third anti-HIV drug approved, and the first under the conditional approval program.

The drug has not been shown to prolong survival, lower the incidence of opportunistic infections or halt HIV progression. Physicians also do not yet know the optimum dose of the drug.

The FDA said it did not approve DDC as monotherapy because it has not proved as effective as AZT alone. DDC is indicated for patients with 300 CD4 cells/mm³ or fewer. Its yearly wholesale price is listed at $1,826. The AZT/DDC combination is expected to cost $3,400 a year.

Marcus Conant, M.D., a clinical professor at the University of California Medical Center in San Francisco, and a proponent of the conditional approval system, said the approval of DDC will allow many patients to stop taking black-market versions of the drug, which often were too strong or too weak. "It provides us with a pharmaceutical-grade drug that we can use on desperately ill patients," he said.

DDC and DDI cause neuropathy, but DDI tends to cause more pancreatitis, he said. DDC also can lower blood-platelet counts and cause abnormal liver function.

Reports of AIDS-like illness baffle researchers

By L.A. McKeown

AMSTERDAM, JULY 21—A string of cases of an AIDS-like illness that occurs in the absence of HIV has baffled researchers, and became the unscheduled focus of the 8th International Conference on AIDS here last month.

After Jeffrey Laurence, M.D., of Cornell University Medical College in New York reported that he had seen five cases of the mysterious disease, researchers at a hastily called press conference during the AIDS symposium came forth one by one to say that they, too, had seen similar syndromes they are reluctant to treat as AIDS cases.

The reports of a total of 26 cases to date raised the possibility of a new, HIV-like virus or even a mutant form of HIV. They also sparked concern about the safety of the nation's blood supply, and whether a new or mutant virus may be able to elude standard HIV screening.

But at least one expert believes the cases that have turned up so far are highly unusual, and not indicative of an unknown, HIV-like transmissible agent.

"This isn't AIDS without HIV," said James Curran, M.D., of the Centers for Disease Control."This is important work, but it isn't AIDS."

Dr. Laurence opened the door to talk of the mysterious virus by announcing that he had seen five cases of patients with typical AIDS symptoms and low or borderline CD4 cell counts, but with negative polymerase chain reaction and ELISA results.

Soon after the New York investigator's revelation, Dr. Curran said that the CDC knows of another six cases in the United States. And Sudhir Gupta, M.D., an immunologist at the University of California at Irvine, reported in the Proceedings of the National Academy of Sciences another two cases, a woman and her daughter.

The announcements prompted Anthony Fauci, M.D., of the National Institutes of Health to urge all doctors with information on similar cases to come forward.

Dr. Laurence, whose report will appear in the Aug. 1 issue of The Lancet, said four of five patients he studied had potential risk factors for AIDS. Two were gay men, one was an elderly Hispanic female who had a blood transfusion in 1978 and one was a male healthcare worker. The remaining

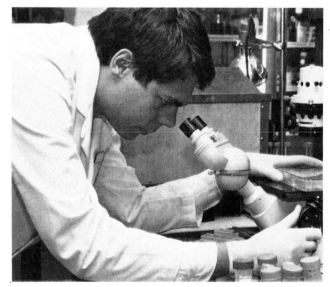

Dr. Laurence's cases all tested negative for HIV and HTLV.

white heterosexual man, who developed Pneumocystis carinii pneumonia and died, had no known risk factors, but had been treated with a one-month course of prednisone for inflammatory bowel disease just prior to presenting with severe CD4-cell depletion.

Dr. Laurence's cases all tested negative for HIV-1, HIV-2 and HTLV-I and -II. Their CD4 counts ranged from 552 to 76 cells/mm³, and clinical disorders included PCP, Kaposi's sarcoma, oral candidiasis, chronic cough, wasting and intractable cutaneous abscess. Two of the patients have died.

The CDC has had reports of six HIV-negative people with moderate to severe CD4 depletion in four states over the past two years, Dr. Curran said. The CD4 counts in these cases were much lower than Dr. Laurence described, ranging from 275 to 50 cells/mm³. Clinical disorders included PCP, cryptococcal meningitis, vaginal candidiasis, molluscum contagiosum and Herpes zoster.

Two of the six had blood transfusions, one related to a kidney transplant. One patient developed Kaposi's sarcoma and another developed PCP. Most of them are alive and still have no evidence of HIV, but continue to have chronic immune depression.

The reports were not made public because the CDC did not want to frighten people before further studies could confirm the findings, Dr. Curran said.

David Ho, M.D., of the Aaron Diamond AIDS Research Center in New York, said that over the last three years, he has seen 11 cases of low CD4 counts in the absence of HIV, some in gay men and a few in people with no risk factors. Three developed opportunistic infections and eventually died.

"As a clinical entity, I think it's real," Dr. Ho said. "We feel very confident, based on the serology, HIV culture and polymerase chain reaction, that these are not the usual cases of HIV-1 or HIV-2."

Highlights of the AIDS meeting

In other papers presented at the AIDS conference, researchers reported that:
• The search for a therapeutic vaccine that could "jump start" depressed immune systems in patients with AIDS continues, but experts warn that there is still a long way to go before approval is seen.

One of the most promising of the therapeutic formulations is composed of gp160, the envelope protein of HIV.

Beginning in 1990, Robert Redfield, Ph.D., of Walter Reed Army Institutes of Research in Rockville, Md., gave the vaccine to 30 HIV-infected patients with CD4 counts of 400 cells/mm^3 or higher. Responders received booster injections of 160 mcg or 640 mcg, depending on initial response, every four months for two years.

Dr. Redfield said that all but one of 28 patients who completed the trials have had sustained antibody responses to selected envelope epitopes.
• People with AIDS whose disease progresses quickly tend to have a mass of cells clumped together that are all infected with the AIDS virus. The conglomerate of cells, known as a syncytium, is a far stronger indication that AIDS will progress more quickly than resistance to AZT.
• A drug that has been used for years to treat blood-vessel disease may improve the benefits of AIDS-fighting drugs. The drug, pentoxifylline (Trental, Hoechst-Roussel), lowers the level of endogenous tumor necrosis factor; TNF blocks the effects of AZT and other anti-AIDS drugs and increases the growth of HIV, according to Boston researchers.
• The overwhelming bulk of funding for AIDS research, prevention and care is spent in the United States, although 60% of AIDS cases occur in Third World countries, Harvard researchers reported. Many Third World countries depend solely on international funding for AIDS care, they pointed out.
Of the total $5.6 billion spent worldwide since 1981, $5.45 billion, or 97%, was spent in industrialized countries.
• Young American doctors are less likely to care for AIDS patients than their counterparts in France or Canada, according to the first such international study. American doctors are more likely to believe that care of patients infected with the AIDS virus is dangerous, and to say they would be reluctant to practice in an area where AIDS is prevalent. —*L.M.*

The latest announcement came from Dr. Gupta, whose findings, to be published Aug. 15, were released early in light of the other reports.

Dr. Gupta believes he may have found a new retrovirus, called human intracisternal retrovirus (HICRV), in a 66-year-old woman with lowered CD4 cells and PCP and in her asymptomatic daughter. Electron microscopy detected particles of the virus in mononuclear cells from both patients; the samples were also HICRV-antibody positive via Western Blot.

Neither woman has any risk factors for HIV, and neither has tested positive for HIV-1, HIV-2 or any of three other human retroviruses associated with T-cell deficiencies.

The reports raise the possibility of a new, HIV-like virus, or mutant forms of HIV that exist undetected in some people, according to AIDS specialists. Another explanation for the syndrome may be an underlying lymphoma or leukemia that suppresses the immune system.

"Back in 1981, almost every unusual case of what we thought at the time was AIDS, turned out to be undetected cancer," Dr. Curran said, adding that the new syndrome "isn't AIDS without HIV."

Dr. Laurence said none of his patients had any malignancies or a family history of cancer, nor was there evidence of a congenital immune deficiency. He also ruled out the possibility of HIV-2 or a similar strain of HIV.

French researcher Luc Montagnier, M.D., acknowledged that he has seen the syndrome in at least two patients. But he later detected a defective form of HIV in urine samples.

Dr. Laurence said he did not do urine testing, and Dr. Curran said he was not aware of its being done in the CDC cases.

The American Association of Blood Banks said that the nation's blood supply is still safe. "The patients in question are considered to be among those at high risk for AIDS, and would, according to the donor screening process in place at U.S. blood banks, be eliminated as blood donors," the association said.

Urine test for HIV called as accurate as current blood tests

AMSTERDAM, JULY 21—A new urine test for the AIDS virus may be less expensive, more convenient and just as accurate as current blood tests, according to University of California at San Francisco researchers who spoke at the 8th International Conference on AIDS.

But researchers warned that if the urine test is approved by the Food and Drug Administration, it could readily, and perhaps secretly, be used by employers or insurers to test for the virus.

"There is a potential to violate the civil rights and confidentiality of patients," said Daniel Berrios, M.D., a research fellow at UCSF's Center for AIDS Prevention Studies.

Dr. Berrios and his team tested 530 people for the AIDS

virus using both conventional blood tests and the experimental urine test developed by Calypte Biomedical Corp. of Berkeley, Calif. Both tests spotted the 36 people infected with HIV.

"This is a replication of other studies," said Douglas Anglin, director of the Drug Abuse Research Center at the University of California at Los Angeles.

"It gives increased confidence that the urine test is as good as blood tests," he said. A urine test would reduce the AIDS infection risk for healthcare workers, he added.

Dr. Berrios said that Calypte is planning to submit a request for approval to the FDA next month, so that the urine test can become a standard diagnostic tool.

Genetic Systems, Seattle, is also in the process of developing an AIDS urine test.

Women at higher AIDS risk than men; poorer survival due to inadequate treatment plans

New York Times/Medical Tribune News Service

AMSTERDAM, JULY 20—By the year 2000, more than half of newly infected AIDS patients will be women, reported a World Health Organization representative at the 8th International Conference on AIDS here. Half of the one million people already infected this year are women, added Michael Merson, head of WHO's Global Program on AIDS.

Women have a poorer chance of survival than men once they are diagnosed, and are less likely to get the drugs they need, according to other specialists at the meeting.

In the United States, women have become the fastest-growing group of AIDS patients, with primary risk factors being intravenous drug use and unprotected sex with drug users, according to the Centers for Disease Control. "The heterosexual epidemic is here, no doubt about it," said Sten Vermund, M.D., chief of epidemiology, Division of AIDS at the National Institute of Allergy and Infectious Diseases.

Nearly 5% of 20- to 29-year old women visiting sexually transmitted disease clinics in the District of Columbia are infected with HIV, according to the Bethesda expert. "It's an astronomical rate for 20-year-olds," Dr. Vermund said.

According to experts meeting at the AIDS conference, not enough attention is being focused on the detection and treatment of AIDS in women. Sally Zierler, M.D., of Brown University in Providence, R.I., said that by lumping the treatment plans for men and women together, gender differences may be ignored.

Women with very low levels of CD4 cells were significantly less likely to get AZT than men with similar levels, according to a study conducted by researchers at the AIDS Research Consortium of Atlanta Inc.

"When women get AZT on time, their survival is equal to men," said researcher Terri Creagh. She found that 80% of HIV-infected men get AZT when their CD4 levels go below 50 cells/mm^3, compared with 59% of women.

She cited social stigmas against female IV-drug users, who account for much of the female AIDS population, as well as the underrepresentation of women, particularly African-American women, in AIDS trials as possible causes for the finding.

Italian researchers at the meeting reported that the age at which a woman is diagnosed with HIV influences disease progression. Women who become HIV-positive after age 25 get AIDS faster than younger women or men the same age.

By 1995, approximately 240,000 to 335,000 people in the United States will have AIDS or will be suffering some type of immunosuppression due to HIV, according to the Centers for Disease Control.

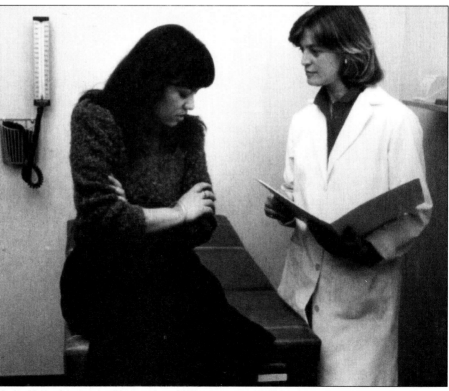

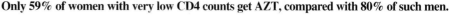

Only 59% of women with very low CD4 counts get AZT, compared with 80% of such men.

CD4 test helps family practitioners in diagnosis

Medical Tribune News Service

JULY 23—A simple, low-cost test for counting CD4 cells may soon enable primary-care physicians to screen patients in the office instead of sending out blood samples for flow cytometry testing.

"The test takes 10 minutes. The only equipment you need is a light microscope and hemacytometer," said Alan Landay, Ph.D., director of clinical immunology at Rush-Presbyterian-St. Luke's Medical Center in Chicago.

Latex beads coated with anti-CD4 monoclonal antibody are mixed for two minutes with a sample of whole blood. To quantitate CD4 cells, a blood smear is made and Wright-stained.

More latex beads coated with CD14 are added to keep CD4 from binding to monocytes in the sample and obscuring the true number of cells. The cell suspension is lysed in Turck's solution, and the CD4 cells counted on a hemacytometer.

In a study of more than 500 healthy and infected people, the new test was 90% as precise "in counting every cell" as laser-operated flow cytometry, said Dr. Landay, who headed a team of researchers from Cornell University, the New Jersey College of Medicine and Dentistry, Case Western Reserve University, and Makerere University, Uganda, in developing the test.

When it was compared in efficacy with standard flow cytometry and hematology counts, the test correlated well, added Thomas Russell, Ph.D., of Coulter Corp., Hialeah, Fla., where the test is being developed.

"A predictive value of 90% accuracy is close enough to assess the patient's stage of disease, choose appropriate HIV therapy, and measure its effectiveness," he said.

Dr. Russell said he receives most inquiries in the United States from areas where there are few AIDS cases and therefore limited testing facilities.

The researchers recently returned from demonstrating the test for medical personnel in Russia and the Ukraine under the auspices of the World Health Organization.

A faster method of obtaining CD4 counts may be especially useful now that the Centers for Disease Control is considering a proposal that would revamp the definition of AIDS by placing more emphasis on the importance of CD4 counts. Under the current definition, last updated in 1988, an AIDS diagnosis requires a CD4 count below 200 cells/mm^3 plus at least one of 23 illnesses that include Kaposi's sarcoma, lymphoma, Pneumocystis carinii pneumonia, wasting syndrome or dementia.

The new definition would classify an HIV-infected person with a CD4 count below 200 cells/mm^3 as having AIDS, regardless of other symptoms.

But AIDS advocacy groups claim that the CDC's proposed definition discriminates against women and intravenous drug users infected with HIV.

Some groups have offered an alternative proposal that would add pulmonary tuberculosis, recurrent bacterial pneumonia and cervical cancer to the current definition.

"It's abundantly clear to me that the CDC's definition is a problem, and that it's resulted in the undercounting of many people who have AIDS," said Theresa McGovern, director of the HIV Law Project in New York, who has spearheaded the drafting of a consensus statement by more than 200 advocacy groups, physicians and legislators.

McGovern and others maintain that the three conditions affect HIV-infected people in disproportionate numbers, and that including them in the definition will alert doctors to test for HIV in patients who have them.

But the CDC has maintained that too few studies have been done to link the conditions to AIDS.

"By adding only T-cell counts and not adding clinical conditions that primarily affect women and drug users, the CDC is going to continue to have skewed surveillance," said Elizabeth B. Cooper, staff counsel of the American Civil Liberties Union AIDS Project in New York.

Another issue in the consensus statement is that the CD4 test should be available to anyone without regard to ability to pay, that the tests be done only by labs that satisfy quality-control conditions and that confidentiality be guaranteed.

Jeffrey Levi, director of government affairs with the AIDS Action Council in Washington, D.C., said that the CD4 tests might compromise confidentiality as laws guaranteeing anonymity of HIV tests do not necessarily cover CD4 tests. He said that anonymous CD4 tests should be available.

The CDC expected to receive further written comments by mid-month. It will then make a final decision on the definition.

More mystery AIDS cases reported; new virus questioned

Axel Springer

AMSTERDAM, JULY 31—In an attempt to bring inferences about a possible new AIDS-like virus closer to scientific reality, the Centers for Disease Control released information it obtained on five more of these puzzling cases, bringing the total to 26.

At press time, experts had slated an emergency meeting at the CDC to discuss the cases. Another meeting by the World Health Organization was tentatively scheduled for September.

The CDC's report coincided with the publication of a report by the New York doctor who kicked off the controversy here at the 8th International Conference on AIDS.

Jeffrey Laurence, M.D., of Cornell University Medical College, reports in tomorrow's The Lancet on four men and one woman with CD4 counts ranging from 552 cells/mm^3 to 76 cells/mm^3 with ELISA and immunoblotting negative for

HIV-1, immunoblotting and competition peptide ELISA negative for HIV-2 and immunoblotting negative for human T-cell lymphotropic virus (HTLV) types I and II.

Peripheral blood mononuclear cell cultures and further ELISAs also were negative for HIV, but particulate reverse transcriptase was detected in the two patients in whom the technique was done. Dr. Laurence said that the nature of the activity and its relation to the clinical syndrome are unclear.

Clinical disorders included Pneumocystis carinii pneumonia, Kaposi's sarcoma, oral candidiasis, chronic cough, wasting and intractable cutaneous abscess.

He said his cases raise the question of the existence of other HIV-like viruses that cause AIDS-like symptoms but are not detectable by current laboratory tests.

Four of the five patients had risk factors for HIV. Two were gay men, one was an elderly Hispanic female who had a blood transfusion in 1978 and one was a male healthcare worker. The remaining white heterosexual man, who developed PCP and died, had no known risk factors, but had received a one-month course of prednisone for inflammatory bowel disease prior to presenting with severe CD4 depletion.

CDC's report of five similar cases includes an elderly man and woman, a male healthcare worker, an older woman with a history of a blood transfusion and a heterosexual middle-aged man with no apparent risk factors.

CD4 counts in the cases were lower than Dr. Laurence described, ranging from 275 cells/mm^3 to 50 cells/mm^3. Clinical disorders included PCP, cryptococcal meningitis, vaginal candidiasis, molluscum contagiosum and Herpes zoster.

"What you're seeing at the moment is just a burst of activity with people reporting patients who have a variety of syndromes," said Jonathan Jacobs, M.D., of New York Hospital-Cornell University Medical College.

He added that while it is possible that a new viral agent is cropping up, other suggestions are just as plausible. One has come from the CDC's James Curran, M.D., who said that with close to 40,000 HIV tests done every year, doctors are looking more closely at the immune system than before, and that these odd cases may previously have been ignored.

French researcher Luc Montagnier, M.D., said that some mutant strains of HIV may not be detectable by traditional tests. He said he had two patients in whom the virus was only detectable in the urine.

"We will take all those suggestions into account and follow up on them but I don't think it will yield HIV, at least not in all of these cases," Dr. Curran said.

It is not the first time that strange cases of immunosuppression in the absence of HIV have turned up. In a January 1991 New England Journal of Medicine article, Drs. Jacobs and Laurence reported on five patients with PCP who had no evidence of HIV infection and no known risk factors. All five were elderly people with normal CD4 counts.

Dr. Jacobs suggested that the five cases may be linked to a case reported by a California doctor who claims to have discovered a new virus.

Sudhir Gupta, M.D., of the University of California, Irvine, reported on a 66-year-old woman who developed PCP and severe immune deficiency with no evidence of HIV and no apparent risk factors. She did have a blood transfusion in 1949 or 1950. Dr. Gupta said he was able to isolate intracisternal viral particles in the woman, as well as in her 38-year-old asymptomatic daughter.

That paper appeared in the Proceedings of the National Academy of Sciences and was rushed to publication because of the media attention surrounding Dr. Laurence. Dr. Gupta has dubbed the condition human intracisternal retrovirus. Of the 26 total cases, 10 or 12 are from the United States, with the remaining coming from Australia, Denmark, England, France, Germany and Spain.

Dr. Gupta's report and the publication of the CDC cases came in response to a plea by Anthony Fauci, M.D., of the National Institutes of Health, that all cases be released immediately rather than await their scheduled publication dates.

Dr. Curran urged physicians to report cases to their state health departments or a special CDC phone line at 404-639-2981. Questions can be directed to the CDC National AIDS Hotline at 800-342-2437.

Resistant tuberculosis spreading in hospitals; HIV-infected patients at 'alarmingly high' risk

By Luba Vikhanski

AUG. 1—Three new reports indicate that multidrug-resistant tuberculosis is spreading through hospitals in the United States, putting patients and healthcare workers at increased risk.

Recent outbreaks involved more and more patients in institutional settings and propagated rapidly, said Samuel Dooley, M.D., of the Centers for Disease Control.

The resistant strains progress quickly, killing up to 89% of infected patients, he said.

Since 1990, CDC has investigated over 200 cases of drug-resistant bacilli, some resistant to at least seven drugs.

Over 80% were in HIV-infected patients, but healthcare workers and other hospitalized patients may also be at risk, according to three studies appearing in the Annals of Internal Medicine. The reports involve outbreaks of multidrug-resistant TB in New York and Florida.

The Florida researchers studied 62 patients with multidrug-resistant TB and 55 patients who had TB caused by single-drug-resistant or susceptible bacilli. Of multidrug-resistant cases, 71% had previous contact with an HIV clinic compared with 27% of single-drug-resistant cases.

"The recent emergence of multiple drug-resistant strains of M. tuberculosis among patients with HIV infection and their close contacts is alarming and has serious public health implications," wrote Margaret A. Fischl, M.D., of the University of Miami School of Medicine.

In a second study, Dr. Fischl and colleagues compared the same groups of patients and found that those with multidrug-resistant disease were sicker than those with single-drug-resistant disease and survived an average of 13 months less.

A third study, conducted at a large unidentified New York City hospital by researchers from the CDC and the New York City Department of Health, found that up to 50% of healthcare workers in wards housing TB patients tested positive for TB, although none had active disease.

In an editorial accompanying the three reports, Dr. Dooley said that at last count, 13 states had at least one patient with multidrug-resistant TB.

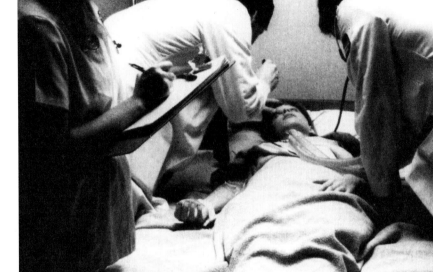

Drug-resistant TB in U.S. hospitals kills up to 89% of infected patients.

"It's not a problem limited to New York and Florida; it potentially exists in other areas and everyone needs to be concerned," Dr. Dooley said.

Michele Pearson, M.D., also of the CDC, said that workers in prisons, hospices, shelters for the homeless and other group settings that may have poor ventilation also are at increased risk of tuberculosis.

The researchers suggest strict implementation of the CDC guidelines on TB prevention, including placing suspected cases of TB in isolated negative-pressure rooms with individual air supply and exhaust systems.

Rooms used to isolate patients with TB or to conduct cough-inducing procedures in the New York hospital were found to have no special ventilation.

Polio pioneer rejects possible AIDS vaccines; says importance of virus-infected cells ignored

SEPT. 15—A preventive or therapeutic vaccine against AIDS will never be successful as long as researchers concentrate purely on eradicating cell-free virus from the body, according to a polio vaccine pioneer.

The importance of virus-infected cells, which are found in high concentrations in the lymph of blood and semen, is being ignored by current vaccine researchers, said Albert Sabin, M.D., developer of the oral polio vaccine.

"The experimental vaccine studies have overlooked the fact that much or most of natural infection with HIV is transmitted not by cell-free virus but rather by cells carrying incompletely expressed virus," Dr. Sabin wrote in the Proceedings of the National Academy of Sciences.

Dr. Sabin said that rectal transmission of HIV introduces

large numbers of virus-infected cells that persistently infect the portal of entry and present one of the biggest challenges to a vaccine.

The researcher pointed to monkey studies in which a vaccine protected against a challenge with cell-free virus, but not virus-infected cells.

Neutralizing antibodies are not effective against intracellular virus and cell-mediated immunity is ineffective against cells in which virus-specific antigens are not expressed on the cell membrane, Dr. Sabin said.

He added that virus-infected cells can transmit viral genome by cell-to-cell contact without the presence of specific HIV receptors.

"In my judgment, the available data provide no basis for

testing any experimental vaccine in human beings or expecting that HIV vaccine could be effective in human beings," he said.

But a government researcher involved in vaccine development said that his feeling is that virus-infected cells are few in number.

Daniel Hoth, M.D., director of the division of AIDS at the National Institute of Allergy and Infectious Diseases, added that despite Dr. Sabin's assertions that virions within cells go undetected, research has shown that they are recognized as foreign invaders by the immune system. "The recipient's immune system has a good chance of knocking them out," he said. "We're just not sure that this 'Trojan horse theory' is right."

Dr. Hoth added that while the medical community respects Dr. Sabin, "We feel that an HIV vaccine is still feasible,

although challenging. His ideas don't form a basis for slowing down research."

Dr. Hoth also took issue with what Dr. Sabin sees as the insurmountable challenge of virus-infected cells clustered at the portal of entry. "This overlooks the fact that the majority of HIV transmission in the world does not occur through anal intercourse."

Dr. Sabin concluded that the main challenge to AIDS researchers is to destroy cells with chromosomally integrated DNA without harming normal cells.

He suggested that this might be done by identifying repressor proteins produced by the integrated cells and using them as targets around which cytotoxic drugs could be developed.

HIV tranfusions risk equals 1 in 60,000 units

Oct. 1—A new report estimates that the risk of contracting HIV from a blood transfusion is about one in 60,000 units of blood, higher than a prior estimate by the American Red Cross of one in 225,000 units.

While the gap between the two estimates may seem large, a Red Cross scientist said that once the differences between the two studies that generated those numbers are taken into account, the risk rates actually are similar.

In the new study, researchers at three hospitals in Baltimore and Houston studied nearly 12,000 surgery patients who required a total of more than 120,000 units of blood. Two patients subsequently became infected with HIV, reported Kenrad Nelson, M.D., in the Annals of Internal Medicine.

When the blood donors for those two patients were contacted, researchers found that in each case one donor had developed HIV after donating blood, although the blood had not tested positive for the virus.

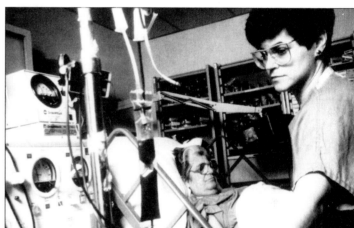

ARC stands by its lower estimate of one in 225,000 units of blood.

The authors suggest that the blood was donated during a "window of time" just after infection when the virus is not yet detectable.

Dr. Nelson, from Johns Hopkins University, said that screening blood and questioning potential donors about risk factors have been successful in excluding most infected people from donating blood.

In addition to interviewing potential donors and giving them educational materials, blood banks also provide a box on the donor's form that can be checked to alert the staff to throw out the blood after the donor leaves the site.

This method reduces the chance that donors will lie about risk factors because no one will know while the donor is at the site whether the blood has been flagged to be discarded, according to Red Cross spokesperson Margaret McCarthy.

But the method is not foolproof. In the new study, one of the donors who initially denied being in a risk group before donating, later admitted to having homosexual contacts.

As a result, more efforts must be made to ensure the safety of the nation's blood supply, Dr. Nelson and colleagues wrote.

Roger Dodd, M.D., who co-authored a Red Cross/Centers

for Disease Control study that resulted in the one-in-225,000 risk estimate, said his study was larger and involved many centers. When those differences are taken into account, the Red Cross risk estimate basically agrees with that of the new study, he said.

Magic scores high for AIDS awareness

Medical Tribune News Service Report

Oct. 3—Basketball legend Earvin "Magic" Johnson's disclosure that he is HIV positive increased AIDS awareness, according to the author of a new study.

A Milwaukee psychologist surveyed Chicago commuters before and after Johnson's announcement last year that he had tested positive for the AIDS virus, and found that the

He pointed out that after Johnson's disclosure that he was infected with HIV, people in Baltimore lined up for blocks and waited for hours to get AIDS testing and counseling.

"The public becomes more aware that testing positive for the AIDS virus does not mean you can't go on living," said Dr. Kalichman. "You can, and with a big raise." Johnson recently signed a $14.6 million one-year contract extension with the Lakers, the largest single-season salary in team sports. [Johnson later changed his mind and retired. —Ed.]

Dr. Kalichman said that one cannot expect people to change their behaviors, including activities such as unprotected sex that put them at high risk for AIDS, unless awareness is first increased.

Earlier this year, a San Francisco researcher found that there was a 20% increase in AIDS testing demand after Johnson's announcement last November.

Calls to the Centers for Disease Control's toll-free AIDS hotline increased from about 200,000 in the month before the announcement to about one million in the following month.

In the new study, 361 men, a little over half of whom were African-American, were asked about their concern about AIDS before and after Johnson's disclosure that he had tested positive for HIV.

More than half of the men said they were very interested in getting more AIDS information after the disclosure, compared with a little over one third before the announcement.

Similarly, more than half said that they talked to friends about AIDS after the announcement, compared with one quarter before.

The disclosure has affected African-Americans the most, Dr. Kalichman said. He rated responses to the question, "Are you more concerned about AIDS since hearing about Magic Johnson?" on a scale of one to four, corresponding to "not at all" to "much more concerned."

The average score of whites was between two and two-and-a-half 10 days after the announcement, compared with a score of almost three-and-a-half for African-Americans.

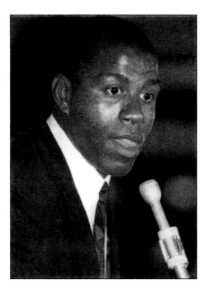

Calls to CDC's toll-free AIDS hotline increased fivefold after basketball star Magic Johnson disclosed that he tested HIV positive.

disclosure sparked significant increases in concern about AIDS. The study appears in the American Journal of Public Health.

"People suddenly felt vulnerable, that this was a disease that could happen to them," said Seth Kalichman, Ph.D., of the Medical College of Wisconsin.

He said that Johnson's decision to play in the Olympics had a similar effect on increasing public awareness, but with one distinct difference.

"This made people think about their attitudes about dealings with people who are HIV positive," Dr. Kalichman said. "If someone with the AIDS virus can participate in a high-contact sport, people will realize you can't catch it from just touching or casual contact," he pointed out.

An AIDS expert at Johns Hopkins in Baltimore agreed. "With such actions from celebrities comes more public awareness and concern," said Thomas Quinn, M.D.

The AIDS orphans: a staggering new challenge

Medical Tribune Report

DEC. 23—By 1995, the nation will need to care for more than 45,000 children and adolescents whose mothers have died of AIDS. And that figure will double by the year 2000 unless the course of the epidemic changes dramatically, predicted epidemiologist David Michaels, Ph.D., of the Sophie Davis School of Biomedical Education/City University of New York.

With their multiple needs for housing, medical and mental health services, the care of these children poses a staggering challenge to America's cities, Dr. Michaels and coinvestigators from the Orphan Project emphasized in their report in The Journal of the American Medical Association. In addition, many of the children will themselves have AIDS.

More than one third of AIDS orphans are in New York City, according to the report. While younger children have the most obvious needs, research by the city's Division of

AIDS Services underlined the problems of adolescents whose parents are dead or dying of AIDS.

Of the seriously ill parents they interviewed, fewer than half had made even a provisional custody plan for their teenage children. And although screening tests of the teens did not point toward diagnoses of depression or anxiety, the bereaved adolescents reported a variety of problems ranging from slipping grades to violent crime.

"As their parents become sicker, adolescents lose not only a loved one but an advocate in dealing with the school, medical and court systems, so problems that should be manageable often get out of control," said Jan Hudis, M.P.H., the city planner who conducted the study. "Professionals working with children and adolescents must recognize that they are often dealing with grieving, traumatized young people who may not know their mother's diagnosis or feel at liberty to disclose it."

COMMENTARY

New AIDS-like illness remains elusive

By Jeffrey Laurence, M.D.

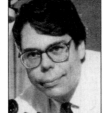

IN JULY 1992, I WAS ONE OF several researchers at the International Conference on AIDS in Amsterdam who presented evidence of an AIDS-like illness in patients who had no evidence of HIV infection.

Many of these patients had typical AIDS symptoms, and all had low CD4 counts. They were negative for HIV-1 and HIV-2 by culture and polymerase chain reaction.

Almost immediately, controversy about the illness began: Was a new etiology for AIDS emerging? Requests for open discussion from government officials, AIDS patients and other researchers with similar findings led to meetings in August at Centers for Disease Control and Prevention headquarters in Atlanta and in September at World Health Organization headquarters in Geneva.

The WHO meeting brought together about two dozen AIDS researchers and representatives from the United States, Russia, India, Africa, Australia and several other countries. At that time it was determined that there were 73 clinical instances of severe immune suppression but no evidence of HIV. Forty-seven cases were from the United States, representing 20 different states. The rest were reported from other countries in attendance at the meeting. There were some surprises: The representative from Russia reported six cases and those from Australia reported eight cases.

The African countries presented a real dilemma. One of their representatives said they did not actually know if they had any cases like ours because they almost never do CD4 counts. If they have a patient who tests negative for HIV but there is a clinical history representative of high-risk behavior, they may assume that they did the test wrong and that they are dealing with an AIDS case.

WHO decided to name the syndrome severe unexplained HIV negative immune suppression, or SUHIS. The CDC has said it will continue to classify its cases as idiopathic CD4-positive T-lymphopenia, or ICL.

WHO has not yet decided whether to use the ICL definition and is working on its own definition. It will include cases where there are progressive falls in CD4 counts and the presence of certain opportunistic infections. While we know that cryptococcal meningitis and pulmonary tuberculosis are associated with AIDS, we also must recognize that these infections can suppress T-cell counts in people without AIDS as well. So it may be best when examining SUHIS cases to concentrate on those instances where there are progressive falls in CD4 counts and presence of such diseases as Pneumocystis carinii pneumonia and Candida albicans.

The WHO conclusion also stated that quite frankly, we don't know that much about CD4 counts. I think this is very important to remember. We have only been looking at this aspect of the immune system in depth for just over a decade, and there is a lot we still have to learn. We really don't have the studies we need on cell counts in "normal" people and certain disease states to be able to judge how the immune system responds to drugs or various infections.

The other important factor here concerns the safety of the blood supply. I agree with WHO officials that it is just not practical to tell every country that it should establish surveillance programs for CD4 cells. But, more important, we believe that there is no reason to fear for the safety of the blood supply, given what we know. Rejecting blood on the basis of low CD4 counts alone does not make sense at this time, and it would waste precious resources.

Last, we believe that there may still be unreported cases of this syndrome, but it is going to take a lot of follow-up, exchange of materials and opening of lines of communication before the syndrome is really understood. Many of us who have seen these cases have our own ideas about what the etiology may be, but we all agree with the conclusions drawn up by WHO. What we have now is a couple of different terms for something that may be all the same thing, may be several different things or may be nothing new at all.

Dr. Laurence is associate professor of medicine and director of the AIDS Virus Research Lab at New York Hospital-Cornell University Medical Center, New York.

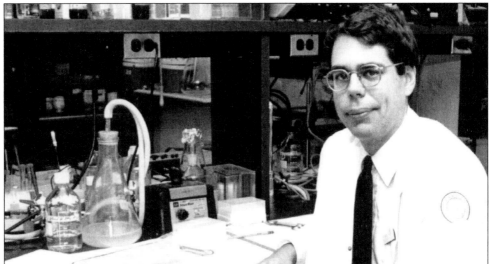

Dr. Laurence's findings led to talk that a new etiology of AIDS was emerging.

Notes

Notes

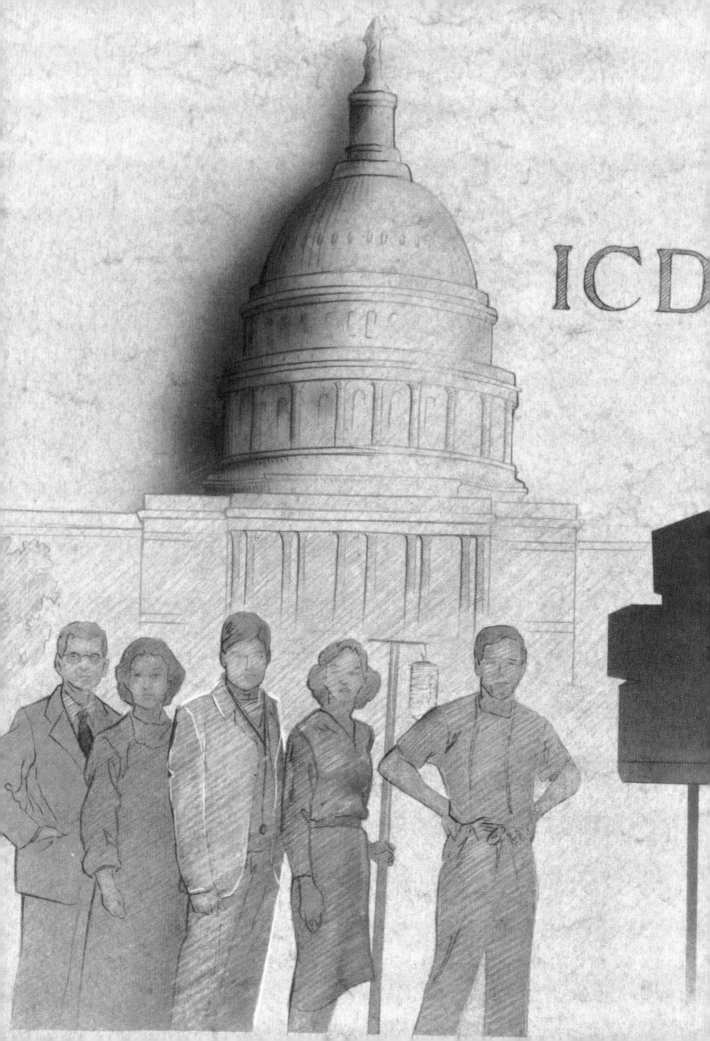

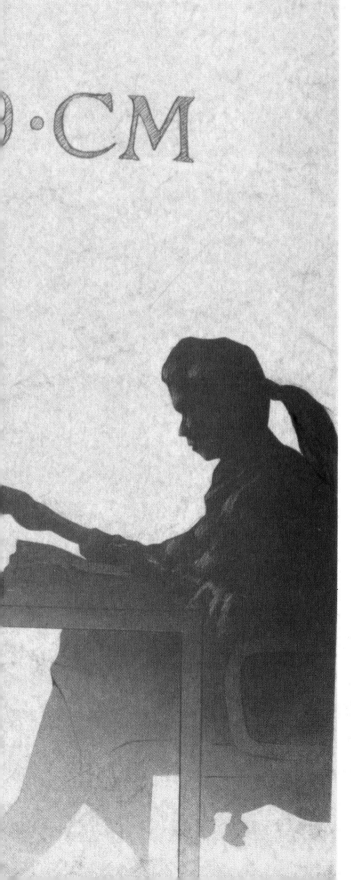

Overview 308
Is healthcare reform a
Gordian knot?

Month-at-a-glance 310

Reported at the Time 322
Dow safety memos on breast
implants…Kevorkian legal roller
coaster…drug-resistant TB…data-
bank leaks and Big
Brotherism…play-or-pay
insurance…rules to track medical
devices…MDs setting own
fees…candidates' pleas for
physician votes…dodging
malpractice with unneeded
tests…generalists protest 2nd-class
Medicare raise…Supreme Court
rulings on abortion…Oregon health
plan…speedier drug
approvals…Medical Tribune
election poll…HCFA's theater
of the absurd

Commentary 335
Three battles to watch in the 1990s
By David M. Eddy, M.D., Ph.D.

Is healthcare reform a Gordian knot?

Tempers flare and suggestions abound on all sides, millions are uninsured, doctors can't afford to treat, patients can't afford treatment...

Lawmakers, physicians, healthcare industry leaders, Presidential candidates and the public grappled all year long with two of the most pressing issues concerning healthcare: spiraling costs and affordable health insurance for all Americans.

Three fourths of all Americans believe that the cost of medical care, insurance and drugs is the main problem facing the U.S. healthcare system, according to a Gallup Organization survey released in June.

Americans are so anxious to obtain adequate health insurance coverage that three fifths of them would be willing to pay $50 extra each month for national health insurance, and two thirds would pay another $50 monthly for a separate long-term-care plan that covered everyone, according to another survey.

Healthcare reform also occupied both Presidential candidates during their fierce 1992 campaign. The cornerstone of President Bush's conservative, free-market plan was a voucher, or credit, that would allow low-income families to buy $3,750 worth of health insurance and higher-income families to take a tax deduction for the same amount. States would be required to develop a health insurance package.

Governor Bill Clinton, who became the President-elect, called for every employer to provide or help subsidize health insurance for every worker. People who do not work would be able to buy health insurance through large, public purchasing co-ops. He also proposed establishing a National Health Board that would institute budget targets to control healthcare costs, and would require insurance companies to insure everyone.

Major medical organizations also unveiled their healthcare reform platforms. Spokespersons for the American Society of Internal Medicine outlined a system that would provide more

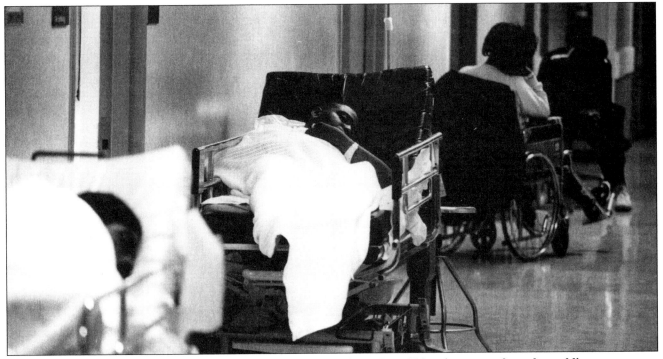

Everyone would be covered under Clinton's plan: those who don't work could buy insurance through a public co-op.

access to care, provided, as much as possible, through employer-based private insurance. The American College of Physicians propounded a stronger role for goverment, with a major focus on the public sector, that would set caps on expenditures.

Having generalists, and not specialists, provide most medical care would be one way to reduce medical expenditures, suggested researchers involved in the Medical Outcomes Study. Family physicians order fewer tests and drugs, charge less for them and hospitalize patients less frequently, they said. They also charge less for their services than do specialists.

Primary-care doctors would agree with that assessment, but with a tinge of bitterness. Medicare allowed them an inflation increase of 0.8%, while increasing surgeons' fees 3.1%. Physicians complained they were being forced to drop their Medicare patients, or were being driven out of practice altogether.

"Downcoding" was another point of contention between policy makers and physicians this year. Reimbursement claims for routine preventive care, diagnoses and decisions that required extensive histories were being downcoded to lower reimbursement levels. The Health Care Financing Administration conceded that more generalists should participate in preparing documentation standards.

In a public health issue that involves pain and dignity as well as costs, Americans are asking for more of a say in how they are treated when they're terminally ill. Most Americans now believe that euthanasia for terminally ill patients should be legalized, according to a study conducted by the Harvard School of Public Health. But while a clear majority believe that doctors should assist patients in irreversible comas, only 52% said they believe they would end their lives if they were terminally ill and in pain, but awake and aware.

While the public seemed clear about their personal views

on the ethics of euthanasia, they were not quite ready to officially sanction physician-assisted suicide. Voters in California—like those in Washington State the year before—rejected a ballot initiative that would have legalized euthanasia and physician-assisted suicide.

Both abetting and sometimes thwarting the cause, according to his detractors, is "suicide doctor" Jack Kevorkian, M.D. Dr. Kevorkian spent stretches of 1992 being arrested and indicted for murder for his participation in the suicides of two chronically ill women. The charges were later dropped.

Although Dr. Kevorkian has brought the issue of physician-assisted suicide into the living rooms of the American people, his participation in the suicides of people who are not terminally ill may be hurting his cause rather than helping it, according to some policy experts.

Political action by persons with AIDS and other life-threatening diseases has resulted in a fundamental change in how drugs are approved. Drug manufacturers will now have the opportunity to speed the Food and Drug Administration approval of their products, but they will have to pay for the privilege.

So 1992 was the year that the healthcare system took center stage in both a Presidential campaign and the consciousness of U.S. citizens. Patients and their families continue to grapple with the sometimes heartbreaking issue of the right to die, with doctors often caught between the suffering of their patients and the legal system. Public policy experts will continue to deal with the effects of an AIDS epidemic that continues to grow, while policymakers have managed to create one solution that hopefully will speed new and powerful drugs to the patients who need them.

Jan. 6

The Food and Drug Administration issued a 45-day voluntary moratorium on the use of silicone-gel breast implants pending a review of information about their safety. The action drew fire both from critics of silicone-gel breast implants, who said they should be banned, and from medical groups that support continued use of the implants.

Jan. 7

A Michigan grand jury heard prosecutors argue that Jack Kevorkian, M.D., should be charged with murder for his role in the October deaths of two women. Neither woman was terminally ill: One had multiple sclerosis, and the other suffered from a painful pelvic disease. Following Dr. Kevorkian's instructions, one woman inhaled carbon monoxide through a mask. The other self-administered a lethal injection from a second-generation suicide machine invented by Dr. Kevorkian after he was barred from using an earlier model by a Michigan court. In November, Dr. Kevorkian's medical license was suspended by the Michigan Board of Medicine.

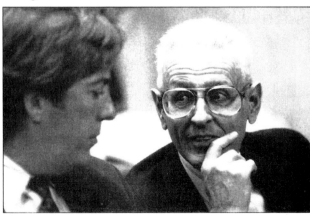

Dr. Jack Kevorkian's (right) second-generation suicide machine landed him in a Michigan courtroom once again.

Jan. 8

As 24,972 Americans waited to receive transplants, a new study revealed that only 37% to 59% of potential donors actually give their organs. Mississippi and South Carolina were among the states with the worst organ donation records in 1989, while Arizona, Iowa, Maine, New Mexico and Nebraska were among the best, according to a report in The Journal of the American Medical Association. Improved procurement systems and public education could boost donations 80%, claimed researchers from the Battell-Seattle Research Center.

• • •

Heroin addicts at half of U.S. drug treatment programs lost their chance at recovery when clinics offered only half the effective dose of methadone or cut off treatment altogether before withdrawal was complete. A 172-center study by the National Institute on Drug Abuse showed that clinics balked at providing ongoing counseling and $7 per day for an adequate dose of methadone. Heroin addiction should be approached more like other chronic illnesses with the potential for relapse if undertreated, addiction experts commented in The Journal of the American Medical Association.

Jan. 13

Officials at Dow Corning Corp. denied that the manufacturer had ignored warnings from its own scientists that silicone breast implants leaked and were of uncertain safety. Company executives claimed to possess 40 years' worth of studies demonstrating that silicone implants are safe and effective, but critics charged that none of the studies dealt with inserting silicone or implants in or under breast tissue.

Jan. 14

Citizens voiced their frustration with the U.S. healthcare system at 285 town meetings across the country. Sponsored by House Democrats, the meetings attracted large numbers of physicians, small business owners and relatives of disabled or chronically ill patients. Some asked for reforms designed to improve access and lower healthcare costs. Others called for a complete overhaul, replacing the U.S. system with single-payer national healthcare modeled on Canada's system.

Jan. 15

Labeling firearms "a national epidemic" causing the deaths of more than 4,000 young Americans every year, the American Academy of Pediatrics called for a ban on handguns. The group recommended the regulation of handgun ammunition, a reduction in the number of privately owned handguns and restrictions on handgun ownership.

Jan. 16

The U.S. Consul General reported that large numbers of Filipino physicians were seeking recertification as nurses in order to get employment visas to work in the United States. Many physicians earn less than $200/month in the Philippines. Filipinos seeking employment in the United States must pass an official nursing examination before being recruited, then pass the board exam of the state in which they will be working.

Jan. 21

Sen. Howard Metzenbaum (D-Ohio) blasted pharma-ceutical manufacturers for using orphan drug laws to block competition and generate windfall profits. Noting that some drugs sell for "an absurdly high" $350,000 per patient per year, he introduced legislation to terminate a company's seven-year orphan-drug monopoly once a drug generates $200 million in sales.

Jan. 22

The Senate Labor and Human Resources Committee told employers to get ready to "play or pay" for their workers' health insurance. If the proposal is adopted by the full Senate and House, most employers would have to provide insurance or pay a payroll tax of 7.5%. The Bush administration warned that most employers would opt for the payroll tax, driving more than 52 million Americans into public insurance.

Jan. 24

The Drug Policy Foundation criticized the federal war on drugs as having its priorities backwards. Instead of spending 70% of its drug war funds on enforcement and 30% on addiction treatment, the government was advised to halt new prison construction and divert those funds into needle-exchange programs and drug treatment. The drug policy group also suggested that seriously ill individuals, such as people with AIDS and cancer, be allowed to use marijuana to alleviate their symptoms.

Jan. 29

The Bush administration announced its 1993 budget proposals. Within an overall 8% increase for Health and Human Services, spending would increase 110% for tuberculosis control, 40% for breast and cervical cancer and 18% for immunizations over 1992 levels.

Footing the bill: Senior citizens earning more than $100,000, who would be required to contribute an additional $60 per month for Medicare coverage.

FEBRUARY

Feb. 3

Fifty former counterintelligence agents joined the FBI's efforts to combat healthcare fraud. The FBI claimed that healthcare fraud is a $50-billion-a-year nationwide problem. The most common scenarios include false billing and kickbacks from equipment suppliers to physicians.

Feb. 5

Jack Kevorkian, M.D., was arrested and indicted for murder for his participation in the suicides of two chronically ill women. Some advocacy groups endorsed the arrest and charged that the actions of the Michigan pathologist thwart the right-to-die movement in its efforts to have doctor-assisted suicide legalized.

• • •

The Food and Drug Administration scrapped plans to issue guidelines that would prevent the pharmaceutical industry from promoting their products to physicians at scientific and educational conferences. The decision came in the face of strong opposition both from the industry, which threatened to stop sponsoring such meetings, and physicians, who said they could make their own decisions about the value of the information presented.

• • •

Low pay, poor working conditions and lack of respect kept physicians away from health clinics for the homeless, leaving the facilities understaffed and able to serve only a fraction of those in need of healthcare, concluded University of California at Los Angeles researchers. Of 157 homeless health clinics receiving federal funds from the McKinney Homeless Assistance Act, 31% had no physicians who worked more than five hours a week, and 10% had no staff doctor at all, the researchers reported in The Journal of the American Medical Association.

Feb. 6

President Bush announced plans to curb Medicare and Medicaid costs. Since the advent of Medicare under the Johnson administration, all five presidents have attempted to halt the growth in spending by trying unsuccessfully to freeze fees, limit the number of in-hospital days, review bills, cajole doctors into accepting what Medicare was willing to pay and this year instituting the resource-based relative value scale.

• • •

A federal appeals court ordered New York State to fill a Medicare gap by paying more to doctors and hospitals for treating impoverished elderly patients who are eligible for both Medicare and Medicaid. Previously, Medicaid had refused to pay the 20% of charges not covered by Medicare for poor elderly patients. The ruling could affect 29 other states with similar payment rules, according to welfare officials.

Feb. 11

To help ease the shortage of donor organs, U.S. Surgeon General Antonia Novello, M.D., urged healthcare workers to gain a better understanding of differing beliefs regarding death and burial. Language and cultural barriers contribute to the failure of many Hispanics and African-Americans to agree to donate a relative's organs when approached by a healthcare worker, she told a meeting of the federal Division of Organ Transplantation.

Feb. 18

Leaking and ruptured silicone-gel breast implants caused joint swelling, fatigue and other signs and symptoms of immune system disorders in some women, physicians told a Food and Drug Administration advisory panel. At the meeting, researchers said more women may have suffered ruptures in their implants than previously thought. New estimates based on several studies ranged from 3% to 6.6%.

Feb. 20

A Food and Drug Administration advisory panel unanimously recommended that breast-cancer patients be permitted to get silicone-gel breast implants, but that only a limited number of participants in tightly controlled clinical trials receive them for cosmetic purposes. The FDA General and Plastic Surgery Devices Advisory Committee concluded that the studies presented did not prove a link

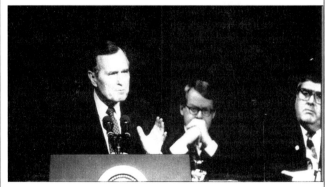

President George Bush announced plans to curb Medicare costs.

between the devices and autoimmune diseases, but that further trials are needed to determine safety.

Feb. 21

A New York City task force called for the quarantine of some people with tuberculosis. In response, experts told Medical Tribune that they sometimes have no other choice if they are to protect the public. The task force fell short of recommending that sanitariums be reopened, but advised quarantining patients in shelters, psychiatric hospitals or special wards in AIDS nursing homes or drug rehabilitation centers.

Feb. 24

Development of an AIDS vaccine could be delayed two to three years because of cuts of more than 20% in the proposed budget of the National Institutes of Health, the assistant director of AIDS research at the NIH warned. The Bush administration submitted to Congress a $873-million request for NIH-supported AIDS research in 1993; the NIH had requested $1.19 billion.

Feb. 27

Critics of the National Practitioner Data Bank warned physicians that Big Brother is watching over their shoulders, and that information on malpractice settlements and physician reviews could be misinterpreted or even made available to the public. An attorney for the American Academy of Family Physicians told Medical Tribune she wants small malpractice settlements excluded from the data bank because they often represent no admission of wrongdoing. Meanwhile, the Public Citizen Health Research Group is lobbying to give the public access to data bank information, while the American Medical Association wants the bank abolished altogether.

Feb. 28

The Health Care Financing Administration released the final version of its CLIA rules, giving physicians with office laboratories three to six months to comply with new regulations governing lab registration and fees, unannounced inspections, proficiency testing and laboratory personnel.

MARCH

March 5

A respiratory infection expert warned that a shortage of antituberculosis drugs poses a life-threatening situation for the rising number of patients with multidrug-resistant TB. Although several drugs were affected, the most prolonged shortages involved two mainstays of TB treatment, streptomycin and aminosalicylate sodium, which were only available from sources outside the United States, a National Jewish Center for Immunology and Respiratory Medicine team reported in The New England Journal of Medicine. Federal agencies met with drug manufacturers to coordinate production in order to confront the problem.

• • •

A government program boosted flu vaccination levels among the elderly from 40% to 60%, Centers for Disease Control epidemiologists announced. The program offered flu vaccine in shopping malls, public clinics and grocery stores, and improved distribution of vaccines from state health departments to private physicians.

• • •

The Department of Health and Human Services released new guidelines recommending more aggressive pain treatment in both adults and children. Saying postoperative patients often do not receive enough pain medication, the federal agency recommended use of opioids continuously for the first 24 hours after surgery.

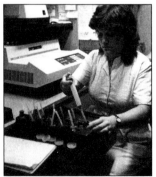

Office-based labs will spend $600 each to meet new federal rules.

March 12

Medical societies told Medical Tribune that the majority of physicians' office laboratories would be able to continue operating after the final version of new rules for clinical labs takes effect September 1. The new federal regulations will cost each lab an estimated $600 per year for the annual user fee, proficiency testing and other paperwork, they estimated.

March 19

Dow Corning, the predominant manufacturer of silicone-gel breast implants, announced that it would no longer make the implants in the United States or abroad. The company also announced a $10-million research fund to be used to study the safety of the implants and a program granting up to $1,200 each to women who decide with their physicians that Dow Corning implants should be removed. The company ceased distribution of its breast implants in January following the Food and Drug Administration's request for a voluntary moratorium.

• • •

Democratic lawmakers told a House subcommittee that the Food and Drug Administration could endanger public health by implementing a plan to streamline the drug approval process. Rep. Ted Weiss (D-N.Y.) questioned whether the Bush administration bowed to industry demands in crafting the reform plan. The reforms would speed the approval time for drugs to treat currently incurable diseases by using drug-evaluation data that some experts consider unreliable.

March 21

An advisory panel to the Food and Drug Administration voted unanimously against approving a new carbon fiber device for repairing anterior cruciate ligaments in the knee. Data from animal and clinical trials submitted by the manufacturer, Plastasil, were insufficient to demonstrate its safety or efficacy, the panel concluded.

March 25

Healthcare in the United States would cost less and be more efficient if most of the care were given by generalists instead of specialists, announced investigators from the Medical Outcomes Study. Family physicians order fewer tests and drugs and hospitalize fewer patients than do cardiologists and endocrin-

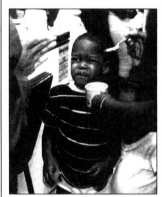

Newark tot swallows TB drug as experts warn of shortage.

ologists, while specialists charged more for their services, the researchers reported in The Journal of the American Medical Association.

March 26

Emergency medical service professionals told Medical Tribune that the Food and Drug Administration's scrutiny of medical devices marketed before 1976 may alter the care they provide. Scientific study is welcome, said the president of the National Association of Emergency Medical Technicians, but not at the expense of potentially life-saving methods. The remarks came as the FDA, in the aftermath of the silicone-gel breast implant controversy, announced plans to look more closely at more

than 100 devices marketed, or "substantially equivalent" to devices marketed before 1976.

• • •

The Health Care Financing Administration told Medical Tribune it is cracking down on physicians who charge patients more than the maximum balance billing limit after several reports of overcharges. The agency has asked Medicare carriers to be more vigilant in identifying potential violations and to assist beneficiaries who think their physicians may have overcharged. This year, physicians can bill up to 120% of Medicare's approved charge; next year and thereafter they will be limited to 115%.

• • •

Two years after decrying patchwork measures to improve access to care, the American College of Physicians told Medical Tribune that it is proposing a health plan that would require employers to pay at least half the cost of health insurance for their workers or pay a combined 6% payroll/3% corporate income tax. Everyone covered by Medicaid or Medicare, plus those between the ages of 60 and 65, would also be covered under the "play or pay" plan.

March 27

Responding to criticism that it had failed to properly oversee the use of medical devices such as heart valves and breast implants, the Food and Drug Administration proposed rules requiring device manufacturers to track patients using their products. The regulations will force companies to maintain data on patients who received dangerous or faulty devices so they can be quickly identified, said the FDA commissioner.

The proposed regulation was limited to permanent implants and devices that sustain life—35 types of devices from more than 370 manufacturers.

April 8

The American Society of Internal Medicine unveiled a new health reform plan allowing physicians to set their own fees using the Resource-Based Relative Value Scale. Physicians would set their own individual conversion factors each year to determine their maximum allowable charges for every service, and insurers would set factors indicating how much they are willing to pay. By looking at the set conversion factors, patients could make an informed choice about their doctor's charges, said the ASIM.

April 9

Vice President Dan Quayle said that the Food and Drug Administration will enact four measures to speed approvals of drugs for life-threatening illnesses. The initiatives include allowing drugs to be approved based on lab tests rather than clinical trials to reduce the time to market by one to three years; a "parallel track" policy that would make experimental drugs available to patients with life-threatening diseases who are unable to participate in trials; accepting safety data from animal trials; and use of outside experts to review certain drugs.

April 10

The American Academy of Family Physicians proposed a new healthcare plan that would provide government incentives to train more primary-care physicians as a way of controlling healthcare costs. The plan calls for up to half of all new U.S. physicians to be generalists; currently, the figure is less than one third. Other provisions of the plan include limiting federal funding to schools that graduate too few primary-care doctors and increasing loans to primary-care residents.

April 13

U.S. Surgeon General Antonia Novello, M.D., renewed her recommendation that the alcohol industry voluntarily eliminate advertising that appeals primarily to youth. Dr. Novello released a report linking teenage drinking to crime.

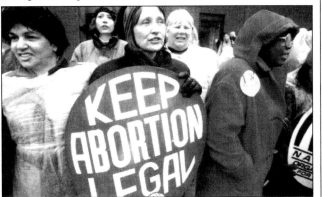

Pro-choicers guarded Buffalo clinics during Operation Rescue.

April 14

The World Health Organization announced that one in every four deaths worldwide in 1991 was due to heart disease. In industrial countries, heart disease causes about half of all deaths annually, while in developing nations it accounts for 16% of the deaths each year, the WHO reported.

April 16

The Association of American Medical Colleges reported that the number of medical school applicants increased for the fourth straight year. Although final figures have not yet been compiled, the association said applications are running about 12.5% ahead of where they were a year ago; last year, they were up about 13.9% over the previous year. The statistics also show continued increases in the number of female and minority applicants.

• • •

The Food and Drug Administration announced it would allow the use of silicone-gel breast implants for all women who want them after breast-cancer surgery but would sharply restrict their use in women seeking breast enlargement.

The decision opened the door for immediate surgery on approximately 9,000 women who had been scheduled for reconstruction when the FDA called a moratorium in January.

April 20

The Coalition on Donations, a group of 50 organizations, launched a national campaign to educate the public about a growing shortage of donor organs.

• • •

Russian physicians, nurses and other healthcare workers went on strike to demand higher wages and better healthcare funding. The physicians said their salaries, averaging about $10 a month, were "ridiculously" low. They also protested against shortages of supplies, including drugs, disposable needles and dialysis machines.

More than half of the healthcare workers, however, stayed away from the strike.

April 23

Presidential candidates George Bush and Bill Clinton accepted an offer from Medical Tribune to present their blueprints for healthcare reform. President Bush presented a comprehensive healthcare proposal that he said builds on the strengths of our current system. Bush suggested health-insurance tax credits and targeted medical malpractice for reform.

Under Clinton's plan, all Americans would be offered a core benefits package, and employers and employees would either purchase private insurance or buy into a public program.

April 29

Rep. John Dingell (D-Mich.) told a hearing of the House Energy and Commerce subcommittee that the Bush administration bungled implementation of new clinical laboratory regulations. Dingell accused the Department of Health and Human Services of delaying the CLIA regulations and of drafting them without consulting experts outside the department. He also added that the final regulations are insufficient to protect the public's health.

April 30

Food and Drug Administration Commissioner David Kessler, M.D., told a House committee that health insurers should not raise rates or cancel coverage for women with silicone-gel breast implants.

Dr. Kessler told a Select Committee on Aging subcommittee that insurers should also continue to pay for reconstructive surgery for breast-cancer patients who want implants following mastectomy.

• • •

Abortion-performing physicians who were targeted by Operation Rescue for a tense two weeks in Buffalo said they were tolerant of the demonstrators, and even those who were picketed said they felt no animosity. A spokesperson for the American Medical Association was more harsh, saying that physicians should not be harassed for performing services they feel are necessary to their patients.

May 1

The Health Care Financing Administration released a report intended to reduce administrative hassles by improving Medicare-physician relations and the Peer Review Organization process. But front-line physicians who are rapidly abandoning the treatment of Medicare patients because of escalating aggravation and diminishing reimbursement immediately derided the report to Medical Tribune. The nonbinding report calls for standardized claim forms, toll-free phone

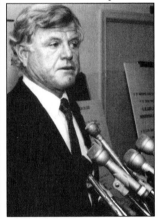

Senator Kennedy: reform urgently needed to help the 200,000 homeless mentally ill.

lines for physicians to reach carriers and better ways to resolve claims disputes.

May 5

Sen. Edward Kennedy (D-Mass.) declared that healthcare reform is urgently needed to help the estimated 200,000 homeless Americans with serious mental illness. At a meeting of the American Psychiatric Association in Washington, Kennedy said Congress was expected to pass a bill sponsored by himself and Sen. Orrin Hatch (R-Utah) to reorganize several federal agencies and create a Center for Mental Health Services.

May 6

The Food and Drug Administration disclosed that it recalled 93 units of blood products from 10 states last November because the donors were not properly screened for HIV infection. The American Red Cross and federal health officials told Medical Tribune that the products were found to be safe and had posed no danger to the public. The red blood cells, platelets and fresh frozen plasma were HIV-negative, but the 47 donors all had tested false-positive for the virus and should have been retested before their donations were accepted, the FDA said.

May 11

The White House announced a public education program designed to cut infant mortality in half by helping pregnant women get prenatal care in the 15 communities with the highest infant death rates.

May 12

Major healthcare reforms are not likely to be enacted by Congress this year or even until the need for change reaches crisis proportions, policy makers said at a forum arranged by the American Medical Association. By 1996, the year he predicted the nation's health system will collapse, annual health expenditures could reach $1.4 trillion, said the editor of The Journal of the American Medical Association. Sen. Bob Kerrey (D-Neb.) told participants that a growing number of Americans cannot afford health insurance for their children or parents.

• • •

Sen. Pete Domenici (R-N.M.) introduced a bill that would guarantee that people with severe psychiatric illnesses get the same health benefits as those with physical illnesses. The bill would be amended to any national health plan passed by Congress, a Yale University physician told Medical Tribune.

May 13

Health insurance plans that do not cover people with certain illnesses or jobs are unethical and are creating a new kind of poverty—medical poverty, reported an expert from the University of Medicine and Dentistry of New Jersey. In The Journal of the American Medical Association, the physician criticized so-called risk-rated plans that he said erode the basic function of insurance—spreading infrequent large losses over a large population.

May 14

A survey of 439 Missouri physicians, conducted by researchers at the University of Missouri-Columbia, found that the wishes of seriously ill patients who have signed a living will may not be heeded if family members request otherwise.

Asked whether they would order a feeding tube for an 89-year-old stroke victim who had signed a living will, half initially said they would not. But two thirds of those doctors said they would change their minds if the family wanted the feeding tube used.

The survey, published in the Journal of the American Geriatrics Society, also found that 42% of physicians who had initially favored using a feeding tube against the living will's dictates said they would change their minds if the family opposed it.

May 15

Three fifths of Americans said they would be willing to pay $50 extra each month for national health insurance, and two thirds would shell out another $50 monthly for a separate long-term care plan that covered everyone. The majority of the 1,004 people surveyed by the Mildred and Claude Pepper Foundation also endorsed raising taxes on liquor and cigarettes but rejected raising taxes on gasoline or on Social Security benefits.

May 18

Eighty-four percent of physicians acknowledged that they order unnecessary tests in order to dodge the threat of malpractice suits, an American Medical Association-Gallup telephone survey found. This percentage is unprecedented, said AMA Executive Vice President James Todd, M.D. He estimated that the extra tests add $20 billion to the annual cost of U.S. healthcare and demonstrate the destructive economic effect that the fear of malpractice suits has on these costs. Replacing the current malpractice system with a no-fault system was favored by more than half of the thousand doctors surveyed.

May 20

A new survey of 1,004 adults found that 63% think physicians should be permitted to end the life of a terminally ill patient if the patient or family makes such a request.

The Harvard survey, published in The Journal of the American Medical Association, also revealed that about 75% of respondents would want life support withdrawn if they were in an irreversible coma, but only 52% would end their lives if they were in a great deal of pain but awake and aware.

May 21

Smoking is on the decline in the United States, announced the Centers for Disease Control. Forty-six million adults, or 25% of the population, smoked in 1990, compared with 29% in 1987, the CDC reported.

May 27

While Medicare plans an inflation increase of only 0.3% next year for primary-care services, surgical fees will increase by 2.6%, announced Health and Human Services Secretary Louis Sullivan, M.D. Primary-care organizations, such as the American Society of Internal Medicine, were angered by the disparity in the increases. They maintained that separate volume standards for primary care and surgery undermined the intent of payment reform.

June 2

A Gallup Organization survey found that nearly three fourths of Americans believe the cost of medical care, insurance or drugs is the main problem facing the U.S. healthcare system. The survey, conducted each year for the American Medical Association, showed that the number of people naming cost as the main problem increased about 8% from last year. About 22% of the 1,514 adults surveyed said they had delayed medical treatment due to cost, and 65% said they would not be able to pay for long-term care.

June 3

An annual survey on preventive health behavior found that more Americans than ever are lowering their intake of fat and cholesterol but still can't control their weight. The 1992 Prevention Index score was 66.5 out of a possible 100, meaning the average American practices about two thirds of the 21 preventive health behaviors tracked. Smoking, Pap smears, self-breast examinations and eating habits were among the topics surveyed, said Secretary of Health and Human Services Louis Sullivan, M.D., in announcing the results.

• • •

The Food and Drug Administration denied a petition asking that the labeling for the oft-prescribed antidepressant fluoxetine (Prozac, Dista) include information about the reputed link between the drug and suicidal tendencies. The Health Research Group, a branch of Ralph Nader's consumer advocate group Public Citizen, petitioned the FDA in 1991 for the warning requirement. The petition denial followed an FDA advisory panel decision that no evidence existed to conclude that fluoxetine or other antidepressants cause violent behavior.

• • •

World Health Organization representatives warned leaders gathered at the Earth Summit in Rio de Janeiro that a deteriorating environment could have disastrous effects on world health, including new epidemics of tropical disease.

Global warming could cause the resurgence of malaria in areas of the world now considered free of the disease, according to a WHO report.

About 30 yet-to-be-discovered drugs would probably be irretrievably lost if, as expected, 62,000 of the current 250,000 known plant species become extinct through habitat destruction by the year 2050, WHO predicted.

June 4

Olympic athletes and spectators planning to attend the Summer Games in Barcelona were advised to consider being vaccinated against a potentially fatal strain of pneumonia that is resistant to penicillin and other standard drugs.

Spain has one of the highest rates of multidrug-resistant Streptococcus pneumoniae, wrote doctors at Boston City Hospital in a letter to the editor in The New England Journal of Medicine. In 1989, 44% of S. pneumoniae was penicillin resistant.

An epidemic could occur if the bacteria were to spread among crowds at the Olympics, they warned, and visitors who contracted the bacteria could bring it home with them.

June 5

The Department of Health and Human Services announced a new national program encouraging doctors and patients to practice preventive care. As part of the program, a clinician's handbook will be distributed through hospitals and medical organizations giving physicians the latest information about a range of preventive services. Physicians will also receive a flow sheet to track what preventive services the patient has had, colored chart stickers to alert physicians to patients who need preventive services and postcards for notifying them. Patients will get booklets to keep track of their health histories and the preventive services they need.

June 10

The American Medical Association took a stand on the issue of violence by mounting a campaign against handguns. In addition, the editor of the association's journal and former U.S. Surgeon General C. Everett Koop drew up a proposal to require all gun owners to be licensed.

A survey by Harvard researchers of 605 gun owners, which appeared in The Journal of the American Medical Association, revealed that guns are present in 46% of households and that more than half of owners keep their guns loaded.

June 15

Charter Suburban Hospital in Paramount, Calif., was ordered to pay more than $45,000 in lawyer's fees to a thoracic surgeon after a judge ruled that the hospital unfairly restricted his medical staff privileges. The hospital appealed the ruling. The case was the first to fall under a recently enacted statute that allows California doctors who have been wrongly punished by peer-review proceedings to reclaim the cost of their appeal, including lawyer's fees.

June 23

The American Medical Association changed its stance on prescription-drug advertising to consumers. At the group's annual meeting, the AMA said it approved of such ads if they included clear health-education or disease-prevention messages and were in patients' best interests.

June 25

American Medical Association officials at the group's annual meeting applauded the recent U.S. Supreme Court ruling allowing those who suffer health effects from smoking to sue tobacco companies for allegedly misrepresenting the dangers of smoking. Antismoking rhetoric dominated a number of sessions and protests at the meeting in Chicago. U.S. Surgeon General Antonia Novello, M.D., led an antismoking rally that focused on the purported negative impact of the cartoon character Joe Camel, prominent in Camel cigarette advertising. The AMA House of Delegates voted to call on R.J. Reynolds and other tobacco companies to refrain from using advertising that targets children.

June 29

The U.S. Supreme Court upheld most of a Pennsylvania law restricting abortion. In its 5-4 ruling on the Pennsylvania abortion statute, the Supreme Court allowed restrictions that do not impose an "undue

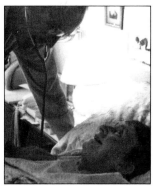

Most Americans say cost of health care is a major problem.

burden" on a woman's right to choose an abortion. The court struck down a provision that required married women to notify their husbands when seeking abortions. But it upheld other provisions, including a 24-hour waiting period, informed-consent requirements and detailed record keeping on abortions.

JULY

July 1

A House Ways and Means subcommittee approved a bill aimed at controlling spiraling healthcare costs and extending health insurance to millions of Americans who lack it. The bill, sponsored by Rep. Pete Stark (D-Calif.) and Majority Leader Richard Gephardt (D-Mo.), would set a national healthcare budget, give states authority to establish hospital and physician cost-containment programs and set national maximum payment rates based on the new Medicare fee schedule. The bill would also extend Medicaid coverage to anyone with an income below 200% of the poverty level, create a government health insurance program for all children under 19 and prohibit physicians from referring patients to any facility in which they have a financial interest.

• • •

A 29-year-old pregnant woman was stopped at Kennedy International Airport as she attempted to bring RU 486 into the country for personal use, and the medication was seized. A 1989 Food and Drug Administration ruling placed RU 486 on an "import alert list," which calls for the drug to be seized upon entry into the United States.

July 7

A New York City law requiring public places or businesses to have special masks and gloves to prevent HIV transmission during cardiopulmonary resuscitation was rescheduled to go into effect in November. The law is intended to increase the likelihood that people will give CPR to strangers by helping to relieve fears of HIV transmission. Some health experts said the law could backfire by encouraging the false belief that the masks are vital to protect against HIV.

July 8

A Boston team noted that the time lag between a medical discovery and experts' recommendation to put it into practice can be as long as 15 years. As one example, thrombolytic therapy was shown to be effective as early as 1973, but was not recommended by experts until 1988, when two major clinical trials showed that the drugs lowered the death rate in acute myocardial infarction. The New England Medical Center report, which appeared in The Journal of the American Medical Association, cited the quantity of medical studies and delays in data analysis as explanations for the time lag.

July 15

A new survey revealed that medical residents planning to go into primary care will have six to 12 job offers to choose from, with salaries ranging from $85,000 to $120,000. And the shortage of primary-care doctors, caused by the ever-increasing specialization of medicine, is likely to continue for a few more years, according to a survey by the Physician Services of America.

Pediatric surgeons were at the top of the demand scale, with a starting salary of $200,000; other specialists getting top offers included hand and spine surgeons, neurosurgeons and medical oncologists, the survey showed.

July 17

The president of the American Osteopathic Association announced a plan designed to improve the image of physicians and possibly shed light on ways to improve access to healthcare. The plan, announced at the group's annual House of Delegates meeting in Dearborn, Mich., would include documentation of any charity care and increased efforts by osteopathic physicians to provide such care, particularly to the chronic poor, the recently unemployed or uninsured middle class and people with long-term illnesses. More emphasis on primary-care education was also strongly recommended.

July 21

Rep. Pat Schroeder (D-Colo.) introduced a bill to reverse a Supreme Court decision and permit a pregnant woman to take the abortion pill RU 486.

Previously, a federal judge had ruled that the government acted illegally in confiscating the drug from a woman at Kennedy International Airport and ordered the drug to be returned immediately, but he did not address the importation issue. The U. S. Court of Appeals for the Second Circuit in Manhattan blocked the judge's order; the appeals court stay was later upheld by Supreme Court Associate Justice Clarence Thomas.

• • •

For the second time, murder charges brought against Jack Kevorkian, M.D., for helping chronically ill patients commit suicide were dropped. There is no law against physician-assisted suicide in Michigan, so the prosecutor opted to forgo legal action against the retired pathologist. His attorney said that the prosecutor "wants to create a law," and added that in another time or place, the repeated legal actions against Dr. Kevorkian would be called persecution.

July 23

President Bush postponed signing an executive order that would have transferred the authority to make assessments of toxic risk from environmental agencies to Vice President Dan Quayle's Council on Competitiveness. The order had been met by a storm of criticism by environmental groups and others who were concerned that the plan could result in dangerous, weaker standards.

July 24

The sponsors of the Mary Immaculate Elder Health Center in Lawrence, Mass., planned to close the clinic because they had run out of money following the federal government's cuts in Medicare payments. The plight of the center raised fears of similar scenes in other urban areas as the full impact of the new Medicare doctor-fee schedule, which took effect Jan. 1, was felt.

July 27

The Pharmaceutical Manufacturers Association launched a campaign to make the free-drug programs of 59 companies more accessible to physicians with indigent patients. The campaign includes a directory of programs that provide prescription drugs free of charge to physicians whose

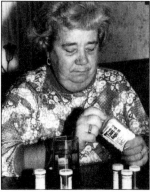

Survey found almost 60% of elderly struggle to pay for drugs.

patients could not otherwise afford them and a toll-free hotline that physicians can call to receive a referral to the appropriate drug company program.

July 30

A survey released by the American Association of Retired Persons found that 58% of Americans aged 65 and older have a problem paying for their prescription medications. Forty-six percent of those between 45 and 64 years of age reported similar difficulty. Ten percent of people 45 and older told the survey they were forced to cut back on such necessities as food or fuel in order to pay for prescription medications.

AUGUST

Aug. 3

The Bush administration rejected the Oregon Health Plan, charging that it violated the Americans with Disabilities Act because its cost-benefit analysis of medical treatments was based on the premise that "the value of a disabled person's life is less than the value of the life of a person without a disability." The president of the Oregon Senate, who is also a physician, called the rejection political. The plan would have eliminated benefits for some indigent Oregonians, but also would have added 130,000 people to the Medicaid rolls.

Aug. 10

An eminent Croatian physician charged that parts of former Yugoslavia may turn into a mass graveyard unless urgent measures are taken to help its refugees. The physician at the Zagreb Medical School told Medical Tribune that hundreds of thousands of people who have been chased from their homes by the war are in danger of freezing to death or dying of starvation this winter.

Aug. 17

Food and Drug Administration Commissioner David Kessler, M.D., told a hearing that food manufacturers need to include labeling information that consumers can readily

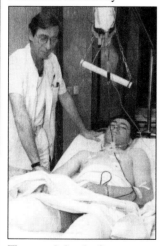

The wounded and refugees urgently need help in Sarajevo.

observe, comprehend and understand in the context of a total daily diet. Representatives for various groups who spoke at the hearing in Bethesda, Md., said that the biggest challenge of the Nutrition Labeling and Education Act is meeting the requirement that labels state the amount of various nutrients in relation to a person's total diet. For example, a label would need to list both how many grams of fat a particular food contains, and how many grams of fat a person should eat in a day.

Aug. 18

Approximately 6,500 healthcare workers are infected with hepatitis B through needle-stick injuries every year, said a Food and Drug Administration researcher at a conference in Washington on the dangers of infection through medical devices.

To prevent such infections, the agency recommended needle-free connectors or permanently sheathed needles for standing intravenous therapy lines. It also recommended self-sheathing, retracting and self-blunting needles for use in syringes.

Aug. 19

Some physician delegates to the Republican National Convention in Houston bristled at the party's staunch antiabortion stand. The party platform called for a constitutional amendment to ban abortion and did not state whether exceptions would be granted in cases of rape, incest or when the health of the mother is threatened. Prochoice Republican physicians said the stand would hurt President Bush's re-election bid.

Aug. 21

Public health system deficiencies, inadequate funding and the inappropriate use of antibiotics were partly blamed for the epidemic of tuberculosis and other infectious diseases by researchers from the Albert Einstein College of Medicine in New York and the Harvard School of Public Health.

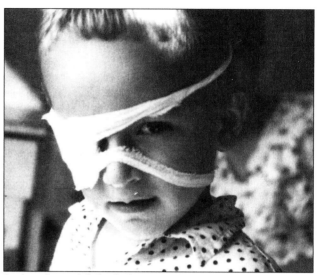

An American ophthalmologist arranged mercy mission to ravaged Ukrainian eye clinic, formerly one of area's best medical institutions.

At a time when the need for TB control has increased, many cities and states have been unable to maintain or improve TB programs, the investigators reported in Science. But if money is not spent to develop vaccines and other prevention efforts, they predicted, the tragedy unfolding in New York City, where one third of TB cases are drug resistant, will repeat itself in other locales.

Physicians can do their part by not prescribing antibiotics inappropriately, the report advised.

Aug. 25

A Ukrainian eye-care clinic received 400 pounds of desperately needed medical supplies from an ophthalmologist at Saint Louis University School of Medicine. The Missouri eye doctor told Medical Tribune that in the University of Ivano Frankivsk clinic— once one of the best eye-care facilities in the former Soviet republic—equipment lies broken, supply cabinets

are bare and paint is peeling from the walls. Donated sutures, solutions, intraocular lenses, bandages, gloves, glasses and an ultrasound machine were delivered, and Ukrainian ophthalmologists were shown how to use the supplies.

Aug. 28

Three studies this month suggested that significant inequities in access to care and medical technology persist between black and white patients.

A study of over 600,000 Americans published in The Lancet found a higher death rate among African-Americans under age 65 compared with whites of the same age and income. A second study, involving 1,184 hospitalized patients and published in the Archives of Internal Medicine, found that elderly African-Americans were more severely ill than whites upon admission to hospitals, yet were hospitalized for fewer days. A third study, in the American Journal of Public Health, found that in a retrospective review of 986 men's medical records, 62% of blacks had died over the 18-year period, compared with 57% of whites.

Sept. 1

The Senate Special Committee on Aging released a report charging that programs to provide free drugs to patients who cannot afford them are being used by only a small number of Americans. The programs often involve long waiting periods before a patient receives the free medications, noted committee chairman Senator David Pryor (D-Ark.).

• • •

Health and Human Services Secretary Louis Sullivan, M.D., announced that total Medicare payments to hospitals for inpatient care will rise 8.5%, to $72.6 billion, for fiscal year 1993, up from $66.9 billion the previous year. More will go to rural hospitals as part of a two-year-old requirement of the Omnibus Budget Reconciliation Act of 1990 to equalize payments for reimbursable services to 2,500 rural hospitals and those to 2,900 urban hospitals.

Sept. 7

The U.S. government announced that all incoming foreign physicians must take one of three U.S. medical exams. The rule change was expected to staunch the flow of Canadian doctors to the United States. In 1991, 524 private Canadian physicians left their country for the United States and other countries, although 275 returned to Canada and resumed practicing in the same year. Nearly 200 Canadian

doctors were granted permanent residence in the United States last year. The number has risen steadily since 1988. Canadian physicians were said to be unhappy because of the fixed-payment reimbursement system and salary caps in some provinces.

Sept. 10

Top doctors in the Bush and Clinton political campaigns made strong appeals for their parties' healthcare reform plans in Medical Tribune. The Bush plan promises to improve access to care through vouchers for the poor and increased deductibility of insurance premiums. Bush would preserve the doctors' role as an integral part of the healthcare system, said the director of the Health Care Coalition for Bush-Quayle. Clinton's universal access plan, which like the Bush plan features malpractice reform and simplified claims, would be directed by cost-capping review boards on which physicians will actively participate, the chairman of the National Health Leadership Council for Clinton-Gore '92 said.

• • •

President George Bush and Gov. Bill Clinton laid their healthcare cards on the table in The New England Journal of Medicine. With less than two months until the election, the presidential candidates seemed to agree on only two things:

that the current system is too costly and care is unevenly distributed, and that the other candidate's plan would only make things worse. Bush's plan called for tax credits to be used to purchase insurance, while Clinton called for a type of play-or-pay system.

Sept. 14

The American College of Physicians threw its hat into the healthcare reform ring as it unveiled its plan to restructure the U.S. healthcare system. The proposal, "Universal Insurance for American Health Care," signals physician support for a play-or-pay plan, also advocated by Democratic

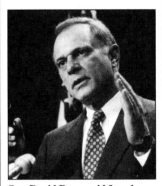

Sen. David Pryor said free drugs reach only a few who need them.

presidential candidate Gov. Bill Clinton. Such a plan would require companies to provide coverage for employees or to pay into a government-sponsored insurance fund. Under the ACP plan, however, the public system would also cover people over age 60, those requiring high-cost care, the unemployed and all retirees. Employees eligible for private insurance would have to pay a maximum of half the cost, based on their ability to pay.

Sept. 23

University of North Carolina researchers found that fewer than half of physicians placed in rural practices by the National Health Service Corps remain in their assigned communities past their service

obligations. And only half of those who do stay remain for more than three years, the investigators stated in The Journal of the American Medical Association.

In an accompanying editorial, a University of Minnesota expert suggested that the poor morale of NHSC physicians could be alleviated by bringing specialists to those physicians' communities to update their knowledge or assist in difficult diagnoses. Giving the rural doctors more time off with coverage by colleagues could also help, he wrote.

• • •

The Oregon Health Services Commission announced that it plans to resubmit the state's request for waivers from Medicaid regulations so that it could go forward with its health reform plan. Under the Oregon plan, which was rejected by the Bush administration in July, medical services were prioritized by ranking 709 medical conditions and their treatments.

Federal officials told the Oregon commission that it must remove "quality of life" factors from its rankings in order to avoid discriminating against the disabled.

Sept. 28

A majority of Americans support using genetic testing in ways that could invade privacy, and a sizable minority support using gene therapy for purposes that could be called eugenic, revealed a 1,000-person poll commissioned by the March of Dimes Birth Defects Foundation. While supporting disclosure of genetic test data to spouses, employers and insurers, a large majority of respondents admitted that they know little or nothing about the techniques. More than 40% of those surveyed expressed support for using gene therapy to improve children's intelligence and physical characteristics. March of Dimes spokespersons said they hoped the data would stimulate debate of the social and ethical issues surrounding genetic medicine.

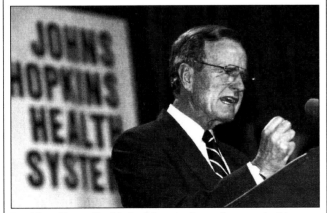

President George Bush's healthcare reform plan promised to improve access to care through vouchers for the poor.

Oct. 1

A bipartisan panel convened by the consumer health group Families USA concluded that it would be easier for an American family to afford healthcare with Gov. Bill Clinton in the White House than it would be if President Bush were re-elected. The panel concluded that by the end of the 1990s, an average family's annual health bill would cost $1,179 more under George Bush's health plan than under Bill Clinton's; that number would rise to a $2,267 difference five years later, the panel said.

Oct. 5

A "report card" issued to mark Child Health Day concluded that healthcare workers and educators are not doing enough to maintain the health of U.S. youth. The report, issued by the American Health Foundation, analyzed immunizations, substance abuse, nutrition and other factors. It found that 3.5 million children suffer from lead poisoning each year, 30% of high-school seniors have five or more alcoholic drinks at one sitting in a two-week period, and 3.5% have used cocaine in the last year. Also, fewer than half of urban children are vaccinated at age two and asthma rates have increased by more than 60% since 1979, the group reported. It recommended that schools hire full-time health-education teachers who will teach drug and alcohol awareness and sexually transmitted disease prevention as early as the preschool years.

Oct. 7

The U.S. Senate paved the way for speeding the Food and Drug Administration's drug-approval process by passing a bill that would require pharmaceutical companies to help pay for reviewing drugs. The Prescription Drug User Fee Act of 1992 had already cleared the House of Representatives,

OCTOBER

and President Bush earlier voiced his commitment to signing the bill. The FDA announced it would concen-

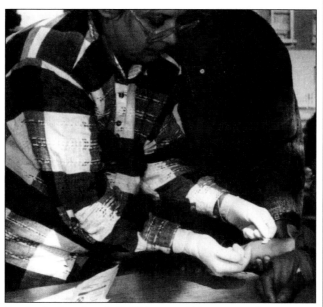

Routine lead testing of all children would be a waste of scarce healthcare resources, according to a panel of experts.

trate on speeding approval of treatments for terminal diseases, such as AIDS and cancer.

The FDA estimated that it will collect about $300 million from drug companies over the next five years. In return, it has agreed to hire 600 new examiners to help speed the approval process and, it is hoped, cutting in half the time for new drug applications to be approved, to six months for drugs for life-threatening conditions and to about a year for others.

Oct. 11

Physicians, scientists and politicians gathered at the Massachusetts Institute of Technology in Cambridge, Mass., were warned that the health of people around the world may deteriorate unless major environmental problems are prevented from getting out of hand. The situation in the former Soviet Union should serve as an example to the rest of the

world of the health disasters that may occur when the environment is ignored in favor of industrial

development, according to a University of Chicago speaker at the symposium on Human Health and the Environment.

Oct. 12

The Health Care Financing Administration huddled with insurance experts and policy makers to formulate a policy and propose national documentation standards for newly revised CPT codes. Revision of the codes earlier this year, which comprise one third of all Medicare bills, was followed by suspension of prepayment screens. About 10% of participating doctors then were notified that they were coding at a level statistically higher than their peers. Doctors feared HCFA would combine documentation standards and utilization review and begin disqualifying claims wholesale.

Oct. 14

A panel of experts concluded that children at high

risk of lead poisoning need to be tested, but that routine lead testing for all children would be a waste of scarce healthcare resources. Instead of screening all children, health authorities should use those resources to screen all houses for lead, said the chief of the lead and toxicology clinic at the Children's Hospital in Boston. He told the American Academy of Pediatrics meeting in San Francisco that high-risk children include those who live in old or substandard homes, especially if the homes are being remodeled. Older homes are likely to have lead-based paint, which was banned in the United States more than a decade ago.

Oct. 23

Former U.S. Surgeon General C. Everett Koop, M.D., told a forum held in Alexandria, Va., that the U.S. healthcare system is obsolete and needs to be overhauled. He recommended a system in which people would pay a flat rate to get a common level of care and pay on a fee-for-service basis if they want additional care. The pediatrician also suggested that more resources be allocated to preventive-care services.

More primary-care physicians should enter practice and there should be fewer specialists, according to other experts at the Institute for Alternative Choices forum. For many conditions, low-tech care should replace less effective high-tech methods, the experts added. Healthcare providers should compete for patients on the basis of quality and service, they said.

Oct. 29

The Centers for Disease Control changed its name to the Centers for Disease Control and Prevention. In enacting the change, Congress specified that the agency continue to use the acronym CDC because of its widespread recognition.

NOVEMBER

Nov. 3

After pledging to voters that he would overhaul the nation's healthcare system—boosting access and reducing costs—Arkansas Gov. Bill Clinton defeated President George Bush for the nation's top executive position.

• • •

Computer manufacturer Unisys Corp. joined a handful of other major corporations, including General Motors and McDonnell Douglas, in gradually eliminating health benefits for its retirees. Surveys have shown that more companies are altering both retiree and active employee health insurance by increasing deductibles and premium contributions or

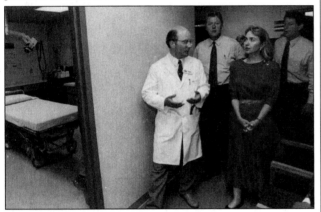

President-elect Clinton pledged to reduce costs and boost access.

changing the level of coverage provided. The changes are designed to counter escalating healthcare costs and soften the impact of new accounting rules that require companies to include future retiree benefit costs on their 1993 balance sheets—a move that can lower profits.

Nov. 9

The Supreme Court refused to hear the case of a Houston man whose medical insurance benefits were slashed from $1 million to $5,000 after he contracted AIDS. Under a 1987 interpretation of the Employee Retirement Income Security Act, even bad-faith actions on the part of self-insured employers are protected from state action or regulation—as long as cost containment is the stated goal of benefit reductions.

Nov. 11

A report in The Journal of the American Medical Association assessed U.S. progress toward a list of health-improvement goals set by a government panel in 1980. Progress was made in the areas of unintentional-injury prevention, high blood pressure control and reduction of cigarette smoking, the Public Health Service report found.

Overall, the panel found that, by 1990, the nation had met or exceeded 32% of its 1980 goals and showed progress in another 30%. Notable failures included attempts to reduce violence, lower the incidence of hepatitis B and syphilis, curb the number of adolescent pregnancies and lessen the gap in infant mortality between whites and African-Americans.

Nov. 12

The Health Care Financing Administration conceded that it should consult the medical profession more closely in preparing documentation standards, Medical Tribune reported. HCFA's failure to hold any real dialogue on documentation is the chief complaint of physicians, according to the report. As a result, doctors are forced to work in the dark to validate visit codes—especially with patients who have multiple chronic problems.

Nov. 13

The Oregon Health Services Commission resubmitted its request for waivers from Medicaid regulations in hopes of winning approval of its Oregon Health Plan. The prioritization of healthcare for Medicaid patients, the core of the plan, would go into effect five months after Medicaid waiver approval. The Bush administration rejected the original waiver request in August.

Nov. 16

The Food and Drug Administration's Oncologic Drugs Advisory Committee voted unanimously to recommend approval of Taxol (Bristol-Myers Squibb) for women whose ovarian cancer does not respond to standard chemotherapy. In clinical trials, about one third of 189 patients with advanced, unresponsive ovarian cancer responded to the drug, the committee noted.

Results from other clinical trials suggest that taxol could also play a role in treating several other types of cancer, including advanced breast cancer, according to the National Cancer Institute.

Nov. 17

San Diego researchers suggested that addressing economic problems may be even more important than patient education in stemming the rise in severity of inner-city asthma. When given no-cost instructions, low-income parents of asthmatic children are more likely than parents with higher incomes to follow guidelines for keeping dust-mite levels low, the doctors from the University of San Diego Medical Center said. However, for many low-income parents it is too costly to comply with dust-mite-avoidance regulations, such as purchasing plastic mattress covers, they told a session at the 50th Anniversary Meeting of the American College of Allergy and Immunology in Chicago.

Nov. 20

Health and Human Services secretary Louis Sullivan, M.D., announced revisions to the 1993 Medicare physician fee schedule. Under the revisions, the conversion factor that determines Medicare payments will be increased by 3.1% for surgical services and by 0.8% for physician services, Secretary Sullivan announced.

Primary-care physicians told Medical Tribune they consider the fee hikes "insubstantial" or "barely noticeable"—and an insulting continuation of the trend by government and other insurers to place a higher value on performing medical procedures than on evaluation and management.

Nov. 21

The Mayo Clinic announced that establishing a smoke-free workplace policy can dramatically increase the number of employees who kick the habit. Within two and a half years after smoking was banned at its medical center in Rochester, Minn., 22.5% of regular smokers had quit—four times the proportion that would have been anticipated based solely on national smoking trends, the researchers reported in the journal Chest.

According to the report, the Mayo policy prohibits smoking not only in all the clinic's buildings, but on its grounds and even in vehicles on the clinic's premises.

Nov. 24

After a sixth ailing woman killed herself yesterday with a "suicide-assist" device invented by Jack Kevorkian, M.D., the Michigan Legislature took steps to ban the practice, with the House passing a bill to make assisted suicide a felony punishable by four years imprisonment. The bill is expected to pass the Senate and be signed by the Governor.

DECEMBER

Dec. 4

The repayment of medical school loans was on the minds of medical school students, residents and young physicians as they met in Nashville prior to the opening of the American Medical Association House of Delegates meeting. A Colorado delegation asked the AMA to explore the feasibility of allowing medical students to wait until graduation before choosing the option of reducing their tuition-related indebtedness through practice in an underserved area.

The current early-choice system is difficult to abide by because many medical students have not made a firm decision regarding specialty and career goals when they first enter medical school, and not all specialty choices readily lend themselves to service in rural and inner-city America, the delegation argued.

Dec. 6

At the American Society of Hematology meeting in Anaheim, Calif., representatives from the House Ways and Means Committee, the Physician Payment Review Commission and the Association of American Medical Colleges debated whether reform plans to control healthcare costs will have a deleterious effect on medical education, academic medicine and access to care.

Dec. 7

The American Medical Association's House of Delegates took up the issue of insurance discrimination against the chronically and seriously ill when they met in Nashville. The New York delegation asked the AMA to take a strong position against insurance companies that manipulate rates in a manner that separates well people from ill and high-risk people, thus increasing the financial burden on the latter group and aggravating the

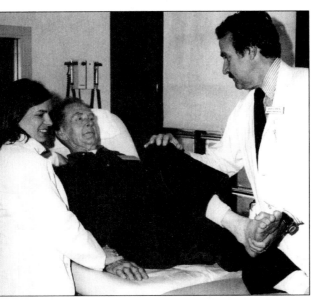

The hospital is fading fast as the center of the healthcare universe, with patients favoring home care and ambulatory treatment centers.

nation's overall health-insurance problem.

Dec. 10

A health industry analyst declared that the hospital is fading fast as the center of the healthcare universe. Within the past five years, the proportion of health revenues expended in hospitals has fallen from 45% to 35%, according to an Oklahoma pathologist who also edits the Reece Report on healthcare issues. Writing in an op-ed piece in Medical Tribune, the analyst credited pressures from government and private payers, as well as improved medical technologies for outpatient surgery, for the dramatic ongoing shift to home care and outpatient delivery sites.

• • •

While the AMA officially calls loudly for changes in laws regarding how self-insurance plans may operate, a Medical Tribune report questioned whether self-insured groups of physicians will put their money where their mouths are—that is, will they peacefully surrender their right to contain costs by

altering benefits midstream. The report also evaluated whether the powerful small-business lobbies are likely to stall any legislative changes in the Employee Retirement Income Security Act, or ERISA.

Dec. 17

A women's-health researcher called on policy-makers to address women-specific problems in drug addiction. Most drug treatment programs were designed for men and only treat women as an afterthought, the author of "The Invisible Epidemic: The Story of Women and AIDS" told Medical Tribune. Programs must confront both the causes of pain that women are trying to numb with drug use, such as sexual abuse, and the practical problems that keep women out of many treatment programs, such as a lack of child-care provisions, the researcher said.

Dec. 20

Two Washington, D.C., attorneys criticized the federal Medicare/Medicaid antikickback statute for

throwing standard business practices into question without offering clear guidance on how manufacturers can comply. The combination of recently issued safe-harbor regulations, state antikickback and antireferral laws and new ethical guidelines for physicians has put marketing plans for many new drugs and devices in limbo, the attorneys stated in the Food and Drug Law Journal.

Dec. 24

A London attorney warned medical-device manufacturers that, for the next several years, those who wish to market their products in the European Community will be required to heed both national regulatory requirements and emerging requirements for the EC as a whole. A directive on active implantable medical devices takes effect in 1993, the attorney reported in the Food and Drug Law Journal. General directives on other devices will allow products to move freely within the EC if they meet certain essential requirements. Eventually, a uniform regulatory system will apply throughout the 12 Member States of the EC and the seven members of the European Free Trade Association, according to the attorney.

Dec. 26

Allergy and immunology experts said expansions in clinical and diagnostic laboratory immunology are needed to meet the challenges of rapidly expanded knowledge in that area. The experts called on diagnostic certification boards to amend their guidelines to include clinical and diagnostic laboratory immunology programs. The authors of the article appearing in the Journal of Clinical Allergy and Immunology also recommended the establishment of immunology workshops at annual meetings of the American Academy of Allergy and Immunology.

Dow safety data did not consider whether silicone leaked from breast implants after insertion

By Saralie Faivelson

JAN. 13—Even as Food and Drug Administration officials review the latest data on breast implants and decide whether to lift the Jan. 6 moratorium, internal Dow Corning Corp. documents have surfaced that show that its own researchers were concerned that safety tests were inadequate.

The silicone-gel implant manufacturer denied the allegations at a press conference in Washington, D.C., while plastic surgeons grappled with new questions and few answers.

"Dow Corning has studied the safety of silicones for almost 40 years," said Robert Rylee, chairman of Dow's Health Care Businesses, at the January 13 press conference. "The conclusion of all those studies is that silicone breast implants are safe and effective."

But according to published reports, Dow scientists did not have sufficient safety data 16 months after a new type of implant began being used in women in 1976. The lack of data left unanswered whether or for how long silicone in implants leaked into the body.

Dow officials did know by 1975 that silicone "bled" through the implants, Rylee said. "Neither we nor our colleagues believed this phenomenon was a safety issue, nor do any of our subsequent studies show this to be a safety issue," he said at the press conference.

But none of the studies dealt with inserting silicone or implants in or under breast tissue, said Norman Anderson, M.D., of Johns Hopkins University, who has been a consultant to the FDA. "I find this omission a peculiar phenomenon which must be unprecedented in the history of medical device evaluation," he said in a letter to David Kessler, M.D., FDA Commissioner.

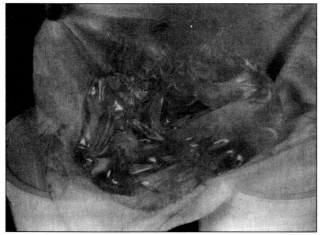

Dow Corning officials admitted they knew silicone "bled" from breast implants, but did not consider this a safety issue.

Concerns about the implants are not limited to how research was conducted, said Melvin Silverstein, M.D., of the Breast Center in Van Nuys, Calif. "Augmentation patients simply cannot get state-of-the-art mammography results. Twenty-five percent of the tissue visible before augmentation is not visible afterwards. Thus, diagnosis will be delayed and survival will drop."

As for the risk posed by silicone leakage, "I can't imagine that silicone in the blood and lymph nodes will be good for you," he said. However, "the data are simply not available."

If silicone does cause problems, "it doesn't do it very often, considering the number of women who have received breast augmentations," Dr. Silverstein said.

Death-with-dignity groups say Kevorkian undermines their cause

By Andrea Kott

FEB. 5—Murder charges against Jack Kevorkian, M.D., may significantly damage the right-to-die movement and hamper the efforts of states trying to legalize doctor-assisted suicide, according to the directors of several patients' rights groups.

"He's really screwing up," asserted Jack Nicholl, campaign director for Californians Against Human Suffering. "He is doing damage to the movement that he claims to be serving."

The charges stem from Dr. Kevorkian's participation on Oct. 23 in the suicides of Sherry Miller, 43, and Marjorie Wantz, 58, two women who were suffering from chronic but not demonstrably terminal diseases.

Critics like Nicholl contend that Dr. Kevorkian's participation in the suicides resulted in the November defeat of Initiative 119, Washington state's measure to legalize doctor-assisted suicide.

Nicholl is lobbying for a similar measure, the California Death with Dignity Act, scheduled for the November 1992 ballot.

"If the Dr. Kevorkians of the world can be stopped, then we can get some kind of law passed that is responsible," said Karen Cooper, of the Washington Citizens For Death With Dignity in Seattle.

In contrast to right-to-die groups who argue for the right of terminally ill patients to choose to die, Dr. Kevorkian has assisted in the suicides of patients not terminally ill.

In his recently published plan, "A Fail-Safe Model for Justifiable Medically-Assisted Suicide," Dr. Kevorkian specifies that candidates for "medicide" may be suffering from incapacitating illnesses such as crippling arthritis, emphysema, severe pneumonia, bronchitis, progressive degenerative neurologic disease or stroke.

But by helping make the means available in Miller's and Wantz's deaths, Dr. Kevorkian crossed the line between doctor-assisted suicide and euthanasia, said Ronald Cranford, M.D., a neurologist from the Hennepin County Medical Center in Minneapolis.

The medical examiner ruled that both deaths were homicides.

Even though the women requested Dr. Kevorkian's help, consent is not a defense, according to George Annas, a medical ethicist at Boston University.

Derek Humphry, president of the Hemlock Society, a right-to-die advocacy group, said that Dr. Kevorkian's plan to help people who are not terminally ill commit suicide cannot be introduced until the law is reformed to permit assisted suicide for the terminally ill.

"He's putting the cart before the horse," Humphry said. "You've got to change the law, and then there are plenty of doctors who will help people to die in the appropriate circumstances. Doctors are not going to be lawbreakers, and why should they be?"

Drug-resistant TB quarantine policy proposed

FEB. 21—In response to a New York City task force recommendation to quarantine people with tuberculosis, experts say they may sometimes have no other choice if they seek to protect the public.

The recommendation, which calls for hundreds of people who may be spreading drug-resistant tuberculosis to be locked up, was made by a task force formed by the City of New York.

"In some situations, quarantines may be the only way to protect the public health," said Craig Studer, coordinator of tuberculosis control for the state of Michigan.

A California TB expert agreed. "If we have an individual who poses a threat to others, then we go the route of incarcerating them, but that's very infrequent," said Tony Paz, director of TB control at the Department of Public Health in San Francisco.

Experts on the New York City task force fell short of recommending that sanitariums be reopened, but said they would quarantine patients in shelters, psychiatric hospitals or special wards to be set up in AIDS nursing homes or drug-treatment programs.

City officials now have a right to detain TB patients, but only if they do not take their medications, and the doctors must try other measures first.

For example, they may give medications on a supervised basis by giving patients an incentive to come to the clinic, like a can of soda or a bus fare, or by using a court order to make them receive treatment. Studer said, "If all that fails, you get a court order to quarantine the patient."

If the City of New York were to go ahead with plans to isolate contagious tuberculosis patients, officials would have to find an appropriate place for them to be detained.

"Where do you hold a person? A hospital? A nursing home? A prison?" Studer asked.

Tuberculosis has been on the rise in the past few years in the United States, particularly among groups of people with weakened immune systems, such as those with AIDS or the homeless who live in overcrowded shelters. There were 25,701 cases of TB nationwide in 1990, according to the latest statistics available.

Perhaps the greatest concern has been caused by the surge in drug-resistant cases of tuberculosis, which is difficult to treat and often is fatal.

Its incidence has increased by 15% nationwide in the past two years, according to the Centers for Disease Control in Atlanta.

In 1991, 13 prison inmates and one guard died in New York City of multidrug-resistant TB, and last April, 23% of patients who were treated in New York City for the first time had drug-resistant disease.

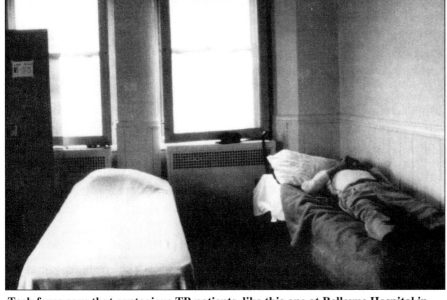

Task force says that contagious TB patients, like this one at Bellevue Hospital in New York City, should be quarantined to protect the public from infection.

Data-bank leaks and Big Brotherism at issue

FEB. 27—Less than two years after the National Practitioner Data Bank began collecting information on the competency of doctors, elements of organized medicine are becoming increasingly outspoken in their opposition to the system.

Saying that it is akin to having Big Brother watching over them, data-bank opponents worry about leaks of information and misinterpretation of data that could harm physicians.

But supporters of the data bank are countering that after millions of queries to the system, confidentiality has been maintained. They concede, however, that it is still too early to tell whether hospitals will be able to use the bank to track incompetent doctors.

The Public Citizen Health Research Group is even lobbying for giving the public access to information in the bank, a prospect that has caused anxieties to balloon.

"There is a tremendous sense of frustration and concern," said John Kelly, M.D., director of quality assurance at the American Medical Association.

In December, the AMA House of Delegates passed a resolution to abolish the nationwide system, which keeps track of malpractice awards and settlements and disciplinary actions taken against physicians. Dr. Kelly said the organization is currently looking at ways to implement the resolution.

"It is quite a reasonable system," countered Fitzhugh Mullan, M.D., director of the Bureau of Health Professionals, which oversees the bank.

"It is important for the medical profession not to deal with it in a hysterical fashion. For physicians to say that they are unwilling to be accountable will not do anything to improve their public image," he said.

Dr. Mullan said the public has demanded a standardized system to insure that medical practitioners "are of the best quality."

The system was established by Congress to collect information on physicians' credentials and to insure that incompetent doctors cannot move from one hospital to another and from one state to another without leaving a record of their misconduct.

Insurance companies do not send the bank information gained from physician profiling, unless it has to do with quality of care, said Peter Kongstvedt, M.D., senior vice president of Blue Cross and Blue Shield of the National Area, in Washington, D.C. "If we take an unfavorable action against a physician because of quality of care, such as incompetence, that would be sent to the bank," he said. "Overutilization is not reported by itself."

Dr. Kongstvedt said, however, that it was too soon to tell whether the data bank will be useful to the insurance company.

The data bank contains information about:
• Medical malpractice payments stemming from a written claim or judgment.
• Licensing actions against a doctor by state medical boards.
• Unfavorable professional reviews by hospitals and other healthcare facilities that affect clinical privileges for longer than 30 days.
• Voluntary surrender or restriction of privileges by a physician in return for not conducting an investigation of possible incompetence or improper conduct.
• Unfavorable actions against a doctor by professional societies.

The data bank has received 25,034 reports since it began operating in Sept. 1990; 84% concerned malpractice payments and 16% actions against a doctor's license, clinical privileges or society membership. More than a million queries have been received by the bank; about 80% of the nation's hospitals have requested information at least once.

Elizabeth Gallup, M.D., assistant general counsel for the American Academy of Family Physicians, criticized the reporting to the data bank of all malpractice payments, no matter how small. A settlement, she pointed out, does not necessarily mean an admission of wrongdoing.

ACP proposes 'play or pay' insurance system

By Jane Anderson

MARCH 26—Two years after decrying "patchwork" measures to improve access to care, the American College of Physicians is proposing a health plan that would require employers to provide health insurance or pay into a public system.

The document resembles "play or pay" plans proposed earlier and was given to several ACP fellows last year for comment.

ACP senior vice president Denman Scott, M.D., said they hope to have a revised version of the plan by early summer.

He stressed that the group wants to preserve "a vigorous private sector" in healthcare that would not offer an incentive to opt "into the public side."

But a fellow in ACP's dissident North Carolina chapter criticized the plan, calling it "national health insurance by the back door. The college is proposing a single payer," said Rodney Hornbake, M.D., of New Bern, N.C. "Government rates would determine the rates for the entire system," he said.

Under the proposed system, employers would either pay at least half the cost of health insurance for their workers, or pay a combined 6% payroll/3% corporate income tax.

In addition to covering workers whose employers do not supply health insurance, the public plan would include everyone now covered by Medicare and Medicaid, plus those between ages 60 and 65.

In addition, the blueprint would "diminish" administrative costs through a single electronic claim and data form per visit.

The plan would cut costs for the private sector by having the government cover catastrophic costs for everyone above a certain amount, Dr. Scott said, adding that the provision would help make private insurance more affordable for employers.

But Dr. Hornbake argued that the ACP plan would make it cheaper for employers to pay into the government plan than to buy even the cheapest private health insurance.

Dr. Hornbake said the ACP plan has fewer incentives for employers to keep private insurance than one proposed by the Pepper Commission, headed by Sen. Jay Rockefeller (D-W.Va.).

Rockefeller said the plan could push the debate toward play or pay.

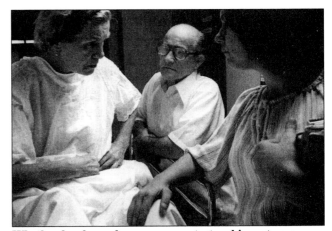

Whether her boss plays or pays, catastrophic costs are picked up by the government, according to the ACP plan.

FDA proposes rules requiring patient-identity tracking for heart valves, other medical devices

WASHINGTON, D.C., MARCH 27—The Food and Drug Administration, following criticism that it has failed to properly oversee medical devices such as heart valves and breast implants, proposed rules requiring device manufacturers to track patients using their products.

The regulations, which Congress mandated in 1990, would help identify patients who receive dangerous or faulty devices so they can be quickly notified, said FDA Commissioner David Kessler, M.D.

"Tracking will help the FDA protect the public by providing the information necessary to quickly remove dangerous and defective devices from the market," Dr. Kessler said.

The public has been given 60 days to comment on the proposal.

The proposed requirement is limited to permanent implants, such as breast implants, and devices that sustain or support life, such as heart valves or defibrillators.

Thirty-five types of devices from more than 370 manufacturers would be affected by the proposed regulation, the FDA said.

Manufacturers would need to ensure that they can trace, identify and report to the FDA the patients' names and locations within three working days of a request. They also would have to set up a system to collect information on the life span of the device.

The FDA rules were issued just two days after a General Accounting Office report asserted that the FDA had failed to enforce regulations on the proper manufacturing of medical devices.

Rep. John Dingell (D-Mich.), chairman of the House Energy and Commerce Committee, criticized the FDA for its putative inability to ensure the health of patients who receive medical devices.

Earlier this week, Dingell's panel heard testimony on a jelly injected into the eye to hold it steady for surgery. The jelly apparently has made some people blind. The panel also heard about radiation machines for cancer patients that gave some patients lethal doses because of faulty computer software.

The new FDA proposals come as Dr. Kessler is considering whether to ban silicone-gel breast implants, used for cosmetic breast augmentation and for breast reconstruction after cancer surgery.

An FDA panel that met in February said that although the implants can leak a small amount of silicone into the body, there is insufficient evidence to show they can cause any diseases.

Dr. Kessler promised a decision on the implants by April 20.

Another medical device causing concern is the Bjork-Shiley 60-degree C-C heart valve, which has cracked in 461 people and caused more than 300 deaths worldwide, according to Pfizer Hospital Products Ltd., the parent company of the valve's manufacturer, Shiley Inc. of Irvine, Calif.

The valve was recalled three times between 1980 and 1983 before being withdrawn from the market in 1986.

About 23,000 patients in the United States and Canada have received the Bjork-Shiley device.

ASIM calls for a way doctors can set own fees

WASHINGTON, D. C., APRIL 8—The American Society of Internal Medicine unveiled a new health reform plan that allows physicians to set their own fees, using the Resource-Based Relative Value Scale (RBRVS).

The plan would create a competitive market for physician

services and health insurance, ASIM said. It is seen as an alternative to proposals in Congress that would base some private insurance payment rates on the new Medicare fees.

Since Congress will likely consider controls on physicians' fees as part of any overall reform package, organized medicine needs to come to the negotiating table with its own plan, said ASIM vice president Robert Doherty.

"Medicine's credibility has been called into question so far by its inability to address questions about the way doctors are paid," Doherty said.

Fees under the new Medicare system are established by taking the relative value of each procedure and multiplying it by a dollar conversion factor. For example, Medicare has adopted a conversion factor of $31, so if an office visit has a relative value of 1, the fee for that visit would be $31.

Under ASIM's proposal, physicians would set their own individual conversion factors each year to determine their maximum allowable charges for every service. Insurers also would set conversion factors to indicate how much they are willing to pay for medical services.

By looking at the set conversion factors, which would be published annually, patients could make an informed choice

about individual physicians' charges, Doherty said. Those doctors who did not deliver good value for the money probably would not do very well, he said.

The plan would place limits on what physicians could charge to low-income patients and would create a national board of physicians, payers, consumers and healthcare experts to set a conversion factor for public programs.

The ASIM supports reforming the healthcare system to require all employers to provide insurance for their workers, and would replace Medicaid with a plan that would cover everyone else.

Separately, the American Medical Association told lawmakers at a hearing early this month that Congress should hold off on proposals setting optional payment rates for private insurers based on the new Medicare fees.

At the House Ways and Means Health Subcommittee, AMA trustee P. John Seward, M.D., said that federal legislation to encourage use of the RBRVS by the private sector is not necessary because insurers already are beginning to use it.

The Physician Payment Review Commission has estimated that physician revenues would drop 15% overall if private insurers adopted Medicare rates and charge limits.

FDA places strict limits on silicone-gel implants

WASHINGTON, D.C., APRIL 16—The Food and Drug Administration has decided to allow the use of silicone-gel breast implants for all women who want them after breast-cancer surgery, but will sharply restrict their use in women seeking breast enlargement.

The decision, which mirrors a recommendation from an FDA advisory panel in February, calls for all women who receive the implants to participate in studies of their safety.

"We know more about the life span of automobile tires than we do about breast implants," said FDA Commissioner David Kessler, M.D. "We're going to acquire, once and for all, the information necessary to establish the safety of these devices."

The FDA will allow approximately 9,000 women who were scheduled for breast reconstruction when the FDA called for a moratorium on the implants in January to receive the implants immediately.

Other women, including up to 2,000 breast-enlargement candidates, will have to wait several months while the FDA and implant manufacturers decide how best to design the clinical trials.

Women who receive silicone-gel implants will be asked to read and sign a six-page agreement informing them of the risks and unanswered questions about the implants.

Manufacturers will be required to follow each patient and keep records on her health experiences, according to Dr. Kessler.

The FDA is also working with former and present implant manufacturers to set up a registry of implant recipients.

Public Citizen Health Research Group director Sidney Wolfe, M.D., said the FDA's decision "means the end of silicone implants."

He criticized the FDA's decision to allow some women to get the implants. "I think the decision to allow further human experimentation, given the known risks, is wrong," he said.

Norman Cole, M.D., president of the American Society of Plastic and Reconstructive Surgeons, said he was pleased with the FDA's decision, and said his group will fund $500,000 in separate studies on implants.

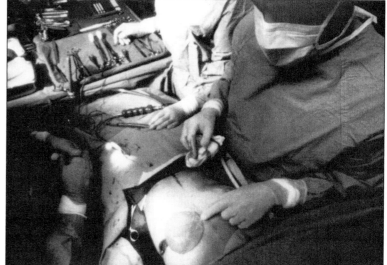

Women seeking cosmetic enlargement must agree to be studied.

Candidates lure MDs with different health plans

APRIL 23—Medical Tribune offered President Bush and his Democratic challenger for the presidency a forum to deliver special health messages to the nation's doctors.

Both took us up on the offer—on an equal-space basis. The statements follow.

For the first time, the candidates' health philosophies and their blueprints for healthcare reform are presented together—pointedly, succinctly and exclusively for health professionals.

It's no surprise that the President and Governor Bill Clinton want to get your attention. Pivotal primaries lie ahead in Pennsylvania, Ohio and California. They also recognize the importance of your cooperation in any future health plan.

While their objectives are the same, their positions on healthcare delivery are far apart. See for yourself. Please read their statements carefully.

Bush: build on the system

By George Bush

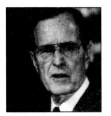

APRIL 23—It is a pleasure to extend warm greetings to our nation's doctors. I firmly believe that the American people share a feeling of admiration and gratitude for the important work you do.

Quality healthcare is absolutely essential to the well-being and happiness of all citizens, and your commitment to healing others makes a uniquely personal difference in our lives.

As you know, I announced my comprehensive healthcare proposal on Feb. 6, 1992. As doctors, you're used to extended debates about healthcare; you probably can't get through a family reunion without such a discussion. But your families also understand something that politicians sometimes forget: America's medical system offers the best care in the world. When people from other countries seek the best possible care, they come here.

My comprehensive proposal builds on the many strengths of our medical care system. I don't want to roll the dice on a nationalized plan that can guarantee only long lines, indifferent service and very high taxes. I want a plan that will work.

My proposal addresses Americans' basic concerns about healthcare: that it costs too much, that too many people lack access to appropriate care, and that you can't be sure of keeping coverage if you lose your job or fall victim to a debilitating injury or illness.

First, we must make healthcare available to all Americans. A health insurance credit on a deduction of up to $3,750 per family would be available to individuals, and two-person and larger families with annual incomes up to $50,000 and $80,000, respectively. These measures will help over 90 million Americans purchase the healthcare they need.

Second, we must improve the efficiency of our system.

One way to do that is through health insurance networks, which will drive costs down, allowing small employers to band together and benefit from the same economies of scale that large employers do.

Third, we must wring out waste and excess—and we start by targeting medical malpractice for reform. The national epidemic of lawsuits has persuaded some doctors to avoid such vital specialties as surgery and obstetrics and encouraged others to perform unneeded procedures that add unnecessary costs. We cannot allow this cycle to continue. Also, we must dramatically reduce the paperwork blizzard associated with current administrative practices.

Finally, we must bring the staggering cost of federal health programs under control and encourage innovation at state and local levels—keeping benefits and taxes as is.

America has the world's best doctors, best hospitals and finest training institutions. My healthcare plan will reward your hard work and free you of red tape. You need the freedom to serve others.

Congratulations on the challenging and noble careers you have chosen. Together, we'll make the world's best healthcare system even better—and we'll show the world once again that there's nothing Americans cannot do.

Clinton: streamline system

By Bill Clinton

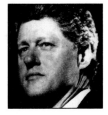

APRIL 23—We are the only advanced nation in the world that doesn't provide national healthcare to all its citizens and doesn't effectively control costs. America spends 30% more of its GNP on healthcare than our major competitors. Every day America spends twice as much on health—$2 billion—as we did for a day of Desert Storm.

In 1980, 12.5% of Americans under 65 had no health insurance. Today, that number is 16%.

In 1980, total spending by federal and state governments on healthcare totaled $105 billion. Today it totals almost $300 billion.

Why, if we insure fewer people and provide less care, are we still spending more than any other nation in the world?

It doesn't have to be this way.

Under the Clinton plan for national health insurance reform, all Americans will have affordable healthcare. Employers and employees will either purchase private insurance or opt to buy into a public program. The poor and the unemployed will have access through the public program, and will be asked, to the extent possible, to share some of the costs.

All Americans will be covered with a core benefit package, and no person will be cut off, canceled, denied or forced to accept low-quality care. We'll bring down costs for middle-class families, maintain a choice of providers and assure comprehensive coverage.

My healthcare plan will:

1. Streamline the 1,500 different insurance underwriting practices and reform the federal and state bureaucracies that regulate health.

2. Establish a National Board including healthcare consumers, providers and payers to set annual budget targets to guide public and private expenditures and to define a core benefit package that businesses will be able to afford for their workers.

3. Eliminate tax breaks for drug companies that raise their drug prices faster than our incomes go up, speed the FDA approval process and limit marketing and lobbying deductions by the pharmaceutical industry.

4. Develop an alternative dispute resolution system to avoid costly legal battles that force up insurance costs; end "defensive medicine."

5. Create group networks to improve quality and control costs.

6. Provide basic coverage for the poor and unemployed via a public program with some form of copayments to discourage overutilization and to encourage shared responsibility. The disabled and the elderly will have access to comprehensive long-term care from Medicare, including inexpensive in-home services designed to foster independence.

7. Protect small businesses by basing premiums on a community-based rating system, allowing small employers to band together to purchase less expensive insurance.

By containing costs and eliminating waste, and by providing a vision of change and a commitment to leadership, we can protect our families' pocketbooks while guaranteeing affordable, comprehensive, high-quality healthcare and long-term care for all.

This guarantee will be the hallmark of the Clinton administration.

Doctors say lawsuit fear leads to unneeded tests

MAY 18—An American Medical Association survey of about 1,000 physicians found that 84%—more than four out of five—increasingly are ordering tests that may be unnecessary as a way of dodging the threat of malpractice suits.

The figure is almost 10% greater than the 75% of physicians who reported practicing "defensive medicine" in 1989, the AMA Gallup telephone survey found.

It also represents the most physicians in history who have tried to protect themselves by ordering extra tests, adding $20 billion to the annual cost of U.S. healthcare and demonstrating the destructive economic effect that the fear of malpractice suits has on those costs, according to AMA Executive Vice President James Todd, M.D.

"The cost is $20 billion annually and rising," Dr. Todd said.

The survey revealed that 93% of family and general practitioners said they ordered the extra tests to avoid the threat of malpractice suits.

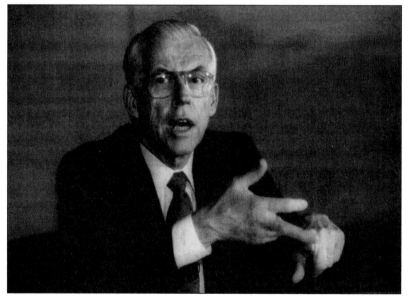

AMA Executive Vice President Dr. James Todd said that many physicians order extra tests to protect themselves from malpractice suits.

However, three out of four doctors aged 65 or older and 70% of doctors working in teaching hospitals said the fear of malpractice was not their reason for ordering more tests.

Replacing the current malpractice system with a no-fault system was favored by more than half of the physicians surveyed.

In a no-fault system juries can award damages for a patient's actual loss, but they cannot award additional, or punitive, damages.

Because the amount of money patients can win in such suits is limited, a no-fault system in theory could lower the number of lawsuits and bring down the cost of malpractice insurance, its supporters say.

The AMA and President Bush also have called for reforming medical malpractice laws.

Gallup also surveyed physicians about Medicare and found that at least 84% treat Medicare patients.

In fact, 12% of physicians said that Medicare patients comprise 61% or more of their total patients.

In addition, about 86% of respondents said they were at least somewhat familiar with the new Resource-Based Relative Value Scale payment system.

Almost as many physicians, 82%, said the medical

profession should negotiate directly with the government regarding physician fees, while approximately 71% said the profession should settle its own fee disputes.

Regarding physician-patient disputes, about 30% of respondents from the general public said that conflicts should be resolved by state licensing boards, while one in four people said that medical societies should resolve the problems.

Generalists protest 2nd-class 0.3% Medicare raise

WASHINGTON, D.C., MAY 27—While Medicare plans an inflation increase of only 0.3% next year for primary-care services, surgical fees will increase by 2.6%, Health and Human Services Secretary Louis Sullivan, M.D., announced.

The disparity in the inflation updates angered physicians and primary-care organizations, including the American Society of Internal Medicine and the American Medical Association, which said that separate volume standards for primary care and surgery undermine the intent of payment reform.

Each year, HHS sets a target, called a volume performance standard, for increases in services in the Medicare program. If physician services exceed that target, HHS then can cut future fee updates, intended to offset inflation.

For example, primary-care fees need to rise by 2.2% next year to keep pace with practice expenses. But Medicare will increase the fees by just a fraction of that because doctors provided more primary-care services in 1991 than Medicare had allowed under its volume performance standard.

Surgical services will receive a 2.6% increase because surgeons did not exceed their 1991 target.

Dr. Sullivan said he is considering other initiatives to help primary care, including speeding up the transition to the new Medicare fee schedule.

But John Hartman, M.D., an internist in Charleston, W.Va., said any help could be too little, too late.

"To not give us even a realistic increase in charges to cover inflation is just another indicator of why primary-care physicians are being driven out of practice," he said.

"Obviously, everything else goes up 3% to 4% a year, most everybody raises their employees 5%, obviously one's overhead goes up and one's income has a ceiling. At some point, one's overhead and ceiling meet, and we can't afford to practice," Dr. Hartman added.

HHS proposed new volume performance standards for 1993, under which the volume of primary-care services will be allowed to increase more than surgical services before future fee increases are jeopardized.

Primary-care physicians will continue to see increases from payment reform, which is separate from the yearly inflation update.

U.S. Supreme Court's abortion ruling could influence doctors' role in counseling patients

WASHINGTON, D.C., JUNE 29—The U.S. Supreme Court's ruling on abortion gives states broad powers to dictate how a doctor should deal with a patient who wants to end her pregnancy, medical experts said.

Today's high court ruling, which upheld most of a Pennsylvania law restricting abortion, likely will lead to waiting periods, parental-consent rules and required doctor-patient counseling in other states, experts said.

"This gives all other states a green light to come up with whatever restrictions they can get away with," said Michael Policar, M.D., Planned Parenthood's vice president for medical affairs.

"Most of them are consent and notification, and they do interfere with the doctor-patient relationship," Dr. Policar said. Many doctors believe the federal government has no right to interfere with that relationship, he said.

In its 5-4 ruling on the Pennsylvania abortion statute, the Supreme Court allowed restrictions that do not impose an "undue burden" on a woman's right to choose an abortion.

The court struck down a provision that required married

women to notify their husbands when seeking abortions. But it upheld other provisions, including parental notification for minors, a 24-hour waiting period, informed-consent requirements and detailed physician recordkeeping on abortions.

The American College of Obstetricians and Gynecologists said in a statement that it will take time to determine the full implications of the high court's ruling.

But the group said it fears that states will interpret the decision as "carte blanche" to approve similar restrictions.

A 24-hour waiting period and doctor-patient counseling on abortion alternatives already are required in 13 states, according to the Alan Guttmacher Institute. Another eight require informed consent but no waiting period. Twenty states have parental-consent or -notification requirements, according to the institute.

Under the Pennsylvania abortion law, doctors must offer to counsel women seeking abortions about the methods of abortion, its physical and emotional risks and the medical risks of childbirth.

They also must provide a booklet of drawings depicting

stages of fetal development at two-week intervals, and a directory of local agencies that provide prenatal care, adoption and financial aid for pregnant women.

Women are free to refuse this counseling. The doctor must note in the patient's medical history that it was offered and either accepted or refused.

Much of the recordkeeping doctors must do under the new Pennsylvania law is not new, a state Health Department spokesperson said. But now, some of it—including the names and office addresses of abortion providers—is subject to public disclosure as long as the providers accept state or federal funds.

Doctors already file individual reports on each abortion they perform, but now they also must include how they determined the gestational age of the fetus and whether a medical emergency existed that made the abortion necessary. The reports already require the patient's age, race and marital status.

Patient names are not required, and the information will not be released to the public, except in summary reports, a Health Department spokesperson said.

The Bush administration is fighting in court to prohibit all medical personnel except doctors from mentioning abortion as an option in federally funded clinics.

Some doctors, and the American Medical Association, have said they fear this so-called "gag rule" could lead to bans on counseling for other medical procedures, especially ones that cost the government money.

After the latest Supreme Court ruling, the AMA said in a statement that it still leaves the decision to support or oppose abortion up to its individual members.

But it warned that requiring parental consent or notification could lead minors to seek abortions from nonmedical facilities, or to attempt abortions themselves.

In contrast to the Supreme Court ruling, Germany recently broadened its abortion law to give women in what was West Germany the more liberal abortion rights of their neighbors in the former East Germany. A German woman now can get an abortion in the first trimester if she says she is in a state of distress, and if she goes through official counseling.

After the first trimester, a woman can get an abortion only if her physician certifies that the pregnancy threatens the woman's life, or if the fetus has serious medical problems.

Before, a woman in West Germany could get an abortion only if a doctor ruled the pregnancy put her health at risk.

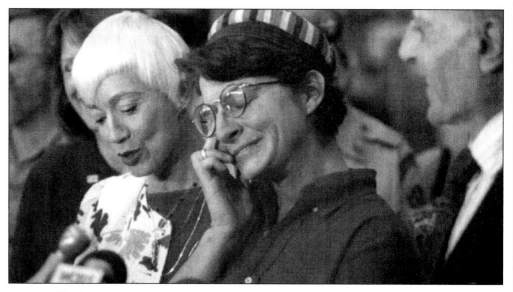

Seizure of French abortion pill upheld

JULY 7—Banned French RU 486 "abortion pills" were seized from pregnant Californian Leona Benten when she arrived in New York City on a flight from London, days after the U.S. Supreme Court ruling upheld Pennsylvania's abortion restrictions that dictated doctors' counseling role.

Lawyers for the Center for Reproductive Law and Policy in New York City challenged the U.S. import ban on RU 486, saying the government did not allow time for public comment before imposing the ban, and thus violated administrative rules. A federal judge then ruled that the government acted illegally in confiscating the drug, but the U.S. Court of Appeals for the Second Circuit in Manhattan blocked the judge's order. The appeals court stay was upheld by the Supreme Court.

RU 486 is being tested as a postcoital contraceptive, as well as for meningiomas, Cushing's disease and several other uses, according to its manufacturer, Roussel-Uclaf. The drug is expected to present an important issue to the Clinton administration.

Bush administration rejects Oregon health plan

By James W. Fiscus

PORTLAND, ORE., AUG. 3—The Bush administration's rejection of the Oregon Health Plan, saying it violates the Americans with Disabilities Act, has shocked and angered many Oregon leaders, and they now must decide whether to amend the plan to try to meet the federal government's demands.

The plan, which prioritized Medicaid payment of medical treatments according to their costs and benefits, required federal waivers from Medicaid laws. While eliminating benefits for some of the indigent, it would have immediately added 130,000 to the Oregon Medicaid rolls, which now number 205,000.

"I regret that I am unable to give your application final approval, particularly given the real possibility that Oregon's general approach will serve as a model for other states," Health and Human Services Secretary Louis W. Sullivan, M.D., wrote in a letter to Oregon Gov. Barbara Roberts.

HHS General Counsel Mike Astrue said that the plan's design was "based in substantial part on the premise that the value of a disabled person's life is less than the value of the life of a person without a disability."

That premise violates the Americans with Disabilities Act, which took effect last month, HHS officials said. Astrue is expected to spend a week in Oregon at the end of this month to help clarify the agency's problems with the Oregon plan.

Amending the Medicaid waivers in any fashion could take over three months, Oregon leaders say, especially if any of the serious underpinnings of the plan are changed.

John Kitzhaber, M.D., president of the Oregon Senate and the driving force behind the Oregon plan, said the denial was political. He called the use of the ADA a "smoke screen," behind which President Bush was avoiding confronting the fundamental issues surrounding the healthcare debate.

"We have been betrayed," agreed Oregon Republican Sen. Bob Packwood, who invested heavy political capital during his re-election campaign to ensure approval of the waivers.

The core of the Oregon Health Plan is a prioritized list of 709 pairs of medical conditions and their treatments. The list would determine—depending on available funding—which procedures are covered by Medicaid.

It also would set minimum standards for employer-paid health plans under a "play or pay" policy mandating health insurance.

Procedures paid for under the plan would include treatment for tuberculosis, cirrhosis of the liver not related to alcohol and spina bifida. Those not included in the plan include therapy for viral hepatitis, chronic bronchitis and acute upper respiratory infections.

AIDS treatment would be paid for unless the patient were thought to be in the last six months of life.

President, Clinton make doctor-to-doctor pitch

By Bill Ingram

SEPT. 10—The top doctors in the Bush and Clinton political campaigns have made strong appeals for their parties' healthcare reform plans, aimed at controlling costs and solving access, portability and malpractice problems.

Bush's plan, based on a tax-credit and deduction scheme and small-company risk pools, would preserve the doctor's role as "an integral part of the most advanced healthcare system in the world," argued Peter Collis, M.D., an emergency physician.

Malpractice damages would be capped and costs contained by a simplified claims system and managed care, but the fee-for-service option would be preserved. "We're really going to empower the strength of the individual doctor," Dr. Collis wrote.

The Bush plan eschews rationing. "Once you start drawing the line on technology, the next thing you know you're delivering second-class healthcare."

Clinton's universal access plan, also featuring malpractice reform and simplified claims, would be directed by cost-capping review boards on which physicians would actively participate, said Irwin Redlener, M.D., a specialist in community pediatrics.

Doctors would also participate in community provider networks formed by physicians, insurers, hospitals and clinics.

"The delivery of care remains in the private sector," asserted Dr. Redlener. And astute doctors "will wind up exerting more control over their professional lives than at any time in the last three decades."

Prevention is another key component of the Clinton plan. His strategy for improving preventive care in schools and expanding community health centers in underserved areas "is an extension of family values that really mean something," Dr. Redlener wrote.

'Universal insurance' plan unveiled by ACP

WASHINGTON, D.C., SEPT. 14—The American College of Physicians, which represents 77,000 internists, introduced a proposal to provide healthcare coverage for all Americans.

The proposal, "Universal Insurance for American Health Care," signals physician support for a "play or pay" plan, also advocated by Democratic presidential candidate Gov. Bill Clinton, which would require companies to provide coverage for employees or to pay into a government-sponsored insurance fund.

Under the ACP plan, however, the public system would

also cover people over age 60, those requiring high-cost care, the unemployed and all retirees. Employees eligible for private insurance would have to pay a maximum of half the cost, based on their ability to afford that.

Funding for the public system would come from Medicare, Medicaid, and other government health programs, payroll taxes from employers not sponsoring private insurance, income-linked premiums from retirees and other tax revenue.

Private insurers would have to accept applicants despite any pre-existing conditions, and calculate premiums based on a community rating.

The proposal would offer guidelines that give doctors more freedom to use their judgment instead of being constrained by what procedure is covered. Actions that went outside the guidelines would be subject to advisory panel reviews.

The proposal also calls for:
- A national cap on health spending.
- A cap on malpractice awards for noneconomic damages.
- Public and private sponsorship of health insurance.
- A national healthcare budget to be determined by Congress, allocated to states and administered at the state level.
- Uniform benefits for everyone, which would include both preventive and long-term care.
- Consolidation of public programs so that they offer the same benefits as private insurance.
- Regulation of the supply of doctors and medical facilities.

Speedier drug approval with makers chipping in

By Fran Kritz

OCT. 7—In a decision that could dramatically change the way prescription drugs come to market, the government and the pharmaceutical industry have agreed on a series of user fees that would be used to hire additional Food and Drug Administration examiners and to speed the drug-approval process.

While the plan may cost drug companies several hundred thousand dollars a year, the FDA and drug manufacturers agree that the decision could help restore the millions companies lose when a drug approval is delayed.

The agreement is intended to avert what government and industry analysts say is a catastrophe waiting to happen: the inability of the FDA to handle the increasing number of new drug applications. With the additional funding and staff, the FDA could cut drug-approval time in half for priority drugs and by eight months for standard drugs.

Under the proposal, manufacturers would pay annual company- and product-registration fees, as well as application fees for each new drug. The money would be used to hire at least 600 additional drug reviewers and pay for other drug-approval-related costs, according to the FDA.

U.S. Rep. John Dingell (D-Mich.) and Sen. Edward Kennedy (D-Mass.) are expected to introduce user-fee legislation. The Health and Environment Subcommittee of the House's Committee on Energy and Commerce held a hearing last month on the proposed bill, whose concept has the approval of both the drug companies and the Bush administration.

User-fee bills were rejected by the pharmaceutical industry in the past because they called for decreasing the FDA's government-allotted funds and supplementing them with user-fee revenue, Gerald Mossinghoff, president of the Pharmaceutical Manufacturers Association, said at last month's hearing.

Mossinghoff and other industry officials, including those from Glaxo Inc., Genentech Inc., Merck & Co., Inc. and the Upjohn Co., said they would support the bill if the fees were added to existing FDA appropriations and used only to pay for the approval of new drugs and biotechnology products.

The manufacturers also stipulated that the fees be reasonable and that the government must promise a long-term commitment to improvements in the drug-approval process.

The average drug approval now takes about 20 months, but it is expected to be shortened to 12 months once the new reviewers are hired. The review time for priority drugs, such as those for treating AIDS and other life-threatening diseases, could be shortened from 12 months to six months. FDA Commissioner David Kessler, M.D., has said that while the agency now approves six to 12 new products each year, it is expecting an eightfold increase in biotechnology product applications. The additional reviewers are expected to address that projected increase.

Dr. Kessler said the plan will neither lower the agency's standards nor compromise the integrity of the review process. "I am simply talking about getting the resources we need to keep pace," he said. "The user-fee system is the only way we could provide an adequate number of reviewers."

The core proposal calls for drug companies to pay an annual $50,000 registration fee, an annual $5,000 fee for each drug on the market and $150,000 for each new drug application. For now, generic and over-the-counter drugs would not be subject to the fees.

The user fees are expected to bring in between $75 million and $200 million each year for FDA use.

"The interest of this committee in authorizing...FDA user fees comes at an opportune moment," Dr. Kessler said, adding that his agency is continually underfunded.

Fees would be waived or reduced for small companies. Although larger companies could end up paying hundreds of thousands of dollars in user fees, however, FDA officials say that companies make an additional $10 million per month, on average, for each month the approval process is reduced.

Upjohn, for example, which has 58 products on the market, would pay yearly fees of at least $340,000, even in a year with no new drug applications.

The AMA supports the user-fee idea. "Even the most casual observer has seen that the FDA can't [currently] do everything it is supposed to do," said M. Roy Schwarz, M.D., senior vice president for education and science. "Anything we can do to speed up the ... review of new products will be very useful and is long overdue."

Bush won in a landslide...

Nov. 12—The problem was the now-lame-duck president chose the wrong forum—the 130,000 primary-care doctors in the United States.

In something approaching the converse of results in the electorate, Bush doubled President Clinton's total when doctors' straw-votes were counted.

At that, Bush took a terrific fall. In the first tally, last June, he garnered 77% of doctors' votes and Clinton trailed at about 11%, pretty much the same as "none of the above."

By July, without saying word one (Remember? Bush and Clinton had each pitched the doctors with 500-word statements), billionaire H. Ross Perot had headed Clinton, gaining 24% of the votes.

Then Perot walked away, Bush consolidated his position at 47% and Clinton limped at 19.4%. Good luck, Bill.

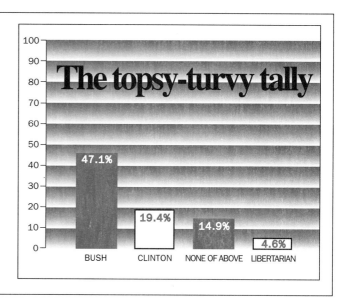

The topsy-turvy tally

BUSH 47.1% CLINTON 19.4% NONE OF ABOVE 14.9% LIBERTARIAN 4.6%

Is HCFA heeding physicians' cries for clarity?

By Bill Ingram and Brant Mittler, M.D.

Nov. 12—Amid bitter protest by many generalists that the specter of downcoding and overutilization is threatening their livelihood at a time when they can scarcely meet their overhead, a wee light has appeared at the end of the tunnel.

The Health Care Financing Administration conceded that it should consult the profession more closely in preparing documentation standards. The American Medical Association acknowledged that "not enough generalists are participating in the [fee-policy formulation] process" with Medicare-carrier directors. And HCFA "refinements" were expected to address inequalities in hospital visit codes.

Disclosing that HCFA is working with the AMA to promulgate national documentation guidelines by next spring, Gary Kavanagh, deputy director of the agency's Bureau of Program Operations, said, "One thing we've learned from the Early Claims Review program is that we've got to sit down and communicate more."

HCFA's failure to hold any real dialogue on documentation is doctors' chief complaint. As a result, especially with patients who have multiple, chronic problems, physicians are forced to work in the dark to validate visit codes.

Their major concerns: rejection or downcoding of claims involving routine preventive care (advice, exams), diagnosis ("comprehensive exam" ill-defined) and decision making (extensive histories demanded).

Voicing the frustration of tens of thousands of family practitioners, Rosemarie Sweeney, an American Academy of Family Physicians vice president, said, "Deeply resentful doctors are saying quite frankly that they are documenting for dollars rather than good medicine."

"Agreed," said Philip Lee, M.D., chief of the Physicians Payment Review Commission, the builder and monitor of the Resource-Based Relative Value Scale.

"The American Medical Association just testified that not enough generalists have been participating in the policy

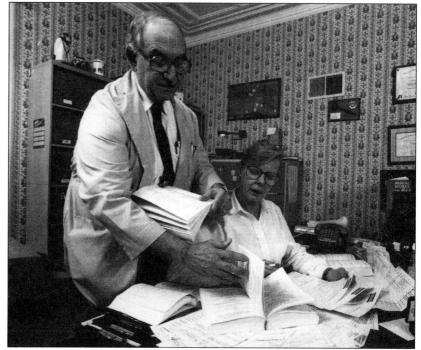

Physicians drowning in a sea of HCFA-rejected and downcoded claims.

process and that recently there has been significant improvement.

"I know. Doctors all over the country are hurting. I've been talking to them. A Seattle internist just told me about five generalists in his area going over to HMOs recently.

"We're all aware that the relative work value is not accurate and must be straightened out. Look at internists. Their conversion factor has been cut 3%. They've lost their specialty differential. Many suffer from the geographic adjustment. Practice costs keep going up."

Some relief may be provided by "refinements" in hospital visit codes, due out next week, Dr. Lee hinted. "The initial hospital visit under RBRVS pays less than subsequent visits. That doesn't make sense," he said.

Medicare fee inequalities are such, he conceded, that "the suggestion has been made [within PPRC] that doctors with [substantial] Medicare practices get a 60% fee bonus."

That prospect scarcely mollifies doctors who have been through HCFA's Early Claims Review grinder. About 12,500 claims were audited nationwide, "less than 1% of the multi-

million Medicare claims," according to the American Society of Internal Medicine's John Hernandez.

In 40% to 50% of cases, HCFA found that doctors failed to substantiate the level of service coded. "But they did not share [a single example] of documentation with actual determinations as to what levels of history, examination and decision making they felt was appropriate," Hernandez said. "So we have no way to judge whether we agree or disagree."

Of 335 Texas claims reviewed, 49% were "nonverified," but Texas Blue Cross gave no downcoding breakdown. In 252 Maryland cases, the carrier said nobody had coded too low. In a New York "focused review" of 40 cases, the Blues found a 79% "disagreement" rate.

"We're making a good-faith effort to achieve [dead-center] accuracy in coding—no doctor upcoding, no carrier downcoding," said Daniel Johnson, M.D., speaker of the AMA House of Delegates. "The worst-case scenario is that HCFA sets up as many hoops as possible. I can tell you one thing. You can look for an AMA thrust against price control."

Behold HCFA's theater of the absurd

Nov. 12—Franz Kafka's *The Trial* "states the problem of the absurd in its entirety," Albert Camus wrote. Ditto downcoding and overutilization.

In the book, Joseph K., a respectable Chief Clerk at a bank, is arrested and goes through hell the rest of his days, sardonically and existentially fighting a charge about which he is told zip.

At the end, when two goons proffer a butcher knife so he can kill himself, and he hesitates, one plunges it into his heart.

For parallelism, behold members of a once-respected profession receiving an empyrean decree via HCFA reviews that they are running amok behaviorally, oututilizing peers and upcoding, only to be denied so much as a glimpse of their peers; and as ASIM's John Hernandez points out, "denied shared examples of documentation with actual determinations as to what levels of history, examination and decision making [HCFA] felt was appropriate."

In other words, convicted like Willie Miranda on the high seas.

It's guilt by association with unbridled greed. Carrier explicators throw up a few slides, cite horrendous "nonverification" results, and now, as a carrier harrier tells us, "it's up to state and county medical associations and specialty societies, locally and nationally, to educate doctors in the appropriate patterns [of utilization and documentation]."

A med-group honcho detachedly adds, "We think we've given doctors the tools [to utilize and document properly] as best we could, but some are just not using them."

So as healers burn with bitterness and balk at bawling mea culpa, some of their own organizations seem to play Josef Goebbels for Herr HCFA, metaphorically beckoning to Joseph K. with a knife.

Granted, working in the wings as the deadly drama debouches, HCFA is actually preparing documentation standards. By trickle-down trajectory, the AMA will catch the hot potatoes next spring, masticate them with ASIM, AAFP and AOA and haggle with HCFA about carbohydrate exchange before they go into effect.

Ultimately, as sure as God made little green apples, there will be a crunch. Doctors will be cited as upcoders until they go down-level and take a lesser fee. Doctors will be cited individually as utilization outliers and their collective volume excesses reckoned, too, wiping out fee increases or even bringing decreases. "They'll be picked up one way or another," says the carrier harrier.

According to a statement by ASIM to HCFA's panel of consultants, the Practicing Physicians Advisory Council, six out of 10 doctors ASIM talks to say, "The new coding system will make it easier for carriers to reduce payments for internists' visits. Many of the results of [HCFA's] monitoring initiatives appear to bear out these fears."

It goes beyond fear. In an interview on the making of the film *The Trial*, the late Anthony Perkins was asked whether he applied Stanislavski in approaching the role of Joseph K., or what. Perkins replied, "You know, I asked Orson Welles [the director] about that. He said, 'Play it like you're guilty as hell.' "

So go get a guilt complex about upcoding, okay? At the same time, as a cunning FP suggests, go to your bag of tricks. Figure the overhead you must meet and the income you anticipate, then add patients and shave the time you see everybody by, say, a minute. Call patients back in 10 days instead of two weeks. Find reasons to do more tests.

Whatever it takes, Dr. K. —*B.I.*

B.I. is Bill Ingram, editor in chief of Medical Tribune and winner of the 1992 Clarion Award for Newspaper Editorial/Opinion Column.

COMMENTARY

Three battles to watch in the 1990s

By David M. Eddy, M.D., Ph.D.

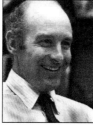

THE YEAR 1992 HAS BEEN A fascinating one for health policy. Buzzwords such as guidelines, outcomes, patient preferences and total quality management came to life. Proposals for healthcare reform were not only being pushed with increasing vigor, but were actually being taken seriously. The seemingly incompatible goals of increasing quality, increasing access and lowering costs almost appear within reach.

Virtually all the activities that took shape in 1992 were bound together by a common theme: The days of laissez-faire, when physicians were free to do as they pleased, are rapidly disappearing. The unit being managed in "managed care" has narrowed from hospitals (e.g., caps on hospital costs, review of hospital admissions), to broad disease categories (e.g., DRGs), to very specific treatments and patient indications (e.g., coverage policies, outcomes management and guidelines).

Because the content of care has traditionally been the exclusive domain of physicians, these trends will encounter increasingly vigorous resistance. There will be three main battles to watch as the decade unfolds. They will be over evidence, costs and physician autonomy.

The battle over evidence. How much evidence is needed to say that a treatment (defined very broadly to include any type of medical intervention) should be used and should be paid for?

Traditionally, physicians have been given very wide latitude to decide how to treat their patients. A decision could be justified by little more than an observation that it was "standard and accepted," or simply that the individual physician believed it was in the patient's best interest. However, as we examine more closely the actual evidence that supports many treatments, the realization grows that decisions about treatments must require more than consensus and testimony; they require support with real empirical evidence. This trend challenges the quality of physician judgment, it threatens physician control and it means that many treatments physicians want to use will not pass muster. Despite the fact that it follows the principle of "First, do no harm," it will be fought.

The battle over costs. Healthcare costs have been a major problem for decades. However, as the need to control costs pushes harder against the view that "cost should play no role in medical decisions," the battle lines are drawn.

Where will this battle be fought? Despite the fact that control of costs was a major stimulus for the new reform proposals, the fact is that none of them actually give operational instructions for how that should be done. Instead, the

proposals describe schemes for routing payments to put pressure on others to figure that out. The proposals acknowledge this with phrases like "decent," or "basic," or "necessary" care, which clearly imply that reducing costs will require retreating from the idea of covering all people for all possible care. And that is where the battleline will be: Just what treatments, for what indications, should be included in this as yet undefined package called "decent," "basic" or "necessary" care?

The battle over physician autonomy. For obvious reasons, many physicians are not going to like current trends in the areas of either costs or evidence. Such trends threaten what has historically been one of the most sacrosanct, untouchable features of medical practice—the autonomy of physicians to do as they please.

Historically, the mandate to physicians has been to apply their best judgment to provide the best possible care to their individual patients. Both components of that mandate are under fire—the quality of their judgments is being questioned, and the idea of maximizing the care of an individual is being replaced by a different set of instructions—to maximize the health of a population. Because a high-cost, heroic treatment for one can deprive hundreds of others of more mundane but more beneficial treatments, physicians will be increasingly asked to act as members of a team and give up to others some of the resources they would prefer to spend on their individual patients. It is easy to see that this will meet resistance; if we really believe that resources are limited and if we really want to allocate them to maximize the health of all patients, physicians will no longer be able to do everything they want to do, and will often be asked to do things they do not want to do.

The future. How will these battles come out? Two things are clear. One is that the people served by healthcare organizations that anchor their decisions to evidence rather than to beliefs, that take costs into account, that allocate resources to achieve the most bang for the buck, and that have physicians who act as a team—those will be the healthiest people. The other is that organizations with those qualities will be able to offer a higher quality of care for a lower cost than organizations that do not. They will be the ones that thrive in the coming decade. The others will struggle to survive.

Dr. Eddy is professor of health policy and management at the Duke University School of Medicine in Durham, N.C., and a senior advisor for health policy and management for the Kaiser Permanente health-maintenance organization in Southern California.

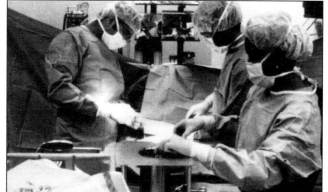

Still under debate: who pays for bone-marrow transplants?

Index

Abdominal compression: 87
Abortifacients (See also individual drug names): 110, 116, 119, 316, 330
Abortion: 108, 110, 112-113, 116, 119, 121, 124, 129-130, 286, 311, 315-317, 329-330
Accidents (See also injuries): 14, 45, 75, 88, 193, 203
ACE deletion polymorphism: 83
ACE inhibitor: 72, 75, 77, 88, 93
Acebutolol: 101
Acetaminophen: 48, 54, 205
Acne: 110,   205, 253, 255-257, 265-266, 271
Acrodermatitis chronica atrophicans: 263
Acupuncture: 24, 259
Acyclovir: 22, 29
Addiction (See also drug addiction and alcoholism): 15, 23, 135-136, 188, 234, 310, 321
Adenosine: 75
Adenovirus: 44, 50, 56
Adrenal medulla graft: 212
Aging: 16, 18, 120, 138, 141, 171, 193, 205, 313, 318
AGT: 83
AIDS
 awareness: 279, 287-288, 301-302
 blood transfusions: 282, 287, 292-293, 295
 cases: 277, 279, 282-285, 288, 292-296, 298-300, 303
 definition: 277, 298, 303
 HIV: 67, 110-111, 114, 131, 188, 190, 225, 252, 276-277, 279, 278-289, 290-302, 303, 314, 316
 non-HIV: 284, 286-287, 295, 298, 303
 resistant tuberculosis: 299
 survival: 279, 279-281, 283-284, 290-291, 295, 297
 test: 277, 279, 278-279, 284, 288, 291-293, 296-298, 303
 transmission: 278-282, 286-289, 292-293, 300-301, 316
 vaccine: 277, 279, 278-284, 286-287, 292, 296, 300-301, 311-312
 women: 276-277, 279, 279-281, 284, 286, 288-289, 293-294, 297-298
Albumin: 42, 50, 61, 147, 157, 197, 257
Albuterol: 44, 259
Alcohol: 13, 14, 19, 21, 28, 34, 75, 75-76, 78-79, 81, 83, 90, 109, 116, 118, 147, 149, 152, 155-156, 160, 165-166, 185, 184, 194, 196, 203, 229, 288, 313, 319, 331
Alcoholism: 75, 90, 288
Allergic dermatitis: 258, 262, 270
Allergies
 airborne: 208, 260, 265
 dust mites: 24, 151, 166-167, 253, 261
 elderly: 16
 food: 254, 259, 261, 262, 263
 latex: 110, 251, 253, 253, 262, 270, 284, 298
Alteplase: 82, 100
Aluminum: 135, 137-138, 139
Alzheimer's disease: 20, 135-141, 188, 190-191, 193, 203-205

Amblyopia: 54
Amitriptyline: 34
Amlodipine: 72, 81, 101
Amniocentesis: 114-115, 117-119, 130
Amniotomy: 111
Amyotrophic lateral sclerosis: 137, 190
Anemia: 19, 28, 53, 65, 129, 151, 174, 214, 245, 279, 291
Angina: 73, 74, 76, 80-83, 86, 95, 98, 100, 102
Angiography: 84-85, 99, 100, 102
Angioplasty: 75, 74-75, 77, 83-85, 86, 88, 95, 98, 102, 173, 213
Anistreplase: 76, 82
Anorexia: 22, 135, 184
Anosmia: 152
Antibiotics (See also individual drugs): 13, 15, 17, 36, 114, 120, 130, 176, 182-184, 186, 191-192, 202, 207-208, 212, 251, 253, 257, 290, 317
Antihistamines (See also individual drugs): 16-17, 258, 262, 264
Antihypertensives (See also individual drugs): 72-73, 79, 83, 95-96, 101, 200
Antimicrobial therapy (See also individual drugs): 110, 184
Antipyretics (See also individual drugs): 54
Anxiety: 14-15, 18, 26, 36-37, 43, 51-53, 60, 66, 77, 135-137, 153, 155, 184, 193, 237-238, 302
Anxiolytics (See also individual drugs): 24, 26, 135, 137,184, 186
Apheresis: 75, 94
Arrhythmias: 21, 74, 78, 81-82, 103, 116, 128, 258
Arterial occlusion: 80
Arterial surgery: 80
Arteriography: 98
Arthritis
 rheumatoid: 120, 165, 251, 252, 255-256, 260-261, 264-265, 269-270
 osteo-: 17, 252, 260, 264
Artificial insemination: 122
Artificial sweeteners: 50, 145, 155, 161, 254
Aspartame: 50, 254
Aspirin: 48, 74, 77, 79-81, 88, 163, 185, 185, 192, 205-206, 232
Astemizole: 258
Asthma: 15, 14-17, 19, 25, 28, 33-34, 43, 44, 47, 52, 54-55, 59, 64-65, 114, 119, 151, 166, 250-251, 253, 252-256, 259-263, 265, 272, 319-320
Atenolol: 96, 200
Atovaquone: 277, 284, 286
Atrial fibrillation: 74, 84
Atropine: 54
Attention deficit disorder: 48
Autoimmune disease: 120, 147, 150, 165, 255, 260, 270, 290
Azathioprine: 263
Azithromycin: 22, 174
AZT, 276, 279, 278-285, 287, 290-292, 294-297
Aztreonam: 17

Back injuries: 22
Back pain: 17, 22-23, 190
Benign prostatic hyperplasia: 173-174, 177

Benzodiazepines: 24, 184, 186
Benzoyl peroxide: 255, 265-266
Beta-agonists (See also individual drugs): 15, 34, 44, 52, 251, 261, 272
Beta-blockers (See also individual drugs): 16, 24, 81, 86, 96, 99, 135-136, 187, 199-200, 272
Beta-carotene: 28, 152, 154, 156-157, 170
Biofeedback: 78
Birth control (See also contraceptives, individual methods): 110, 124, 127, 131
Birth rate: 49
Bjork-Shiley valve: 92
Bladder cancer: 161, 237, 241
Blood
 pressure (See hypo-, hypertension)
 storage: 154, 212
 transfusion: 225, 278, 282, 287, 293, 295, 299, 301, 314
Body fat, abdominal: 18
Body temperature: 16, 22-23, 128-129
Bone cancer: 231
Bone marrow transplant: 224-225, 230, 258
Borrelia burgdorferi: 36, 135, 184, 257, 267
Borreliacidal antibody: 18, 33
Botulinum: 42, 45, 45, 56-57
Bowen's disease: 259
Brain cancer: 226, 229, 232
Breast cancer: 17, 25, 30, 76, 85, 90-91, 108-109, 111, 113-116, 119, 121, 126-127, 131, 151, 155, 157, 170, 195, 222-223, 224-235, 236-237, 240-246, 247, 310-311, 313, 320
Breast enlargement: 313, 326
Breast-feeding: 45, 113, 117, 147-149, 151, 166, 254
Breast implants: 17, 25, 108-109, 115, 120, 131, 213, 226, 260, 311, 310-313, 322, 325-326
Breast self-examination: 120-121
Breast surgery (See also mastectomy): 111, 114, 226-227, 233, 240
Bronchodilators (See also individual drugs): 28-29, 34, 54, 272
Budesonide: 52
Bulimia: 136, 188
Bush, George: 90, 123, 186, 198, 255, 276-277, 283, 308, 310-313, 316-320, 327-328, 330-333
Buspirone: 13, 15, 26-27, 135, 137

Caesarean section: 109, 111-113, 117-118
Calcitonin: 22, 120, 201, 211
Calcium: 15, 19, 22-23, 50, 65-66, 80, 96, 120, 147, 149, 156, 160, 201, 211
Calcium antagonists (See also individual drugs): 80-81, 101
Calcium-channel blockers (See calcium antagonists)
Cancer (See also individual cancers): 12-13, 15, 14, 17, 25, 30-31, 44, 46, 48, 75-76, 85, 88, 90-91, 108-109, 111-116, 119, 121, 125-127, 131, 136, 144-145, 146-149, 151-157, 158-161, 169-170, 171, 172-174, 175-177, 184, 195, 201, 212, 218, 222-223, 225, 224-235, 236-246, 247, 250, 253-260, 266, 268-269, 271, 280, 284-286, 288, 296, 298, 310, 319-320, 325
Cancer prevention: 144, 154, 169-170, 223, 232, 246
Cancer statistics: 236
Candida esophagitis: 287
Candidiasis: 148, 295, 299, 303
Capsaicin:, 253, 252, 264
Captopril: 72-73, 77, 82, 88, 93, 96-97, 99, 200
Carcinoma (See cancer, individual cancers)
Carbamazepine: 138, 139-140
Carbon monoxide: 18, 136, 194, 232, 310
Cardiac arrest: 74-75, 78-79, 83, 87, 89, 94-95
Cardiopulmonary resuscitation: 45, 74-75, 84, 87, 89, 94-95, 102, 282, 316
Cardiovascular disease: 45, 74-76, 78-80, 82, 84, 88, 90, 101, 148, 165-166, 185, 189, 203, 206, 245, 254, 313
Carpal tunnel syndrome: 15, 17, 27, 214
Cataracts: 21, 153
Cefamandole: 111
Ceftriaxone: 55, 135
Cefuroxime: 37, 55
Cephalosporins: 55
Cerebral palsy: 42, 45, 45, 47, 56
Cerebral transluminal angioplasty: 213
Cervical cancer: 112-113, 115, 146, 158-159, 223-224, 286, 288, 298, 310
Chemical peels: 263
Chemical pollution: 174
Chemotherapy: 44, 46, 121, 187, 193, 195, 201, 223, 224-226, 229-230, 232, 234-235, 236-237, 247, 320
Chicken pox: 110
Chlamydia: 22, 110, 114, 120-121
Chlorthalidone: 101
Cholecystectomy: 148, 189, 193, 213-214, 215-218
Cholera: 15, 22, 38, 147, 185, 194, 210
Cholesterol: 12, 20, 73, 74-76, 78-80, 82-85, 86, 89-90, 94-96, 101, 141, 145, 147-151, 155-157, 159-163, 165-166, 168, 189, 203, 211, 225, 315
Chorionic villus sampling: 118-119, 130
Chronic fatigue syndrome: 53, 191, 205, 252, 257
Chronic mitral regurgitation: 85
Chronic obstructive pulmonary disease: 189
Cigarettes (See also passive smoke, smoking): 21, 26-27, 44, 112-114, 157, 227-228, 314
Cimetidine: 184
Circadian rhythm: 23
Cisplatin: 225
Clarithromycin: 290
CLIA rules: 39, 311-313
Clindamycin: 111, 130
Clinton, Bill: 108, 120, 131, 308-309, 313, 318-320, 327-328, 330-331, 333
Clozapine: 135-136, 184
Coarctation of the aorta: 80

Cocaine: 77, 136, 189, 319
Coffee: 75, 112, 145, 155, 158, 200
Color blindness: 20
Colorectal cancer: 146, 149, 153, 156, 170, 222, 224, 227, 230, 233, 236, 241
Colposcopy: 113, 115
Computer software, medical procedures information: 23
Congenital defects: 47, 77
Contraceptives (See also birth control, individual methods): 25, 27-28, 65, 120-121, 126
Coronary artery bypass surgery: 83, 86
Coronary artery disease: 75-76, 79-81, 83, 95, 102, 145, 155, 226
Corticosteroids (See also individual drugs): 15, 16, 19, 29, 33-34, 52, 128, 185, 187, 196-197, 211, 225, 251, 253
Craniofacial deformities: 51
Crohn's disease: 146-147, 158, 218, 263
Cromolyn: 16, 25, 29, 251, 272
Croup: 52
Cryptococcal meningitis: 278, 290, 295, 299, 303
Cyoctol: 253
Cystic fibrosis: 42, 44-46, 56, 108, 114, 118, 129-130, 185, 186-187, 193, 199, 213
Cytarabine: 228
Cytomegalovirus: 46, 258

Daycare centers: 46, 61
Defibrillation: 78-79, 81, 89, 94, 102
Dementia:137, 141, 191, 204, 298
Dengue fever: 23
Depression: 14-15, 18-19, 27, 31, 35, 52, 75, 81, 98, 112, 119, 123, 135-136, 138, 153, 155, 168, 184, 187-188, 194-195, 199-200, 205, 237-238, 295, 302
Dermatitis: 253, 255, 257-258, 262-263
Dermatomyositis: 253
Diabetes: 13, 20, 28, 32, 38, 42, 45, 47-50, 61, 65-66, 77-78, 80, 84, 101-102, 118, 146-147, 150, 157, 184-185, 187-190, 192-193, 203-206, 252, 264
Dialysis:, 184, 194, 313
Diarrhea: 17-18, 31, 35, 37-38, 50, 137, 147-151, 155, 158, 167-168, 190, 205, 210, 215, 279, 291
Dideoxycytidine: 278-279, 281, 283, 285, 290-291, 294
Dideoxyinosine: 281, 290, 292
Diet and Nutrition
 bingeing: 54
 liquid diet: 152, 167
 nutritional supplements: 153, 157, 167-168
Dietary fat: 14, 146-149, 155, 163, 170, 225, 236
Dietary fiber: 19, 146-147, 149, 155, 157, 163
Digital rectal exam: 173, 175, 222, 228
Digoxin: 80
Dihydroergotamine: 137
Diltiazem: 73, 83, 96
Dipyridamole: 75
Diuretics: 79, 95-96

DNA markers: 82
Dobutamine: 75
Domestic violence: 14, 19
Down's syndrome: 117
Doxazosin: 101
Doxycycline: 22, 37, 111, 114, 135, 174, 291-292
Drowning: 48, 333
Drug addiction (See also addiction, alcoholism): 15, 21, 23, 77, 135-136, 321
Drug testing: 24, 80
Dust mites: 24, 151, 166-167, 253, 261
Dwarfism: 212
Dysentery: 38, 183
Dyskaryosis: 115
Dyslexia: 44, 110
Dysplastic nevi: 271-272

Earlobe creases: 254
Earthquake: 15, 21, 36
Echocardiography: 75, 91, 111-112
Ecstasy: 21
Eczema: 43, 151, 166, 253-255, 257, 263
Electrocardiograms: 80, 82, 93
ELISA test: 33, 183
Enalapril: 72, 99, 101
Encephalitis: 18, 190
Endarterectomy: 75
Enhanced external counterpulsation: 83, 95
Epilepsy: 136, 138, 139-140, 187-188, 214
Epinephrine: 83, 259
Episiotomy: 116
Erectile dysfunction: 173
ERISA: 321
Erythema nodosum: 263
Erythromycin: 65, 114, 130, 184, 258
Esophageal cancer: 153, 247
Estrogen: 65, 113, 150, 210, 240
    patch: 19, 24, 54, 116, 211, 263
    replacement therapy: 15-16, 19, 27, 75-76, 90-91, 111, 114, 119, 211
Ethambutol: 262
Euthanasia: 309-311, 314, 316, 322-323
Exercise
    and diabetes: 84, 203
    during pregnancy: 27-28, 46, 109, 111-122, 124, 130, 187
Eye injuries: 17
Eye surgery: 17

Family history: 13, 14, 25, 28, 32, 45, 53, 119, 121, 125, 137, 151, 170, 191, 228, 230, 243, 246, 255, 296
Falloscope: 120
Famotidine: 184
Fast food: 146-147, 158
Fenfluramine: 18, 31
Fertility: 16, 28, 64, 110-111, 116, 120, 122-123, 126, 129, 172, 174, 175, 186, 194
Fertility drugs: 110, 116
Fibrinogen: 76, 81-82
Fibrinolytic therapy: 85
Fibromyalgia: 15, 27
Finasteride: 173-174, 177
Fire ants: 254
Fish oil: 113, 150, 187

5-hydroxytryptophan: 156
FK-506: 214, 217-218, 252
Fluconazole: 278, 287, 290
Fluoroquinolones (See also individual drugs): 19, 186
Fluoxetine: 22, 117, 136, 138, 187, 315
Folic acid: 28, 42, 131, 145-147, 150-152, 154, 158, 168-169
Food,
    labeling: 146-147, 156-157, 290, 310, 315, 317
    poisoning: 24, 43, 47, 49, 55, 64, 146, 150-151, 155, 194, 319
Fractures: 15, 22-23, 50, 84, 92, 114, 116, 120, 153, 165, 191-192, 201, 212
Framingham heart study: 74
Fundoplication: 212, 215
Fungal infections: 260, 271-272

Gallbladder disease: 13, 32, 148, 184, 188, 193
Ganciclovir: 229, 247
Garlic: 145, 147, 149, 153, 157, 162-163
Gastroesophageal reflux: 212, 215
Gemfibrozil: 12, 86
Gender studies: 75, 78-79, 102, 245
Gene therapy: 44, 56, 227, 247, 318
Genetic diseases: 118, 129
Genetic immunization: 254
Gestrinone: 110
GISSI: 80, 97
Goiters: 146
Gonorrhea: 120, 183
Graves' disease: 186, 198-199
Guns: 45, 49, 174, 231, 245, 315
GUSTO: 98

Hair loss: 74, 253, 260
Hair transplants: 260
Hansen's disease: 253
Head injury: 136, 188
Headache, migraine: (See migraine)
Healthcare
    Cost: 282, 285, 295, 308, 312, 314-315, 318-320, 324, 327-328, 330, 332, 335
    Fraud: 111, 122, 168, 311
    Reform: 312-314, 318, 321, 325-329, 331, 335
Hearing aids: 192
Heart disease (See also cardiovascular disease): 12-13, 20, 32, 45, 65, 73, 74-76, 78-80, 83, 87-90, 102, 141, 144, 148, 155-156, 160, 165-166, 170, 173, 186, 189, 203, 206, 227, 232, 254, 313
Heart attack (See also myocardial infarction): 73, 74, 76-77, 81-82, 84, 86-89, 92-93, 95, 99, 102, 149, 163, 184, 205
Heart valves: 81, 312, 325
Helicobacter pylori: 150, 183, 191-192, 207
Hemochromatosis: 146
Hemophilia: 28, 118, 129, 278, 286
Hemorrhoids: 213
Heparin: 80, 185, 197

Hepatitis A: 43, 51, 61-62, 152, 192
Hepatitis B: 43, 47, 51, 57-58, 60, 62, 67, 108, 114, 183, 186, 188, 190, 252, 288-289, 317, 320
Hepatitis C: 183, 186, 188, 191, 281
Herbal medicine: 45, 258
Herpes simplex: 16, 29, 48, 111, 260, 279, 286
Herpes zoster: 288, 295, 299
Hiccups: 24
High-density lipoproteins: 76, 79, 83, 85-86, 90, 151, 189, 203
Histamine H_2 receptor antagonists (See also individual drugs): 184
Hodgkin's disease: 225-226, 235
Holter monitor: 77
Home uterine-activity monitoring: 110, 122
HTLV-I and II: 279, 295, 299
Human papillomavirus: 115, 146-147, 226
Huntington's disease: 194
Hurricane Andrew: 15, 21, 37, 260
Hydrochlorothiazide: 96
Hyperactivity: 17, 52, 54, 256
Hyperbilirubinemia: 263
Hypertension: 13, 20, 28, 31-32, 49, 73, 75, 76, 78-81, 83-84, 95-97, 101-102, 145, 149, 155-156, 159, 173, 177, 200, 205
Hypnosis: 19-20, 24, 34
Hypoglycemia: 19, 146, 154, 189
Hypotension: 14, 79

IL-1 receptor: 193, 252
Ileocolic intussesception: 54
Immunizations (See also individual diseases, vaccination): 42-43, 44, 49, 60-61, 310, 319
Impotence: 174, 177, 215
In-vitro fertilization: 52, 63, 108, 114-115, 118, 120-121, 123, 126, 129-130
Infant carriers: 47
Infant formula: 43, 45, 54, 117, 146-149, 151, 154, 164
Infant mortality: 46, 50-51, 127, 314, 320
Inflammatory bowel disease: 218, 252, 295, 299
Influenza: 14, 16, 23, 48, 55, 252
Injuries: 14-17, 19, 22, 25, 33, 44-45, 48-50, 52, 54, 101, 111, 136, 188-189, 202, 213, 215-218, 261, 317
Insulin: 13, 18, 32, 49, 147, 159, 184, 187, 189, 191-193, 204
Insurance: 14, 39, 44, 76, 92, 94, 112, 124, 129, 289, 308-309, 311, 310, 312-316, 318-321, 324-328, 331-332
Interferon: 35-36, 183, 190, 237, 256, 279
Intrauterine device: 112, 124-125, 127
Iodine: 146, 151
IQ scores: 147
Iron: 28, 49-50, 53, 146, 151, 153
Irritable bowel syndrome: 19-20, 34
Ischemia: 78, 81-82, 98-99, 103, 123
ISIS-2: 80, 97

ISIS-4: 88, 97
Islet cell transplant: 187, 191
Isosorbide mononitrate: 73, 76, 88
Isotretinoin: 257, 265, 271

Jaw implants: 213
Johnson, Earvin "Magic": 278, 287
Joint pain: 59, 192, 208, 251, 255, 261

Kaposi's sarcoma: 295, 298-299
Keratitis: 185
Kessler, David: 126, 285, 313, 317, 322, 325-326, 332
Ketoconazole: 258, 287
Kevorkian, Jack: 232, 309, 311, 310-311, 316, 320, 322-323
Knee injury: 213
Knee replacement: 259-260

L-nitroarginine: 174
Labor: 110, 115-116, 118
    preterm: 122, 127
Lactase deficiency: 150
Laparoscopic surgery: 213-214, 216
Laser photorefractive keratectomy: 214
LATE: 99-100
Lead: 22, 43, 47-48, 52, 55, 64, 112, 146, 319
Left-ventricular dysfunction: 72, 80, 82, 99, 102
Leg cramps: 192
Legionnaires' disease: 17
Leishmaniasis: 209
Leprosy: 186, 253
Leukemia: 48, 187, 224-225, 227, 230-232, 234, 241-242, 244-245, 296
Leukoplakia: 257
Leuprolide: 113
Levonorgestrel: 127
Lindane: 258
Lipidemia: 94-95
Lipoproteins (See also High-, low-density lipoproteins): 75-76, 79, 83, 85, 90, 94-95, 150-151
Listeriosis: 113
Lithium: 39, 111
Lithotripsy: 193
Liver cancer: 226-227
Liver transplant: 53, 209-210, 286
Liver, artificial: 48
Loneliness: 74
Lovastatin: 94
Low birthweight: 47
Low-density lipoproteins: 78, 85-86, 94, 148, 150
Lung cancer: 13, 14, 152-153, 173, 225, 232, 234, 236-237, 247
Lupus, neonatal: 263
Lyme disease: 13, 15, 18, 21, 33, 37, 135, 184, 186, 253, 257-258, 263, 267-268
Lymph node cancer: 241
Lymphoma: 225, 230, 265, 270, 296, 298

Magnesium: 75, 78-79, 88, 96-97, 156
Magnetic resonance imaging: 85, 137, 213
Malaria: 45, 183, 186, 257, 267, 276, 287, 315
Malpractice: 23, 25, 26, 115, 311, 311, 313-314, 318, 324, 327-328, 331-332

Mammography: 17, 30, 114, 131, 222-223, 225, 224, 227-228, 230, 242-244, 246, 322
Manic-depression: 111
Marijuana: 172-173, 187, 310
Mastectomy: 226-227, 232-233, 235, 240, 313
Measles: 45, 47, 52, 59-60, 182, 257, 279-280
Medicaid: 52, 64, 112, 124, 135-136, 187, 199, 202, 311-312, 316-318, 320-321, 324, 326, 331-332
Medical education: 25, 87, 313, 321
Medical histories (See also family histories): 20
Medicare: 14, 26, 76, 84, 124, 176, 189, 194-195, 309, 311, 310-312, 314, 316, 318-321, 324, 326, 328-329, 332, 334
Medroxyprogesterone: 113, 115, 126-127
Megestrol acetate: 228
Melanoma: 224, 227, 231, 233-235, 250, 252, 255-256, 266, 271
Meningitis: 52, 55, 67, 113, 130, 183, 280, 290, 295, 299, 303
Menopause: 19, 27, 46, 91, 120, 126, 145, 150, 201, 211, 232
Methadone: 310
Methotrexate: 110, 121, 229, 251, 255
Methylphenidate: 51
Metyrapone: 112
Midwives: 112, 117, 128
Migraine: 14, 16, 19, 135, 137, 185, 196
Milk: 42-43, 45, 45, 50, 52-53, 61, 65-66, 144, 147, 147-154, 157, 160, 164-166, 255, 259
Miscarriage: 63, 111, 115, 119, 121, 286
MITI: 75, 92
Molluscum contagiosum: 295, 299
Monoclonal antibodies: 227, 229, 241, 251, 260, 269-270
MRFIT: 189, 203
Multiple births: 116, 130
Muscular dystrophy: 50, 114, 118, 129
Mycobacterium avium infection: 290
Mycoplasma: 121, 281
Mydriasis: 186
Myocardial infarction: 73, 74-75, 77, 80-85, 86, 88, 92-93, 97-100, 166, 192, 205-206, 316
Myopia: 214
Myotonic dystrophy: 185
Myringotomy: 46

Nadolol: 200
Naproxen: 20, 35
National Practitioner Data Bank: 311, 324
Nausea: 18, 22, 115, 119, 136-138, 155-156, 187, 190, 194, 196, 205, 270, 279, 291
Neural-tube defects: 28, 128, 131, 145, 150, 154, 168-169
Neurosurgery: 184, 214
Nicardipine: 73
Nicotine: 13, 15, 21, 24, 26, 79, 135
Nightmares: 18-19, 136
Nitric oxide: 72-73, 84, 101, 174
Nitrogen dioxide: 18, 136

Non-steroidal anti-inflammatory drugs (See also individual drugs): 185
Nonoxynol-9: 110, 279
Norgestimate/ethinyl estradiol: 119
Nosocomial infections: 152, 167, 229
Novello, Antonia: 13-14, 156, 311, 313, 315
Nurses' Health Study: 21, 144, 147, 148, 153, 155-156, 170
Nursing home care: 16, 20

Obesity: 13, 17, 31, 148, 151, 154, 159, 185, 203-204, 229, 241
Ofloxacin: 253
Olympics: 45, 80, 302, 315
Omeprazole: 191, 207, 215
Oocyte donation: 109, 118
Optic neuritis: 15
Oregon plan: 318, 331
Organ donors: 311, 313
Organ rejection: 217-218, 254
Organ transplant (See transplantation)
Osteopathy: 316
Osteoporosis: 15, 19, 22, 45, 90, 109, 116, 120, 153, 185, 188, 201-202, 211, 227
Otitis media: 55, 288
Ovarian cancer: 109, 125-126, 223, 224, 226, 235, 238, 253, 320
Ovarian cysts: 118
Oxazepam: 186
Oxytocin: 111
Oysters: 152
Ozone depletion: 233, 257

Pancreatic cancer: 230
Pap test: 113, 115, 117, 224
Parkinson's disease: 136, 187
Passive smoke: 48, 52, 121, 231
Peak-flow monitoring: 16, 28
Pediculosis: 258
Pelvic inflammatory disease: 111, 113, 124-125
Penicillamine: 265
Penile cancer: 226
Pentamidine: 290
Pentoxifylline: 296
Peptic ulcer disease: 150
Perchloroethylene: 20
Percutaneous transluminal coronary angioplasty: 85
Peroxidase: 285
Phentermine: 18, 31
Phenylketonuria: 28, 50
Phobia: 51
Photopheresis: 252-253, 264-265
Phototherapy: 19, 23, 136, 188, 263
Physicians' fees: 325-326, 333-334
Physicians' Health Study: 12, 21, 80, 189, 192, 203, 206
Plague: 192-193
Pneumonia: 130, 167, 183, 186, 225, 229, 277, 278, 280-281, 284, 286, 288, 290, 295, 298-299, 303, 315, 323
   Pneumocystis carinii: 225, 277, 278, 280-281, 284, 286, 290, 295, 298-299, 303
   Streptococcus: 183
Poison: 24, 49, 55
Polymerase chain reaction: 50, 82, 114-115, 118, 129, 135, 184, 188, 190, 281, 286, 295-296, 303

Polymyositis: 253
Positron Emission Tomography: 136, 188, 234
Potassium: 78, 253
Pravastatin: 94
Prazosin: 73, 96
Preconception counseling: 15, 27
Prednisolone: 52, 185, 196-197
Prednisone: 15, 165, 253, 255, 262, 295, 299
Pregnancy
   asthma: 119
   complications of: 113, 117, 147, 157
   diabetes:118
   diet during: 113, 117
   driving during: 113
   ectopic: 110, 120, 286
   exercise during: 112, 114
   maternal morbidity: 127
   smoking during: 114, 116, 120-121
   swimming with dolphins: 117-118, 128
   weight gain during:, 109, 116-117
Premenstrual syndrome: 117, 168
Prenatal care: 111, 113, 119, 121, 124, 128, 130, 152, 314, 330
Priapism: 174
Progesterone: 19, 108, 110, 115-116, 126
Prolotherapy: 23
Prostate cancer: 172-174, 175-177, 222, 224, 226, 228-229, 236, 238-240
Prostate specific antigen: 172-173, 175-177, 195, 222, 225, 228, 239-240
Prostratin: 286
Prostaglandin: 35, 174, 272
Psoriasis: 252, 264
Psychotherapy: 15, 74, 135, 154, 237
Pyoderma gangrenosum: 252, 263

Quarantine: 187, 200, 280, 311, 323
Quinine: 192

Radar guns: 174, 231, 245
Radiation-induced immune suppression: 257
Ranitidine: 183, 184-185, 207, 215
Recombinant human deoxyribonuclease I: 186, 199
Reconstructive surgery: 313
Renal disease: 184, 194
Repetitive motion disorder: 15
Respiratory distress syndrome: 43, 128, 150
Retinopathy: 17, 47, 58-59, 150, 184, 192, 206
Reye's syndrome: 48
Rhinovirus: 20, 35-36
Rifampin:182, 200, 253, 262, 278
Ritodrine: 116, 127-128
Roe v. Wade: 110, 112, 124
RU 486: 108, 110, 116, 119-120, 316, 330

Saccharin: 147, 149, 161
Salbutamol: 52
Salmonella: 150, 186
SAVE: 72, 77, 82, 88, 93, 99

Schizophrenia: 20, 135-136, 138, 184
Scleroderma: 120, 252-253, 264
Seasonal affective disorder: 19, 136
Seizures, febrile: 53
Septic shock: 193
Serum CA-125: 108, 113, 125-126
Sexual abuse: 46, 53, 110, 153, 321
Sexual activity: 14, 67, 78, 155, 289
Sexually transmitted diseases (See also individual diseases): 16, 22, 174, 279, 285, 319
Skin cancer: 14, 184, 232-233, 240, 250, 255, 257, 259, 266, 268-269
   Basal cell carcinoma: 252, 257-260, 269
   Squamous cell carcinoma: 225-226
Skin grafts: 260
Skin sun-damaged (See also sunscreen): 263, 266
Sleep
   apnea: 185, 188
   disorders: 15, 19, 136
   infants: 54, 66
Smoking (See also cigarettes, passive smoking): 13, 24, 26, 44, 46, 50, 73, 79, 81, 112-113, 116, 120, 135, 157, 212, 227-228, 231, 234, 314, 320
   cessation: 14-15, 21, 320
SOLVD: 72, 75, 99
Sotalol: 77, 81
Sperm donation
   microinjection of: 111
Spermicide: 100, 110, 279
Spina bifida: 42, 152, 168, 331
Spine densitometry: 19
Sports: 16, 22, 48-50, 115, 256, 262, 302
Staphylococcus aureus: 257
Step-care treatment: 200
Steroid: 52, 185, 196
Stomach cancer: 230
Strabismus: 57, 120
Streptococcus B infections: 120
Streptokinase: 76, 80, 85, 97-98, 100
Stress:, 112, 209
Stroke: 12, 73, 74-76, 78-79, 81, 84-85, 88-89, 97-98, 100-101, 137, 185, 205, 314, 323
Subdermal implants: 263
Sucralfate: 215
Sudden infant death syndrome: 43, 45, 48, 50, 53, 66, 121
Suicide: 46
   assisted (See also Kevorkian): 232, 320, 322-323
Sullivan, Louis: 114, 283, 314-315, 318, 320, 329, 331
Sumatriptan: 16, 135, 185, 196
Sunscreen: 14, 224, 250, 256-257, 259, 269
Swimming: 14, 45, 48, 109, 117-118, 128, 256
Syphilis: 33, 114, 279, 320
Systemic lupus erythematosus: 150, 165, 255

Tacrine: 137-138, 141, 185, 190, 193, 204-205
Tamoxifen: 85, 121, 195, 201,

223, 225, 224, 226-227, 229, 231, 233, 236-237, 241, 245-246
Tattoos: 252
Taxol: 223, 225, 224, 226, 235, 238-239, 247, 320
Taxotere: 235
Temafloxacin: 19
Temporomandibular joint disorder: 213
Tenosynovitis: 254-255
Terazosin: 173, 177
Terfenadine: 16, 258
Testicular cancer: 174, 237-238
Testosterone: 79, 127, 177, 189
Thalidomide: 253
Theophylline: 45, 48, 52, 59-60, 64-65, 119
Thoracoscopic lobectomy: 213
Thrombocytopenia: 151
Thromboembolism: 85, 185, 197
Thrombolytic therapy: 73, 74-75, 77, 80, 82, 88, 92-93, 97-99, 316
Thrombosis: 85, 185, 185, 197-198
Thumb-sucking: 49
Thyroid: 48, 151, 185, 186, 198, 205, 230, 233
TOMHS: 73, 75, 83, 101
Toxic risks: 316
Toxins: 47, 77, 136, 138, 174, 198, 252
tPA: 76, 78, 97-98, 100
Transplantation: 184, 193-194, 209, 212-213, 216-218, 224-225, 227, 232, 244-245, 252, 311
Tretinoin: 250, 253, 255, 265-266
Triazolam: 14, 18, 136, 186
Trichloroethylene: 23, 138
Trichophyton tonsurans: 260
Triglycerides: 74, 83, 85, 86-87, 147, 159
Trimethoprim sulfamethoxazole:, 284, 286, 290
Tuberculosis: 43, 46, 57, 182-183, 186-188, 190-191, 200-202, 252, 276-277, 278, 282-283, 285-288, 298-300, 303, 310-311, 317, 323, 331
Tuberculous meningitis: 280
Type A behavior: 46
Tyrosinemia: 53

Ulcerative colitis: 146, 158, 187, 263
Ulcers: 150, 183, 185, 191-192, 207-208, 279
Ultrasound
   transvaginal: 109, 113, 118, 125
Umbilical cord: 244
Urinary incontinence: 213
Urinary-tract infection: 151
Ursodiol: 18, 188
Uterine monitoring: 122

Vaccination (See also immunization, individual diseases): 44, 47-49, 51-52, 55, 57, 59-62, 311, 319
   acellular pertussis vaccine: 44, 47
   AIDS vaccine: 277-278, 281-282, 292, 311
   Bacille Calmette Guerin vaccine: 283
   cholera vaccine: 185, 194, 210
   flu vaccine: 48, 252, 312

hemophilus influenza B vaccine: 67
hepatitis A vaccine: 43, 51, 61-62
hepatitis B vaccine: 58, 62, 67
Lyme disease vaccine: 253
malaria: 257
MMR 43, 52, 257
pneumonia: 315
polio: 280
urinary tract infections: 173, 176
varicella zoster: 259
VA Cooperative Study of Monotherapy in Hypertension: 73, 75, 79
Valproate: 138, 139-140
Valvuloplasty: 75, 77, 84, 91
Varicella: 22, 110, 259
Varicose veins: 25, 185
Vasectomy: 39, 172-173, 194, 225, 226, 238, 282
Vasospasm: 213
Vegetables: 17, 22, 38, 66, 75, 144-145 146-147, 149, 151-154, 157, 160, 163-164, 166, 168-170, 233
Ventricular arrhythmia: 78
Ventricular tachycardia: 77, 81
Verapamil: 81, 163, 247
Vertigo: 187
Vitamin A: 28, 146, 152-154, 165, 168
Vitamin C: 147, 151, 153-154, 157, 170
Vitamin D: 19, 66, 120, 147, 149, 153, 164-165, 168, 201-202, 210, 211
Vitamin E: 156, 192, 245
Vitamin K: 48, 231

Warfarin: 84
Weight lifting: 18
Weight loss: 15, 22, 31-33, 138, 144-145, 147-148, 153, 155-156, 164, 258, 290
Women's Health Initiative: 170, 232
Women's Health Study, 232

Xenografts: 213-214, 216-217
Xeroderma pigmentosum: 255, 266

Zinc: 147, 149, 162

Credits

Notes

Notes

Notes

Notes

Notes

Notes

Notes

Notes

Notes

Notes

Notes

Notes

Notes